· A N · E R A · I N ·

CARDIOVASCULAR MEDICINE

·An·Era·In·
CARDIOVASCULAR MEDICINE

EDITED BY

SUZANNE B. KNOEBEL, MD
Indiana University School of Medicine
Krannert Institute of Cardiology
Indianapolis, Indiana

SIMON DACK, MD
Division of Cardiology
Mount Sinai School of Medicine
New York, New York

◆

Published for the
AMERICAN COLLEGE OF CARDIOLOGY

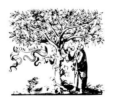

ELSEVIER
NEW YORK • AMSTERDAM • LONDON

Elsevier Science Publishing Co., Inc.
655 Avenue of the Americas
New York, New York   10010

Sole distributors outside the United States and Canada:
Elsevier Science Publishers B.V.
P.O. Box 211, 1000 AE Amsterdam, The Netherlands

© 1991 by the American College of Cardiology

This book has been registered with the Copyright Clearance Center, Inc.
For further information, please contact the Copyright Clearance Center, Inc., Salem, Massachusetts.

This book is printed on acid-free paper.

Library of Congress Cataloging-in-Publication Data

An era in cardiovascular medicine / edited by Suzanne B. Knoebel, Simon Dack.
        p.   cm.
    A collection of articles reprinted from the Journal of the
 American College of Cardiology, in celebration of the 40th
 anniversary of American College of Cardiology.
    Includes index.
    ISBN 0-444-01580-9 (hardcover : alk. paper)
    1. Cardiology—Congresses. 2. Heart—Diseases—Congresses.
  3. American College of Cardiology—Congresses.
    [DNLM: 1. Cardiology—trends—collected works.   2. Cardiovascular Diseases—collected works.   WG 100 E65]
RC681.A2E73 1991
616.1′2—dc20
DNLM/DLC   91-6525
for Library of Congress   CIP

Current printing (last digit):
10 9 8 7 6 5 4 3 2 1
Manufactured in the United States of America

◆ CONTENTS ◆

◆ PREFACE ◆

For cardiovascular medicine, the period between the approximate years of 1950 and 1990 merit designation as an era or epoch—a period of time characterized by a memorable series of events. More new knowledge about mechanisms of cardiovascular disease, its diagnosis, therapy, and prevention was created in these four decades than in the whole of human history. Cardiovascular medicine became a discipline that attracted creative minds and compassionate physicians.

In 1948, Congress passed the National Heart Act, which established the National Heart Institute by adding a new section to the Public Health Service Act. The impetus given to cardiovascular research and the training of cardiovascular scientists cannot be overstated. The achievements toward the conquering of cardiovascular disease during the ensuing years were, in the parlance of the 1980s, awesome.

In 1989, the American College of Cardiology celebrated its 40th anniversary by sponsoring a symposium designed to highlight some of the major advances in cardiovascular knowledge and their application in patient care that occurred during the 40-year period following its founding. The intent of the symposium, however, was not just to document the events of that era but to suggest in addition that a new era was in the making—the era of molecular cardiology, an understanding of dynamic patterns of disease made possible through the study of nonlinear systems, and decision-making based in probability theory.

The articles comprising the 40th Anniversary Symposium of the American College of Cardiology were published over a year's period in the *Journal of the American College of Cardiology*. Because of the quality and comprehensiveness of the material there was considerable interest in gathering the scientific articles from the symposium into a single volume so as to make them more readily accessible. The single volume format also gave the editors somewhat more leeway in structuring the content. Articles not in the original symposium because of space limitations have been added to *An Era in Cardiovascular Medicine*.

The basic tone of the original symposium was clinical in keeping with the long-standing orientation of the *Journal of the American College of Cardiology*, which makes relevance for optimal patient care its guiding principle. Research leading to improved diagnosis, therapy, and prevention through an understanding of disease mechanisms, an integral part of clinical progress, is woven into the presentations.

The Editor of the *Journal of the American College of Cardiology* and the Guest Editor of the 40th Anniversary Symposium of the American College of Cardiology are pleased to have had the opportunity to prepare this volume dedicated to a remarkable era in cardiovascular medicine. The value of its content as a reference to current patient care principles and practices and as a preview of the future are the result of the masterful approaches of the contributors. The editors thank them for their dedicated effort.

Suzanne B. Knoebel, MD
Guest Editor, 40th Anniversary Symposium

Simon Dack, MD
Editor, Journal of the American College
of Cardiology

◆ CONTRIBUTORS ◆

Walter H. Abelmann, MD
Professor of Medicine
Harvard Medical School
Senior Physician
Beth Israel Hospital
Boston, Massachusetts

Marvin L. Appel, MS
M.D., Ph.D. Candidate
Harvard-MIT Division of Health Sciences and Technology
Cambridge, Massachusetts

Juan J. Badimon, PhD
Assistant Professor of Medicine
Mount Sinai Medical Center
New York, New York

Lina Badimon, PhD
Associate Professor of Medicine
Mount Sinai Medical Center
New York, New York

George L. Bakris, MD
Director of Renal Research
Ochsner Medical Foundation
Staff Nephrologist
Ochsner Clinic
Assistant Professor of Medicine and Physiology
Tulane University School of Medicine
New Orleans, Louisiana

Nils U. Bang, MD
Senior Clinical Pharmacologist
Lilly Research Laboratories
Professor of Medicine and Pathology
Indiana University School of Medicine
Indianapolis, Indiana

Ronald D. Berger, MD, PhD
Cardiology Fellow
Johns Hopkins Hospital
Baltimore, Maryland

Eugene Braunwald, MD
Chairman, Department of Medicine
Brigham and Women's Hospital
Harvard Medical School
Boston, Massachusetts

Pedro Brugada, MD
Staff Cardiologist
Onze Lieve Vrouwe Ziekenhuis
Department of Cardiology
Aalst, Belgium

Bruce H. Brundage, MD
Professor of Medicine & Radiological Sciences
UCLA School of Medicine
Chief, Division of Cardiology
Harbor-UCLA Medical Center
Director of Research
St. John's Cardiac Research Center
Torrance, California

Robert M. Califf, MD
Associate Professor of Medicine
Duke University Medical Center
Durham, North Carolina

James H. Chesebro, MD
Professor of Medicine
Consultant in Cardiovascular Disease
Mayo Clinic and Mayo Foundation
Rochester, Minnesota

Michael D. Clayman, MD
Director, Internal Medicine Division
Lilly Research Laboratories
Assistant Professor of Medicine
Indiana University School of Medicine
Indianapolis, Indiana

Marc Cohen, MD
Associate Professor of Medicine
Mount Sinai Medical Center
New York, New York

Richard J. Cohen, MD, PhD
Hermann von Helmholtz Associate Professor
Harvard-MIT Division of Health Sciences and Technology
Director, Harvard-MIT Center for Biomedical Engineering
Cambridge, Massachusetts

Donald W. Dixon, MD
Associate Professor of Clinical Medicine
Stritch School of Medicine
Loyola University
Maywood, Illinois
Medical Director, Section of Cardiology
MacNeal Hospital
Berwyn, Illinois

Mary Allen Engle, MD
Stavros S. Niarchos Professor of Pediatric Cardiology
Professor of Pediatrics
Director of Pediatric Cardiology
The New York Hospital—Cornell Medical Center
New York, New York

Charles Fisch, MD
Distinguished Professor of Medicine
Indiana University School of Medicine
Krannert Institute of Cardiology
Indianapolis, Indiana

Edward D. Frohlich, MD
Alton Ochsner Distinguished Scientist
Vice President for Academic Affairs
Alton Ochsner Medical Foundation
Professor of Medicine/Physiology
Louisiana State University School of Medicine
Clinical Professor of Medicine and Adjunct Professor
    of Pharmacology
Tulane University School of Medicine
New Orleans, Louisiana

Robert L. Frye, MD
Professor of Medicine
Chairman, Department of Medicine
Rose M. and Maurice Eisenberg Professor of Medicine
Mayo Clinic
Rochester, Minnesota

Valentin Fuster, MD
Arthur M. & Hilda A. Master Professor
Chief, Division of Cardiology
Mount Sinai Medical Center
New York, New York

Steven Georgeson, MD
Temple University Hospital
Cardiology Department
Philadelphia, Pennsylvania

Bernard J. Gersh, MD
Cardiovascular Diseases and Internal Medicine
Mayo Clinic
Rochester, Minnesota

Raymond J. Gibbons, MD
Cardiovascular Diseases and Internal Medicine
Mayo Clinic
Rochester, Minnesota

Rolf M. Gunnar, MD
Professor and Chairman
Department of Medicine
Stritch School of Medicine
Loyola University
Maywood, Illinois

Frank E. Harrell, Jr., PhD
Associate Professor of Biometry & Medical Informatics
Duke University Medical Center
Durham, North Carolina

David R. Hathaway, MD
Professor of Medicine
Chief, Cardiovascular Division
Director, Krannert Institute of Cardiology
Indiana University School of Medicine
Indianapolis, Indiana

Mark A. Hlatky, MD
Associate Professor of Health Research and Policy and
    of Medicine
Stanford University School of Medicine
Stanford, California

Douglas H. Israel, MD
Research Fellow
Mount Sinai Medical Center
New York, New York

Arnold M. Katz, MD
Professor of Medicine
Head, Cardiology Division
University of Connecticut Health Center
Farmington, Connecticut

Kerry L. Lee, PhD
Associate Professor of Biometry & Medical Informatics
Duke University Medical Center
Durham, North Carolina

Beverly H. Lorell, MD
Associate Professor of Medicine
Harvard Medical School
Co-Director, Hemodynamic Research Laboratory
Beth Israel Hospital
Boston, Massachusetts

Keith L. March, PhD, MD
Assistant Professor of Medicine
Indiana University School of Medicine
Krannert Institute of Cardiology
Indianapolis, Indiana

Daniel B. Mark, MD, MPH
Assistant Professor of Medicine
Duke University Medical Center
Durham, North Carolina

Henry D. McIntosh, MD
Adjunct Professor of Medicine
Baylor College of Medicine
Houston, Texas
Clinical Professor of Medicine
University of Florida School of Medicine
Gainesville, Florida
Watson Clinic
Lakeland, Florida

Klemens B. Meyer, MD
Assistant Professor of Medicine
Tufts University School of Medicine
Boston, Massachusetts

Michael B. Mock, MD
Cardiovascular Diseases and Internal Medicine
Mayo Clinic
Rochester, Minnesota

Lawrence H. Muhlbaier, PhD
Assistant Professor of Biometry & Medical Informatics
Duke University Medical Center
Durham, North Carolina

Edmond A. Murphy, MD, ScD
Professor of Medicine
Johns Hopkins University School of Medicine
Baltimore, Maryland

John L. Myers, MD
Associate Professor of Surgery
Division of Cardiothoracic Surgery
Department of Surgery
The Milton S. Hershey Medical Center
The Pennsylvania State University
Hershey, Pennsylvania

John H. Newman, MD
Associate Professor of Medicine
Vanderbilt University Medical Center
Chief, Pulmonary Medicine
St. Thomas Hospital
Elsa S. Hanigan Chair in Pulmonary Medicine
Nashville, Tennessee

Robert A. O'Rourke, MD
Professor of Medicine
Director of Cardiology
The University of Texas Health Science Center
    at San Antonio
San Antonio, Texas

Walter E. Pae, Jr., MD
Associate Professor of Surgery
Division of Cardiothoracic Surgery
Department of Surgery
The Milton S. Hershey Medical Center
The Pennsylvania State University
Hershey, Pennsylvania

William W. Parmley, MD
Professor of Medicine
University of California, San Francisco
Chief of Cardiology
Moffitt/Long Hospital
San Francisco, California

Stephen G. Pauker, MD
Professor of Medicine
Tufts University School of Medicine
Boston, Massachusetts

William S. Pierce, MD
Evan Pugh Professor and Jane A. Fetter
Professor of Surgery
Chief of the Division of Artificial Organs
Department of Surgery
The Milton S. Hershey Medical Center
The Pennsylvania State University
Hershey, Pennsylvania

David B. Pryor, MD
Associate Professor of Medicine
Duke University Medical Center
Durham, North Carolina

Reed E. Pyeritz, MD, PhD
Professor of Medicine and Pediatrics
Johns Hopkins University School of Medicine
Clinical Director, Center for Medical Genetics
Johns Hopkins Hospital
Baltimore, Maryland

Shahbudin H. Rahimtoola, MD
George C. Griffith Professor of Cardiology
Professor of Medicine
Chief, Section of Cardiology
University of Southern California
Los Angeles, California

Stuart Rich, MD
Associate Professor of Medicine
Chief, Section of Cardiology
University of Illinois at Chicago
Chicago, Illinois

Wayne E. Richenbacher, MD
Assistant Professor of Surgery
University of Utah
School of Medicine
Salt Lake City, Utah

Joseph C. Ross, MD
Professor of Medicine
Associate Vice Chancellor for Health Affairs
Vanderbilt University Medical Center
Nashville, Tennessee

J. Philip Saul, MD
Assistant Professor of Pediatrics
Harvard School of Medicine
Pediatric Cardiologist
Children's Hospital
Boston, Massachusetts

Hartzell V. Schaff, MD
Division of Thoracic and Cardiovascular Surgery
Mayo Clinic
Rochester, Minnesota

Joseph M. Smith, MD, PhD
Cardiology Fellow
Brigham and Women's Hospital
Boston, Massachusetts

Bernardo Stein, MD
Research Fellow
Mount Sinai Medical Center
New York, New York

Borys Surawicz, MD
Professor Emeritus of Medicine
Indiana University School of Medicine
Senior Research Associate
Krannert Institute of Cardiology
Indianapolis, Indiana

Ronald E. Vlietstra, MD
Watson Clinic
1600 Lakeland Hills Blvd.
P.O. Box 95000
Lakeland, Florida

John A. Waldhausen, MD
John W. Oswald Professor of Surgery
Chairman, Department of Surgery
The Milton S. Hershey Medical Center
The Pennsylvania State University
Hershey, Pennsylvania

Bruce F. Waller, MD
Clinical Professor of Pathology and Medicine
Indiana University School of Medicine
Director, Cardiovascular Pathology Registry
St. Vincent Hospital
Indianapolis, Indiana

Sylvan L. Weinberg, MD
Clinical Professor
Department of Medicine
Wright State University School of Medicine
Chairman of Cardiology
Good Samaritan Hospital
Dayton, Ohio

Hein J. J. Wellens, MD
Professor and Chairman
Department of Cardiology
Academic Hospital Maastricht
University of Limburg
Maastricht, The Netherlands

Olaf G. Wilhelm, MD
Postdoctoral Fellow
Lilly Laboratory for Clinical Research
Lilly Research Laboratories
Indianapolis, Indiana

◆ CHAPTER 1 ◆

The Golden Age of Cardiology

EUGENE BRAUNWALD, MD

The rhythm of many human activities in which periods of rapid forward motion alternate with periods of relative quiescence and recovery resembles the alternate contraction and relaxation of the heart. In the history of cardiology, the last 40 years might be described as a "systolic phase." During this period, the entire field has been transformed so radically that even the most enlightened cardiologist in 1950, if transported in a time capsule to the present, would be shocked and confused. Between 1950 and 1990, the safe accurate diagnosis and effective treatment of most forms of heart disease became possible and the age-adjusted mortality rate for cardiovascular disease declined by more than 40%.

Major Developments Between 1950 and 1990

In 1950, the outlook for the majority of patients with congenital heart disease, particularly cyanotic infants, was poor. Although diagnosis by cardiac catheterization and angiocardiography was feasible, these procedures were sometimes risky, and surgical treatment was limited to a few extracardiac operations. Today, invasive diagnostic procedures are relatively safe even in critically ill neonates with congenital heart disease, but are often unnecessary because echocardiography and other noninvasive studies now provide valuable diagnostic information in many patients. Although most congenital cardiac malformations now can be corrected surgically, an increasing number can also be treated definitively in the catheterization laboratory by the relief of obstructive lesions and closure of intracardiac and intravascular communications.

Forty years ago, rheumatic heart disease was among the most common causes of death among school-age children and adolescents. Treatment of acute rheumatic fever was largely symptomatic and consisted primarily of bed rest and aspirin. For the most part, complications of valvular heart disease were treated expectantly, with the exception of closed mitral valvotomy for stenosis—a procedure that was still in its infancy and, in the majority of patients, of limited efficacy. Today, with prompt treatment of streptococcal infections and attention to penicillin prophylaxis, acute rheumatic fever occurs only sporadically in the United States. Essentially all severe valvular deformities, regardless of etiology, are now amenable to corrective surgery. Valve replacement, although not curative, has proved to be a successful therapeutic option for most patients with advanced valvular heart disease.

Clinicians in 1950 did not yet appreciate the importance of

hypertension as a risk factor for the development of atherosclerosis. The mechanisms underlying blood pressure elevation were not well understood, potentially curable forms of secondary hypertension were rarely recognized during life and pharmacologic treatment of patients with essential hypertension was not effective or practical. Today, the diagnosis of secondary curable forms of hypertension is rarely missed. Effective control of arterial pressure has been shown to reduce the mortality rate not only in patients with severe hypertension, but also in those with moderately and even mildly elevated blood pressure, providing a strong impetus to attempts to control hypertension. Therefore, the importance of treating hypertension to prevent atherosclerosis and its complications is now widely appreciated, and an array of effective, well-tolerated, safe antihypertensive agents is available.

In 1950, conflicting theories concerning the pathogenesis of atherosclerosis abounded. A variety of causes were considered, including nutritional, toxic and postinfectious etiologies. Today, we appreciate the importance of low density and other lipoproteins, such as Lp(a), as well as the protective role of high density lipoproteins, the damaging effects of hypertension and hyperlipoproteinemia on the arterial endothelium, the elaboration of growth factors and the mitosis and migration of vascular smooth muscle cells in this process.

Four decades ago, acute myocardial infarction was managed by bed rest, with relatively ineffective pharmacologic therapy for certain complications. Today, in-hospital death due to primary arrhythmias—previously the most important cause of such deaths—is almost unheard of. Often, the evolution of an infarct can be interrupted by thrombolytic therapy, which is sometimes administered in the home, workplace or ambulance before the patient is admitted to the hospital. Many complications of myocardial infarction can be managed using modern revascularization techniques. As a result of these developments, both the mortality rate and hospital stay have been reduced to about one-fifth of what they were in 1950. Forty years ago, the treatment of chronic coronary artery disease consisted of limiting physical activity and administering sublingual nitroglycerin. Today, a wide variety of effective antiischemic drugs is available; if these fail, mechanical revascularization is usually effective.

At the start of this era, no treatment was available for the large number of sudden deaths due to ventricular fibrillation (outside the operating room). Deaths secondary to complete atrioventricular block were common and could not be prevented. Now, modern techniques of cardiopulmonary resuscitation are life-saving when applied rapidly and appropriately. The implantable automatic cardioverter-defibrillator is also often useful for the immediate treatment of ventricular fibrillation and the prevention of its recurrence. Clinical electrophysiologic studies have helped unravel complex arrhythmias and can be of value in selecting appropriate antiarrhythmic drugs and devices. A wide range of pacemakers has become available to treat a variety of brady- and tachyarrhythmias.

In 1950, the management of congestive heart failure was expectant and not very effective. The patient's physical activity was limited, and sodium and water intake were reduced. The drugs administered—digitalis glycosides and parenterally administered mercurial diuretic agents—were only modestly effective. Since then, several new groups of agents have been introduced for the treatment of heart failure, including potent, orally active diuretic drugs and vasodilators; the latter have been shown to improve survival in selected patients. When these pharmacologic measures fail, cardiac transplantation and various forms of assisted circulation—used separately or in tandem—may be effective in properly selected patients.

Genesis of the Golden Age

In this volume, leading figures, many of whom have left their strong personal imprints on the field, describe the important advances that have radically transformed cardiology since 1950. It may be of interest to speculate on what led to this transformation. The principal forces responsible for what might be termed this ''golden age'' may be seen as separate threads woven together to create the fabric that is contemporary cardiology.

The heritage of basic science. Modern cardiology did not materialize suddenly out of a vacuum. Rather, the rapid developments after 1950 were preceded by more than a century of research in the basic cardiovascular sciences. By 1950, the pathophysiologic basis of most forms of heart disease had already been established. Giants of cardiovascular physiology of the late 19th and early 20th centuries, such as Frank and Starling in Europe and Wiggers in the United States, had provided a framework that allowed clinical investigative techniques, such as electrocardiography, cardiac catheterization and angiocardiography, to be used to elucidate the pathophysiologic changes in cardiovascular disorders. In addition, the development of open heart surgery would have been impossible without earlier advances, including blood transfusion, modern anesthesia, inhalation therapy, the blood oxygenator and electrical defibrillator and drugs such as norepinephrine, penicillin, heparin and protamine.

Early developments in cardiology. Unlike many other subspecialties, cardiology had already become a distinct clinical discipline by 1950. It became established as a result

of three seminal advances: 1) the development of electrocardiograph by Waller and Einthoven and then applied by Lewis, White, Wilson and others; 2) the discovery of x-rays by Roentgen, and the application of radiology to cardiology by Parkinson and others; and 3) the introduction of cardiac catheterization by Forssman, Cournand and Richards. Consequently, by 1950, a small but enthusiastic group of clinical cardiovascular investigators was already present and poised to advance the field rapidly.

Technical and surgical developments during World War II. The Second World War greatly accelerated several technical and engineering developments that were later applied successfully to cardiovascular research and the clinical care of patients with heart disease. Tools such as the cathode-ray oscilloscope, multichannel oscillographic recorder, strain-gauge arch, television, fluoroscopic image intensifier, ultrasonography and other imaging techniques, radioisotopes, and calculating machines (the forerunners of modern computers) whose development was greatly stimulated by the war effort revolutionized cardiovascular science and cardiology during the post-war years. During World War II, the successful surgical treatment of cardiac trauma, including the removal of foreign bodies from the heart under battlefield conditions, served as a powerful stimulus to thoracic surgeons to cross the frontier into cardiac surgery.

Federal support for cardiovascular research. It was no coincidence that the golden age of cardiology began soon after the National Heart Institute (now the National Heart, Lung and Blood Institute [NHLBI]) was established in 1948. The federal commitment to biomedical research grew progressively, especially at the beginning of this period, and the Institute's annual budget rose from 16 million dollars in 1950 to more than 1 billion dollars in 1990. The government's wise and far reaching decision to invest in research and research training provided the vital resources that accelerated the pace of discovery. Moreover, the Institute has not served simply as a conduit of funds from the taxpayer to the research community. Rather, it has displayed vigorous and imaginative leadership in identifying scientific opportunities and matching them to the available resources. Where appropriate, it has played a key role in the assessment of various modes of cardiovascular therapy as well as in public education.

The importance of the basic sciences to cardiology. In the 1950s, it became evident that the preclinical sciences—particularly physiology, biophysics, biochemistry and pharmacology—were of fundamental importance to clinical cardiology. Cardiovascular surgeons and radiologists became experts in hemodynamics. Pediatric cardiologists learned about cardiac embryology to understand more fully the congenital cardiovascular lesions they encountered, whereas adult cardiologists became well versed in basic electrophysiology and applied it to the treatment of arrhythmias. Enzymes involved in the biosynthesis of cholesterol, events in the cell membrane that control the transport of ions, details of the coagulation pathway, Laplace's law, the compartmentalization and kinetics of drugs, the intrapulmonary shunting of blood and a wide variety of biostatistical techniques are just a few of the many subjects that had previously been of little interest to clinical investigators and clinicians, but that suddenly acquired vital significance.

Attraction of the "Best and the Brightest." In any field, the rate of progress depends on the talent, enthusiasm, dedication and vigor of the individuals it attracts. From 1950 onward, cardiology became the subspecialty of choice for a disproportionate share of the most capable, gifted and intellectually motivated medical school graduates. One powerful attraction was the ability to establish both an anatomic diagnosis and a physiologic assessment of heart disease by means of cardiac catheterization and angiocardiography within 1 or 2 h of the clinical examination—a feat unprecedented in clinical medicine. The immediate feedback supplied by these and other laboratory techniques, such as phonocardiography, echocardiography and other imaging modalities, actually heightened interest in careful bedside examination.

Not only clinicians, but also scientists excited by these informative diagnostic and physiologic tests began to direct their attention to the cardiovascular system. Funds for the training of additional cardiovascular investigators were made available early during this era by both the federal government and private agencies. Standards for research training were raised and accrediting boards spelled out rigorous requirements for certification of cardiovascular specialists in medicine, pediatrics and surgery. Finally, once an individual entered the field, opportunities to obtain an academic position or practice the specialty were abundant.

Early successes. Nothing breeds success like success. In the 1950s, several spectacular advances in clinical cardiology had an enormous impact on the future of the specialty. Among these, four stand out: 1) the discovery and application of penicillin prophylaxis of acute rheumatic fever, which has almost eliminated this important disease; 2) the development of orally effective thiazide diuretic drugs, which simplified and enormously improved the management of patients with hypertension and heart failure; 3) the development of open heart surgery, which has allowed the successful treatment of many forms of congenital heart disease, then of acquired valvular disease and finally of ischemic heart disease; and 4) the development of the coronary care unit, which almost immediately reduced by half the number of in-hospital deaths from acute myocardial infarction. These early triumphs not only attracted a great deal of public attention, but also contributed to enticing the most talented young physicians and surgeons into cardiology.

Contributions by organized cardiology. By enlisting the aid of tens of thousands of volunteers, both professional and lay, the American Heart Association (AHA) has obtained private funds to help support cardiovascular research of the highest quality. The AHA has also established innovative

programs for the career development of scientists (such as the Established Investigator program), which have served as models for much larger federally sponsored efforts. The Association has developed effective programs for both professional and public education. Another important contribution of the AHA has been to heighten the public's awareness of heart disease and of the important advances that have been made in cardiovascular research. This has heightened the public's expectation for high quality, up to date cardiovascular services and facilities, which in turn has stimulated institutions to provide such services.

The American College of Cardiology has provided a powerful and effective organizational framework for the professional activities of a wide variety of cardiovascular specialists and investigators. It has been conspicuously effective in enhancing postgraduate education of cardiovascular specialists. The College has been instrumental in setting standards for practice, training and facilities for cardiology and has articulated clearly to political leaders the views of the profession and the needs of the patients it serves.

Cardiovascular disease knows no national boundaries; people on all continents and in all countries are afflicted. The International Society of Cardiology and the several continental societies of cardiology have met regularly since 1950 and have contributed to progress in the field by rapidly disseminating important information worldwide, providing a framework for carrying out international projects and, perhaps most important, establishing professional ties among cardiovascular scientists and clinicians around the world.

Contributions by industry. In our society, the fruits of research must usually be commercialized before they can be made widely available to the public. Recognizing the high incidence of cardiovascular diseases and their enormous human and economic costs, as well as the enormous potential opportunities for progress, the private sector has begun to focus its attention on these conditions and has unleashed enormous resources in the effort to improve cardiovascular health. Industry has supported cardiovascular research, ranging from fundamental to applied, both within its own laboratories and in universities. New effective drugs and innovative devices developed by the private sector—often in close collaboration with university-based scientists—have revolutionized both the diagnosis and treatment of heart disease.

Contagious excitement. Beginning in nonuniversity settings, artificial administrative boundaries were removed so that interdepartmental, interdisciplinary collaborative approaches to cardiovascular research and cardiac care could be tried. The obvious success of these new organizational arrangements led many university medical centers to adopt similar approaches. As all of the individual threads just mentioned began to be woven together, excitement about the discoveries and changes taking place in cardiology became contagious. Those who attended the major cardiology meetings were invigorated by the pace of progress, and the latest issues of cardiology journals were eagerly anticipated and rapidly devoured.

Future Directions

As interesting as it may be to review past accomplishments, it is more exciting to contemplate the future. Although further advances of the kind similar to those made in the past four decades are still possible, they are likely to yield only refinements. Today, the challenge is to elucidate the fundamental mechanisms underlying cardiac disorders in an effort to eliminate or prevent them. To reach this ambitious goal, we must investigate questions that transcend the boundaries of what has traditionally been considered to be cardiovascular science.

It is now clear that many cardiovascular diseases result ultimately from abnormalities in membrane receptors, transmembrane ion fluxes, the production of and response to a variety of growth factors and the synthesis of apoproteins and contractile proteins. Such abnormalities involve not only cardiac cells, but perhaps even more importantly a variety of noncardiac cells, including endothelial cells, macrophages, hepatocytes and platelets. In the case of congenital heart disease, the fundamental causes—be they chromosomal disorders, single gene mutations or maternal viral infections such as rubella—must be unraveled to prevent and eventually eliminate these disorders. Much remains to be learned at the molecular level about the pathogenesis of viral and other forms of myocarditis. If the fundamental cause or causes of essential hypertension could be elucidated, perhaps this condition could be prevented entirely. We are now moving toward a more comprehensive theory of the pathogenesis of atherosclerosis. In turn, this could lead to interventions designed to prevent, interrupt and reverse this process.

As the focus of cardiovascular research is redirected toward the molecular and cellular biology of the normal and diseased cardiovascular system, perhaps the golden age of cardiology will be extended to an even greater "platinum age."

◆ CHAPTER 2 ◆

Evolution of the Clinical Electrocardiogram

CHARLES FISCH, MD

As a laboratory procedure, the electrocardiogram (ECG) is unique, having been in continuous and ever-increasing use since its introduction nearly 90 years ago by Willem Einthoven. Some would suggest that, conservatively speaking, a volume of approximately 100 million ECGs recorded annually at a cost approaching $5 billion attests to the importance of the procedure. Others would point to the capability and versatility of the ECG as far more important measures of its contribution to the care of patients with and without heart disease. Electrocardiography, the only practical method of recording the electrical behavior of the heart, has the potential to reflect anatomy, blood flow, hemodynamics, transmembrane ionic fluxes and effect of drugs, each of these often the single goal of other noninvasive techniques (1–4).

To place this unique noninvasive technique in its proper perspective, it would seem appropriate that this review begins with the history of electrocardiography and includes comments regarding its sensitivity and specificity, its role as a marker for heart disease as a clue to anatomic, metabolic and hemodynamic abnormalities, its role as the reference standard for the diagnosis and study of arrhythmias, its contribution to research and the issues facing electrocardiography.

Historic Notes

The origin of the ECG can be dated to the observation made by Aloysio Luigi Galvani in 1794. Galvani (5) placed the nerve of a nerve-muscle preparation on an injured muscle and noted contraction of the muscle of the nerve-muscle preparation. Some 50 years later, Matteucci (6) observed that if the nerve of the Galvani nerve-muscle preparation was laid across the beating heart, the muscle of the nerve-muscle preparation contracted in synchrony with the beating heart. In 1855, Kolliker and Muller (7) also placed the nerve of the Galvani nerve-muscle preparation on the beating heart and noted that not only did the muscle contract synchronously with the contraction of the heart, but two contractions were also evident on occasion. The first contraction of the muscle of the nerve-muscle preparation occurred just before the cardiac systole—the R wave—and was followed by a second feeble late diastolic twitch—the T wave. The next important landmark in the evolution of the ECG was the Lipmann capillary manometer (8). With this instrument, it was possible to record from the body surface voltage changes generated by the beating heart. The instru-

ment consisted of a finely drawn glass tube filled with mercury and immersed in sulfuric acid. The surface of the mercury moved as the potential difference between the mercury and sulfuric acid changed, and this motion was recorded on photographic paper. In 1887, Waller (9,10), using the Lipmann manometer, was the first to record voltage changes generated by the human heart. The frequency response of the Lipmann capillary manometer, however, was poor and its use short-lived.

Einthoven, realizing the potential of the string galvanometer developed by Ader (1) for use with transatlantic cable, modified the instrument, greatly improved its sensitivity and applied it to recording the electrical activity of the heart. A preliminary report (11) describing the instrument appeared in 1901 and a more detailed description (12) including ECG tracings in 1903. Einthoven discussed the theory of the ECG and its application to the study of heart disease in two classic works, "Le Telecardiogramme" published in 1906 (13) and "Weiteres uber das Electrokardiogramm" published in 1908 (14). Einthoven was interested in the ECG not only as a tool for the study of physiology, but also for its potential application to clinical cardiology. In fact, his galvanometer, while housed in the physiology laboratory in Leiden, was connected by telephone wires to the clinic at the Academic Hospital located more than a mile away.

The early years of electrocardiography were dominated by Einthoven and Sir Thomas Lewis. The two introduced the ECG into clinical medicine and brought it to the bedside. Einthoven made his major contributions by the year 1913, whereas Lewis continued his studies of arrhythmias until 1920 when he concluded that no further important information could be gained from the study of the ECG and turned his attention to peripheral vascular disease, effectively ending the period dominated by studies of arrhythmias. Lewis (15) summarized his work in the 1920 edition of *The Mechanism and Graphic Registration of the Heart Beat*. Commenting on the role of graphic records as an investigative and clinical laboratory tool he wrote: "Of the immediate value of graphic methods to practical medicine, it is my desire to speak, but briefly. These records had placed the entire question of irregular or disordered mechanism of human heart upon a rational basis, so giving to the works the confidence of knowledge; they have influenced prognosis, rendered it more exact; they have potentially abolished the promiscuous administration of certain cardiac poisons, and have clearly shown the lines which therapy must follow. The new clinical observations have stimulated and directed a host of valuable laboratory researches, anatomical, physiological, pathological, and pharmacological. The records constitute the most exact signs of cardiac affections which we possess.''

The period after 1920 was dominated largely by Frank N. Wilson and his group. According to Burch and DePasquale (16), although many contributed to our knowledge of electrocardiography ''. . . none did as much to advance electrocardiographic knowledge as did Frank N. Wilson.'' The interest shifted from arrhythmias to the theory of the ECG, to ECG leads and abnormalities of waveforms. In 1944, shortly before the founding of our College, Wilson et al. (17) published the study entitled ''The Precordial Electrocardiogram.'' They described the utility and contribution of the unipolar precordial leads to clinical cardiology and, for all practical purposes, ushered in clinical electrocardiography as we know it today (18).

Although it is unlikely that any one individual or, for that matter, any group of individuals can appropriately identify and properly evaluate the contributions of the many early ECG investigators, I propose that the list compiled by Burch and DePasquale (16) is representative and reasonably inclusive. Burch, himself a serious student and contributor to electrocardiography and one who was familiar with many of the early investigators, published in 1962, in collaboration with DePasquale, an elegant volume on the history of electrocardiography (16). In chapter III, entitled ''Great Men of Electrocardiography,'' they list: Willem Einthoven, Aloysio Luigi Galvani, Carlo Matteucci, Emil DuBois-Reymond, Hermann L. F. von Helmholtz, Sir John S. Burdon-Sanderson, Julius Berstein, Gabriel Lipmann, Walter H. Gaskell, Sir James Mackenzie, Augustus D. Waller, Fredrick Kraus, Sir William M. Bayliss, James B. Herrick, Augustus Hoffmann, Karel F. Wenckebach, Heinrich E. Hering, Horatio B. Williams, Alfred E. Cohn, Sir Thomas Lewis, George E. Fahr, Harold E. B. Pardee, Frank N. Wilson, Fritz Schellong, Hubert Mann and W. H. Craib.

With the development of direct writing equipment in the late 1940s, the ECG became, as it continues to be, the most commonly used cardiovascular laboratory procedure. It is noninvasive, simple to record, highly reproducible and can be applied serially. The cost of the equipment and of recording is minimal compared with that of other cardiovascular laboratory procedures. It is the only practical method of recording the electrical activity of the heart and arrhythmias and, importantly, it is usually the first laboratory test performed in a patient with chest pain, syncope or presyncope, the two major markers of potential cardiovascular catastrophe.

Sensitivity and Specificity of the ECG

For proper interpretation of the ECG, it is imperative that the physician be familiar with the sensitivity and specificity of the techniques because as with other laboratory proce-

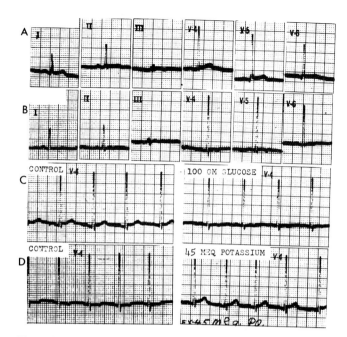

Figure 2.1. The labile nature of the T wave recorded in a 21 year old healthy student. The T waves are normal in **A** and inverted in **B**. In **C**, the normal T waves become inverted after oral administration of 100 g of glucose, whereas in **D**, the inverted T waves become upright after administration of 45 mEq of potassium.

dures, these are often the critical determinants of the clinical utility of a procedure. These are by far more complex for the ECG than for other procedures that are developed for a single purpose (2). The ECG consists of a number of waveforms that differ in origin and are influenced differently by a variety of factors and by the sequencing of those factors. At times, it is difficult if not impossible to identify a single or specific cause of an ECG change. Most often, identification of a specific cause of an ECG abnormality is possible only because of the information that has been derived from extensive and detailed correlation of the ECG with clinical, autopsy and experimental findings.

The sensitivity and specificity of a given ECG abnormality are to a large extent dependent on the setting in which the ECG is recorded, the question asked, use of appropriate recording technique and sequencing of the tracings, recognition of subtle changes and, importantly, the skill with which the ECG is interpreted.

The low specificity of an ECG waveform is exemplified by T wave changes. Although a T wave change is the most common ECG abnormality, recorded in approximately 50% of all abnormal tracings and 2.4% to 4.5% of all tracings (19), it is also the most labile of all the ECG waveforms (Fig. 2.1). A decrease in the duration of the monophasic action potential by only 12 to 18 ms involving an area of the myocardium of only ≤8% will alter the T wave (20,21). Abnormal T waves can be seen in the absence of heart disease and can be induced by a variety of physiologic and pharmacologic interventions, extracardiac disorders, primary myocardial

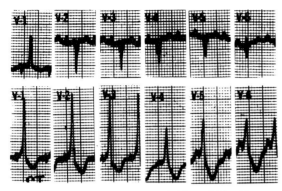

Figure 2.2. Precordial Q waves recorded in a child with an anomalous coronary artery (**upper tracing**) are obscured during conduction through an anomalous pathway (Wolff-Parkinson-White) (**lower tracing**).

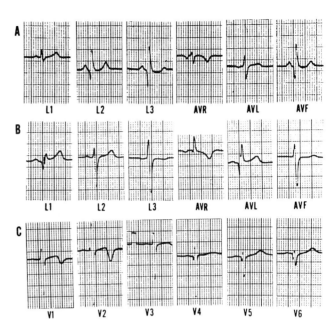

Figure 2.3. Simulation of inferior (**A**), high lateral (**B**) and lateral (**C**) myocardial infarction in three cases of idiopathic hypertrophic cardiomyopathy.

disease, secondary forms of heart disease and ischemic heart disease. Thus, the most sensitive component of the ECG is also the least specific. The labile and sensitive but nonspecific nature of the T wave was clearly recognized by Wilson and Finch (22) in 1923 when they recorded T wave inversion after ingestion of cold water.

Similarly, but to a lesser degree, the limitation of specificity is applicable to the QRS complex, the ST segment and the U wave. For example, although myocardial infarction is the most common cause of an abnormal Q wave, an abnormal Q wave may be associated with a variety of anatomic and functional abnormalities, including congenital heart disease (Fig. 2.2), pulmonary disease, nonischemic myocardial disease, left ventricular hypertrophy, idiopathic hypertrophic cardiomyopathy (Fig. 2.3), intraventricular conduction defects, Wolff-Parkinson-White syndrome, coronary embolism and metabolic and neurogenic abnormalities (23). This variety is hardly surprising because the ECG as a record of an electrical phenomenon can be altered identically by many functional and anatomic abnormalities, the common denominator being a transient or permanent loss of electrically functioning myocardium.

An example of a subtle but clinically significant change is a negative U wave. The genesis of the U wave is unclear. Some investigators believe that the U wave represents repolarization of the Purkinje fibers, whereas others believe that it reflects a myocardial diastolic event. A number of physiologic variables, including metabolic and electrolyte abnormalities, and drugs alter the duration, direction and amplitude of the U wave. A negative U wave is rarely if ever recorded in the absence of heart disease. Although the most common cause of a negative U wave is hypertension, a negative U wave may be the only ECG evidence of acute myocardial ischemia (Fig. 2.4).

Skillful ECG interpretation with particular attention to the limitations of the technique enhances its sensitivity and specificity. For example, although the first ECG recorded in the course of evolution of acute myocardial infarction is normal in 10% of patients, abnormal but not diagnostic in 40% and "typical" of myocardial infarction in 50%, serial tracings increase the sensitivity to approximately 95%. Similarly, attention to subtle ST segment and T wave changes, recognition of the fact that a large number of cases of myocardial infarction are manifested by T wave changes only, a careful search for negative U waves, awareness of transient normalization of the ECG in the course of evolution of infarction and recognition of "silent" areas of infarction (Fig. 2.5), masking (Fig. 2.2 and 2.6) and simulation of myocardial infarction by intraventricular conduction abnormalities and recurrent infarction enhance the sensitivity of the ECG. In general, although the T wave is the most sensitive indicator of infarction, it is also the least specific. Conversely, a new Q wave, although the most specific finding for myocardial infarction, is much less sensitive than a T wave change.

The ECG as an Independent Marker of Heart Disease

Occasionally, the ECG is the first and sometimes the only finding of a clinically or potentially significant cardiac abnormality. This is true for congenital and acquired disorders, with anomalous coronary artery and Wolff-Parkinson-White syndrome being examples of the former (Fig. 2.2) and acceleration-dependent bundle branch block an example of the latter (Fig. 2.7). Acceleration-dependent aberration, a relatively frequent but often overlooked abnormality, is nearly always a sign of heart disease, even though clinical signs of heart disease may be absent. This form of aberration

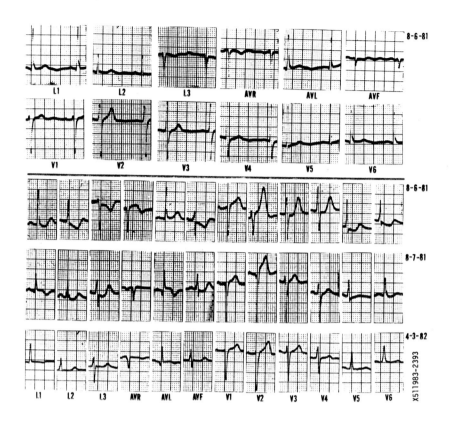

Figure 2.4. In the **upper panel** (8-6-81), the negative U wave in leads I, aVL, V₄, V₅ and V₆ is the only evidence of an acute ischemic process. Evolution of a septal and lateral infarction is recorded in the **next two lower panels** (8-6 and 8-7-8). Eight months later (4-3-82), only isolated high lateral infarction is evident, with T wave changes localized to leads I and aVL.

differs from physiologic aberration. In the latter, the block is most often a right bundle branch block, and the aberration is a result of attempted conduction during the period of physiologic recovery, namely, during the voltage-dependent refractory period. In contrast to physiologic aberration, the pattern of acceleration-dependent aberration is most often that of left bundle branch block, frequently appearing at slow rates and occasionally only after a number of cycles of the accelerated rhythm. These features of aberration point to abnormal function with a longer refractory period of the left

bundle branch than of the right bundle branch and with the refractory period exceeding the duration of the physiologic electrical recovery (the voltage-dependent refractoriness) and extending well into diastole. The period of diastolic refractoriness is referred to as time-dependent refractoriness (Fig. 2.8). The appearance of bundle branch block after a number of regular cycles of an accelerated rhythm indicates an abnormal prolongation of the refractory period in response to acceleration of the heart rate.

A model of the ECG as an independent marker for heart

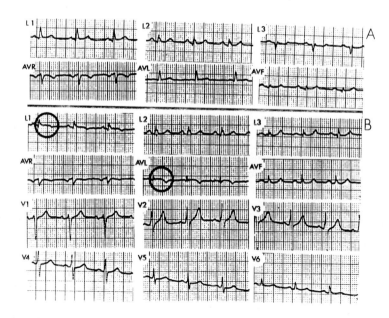

Figure 2.5. Subtle early electrocardiographic changes of acute myocardial infarction. **A,** At the onset of myocardial infarction, subtle ST elevation is seen in leads I and aVL and a reciprocal concavity of the ST segment in lead III. **B,** Evolution of an isolated high lateral infarction manifested by T wave inversion confined to leads I and aVL. The left axis in **A** is probably the result of conduction delay due to ischemia.

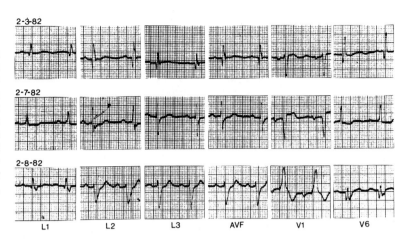

Figure 2.6. Masking of the Q waves of myocardial infarction (**top panel**) by intraventricular conduction delays. An inferior and lateral infarction manifested by a Q wave in leads II, III, aVF and V_6 is recorded on February 3, 1983. Incomplete left bundle branch block recorded on February 7, 1982 obscures the inferior as well as the lateral infarction. On February 8, 1982, the pattern is that of right bundle branch block and left anterior fascicular block. The latter obscures the inferior infarction. The right bundle branch block, in contrast to the incomplete left bundle branch block, does not obscure the lateral infarction.

disease is the ECG in the aged. In these patients, whose history is often unreliable and physical examination difficult, the ECG carries a different connotation from that in other age groups. The ECG abnormality is nearly always acquired, as suggested by comparison of the consecutive observations made in 776 individuals <25 years of age admitted to a psychiatric hospital with the findings in 671 individuals >65 years old residing in a nursing home (24). In the young group, nonspecific ST-T changes, left anterior fascicular block, first degree atrioventricular (AV) block, right bundle branch block, left bundle branch block, intraventricular conduction defect, myocardial infarction, right-axis deviation >+120°, left ventricular hypertrophy and Wolff-Parkinson-White conduction were present in 0.0%, 1.4%, 0.3%, 0.3%, 0.0%, 0.1%, 0.0%, 2.1%, 0.1%, 0.0% and 0.3%, respectively. In the aged, the respective values were 15.7%, 11.0%, 9.9%, 7.1%, 4.9%, 1.9%, 4.4%, 0.9%, 0.9%, 5.0% and 0.4%. In the group of aged patients, ST segment and T wave changes, intraventricular conduction defect, left bundle branch block and atrial fibrillation showed a high and significant correlation with clinical heart disease. Therefore, it appears that even in the absence of clinical signs of disease, these ECG abnormalities are indicative of heart disease. Interestingly, in a large number of the aged, the ECG pattern of myocardial infarction failed to correlate with either symptoms or signs of coronary disease, further sup-

porting the value of the ECG as an independent marker for heart disease.

ECG in epidemiologic studies. The ECG is used widely in epidemiologic studies designed to determine the prevalence of ischemic heart disease, identify latent heart disease and assess physical fitness and appropriateness of employment in sensitive occupations. However, the rest ECG is not a very sensitive or specific marker for occult heart disease, and prognostic value of many of the ECG abnormalities is unclear. The diagnostic and prognostic implication of a given ECG abnormality differs greatly, depending on the patient group studied and the reason for which the ECG is recorded. An ECG abnormality recorded in a population with a low prevalence of cardiac disease is likely to be a false-positive finding for clinically significant heart disease and indicates a low risk for future cardiac events. In contrast, the same ECG abnormality recorded in a population with a high prevalence of heart disease is very likely to be a true-positive finding and of considerable prognostic significance. It has been shown (25) that an ECG abnormality identified during a clinical evaluation is associated with a two to four times greater incidence of new cardiovascular events than if the abnormality is discovered during a screening procedure. Failure to consider the characteristics of the population studied, the clinical picture and the sensitivity and specificity of the abnormality may result in crippling iatrogenic heart disease.

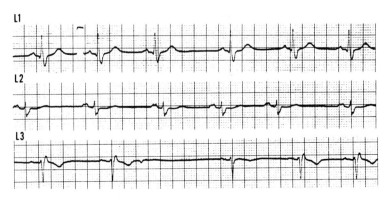

Figure 2.7. Acceleration-dependent aberration due to marked prolongation of the time-dependent refractoriness. In lead 2, right bundle branch block is recorded at an RR interval of 1,230 ms, a rate of approximately 50/min. In lead 3, the blocked atrial premature complex after the second beat is followed by a return cycle of 2,000 ms and a normally conducted QRS complex. The duration of the right bundle branch refractory period is somewhere between 1,230 and 2,000 ms.

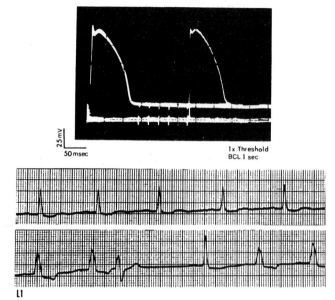

Figure 2.8. Acceleration-dependent left bundle branch block at a cycle length of 960 ms (**bottom trace of lead I**), with normalization at a cycle length of 1,120 ms (**upper trace of lead I**). The **upper panel** illustrates failure to respond to stimulation during diastole after the recovery of the transmembrane action potential. A response is elicited only after the sixth stimulus. This diastolic refractoriness is referred to as time-dependent refractoriness. BCL-basic cycle length. Reproduced with permission from Fisch (34).

Prognostic significance of ECG abnormalities. In patients with known heart disease, ST segment and T wave changes and abnormal Q waves reach statistical significance as independent prognostic markers. However, there are no data that permit a separation of the prognostic significance of the ST segment and T wave changes observed in an individual with heart disease from that of ST-T changes observed in an individual without heart disease. The limited data that are available suggest that the prognostic significance of an abnormal ST segment or T wave is dependent primarily on the absence or presence and severity of heart disease. Moderate T wave inversion has a 1 year mortality rate of 21% when associated with a history of heart disease compared with a rate of only 3% when heart disease is absent (25).

The information relating the ECG to future events such as angina, myocardial infarction, cardiovascular and sudden death, presence or absence of clinical heart disease and severity of myocardial impairment, although meager, does at times prove useful (25–28). For example, even though right bundle branch block is an acquired abnormality and thus undoubtedly associated with some form of cardiac disease, the long-term survival of patients with right bundle branch block is no different from that of patients without such block (28). This outcome might be expected because it is the cardiac function that is the primary determinant of prognosis, and cardiac function as such is rarely reflected on the ECG.

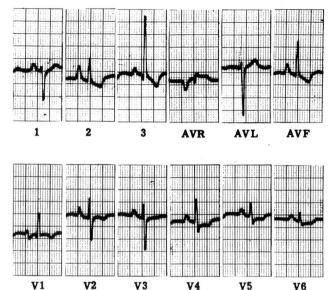

Figure 2.9. Electrocardiogram recorded in a patient with congenital pulmonary stenosis. The qR pattern in lead V$_1$ indicates that right ventricular pressure exceeds left ventricular pressure.

The major contribution of the ECG in epidemiologic studies is as an aid in identifying the individual with ischemic heart disease, the most prevalent form of heart disease in the Western world and the most common matrix for sudden death (29).

The ECG and Anatomic, Metabolic and Hemodynamic Changes

As noted previously, the ECG reflects an electrical event, and extrapolation to an anatomic or hemodynamic diagnosis is based on correlation of the ECG changes with experimental, clinical and autopsy findings.

Electrocardiographic changes may give a clue as to the severity of a hemodynamic abnormality. Such clues, however, are only indirect evidence because the ECG reflects anatomic changes secondary to altered hemodynamics and not the altered hemodynamics as such. For example, in patients with congenital heart disease, tracings showing incomplete right bundle branch block, a prominent R wave with a slur on the upstroke and a qR pattern reflect, respectively, a left ventricular pressure that exceeds the right ventricular pressure (as in atrial septal defect), right ventricular pressure that equals left ventricular pressure (as in tetralogy of Fallot) and right ventricular pressure that exceeds left ventricular pressure (as in pulmonary stenosis with an intact intraventricular septum) (Fig. 2.9) (30). However, identical ECG abnormalities may be due to a variety of disorders. For example, the ECG pattern of left ventricular hypertrophy may be due to hypertension, aortic stenosis, coarctation of the aorta or idiopathic hypertrophic subaortic stenosis. Similarly, ST segment elevation may be due to

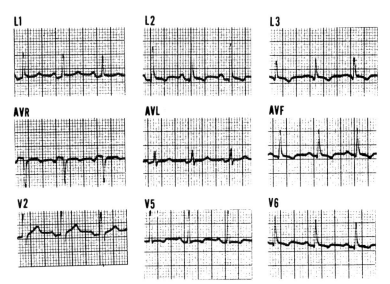

Figure 2.10. The elevated Ta segment in lead aVR and the depressed Ta segment in leads I, aVL and V₅ are the only evidence of acute pericarditis. The T wave changes are nonspecific. Reproduced with permission from Fisch C. Electrocardiography and vectorcardiography. In: Braunwald E, ed. Heart Disease, 3rd ed. Philadelphia: WB Saunders, 1988:180–222.

early repolarization, be a normal finding or reflect acute ischemia, pericarditis or hyperkalemia. Despite these limitations, occasionally an ECG abnormality is the only clue to a correct diagnosis (Fig. 2.10).

The ECG and Arrhythmias

More than 85 years after introduction of the ECG by Einthoven (11) and 70 years after Lewis (15) summarized its early contributions to clinical cardiology, the role of the ECG in the diagnosis of arrhythmias remains unique as the only practical method of recording cardiac rhythm. Free of theoretical assumptions that are important in the analysis of ECG waveforms relative to the diagnosis of myocardial structural abnormalities, arrhythmias recorded from the surface of the body can be said, with some exceptions, to directly reflect the intracardiac events responsible for the ECG manifestations of cardiac arrhythmias (31).

It is important to recall that whereas the ECG reflects the voltage generated by the atrial and ventricular myocardium, arrhythmias are frequently the result of abnormalities of impulse formation or conduction, or both, of the specialized conduction tissue. Because the activity of the specialized tissue is not recorded on the ECG, its function must be extrapolated from the temporal relations of the waveforms generated by the myocardium. Such deductive analysis is facilitated by recognition of electrophysiologic concepts, many of which were described during the early years of electrocardiography. Thus, the aberrations that later became known as the Ashman phenomenon, electrical alternans, acceleration-dependent aberration, ventricular fusion, reciprocation, parasystole, exit block, supernormality and concealed conduction were clearly described and understood by the year 1925. In the diagnosis of complex arrhythmias, recognition and proper interpretation of the behavior of specialized tissue are important and must be derived from the behavior of myocardium by the process of deductive reasoning.

Although many investigators contributed to the understanding of the mechanisms that make the ECG diagnosis of complex arrhythmias possible, it was largely Katz, Langendorf and Pick (32,33) who gave structure to the diagnostic process. Through deductive reasoning, they coupled the surface ECG with electrophysiologic principles to achieve a mechanistic as well as a clinical diagnosis. Their systematic contributions to the ECG literature over more than four decades and their enthusiasm as teachers firmly established the major role of this analytic approach to the accurate diagnosis of arrhythmias (34).

ECG clues to electrophysiologic mechanisms of arrhythmias. In general, the currently recognized electrophysiologic mechanisms of clinical arrhythmias include automaticity, reentry and, possibly, "triggered" automaticity. Although recognition of these mechanisms from the ECG is often difficult or impossible, occasionally there are ECG clues that point to one or another of these mechanisms. Thus, gradual acceleration, long coupling intervals, variable coupling, gradual emergence of an arrhythmia and the appearance of a fusion complex as the first complex of an emerging arrhythmia point to automaticity. Such automatic rhythms include, among others, a slow dominant pacemaker, parasystole, escape rhythm, nonparoxysmal junctional tachycardia, fascicular ventricular tachycardia and accelerated idioventricular rhythm. Reentry is suspected in the presence of fixed coupling, abrupt termination of an arrhythmia by an extraneous impulse and emergence of an ectopic rhythm in the setting of abnormally prolonged conduction. Electrocardiographic evidence is less convincing for "triggered" automaticity than for either automaticity or reentry. It should be suspected when an accelerated escape or escape tachycardia occurs after a "triggering" impulse or impulses (Fig. 2.11). These arrhythmias follow the rules

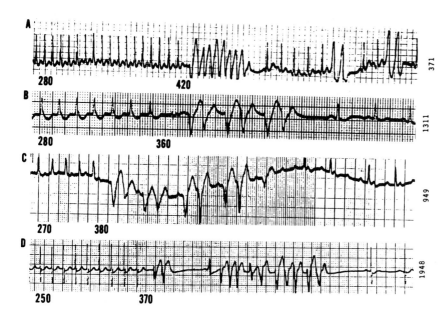

Figure 2.11. Ventricular tachycardia after supraventricular tachycardia recorded in four patients treated with digitoxin. The ventricular tachycardia was possibly "triggered" by the supraventricular tachycardia. The **first number in each panel** denotes the RR cycle of the supraventricular tachycardia and **the second number** denotes the coupling interval between the ventricular ectopic beat and the last complex of the supraventricular tachycardia. Reproduced with permission from Fisch and Knoebel (35).

described for "triggered" automaticity at the cellular level and may be the clinical counterpart of the cellular phenomenon of depolarization (35).

Limitations of the ECG in interpretation of arrhythmias. Despite the high sensitivity and specificity of the ECG for arrhythmias, as with any other laboratory procedure, there are limitations. These limitations fall into two groups and, when recognized, do not interfere with interpretation of the ECG. One, for lack of a better term, is referred to as "inherent," and the other reflects technical limitations of the equipment, including failure to recognize small changes of voltage (Fig. 2.12), and of time intervals (Fig. 2.13). The "inherent" limitations are the result of the inability to record the activity of the specialized tissue and include dependence on deductive analysis, occasional inability to make a definitive diagnosis, the possibility of multiple diagnoses and multiple mechanisms and, on occasion, failure to identify any mechanism (Fig. 2.14). Because the ECG is insensitive to small but physiologically significant changes, an interval change should be assumed when suggested by a changing ECG pattern, even if the interval change is not measurable (Fig. 2.13). Such an assumption is valid and is supported by intracardiac studies demonstrating that small changes in conduction or cycle length, often on the order of only a few milliseconds, may be the critical determinant of whether an impulse will conduct, be delayed or blocked.

The ECG and Research

From the time of its introduction, the ECG stimulated an exchange of ideas between the clinical electrocardiographer and the basic and clinical investigator. Many electrophysiologic concepts derived by deductive analysis of the surface ECG have been ultimately confirmed in the laboratory. Similarly, concepts initially derived from animal studies

have been identified in humans by the clinical electrocardiographer. Importantly, as a result of such interaction, electrocardiography, at first largely an empiric body of knowledge, was gradually and continuously placed on a firm experimental foundation. This interaction, particularly in the field of arrhythmias, has been so successful that a task force

Figure 2.12. Failure of the surface electrocardiogram to record small changes in voltage. Atrial activity recorded in low right atrial lead (LRA) is not evident in leads III and V₁. From Fisch C. The electrocardiogram and arrhythmias: limitations of a technique. Circulation 1987;75(suppl III):III-48–53. Reproduced with permission from the American Heart Association, Inc.

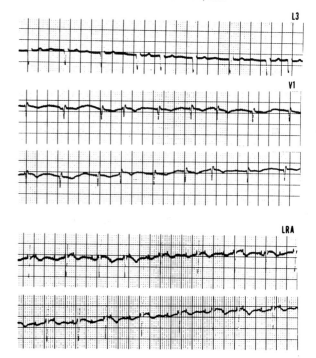

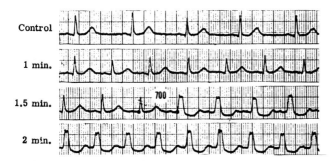

Figure 2.13. Failure to record small but physiologically significant changes in duration of the cardiac cycle, which is manifested by acceleration-dependent left bundle branch block. There is no measurable difference between the critical RR interval of 700 ms initiating the bundle branch block (at 1.5 mm) and the preceding RR interval. Despite failure to note a difference between the two RR cycles, the critical RR cycle is no doubt the shorter of the two. Reproduced with permission from Fisch (34).

of the American College of Cardiology at the Bethesda Conference on Optimal Electrocardiography (31) addressed the current status of intracardiac electrocardiography and concluded that a "careful assessment of the surface ECG often eliminates the need for intracardiac electrocardiography."

The list of concepts and mechanisms deduced by careful painstaking analysis of the clinical ECG that stimulated fundamental laboratory studies is lengthy, as is the list of observations made initially in the basic laboratory that in turn encouraged electrocardiographers to search for the clinical counterpart (36).

An example of how such an interchange between the basic and clinical investigators lead to laboratory confirmation of a concept first derived by deductive analysis of the clinical ECG is presented by concealed His bundle discharge. In 1947, Langendorf and Mehlman (37) proposed that nonconducted AV node premature systoles can imitate first and second degree AV block. Many years later, the validity of this concept was proved by recording directly from the His bundle in an animal (38) and ultimately from the His bundle in humans (Fig. 2.15) (39). Similar interchanges of ideas between the clinical electrocardiographer and the investigator have contributed significantly to our understanding of the ECG waveform.

Present and Future Issues Facing Clinical Electrocardiography

Problems facing electrocardiography are the result of, among other factors, the shortage of experienced human resources, efforts at cost containment, the advent of new noninvasive procedures and, paradoxically, the widespread acceptance and utility of the procedure.

Training and human resources. There is the ever-increasing competition with other procedures for the attention of the bright young clinician and clinical investigator. If research is to continue and a high level of individual ECG competence maintained, both of which are essential for excellence of cardiologic care, an ample number of future electrocardiographers must be trained. Human resource problems generated by the growth of electrocardiography are not new. Carl J. Wiggers (40) in the preface to his text *Principles and Practice of Electrocardiography* published in 1929, stated that ". . . unfortunately, the training of medical manpower in the use of such apparatus and the intelligent interpretation of the electrocardiogram has not kept pace with the increased demand. Few courses in electrocardiog-

Figure 2.14. The inherent limitations of the electrocardiogram resulting from inability to record the activity of the specialized conduction tissue. In the **top trace**, the paradoxic normalization of the QRS complex at the short RR interval can be explained by supernormal conduction of the right bundle branch, equal delay in the two bundle branches, ventricular escape or deceleration-dependent aberration. The correct diagnosis (**lower four tracings**) is ventricular escape and ventricular escape rhythm after an atrial premature systole with right bundle branch block pattern. From Fisch C. The electrocardiogram and arrhythmias: limitations of a technique. Circulation 1987;75(suppl III):III-48–53. Reproduced with permission from the American Heart Association, Inc.

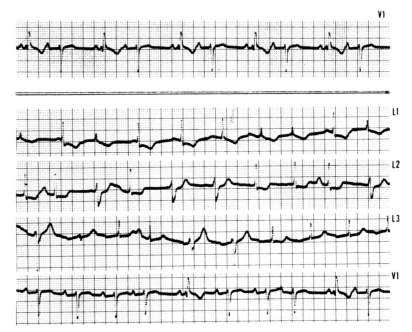

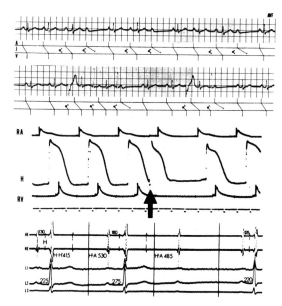

Figure 2.15. The interplay between the electrocardiographer and the basic and clinical investigator. The electrocardiogram in the **top panel** demonstrates atrioventricular (AV) block due to a concealed junctional discharge. The **middle panel** illustrates AV block due to a premature isolated His discharge at the cellular level. The **bottom panel** demonstrates a concealed His potential (H') recorded in a human subject. Reproduced with permission from Fisch (36).

raphy are included in undergraduate and postgraduate curricula in medical schools, so that opportunity for systematic instruction is decidedly restricted.'' Sixty years later, the problems addressed by Wiggers show no signs of relenting.

The widespread availability of ECG equipment and the ease of recording are equated by many with ease of interpretation and lack of sophistication of the ECG as a diagnostic tool. Whereas such assumptions are obviously incorrect, they do result in complacency, and frequently the interpretation of the ECG is relegated to individuals with limited experience. The large volume of tracings and the shortage of properly trained electrocardiographers force a search for alternate approaches to interpretation, processing, storage and retrieval of the ECG. The computer is a widely accepted and, in part, a logical approach to the problem.

Computer analysis of the ECG. There is little question about the usefulness of computers for data storage and retrieval in epidemiologic and large-scale studies of heart disease. To date, however, the role of the computer in sophisticated analyses of the clinical ECG is limited. Computer programs, although reliable for the diagnosis of the normal ECG and reasonably accurate in analysis of ECG waveforms, have serious limitations when applied to the diagnosis of arrhythmias. The programs lack sensitivity, accuracy and reproducibility. The early hopes for improvement of the diagnostic criteria, for "stand alone" programs for interpretation and for cost containment are yet to be realized. In fact, I suggest that because of the availability of

computer interpretation, the intellectual process necessary to arrive at an ECG diagnosis is often circumvented, and the computer may be an obstacle to acquisition of ECG skills. Irrespective of the potential impact of the computer on interpretation of the 12 lead ECG, significant numbers of records require confirmation and interpretation by well-trained electrocardiographers. Not all ECG changes can or should be programmed because such programs would prove complex, difficult or impossible to develop and economically inappropriate.

The future of electrocardiography. Despite the problems faced by electrocardiography, until a better method of recording the electrical potential is developed, the future of this discipline is assured. There is a renewed interest in arrhythmias stimulated by the increased use and complexity of cardiac pacemakers, the development of implantable cardioverters and defibrillators, heart surgery, the ever present problem of sudden death, the search for new antiarrhythmic drugs and new approaches to surgical therapy of arrhythmias. Similarly, new and aggressive approaches to ischemic heart disease have rekindled interest in the ECG as an anatomic, qualitative and occasionally quantitative marker of myocardial ischemia, injury and infarction. Cellular electrophysiology, His bundle electrocardiography, intracardiac pacing, intracardiac mapping, surface mapping, ambulatory ECG monitoring, stress testing, computer science and other noninvasive procedures will continue to have an impact on the clinical ECG.

It is proper to conclude by stating that nearly 90 years after its introduction, the ECG is "of recognized value," "serves as a standard of excellence," is "traditional, enduring" and "in fashion year after year" and thus fulfills Webster's definition of a classic (2).

References

1. Macfarlane PW. The coming of age of electrocardiography. In: Macfarlane PW, Lawrie TDV, eds. Comprehensive Electrocardiography, vol. 1. New York: Pergamon, 1988:3.
2. Fisch C. The clinical electrocardiogram: a classic. Circulation 1980; 62(suppl III):III-1–4.
3. Wellens HJJ. The electrocardiogram 80 years after Einthoven. J Am Coll Cardiol 1986;7:484–91.
4. Krikler DM. Electrocardiography then and now: where next? Br Heart J 1987;57:113–7.
5. Katz LN, Hellerstein HK. Electrocardiography. In: Fishman AP, Richards DW, eds. Circulation of the Blood: Men and Ideas. Bethesda, MD: American Physiological Society, 1964;5:265(ref 91).
6. Katz LN, Hellerstein HK. Electrocardiography. In: Fishman AP, Richards DW, eds. Circulation of the Blood: Men and Ideas. Bethesda, MD: American Physiological Society, 1964;5:346(ref 158).
7. Katz LN, Hellerstein HK. Electrocardiography. In: Fishman AP, Richards DW, eds. Circulation of the Blood: Men and Ideas. Bethesda, MD: American Physiological Society, 1964;5:345(ref 139).
8. Lipmann G. Relations entre les phenomenes electriques et capillares. Ann Chim 1875;5:494.
9. Waller AD. A demonstration on man of electromotive changes accompanying the heart's beat. J Physiol 1887;8:229–34.
10. Burchell HB. A centennial note on Waller and the first human electrocardiogram. Am J Cardiol 1987;59:973–83.

11. Einthoven W. Un nouveau galvanometre. Arch Neerl Sci Exactes Nat 1901;6:625–33.

12. Einthoven W. Die galvanometrische Registerung des Menschlichen Elektrocardiogramms, Zugleich eine Beurtheilung der Anwedung des Kapillar-Electrometers in Physiologie. Pflugers Arch 1903;99:472–80.

13. Einthoven W. Le telecardiogramme. Arch Intern Physiol 1906;4:132–64.

14. Einthoven W. Weiteres uber das Elecktrokardiogramm. Pflugers Arch 1908;122:517–84.

15. Lewis T. The Mechanism and Graphic Registration of the Heart Beat (preface). London: Shaw and Sons, 1920.

16. Burch EG, DePasquale NP. A History of Electrocardiography. Chicago: Year Book Medical, 1964:164.

17. Wilson FN, Johnston FD, Rosenbaum F, et al. The precordial electrocardiogram. Am Heart J 1944;27:19–85.

18. Kossmann C. Unipolar electrocardiography of Wilson: a half century later. Am Heart J 1985;110:901–4.

19. Friedberg CK, Zager A. A "nonspecific" St and T wave changes. Circulation 1961;23:655–61.

20. Autenrieth G, Surawicz B, Kuo CS, Arita M. Primary T wave abnormalities caused by uniform and regional shortening of ventricular monophasic action potential in dog. Circulation 1975;51:668–76.

21. Surawicz B. ST-T abnormalities. In Ref 1:523.

22. Wilson FN, Finch R. The effect of drinking iced water upon the form of T deflection of the electrocardiogram. Heart 1923;10:275–8.

23. Goldberger AL. Myocardial Infarction: Electrocardiographic Differential Diagnosis. St. Louis: CV Mosby, 1984.

24. Fisch C. The electrocardiogram in the aged. Cardiovasc Clin 1981;12:65–74.

25. Rose G, Baxter PJ, Reid DD, McCartney P. Prevalence and prognosis of electrocardiographic findings in middle aged men. Br Heart J 1978;40:636–43.

26. Kannel WB, Gordon T, Offutt D. Left ventricular hypertrophy by electrocardiogram: prevalence, incidence, and mortality in the Framingham Study. Ann Intern Med 1969;71:89–105.

27. Cullen K, Steinhouse NS, Wearne KL, Cumpston GN. Electrocardiograms and 13 year cardiovascular mortality in Brusselton Study. Br Heart J 1982;47:209–12.

28. Blackburn H. The prognostic importance of the electrocardiogram after myocardial infarction. Ann Intern Med 1972;77:677–89.

29. Spain DM, Bradess VA, Mohr C. Coronary atherosclerosis as a cause of unexpected and unexplained death: an autopsy study from 1949–1959. JAMA 1960;174:384–8.

30. Burch GE, DePasquale NP. Electrocardiography in the Diagnosis of Congenital Heart Disease. Philadelphia: Lea & Febiger, 1967.

31. American College of Cardiology Tenth Bethesda Conference: optimal electrocardiography. Am J Cardiol 1978;41:111–91.

32. Katz LN, Pick A. Clinical Electrocardiography. Part I: The Arrhythmias. Philadelphia: Lea & Febiger, 1967.

33. Pick A, Langendorf R. Interpretation of Complex Arrhythmias. Philadelphia: Lea & Febiger, 1979.

34. Fisch C. Electrocardiography of Arrhythmias. Philadelphia: Lea & Febiger, 1990.

35. Fisch C, Knoebel SB. Accelerated junctional escape: a clinical manifestation of "triggered" automaticity? In: Zipes DP, Jalife J, eds. Cardiac Electrophysiology and Arrhythmias. Orlando, FL: Grune and Stratton, 1984:467–73.

36. Fisch C. Electrocardiography of arrhythmias: from deductive analysis to laboratory confirmation—twenty-five years of progress. J Am Coll Cardiol 1983;1:306–17.

37. Langendorf R, Mehlman JS. Blocked (nonconducted) A-V nodal premature systoles imitating first and second degree A-V block. Am Heart J 1947;34:500–6.

38. Moore EN, Knoebel SB, Spear JF. Concealed conduction. Am J Cardiol 1971;28:406–13.

39. Rosen KM, Rahimtoola SH, Gunnar RM. Pseudo A-V block secondary to nonprogagated His bundle depolarization: documentation by His bundle electrocardiography. Circulation 1970;42:367–73.

40. Wiggers CJ. Principles and Practice of Electrocardiography. St. Louis: CV Mosby, 1929:9.

CHAPTER 3

The Current and Future Usefulness of Noninvasive Techniques in Cardiology

ROBERT A. O'ROURKE, MD

The marked decrement in age-adjusted mortality from cardiovascular disease during the past 30 years is multifactorial (1–4). Improvements in patient education, primary and secondary prevention and the available diagnostic and therapeutic options are all contributing factors. The many noninvasive techniques that have been developed and used for the evaluation, treatment and serial assessment of patients with cardiovascular disease during the past three decades have contributed importantly to better health care delivery. Among these are electrocardiographic (ECG) stress testing, ambulatory ECG recordings, transthoracic and transesophageal two-dimensional echocardiography, Doppler velocity recordings and color flow imaging, myocardial perfusion imaging, radionuclide cineangiography and several other nuclear medicine techniques (5–11). Recently introduced noninvasive methods that provide useful information include positron emission tomography, cine computed tomography, nuclear magnetic resonance imaging and spectroscopy and signal-averaged electrocardiography (12–17).

The important uses of noninvasive cardiology methods are listed in Table 3.1. In general, they concern the detection of cardiovascular disease, the quantitation of the severity of disease and the evaluation of medical and therapeutic interventions. A description of the use of these techniques in the diagnosis of congenital heart disease and peripheral vascular disease is beyond the scope of this discussion.

Detection of Cardiac Disease

The availability of accurate noninvasive techniques has greatly enhanced the ability of clinicians to diagnose cardiac disease with certainty earlier in its natural history than was previously possible. Multiple noninvasive methods have been utilized for the detection of myocardial ischemia and necrosis; the identification of impaired function or anatomy, or both, involving the endocardium, myocardium or pericardium, or a combination of these areas; and the detection of various cardiac arrhythmias and abnormalities involving the coronary arteries.

Detection of Myocardial Ischemia and Necrosis

Noninvasive methods utilized to detect myocardial ischemia can record the ECG during normal activity and progressive exercise (ambulatory ECG recordings, exercise ECG testing), evaluate regional and global left ventricular function at rest and during various types of stress (two-dimensional echocardiography, radionuclide cineangiography) and determine the presence of myocardial perfusion abnormalities occurring spontaneously or during stress (thallium-201 imaging, technetium isonitrile scintigraphy) (18–32). Types of stress used to increase the disparity between myocardial oxygen demand and supply include treadmill, bicycle and arm crank ergometry, intracardiac or esophageal cardiac pacing, intravenous dipyridamole or adenosine and intravenous positive inotropic agents such as dobutamine (33–38). The myocardial ischemic cascade has been defined from studies (39–44) in animals and patients undergoing coronary angioplasty. Inadequate perfusion to contracting myocardium results in abnormal regional wall motion during systole and diastole and hemodynamic abnormalities often before and many times without subsequent ECG changes or angina (Fig. 3.1). Thus, exercise-induced myocardial perfusion defects by planar or single photon emission tomographic thallium imaging and regional wall motion abnormalities during stress by two-dimensional echocardiography or radionuclide angiography are more sensitive and more specific indicators of myocardial ischemia than exercise ECG ST segment changes, particularly when ECG abnormalities at rest are already present. Furthermore, ambulatory ECG recordings are less sensitive and specific than exercise ECG tests for determining the presence or absence of ischemic myocardium (22).

Recently (12), metabolic imaging utilizing positron emission tomography has been used to define areas of viable myocardium that metabolize glucose ^{18}F 2-deoxyglucose (FDG-18) despite hypoperfusion as indicated by imaging with nitrogen-13 ammonia. The identification of viable myocardium in areas of abnormal wall motion indicate that reperfusion (coronary surgery or angioplasty) is likely to result in improved cardiac function. Quantitative planar and single photon emission tomography thallium imaging are more sensitive than qualitative imaging and single photon emission tomography is somewhat better than planar imaging for detecting ischemic zones, particularly in the distribution of the left circumflex coronary artery (45–47). New radionuclide agents are needed that are better than thallium-201 for determining myocardial perfusion defect. Higher resolution can be obtained by using agents with short half-lives, permitting high doses and with energy spectra that

Table 3.1. Usefulness of Noninvasive Techniques

Detection of cardiac disease
   Detection of myocardial ischemia and necrosis
   Detection of impaired cardiac function and structure
      Endocardium
      Myocardium
      Pericardium
   Detection of cardiac arrhythmias
   Detection of diseased coronary arteries
Quantitation of the severity of cardiac disease
Assessment of the effects of therapeutic interventions

Table 3.2. Comparison of Thallium-201 Imaging and Technetium-99m Hexakis Methoxyisobutylisonitrile

	Thallium-201	Technetium-99m Isonitrile
Availability	Cyclotron produced Ordered from vendor	Generator produced Available 24 h
Energy for gamma cameras	Lower than optimal energy with <resolution >scatter and attenuation	Optimal energy with >resolution < scatter and attenuation
Radiation and dosimetry	Longer half-life and lower administered dose; no gating and only "equilibrium" study	Shorter half-life and greater administered dose; cardiac gating and first pass study (perfusion and function)
Redistribution	Present, permitting viability assessment	Not sufficient for clinical use

Modified from Berman D. Perspectives on the future of nuclear cardiology. In: Pohost GM, O'Rourke RA. Cardiovascular Imaging. Boston: Little, Brown 1991, p. 320.

yield better images using the gamma scintillation camera (48–51). Although the technetium isonitrile compounds hold considerable promise for imaging patients with acute coronary artery syndromes, particularly before and after early reperfusion therapy, they redistribute poorly and two injections are required to compare rest and exercise images in patients with stress-induced myocardial ischemia (Table 3.2).

Left ventricular diastolic dysfunction often occurs before impaired systolic function in patients with ischemic or hypertensive heart disease, or both. Current noninvasive techniques including M-mode echocardiography, Doppler echocardiography (transmitral valve diastolic velocity waves) and radionuclide cineangiography (time to peak rapid left ventricular filling and rate of peak rapid filling) have been used clinically (52–57), but are yet to be proven as accurate reproducible methods for assessing diastolic function. Furthermore, these measurements are affected by many factors that are altered variably during exercise, even in the absence of myocardial ischemia. The presence of bibasal pulmonary rales de novo during exercise, evidence of pulmonary venous congestion by chest x-ray study or increased lung uptake of thallium during myocardial perfusion imaging (58)

provides indirect data indicating the presence of left ventricular diastolic dysfunction.

Prospective blinded studies (59) comparing the sensitivity and specificity of exercise-induced wall motion abnormalities (two-dimensional echocardiography or radionuclide cineangiography) with areas of decreased thallium uptake during exercise as indicators of ischemic myocardium in large enough numbers of patients have not yet provided conclusive data. Two-dimensional echocardiography during or immediately after exercise is being used with increased

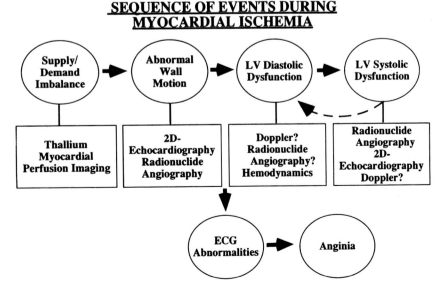

Figure 3.1. Schematic representation of the sequence of events occurring after acute coronary artery occlusion and tests that may reveal the presence of myocardial ischemia. 2D = two-dimensional; ECG = electrocardiogram; LV = left ventricular; ? = questionably accurate.

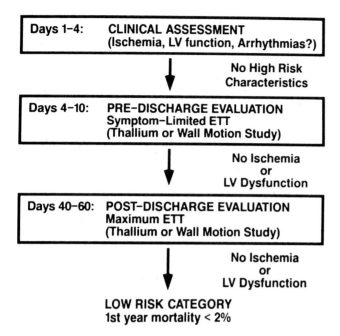

Figure 3.2. One of several potential methods for the use of noninvasive methods in risk stratification of patients with clinically uncomplicated myocardial infarction. ETT = exercise treadmill test; LV = left ventricle.

frequency for risk stratification of patients with suspected myocardial ischemia, particularly after recovery from an uncomplicated myocardial infarction (60). Alternatively, many such patients undergo exercise thallium perfusion imaging for secondary risk stratification (61). Although thallium-201 imaging is applicable to more patients with chronic ischemic heart disease, exercise echocardiography can be performed in the physician's office, does not require the injection of radionuclide material and permits a beat to beat analysis of wall motion in the patients in whom adequate images are obtained.

The scheme used at my institution for the further risk stratification of patients recovering from infarction without high risk characteristics during in-hospital clinical observation is shown in Figure 3.2. A low level, symptom-limited exercise test, often with myocardial perfusion imaging or echocardiographic wall motion assessment, is performed before discharge. A maximal treadmill test is subsequently used 4 to 6 weeks later to evaluate patients with a negative predischarge result.

Technetium-99m (stannous) pyrophosphate has been used for myocardial infarct avid imaging because it localizes in regions of recently infarcted myocardium, with the most intense visualization usually occurring 48 to 72 h after infarction (9,62). Although usually not necessary for establishing the diagnosis, infarct avid imaging is most useful in patients presenting >24 h after the onset of chest pain when enzymes and the ECG may be more difficult to interpret (9). The use of labeled antibody fragments directed against

myosin for the scintigraphic detection of acute myocardial necrosis is currently an investigational technique (63). The sensitivity, specificity and clinical utility of this approach for the diagnosis of acute myocardial infarction remains to be demonstrated (9).

Detection of Impaired Cardiac Function and Structure

The development of noninvasive cardiac imaging techniques has markedly improved the diagnosis, treatment and follow-up evaluation of patients with diseases involving the endocardium, myocardium and pericardium.

Echocardiography is the most common noninvasive method for evaluating patients with disease involving the endocardium. Two-dimensional echocardiography is utilized to detect abnormalities of valve leaflet movement, as well as thickening, redundancy or disruption of the structural components of the four valves; it is useful for assessing the consequences of valvular stenosis and regurgitation, as well as cardiac chamber size (7,64). Echocardiography commonly is used to quantitate the severity of valvular stenosis and regurgitation, with Doppler echocardiography and color flow imaging adding importantly to the two-dimensional echocardiographic assessment of valvular heart disease (65–73). Importantly, two-dimensional echocardiography is the technique of choice for detecting vegetations in patients with suspected endocarditis, and the transesophageal echocardiographic assessment of the left-sided valves has greatly improved the sensitivity for detecting vegetations as compared with the transthoracic method. Complications of endocarditis, including fistulae and abscess formation, are much better detected with transesophageal echocardiography (7,8,74,75). Endocardial tumors are also well delineated by two-dimensional echocardiography (76), as is involvement of the leaflets by other diseases such as lupus erythematosus. In the future, better imaging techniques likely will be developed to detect valvular vegetations with even greater sensitivity and specificity. Ventricular thrombi are also best detected with two-dimensional echocardiography (77), and most atrial thrombi can be visualized with properly applied transesophageal echocardiography (78).

Noninvasive methods often are used to measure left ventricular chamber size and wall thickness in patients with cardiovascular disease, particularly in those with hypertension or valvular heart disease. Calculations of left ventricular wall stress are often made from these measurements (79). M-mode echocardiography remains the most common noninvasive method for the quantitative measurement of wall thickness because of its better resolution, but cine computed tomography and magnetic resonance imaging also provide accurate determinations of wall thickness (13,80,81).

The diagnosis of hypertrophic cardiomyopathy is best determined by echocardiography techniques, specifically two-dimensional echocardiographic delineation of regional left ventricular wall thickness and Doppler measurement of left ventricular outflow tract gradients (82). Two-dimensional echocardiography and radionuclide cineangiography are commonly used to diagnose dilated cardiomyopathy and distinguish regional from global left ventricular dysfunction.

Measurement of ultrasound backscatter has been used as a research tool for myocardial tissue characterization for many years (83,84). Although positive results for differentiating ischemic, infarcted, hypertrophied and normal myocardium have been reported, the clinical utility of ultrasound tissue characterization has not yet been decided. Future advances in the noninvasive differentiation of normal from diseased myocardium and for identifying different myocardial infiltrative processes (inflammation, amyloid, sarcoid, hemochromatosis, tumor) are both likely and important. Two-dimensional, Doppler and color flow echocardiography are useful techniques for detecting complications of acute myocardial infarction, including ventricular septal rupture, mitral regurgitation and pseudoaneurysm formation (9,85–88).

M-mode echocardiography initially was introduced for the diagnosis of pericardial effusion (89), and two-dimensional echocardiography remains the best noninvasive method for this purpose and for demonstrating right atrial and right ventricular compression with pericardial tamponade (90–93). Changes in pericardial thickness and structure can also be assessed by magnetic resonance imaging, computed tomography and other imaging techniques (81). Alterations in transmitral and transtricuspid Doppler velocity recordings during the respiratory cycle have been used successfully to distinguish patients with restrictive cardiomyopathy from those with constrictive pericarditis (94); however, some patient overlap exists. Newer noninvasive techniques with improved sensitivity and specificity for detecting acute pericarditis, metastatic pericardial disease and early pericardial constriction remain to be developed and applied.

Although urgent aortography is commonly utilized for the accurate diagnosis of aortic dissection and the extent of affected aorta and its branches, screening with one of several available noninvasive methods is frequently employed in patients in whom the diagnosis is possible but improbable (95). However, computed tomography, magnetic resonance imaging and echocardiography all have advantages and disadvantages (Table 3.3) (14,95–98).

Detection of Cardiac Arrhythmias

During the past several decades, there has been great emphasis on developing and improving the technology for recording and interpreting various cardiac arrhythmias (6,99–103). However, the need to identify better patients at high risk of sudden cardiac death and determine the favorable or detrimental effects of medical or surgical therapy in patients with depressed left ventricular function and com-

Table 3.3. Usefulness of Several Diagnostic Tests for Aortic Dissection

	Aortic Angiography	CT Scanning	MRI	Echocardiography
Accurate detection	+++	+++	+++	++
Extent of dissection	+++	++	++	+
Site of tear	+++	+	++	+
Presence and severity of AR	+++	0	+	+++
Major branches involved	+++	+	++	0
False channel thrombosis	+++	++	++	0
Pericardial or pleural leak	+	+++	+++	++

AR = aortic regurgitation; CT = computed tomographic; MRI = magnetic resonance imaging; 0 = poor; + = fair; ++ = good; +++ = excellent. Modified from Eagle and DeSanctis (95).

plex cardiac arrhythmias remains. Ambulatory ECG recordings often detect high risk patients among those with hypertrophic or dilated cardiomyopathy and define the mechanisms in many patients with arrhythmia-induced syncope. The utility of ambulatory ECG recordings compared with serial electrophysiologic testing in determining the need and results of antiarrhythmic therapy is being assessed in multicenter clinical research studies.

More recently, the signal-averaged ECG has been used to detect late potentials in patients with myocardial ischemia or depressed left ventricular function, or both. The identification of late potentials appears useful in the overall risk stratification of patients recovering from myocardial infarction (16,17). The presence of late potentials appears to indicate a higher risk in patients recovering from infarction with recurrent myocardial ischemia or depressed left ventricular function. Conversely, the absence of late potentials in these patients with depressed left ventricular function or myocardial ischemia indicates a relative diminished risk for subsequent fatal ventricular tachyarrhythmias (16,17). Further studies assessing the importance of the signal-averaged ECG in the overall assessment of patients with acute and chronic ischemic heart disease and in those with other diseases frequently associated with ventricular arrhythmias such as hypertrophic and dilated cardiomyopathies are necessary before definite conclusions can be made about its clinical utility.

Detection of Diseased Coronary Arteries

The inability of noninvasive methods to assess accurately and completely the anatomy of the coronary arteries is the only reason why many patients undergo cardiac catheterization and selective coronary arteriography. Although several methods have been used to determine the presence or absence of coronary artery stenosis and detect coronary artery anomalies in various subgroups of patients, none has been sufficiently sensitive or accurate to replace invasive arteriography for this purpose. The promising clinical techniques of coronary angioscopy and intracoronary echocardiography are both invasive procedures.

The large epicardial coronary arteries are often visualized in their proximal course by transthoracic and transesophageal echocardiography, magnetic resonance imaging and cine computed tomography (14,15,104). However, none of these has been developed or modified to the point where presurgical coronary arteriography need not be performed in patients with other cardiac disease who are in the high risk age group or in whom congenital abnormalities of the coronary circulation are suspected. The development of a noninvasive technique for defining coronary artery anatomy would revolutionize the practice of cardiology, with coronary arteriography reserved for those likely to undergo interventional procedures at the time of invasive study. Decisions on the development of out-patient versus in-hospital cardiac catheterization laboratories would be greatly influenced by such an advance.

Quantitating the Severity of Cardiovascular Disease

Several noninvasive methods are widely applied for quantitating or semiquantitating the severity of cardiovascular disease. When detecting myocardial ischemia, it is common to assess the amount of exercise or other stress necessary to provide evidence of ischemia. For example, during exercise testing, the development of ST segment depression at a low workload (heart rate-blood pressure product) and in multiple ECG leads and that persists for several minutes after exercise indicates relatively severe myocardial ischemia. Also, a subnormal increase or actual decrease in the systolic blood pressure response during exercise often indicates severe coronary artery disease (5). Likewise, a subnormal increase or a decrease in the *global* left ventricular ejection fraction as determined by radionuclide angiography or two-dimensional echocardiography during exercise is consistent with severe myocardial ischemia, but has several other causes (9). Exercise-induced new or worsening *regional* left ventricular wall motion abnormalities determined by these two techniques is more specific for myocardial ischemia, the severity of the ischemia correlating with the severity and extent of stress-induced left ventricular asynergy. Indicators of severe myocardial ischemia during stress thallium-201 myocardial imaging include multiple regions with reversible thallium defects, dilation of the left ventricular during exercise and increased lung uptake of thallium-201 indicating pulmonary venous hypertension (10). With the development of better imaging techniques and superior radioisotopes for myocardial perfusion imaging, the ability to detect and quantify ischemic myocardium should improve considerably. Furthermore, the use of metabolic imaging with simul-

taneous perfusion imaging for determining the amount of viable but hypoperfused and hypofunctioning myocardium will be simplified and more assessable to a larger number of patients undergoing treatment for ischemia. A major clinical objective is the ability to define regions of viable myocardium in areas of "hibernating" impaired left ventricular function; such regions are likely to improve after myocardial revascularization.

In patients with endocardial disease, Doppler velocity recordings can accurately quantitate the severity of valvular stenosis. For example, echocardiographic measurements of aortic valve cross-sectional area by the continuity equation or the extent of mitral valve stenosis by the pressure-half time Doppler method correlate well with the same measures obtained by cardiac catheterization and cineangiography. Several methods have been developed for using Doppler echocardiography and color flow imaging to assess the extent of valvular regurgitation (105). Although currently less accurate and more time-consuming than echocardiographic measurements of valvular stenosis, future advances in imaging techniques should permit the more rapid and accurate quantitation of valve regurgitation.

The measurement of left ventricular ejection fraction by radionuclide cineangiography or two-dimensional echocardiography has become the most common clinically applied method for determining the presence of normal or abnormal left ventricular systolic function at rest or during exercise. Because of the ease of data analysis and the applicability to more patients, the radionuclide technique is used more commonly. The measured ejection fraction by both noninvasive methods correlates well with the same measurement by contrast ventriculography (106).

Measurements of right ventricular systolic function by both echocardiography and radionuclide cineangiography provide useful information, with right ventricular ejection fraction best quantitated by "first pass" radionuclide cineangiography (9,10). Although the correlation of noninvasive measures with a "gold standard" for right ventricular systolic function has not been well documented, continuous wave Doppler velocity recordings of tricuspid valve regurgitation permit the accurate noninvasive measurement of the right ventricular systolic pressure (107).

As already mentioned, quantitation of left ventricular diastolic function by noninvasive techniques is less commonly used and poorly validated, particularly during the hemodynamic alterations accompanying exercise. New noninvasive methods for the quantitative evaluation of ventricular diastolic function at rest and during stress would greatly enhance the clinical assessment of patients with cardiac disease who frequently present initially with isolated left ventricular diastolic dysfunction. The accuracy of two-dimensional echocardiographically determined left ventricular volume measurements has been verified and is often used with M-mode echocardiographic measurements of wall thickness to calculate left ventricular wall stress (79).

Nuclear magnetic imaging spectroscopy provides a noninvasive method for assessing high energy phosphate spectra (108), which are often altered before left ventricular systolic function in patients with various types of heart disease (hypertension, ischemic heart disease, valvular heart disease). This approach likely will become useful in the early detection and subsequent therapy of patients with subclinical or difficult to document disease affecting the myocardium. Methods for measuring high energy phosphate spectra from the heart in closed chest animals, without reflecting spectra from chest skeletal muscle or the cardiac blood, continue to be developed.

Echocardiography has been used for quantitating the extent of pericardial effusion and estimating its hemodynamic consequences in patients with pericardial disease. It remains the noninvasive technique of choice for determining the presence or absence of cardiac tamponade, particularly when assessing the effects of cardiac compression on the dimensions of the right atrium and ventricle during the cardiac cycle.

Noninvasive methods have been used for determining the frequency, duration and type of cardiac arrhythmias, usually by a prolonged period of continuous ambulatory ECG recording (100–103). However, the normal variability in the incidence and duration of arrhythmias during 24 to 48 h of continuous recording is great, and the consequences of a documented arrhythmia often are variable. Better noninvasive approaches for quantitating arrhythmias, their effects on ambulatory ventricular function or hemodynamics and the favorable or nonfavorable effects of therapy would be useful.

Presently, there is no noninvasive technique for assessing the severity of coronary artery stenosis, except indirectly by the effect on regional or global ventricular function and other indicators of myocardial ischemia (see previous discussion). Coronary artery disease affecting the left main coronary artery will often be visualized by noninvasive techniques such as transthoracic and transesophageal echocardiography or nuclear magnetic resonance imaging. The development of invasive imaging methods for the detection of atherosclerosis involving the main coronary arteries and their branches is a prerequisite for quantitation of the severity of coronary artery stenosis. The usefulness of a noninvasive imaging technique that accurately quantitates the extent of coronary artery disease is self-evident and would alter the practice of clinical cardiology.

Assessing the Effects of Therapeutic Interventions

One of the major uses of these noninvasive methods has been the serial assessment of patients with cardiac disease to detect progression of disease or determine the effect of medical or surgical therapeutic interventions. For example, ECG exercise testing, rest and exercise thallium imaging, exercise echocardiography and exercise radionuclide cine-angiography are commonly performed before and after therapeutic interventions designed to decrease exercise-induced myocardial ischemia and are often used to assess the results of revascularization by coronary angioplasty or bypass graft surgery. Imaging techniques that identify regions of decreased thallium uptake or abnormal wall motion provide information concerning regional myocardial ischemia in areas supplied by coronary arteries that have been treated with dilation or bypass grafts. The response of ventricular function, as assessed by radionuclide cineangiography or two-dimensional echocardiography, to therapeutic interventions (vasodilator therapy, positive inotropic agents and potential myocardial depressants) is frequently used to define the positive or negative effects on ventricular performance. Echocardiography commonly is utilized intraoperatively to guide cardiac surgery, particularly in patients undergoing mitral valve repair or treatment of congenital heart disease. Transesophageal echocardiography will be used with increasing frequency to monitor cardiac function in high risk patients undergoing noncardiac surgery. Two-dimensional, Doppler and color flow echocardiography will continue to be used as the methods of choice for the serial evaluation of patients after correction of valvular or congenital heart disease. Transthoracic two-dimensional echocardiography of the ventricle and transesophageal two-dimensional echocardiography of the left atrium to determine the effects of interventions such as anticoagulation on thrombi are common and likely to become even more frequent in the future.

Conclusions

During the past three decades, the development of noninvasive imaging techniques has played an important role in the decrease in age-adjusted mortality from cardiac disease. The emergence of various imaging methods for the accurate demonstration of cardiac disease and its consequences has been a very important factor in better diagnosis and therapy. With improving technology, further important advances are likely. Foremost among these will be the development of a noninvasive method for determining the presence or absence of coronary atherosclerosis and subsequently the quantitative assessment of the extent of coronary artery disease without the need for cardiac catheterization. Also important will be the use of noninvasive techniques for the quantitative assessment of left ventricular diastolic function at rest and during stress so that specific treatment can be developed for this early manifestation of myocardial disease.

References

1. Sytkowski PA, Kannel WB, D'Agostino RB. Changes in risk factors and the decline in mortality from cardiovascular disease. N Engl J Med 1990;322:1635–41.
2. Thom T, Kannel WB. The downward trend in cardiovascular disease mortality. Ann Rev Med 1981;32:427–34.

3. Gillium RF, Blackburn H, Feinleib M. Current strategies for explaining the decline in ischemic heart disease mortality. J Chronic Dis 1982;35:467–74.

4. Goldman L, Cook EF. The decline in ischemic heart mortality rates: an analysis of the comparative effects of medical interventions and changes in lifestyle. Ann Intern Med 1984;101:825–36.

5. Schlant RC, Blomquist CG, Brandenburg RO, et al. Guidelines for exercise testing: a report of the Joint American College of Cardiology/American Heart Association Task Force on Assessment of Cardiovascular Procedures (Subcommittee on Exercise Testing). Circulation 1986;74:653A–67A.

6. Knoebel SB, Crawford MH, Dunn MI, et al. Guidelines for ambulatory electrocardiography: a report of the American College of Cardiology/American Heart Association Task Force on Assessment of Diagnostic and Therapeutic Cardiovascular Procedures (Subcommittee on Ambulatory Electrocardiography). J Am Coll Cardiol 1989;13:249–58.

7. Ewy GA, Appleton CP, DeMaria AN, et al. Guidelines for the clinical application of echocardiography. J Am Coll Cardiol (in press).

8. Bansal RC, Shah PM. Transesophageal echocardiography. Curr Probl Cardiol 1990;15:643–720.

9. O'Rourke RA, Chatterjee K, Dodge HT, et al. Guidelines for clinical use of cardiac radionuclide imaging: a report of the American College of Cardiology/American Heart Association Task Force on Assessment of Cardiovascular Procedures (Subcommittee on Nuclear Imaging). J Am Coll Cardiol 1986;8:1471–83.

10. Beller G. Nuclear cardiology: current indications and clinical usefulness. Curr Probl Cardiol 1985;10:1–76.

11. Gibbons RJ. The use of radionuclide techniques for identification of severe coronary artery disease. Curr Probl Cardiol 1990;15:303–52.

12. Tillisch J, Brunken R, Marshall R, et al. Reversibility of cardiac wall motion abnormalities predicted by positron tomography. N Engl J Med 1986;314:884–8.

13. Cipriano P, Nussi M, Brody WR. Clinically applicable gated cardiac computed tomography. Am J Radiol 1983;140:604–10.

14. Bateman TM. X-ray computer tomography. In: Pohost GM, O'Rourke RA, eds. Principles and Practice of Cardiovascular Imaging. Boston: Little, Brown, 1991, pp 423–54.

15. Council on Scientific Affairs. Report of the Magnetic Resonance Imaging Panel. Magnetic resonance imaging of the cardiovascular system: present state of the art and future potential. JAMA 1988;259:253–9.

16. Kuchar DL, Thorburn CW, Sammel NL. Prediction of serious arrhythmic events after myocardial infarction: signal-averaged electrocardiogram, Holter monitoring and radionuclide ventriculography. J Am Coll Cardiol 1987;9:531–8.

17. Gomes JA, Winters SL, Stewart D, et al. A new noninvasive index to predict sustained ventricular tachycardia and sudden death in the first year after myocardial infarction based on signal-averaged electrocardiogram, radionuclide ejection fraction and Holter monitoring. J Am Coll Cardiol 1987;10:345–57.

18. Berman DS, Rozanski A, Knoebel SB. The detection of silent ischemia: cautions and precautions. Circulation 1987;75:103–5.

19. McNeer FJ, Margolis JR, Lee KL, et al. The role of the exercise test in the evaluation of patients for ischemic heart disease. Circulation 1978;57:64–70.

20. Goldschlager N, Selzer A, Cohn K. Treadmill stress tests as indicators of presence and severity of coronary artery disease. Ann Intern Med 1976;85:277–86.

21. Ellestad MH, Wan MKC. Predictive implications of stress testing: follow-up of 2700 subjects after maximum treadmill stress testing. Circulation 1975;51:363–9.

22. Crawford MH, Mendoza CA, O'Rourke RA, et al. Limitations of continuous ambulatory electrocardiogram monitoring for detecting coronary artery disease. Ann Intern Med 1978;89:1–5.

23. O'Rourke RA, Miller DD. Detection of viable myocardium within the ischemic risk area after myocardial infarction. Emory Univ J Med 1988;2:80–101.

24. Pohost GM, Zir LM, Moore RH, et al. Differentiation of transiently ischemic from infarcted myocardium by serial imaging after a single dose of thallium-201. Circulation 1977;55:294–302.

25. Berger BC, Watson DD, Burwell LR, et al. Redistribution of thallium at rest in patients with stable and unstable angina and the effect of coronary bypass surgery. Circulation 1979;60:1114–25.

26. Limacher MC, Quinones MA, Poliner LR, et al. Detection of coronary artery disease with exercise two-dimensional echocardiography. Circulation 1983;67:1211–8.

27. Armstrong WF, O'Donnell J, Dillon JC, et al. Complementary value of two-dimensional exercise echocardiography to routine treadmill exercise testing. Ann Intern Med 1986;105:829–35.

28. Armstrong WF, O'Donnell J, Ryan T, et al. Effect of prior myocardial infarction and extent and location of coronary disease on accuracy of exercise echocardiography. J Am Coll Cardiol 1987;10:531–8.

29. Ryan T, Vasey CG, Presti CF, et al. Exercise echocardiography: detection of coronary artery disease in patients with normal left ventricular wall motion at rest. J Am Coll Cardiol 1988;11:993–9.

30. Rozanski A, Diamond GA, Berman DS, et al. The declining specificity of exercise radionuclide ventriculography. N Engl Med 1983;309:518–22.

31. Hecht HS, Hopkins JM. Exercise-induced regional wall motion abnormalities on radionuclide angiography: lack of reliability for detection of coronary artery disease in the presence of valvular heart disease. Am J Cardiol 1981;47:861–5.

32. Kerber RE, Marcus ML, Wilson R, et al. Effects of acute coronary occlusion on the motion and perfusion of the normal and ischemic interventricular septum: an experimental echocardiographic study. Circulation 1976;54:928–35.

33. Younis LT, Chaitman BR. Update on intravenous dipyridamole cardiac imaging in the assessment of ischemic heart disease. Clin Cardiol 1990;13:3–10.

34. Iskandrian AS, Heo J, Askenase A, et al. Dipyridamole cardiac imaging. Am Heart J 1988;115:432–43.

35. Chapman PD, Wann LS. Two-dimensional echocardiography during transesophageal pacing. Pract Cardiol 1987;13:105–9.

36. Leppo J, Boucher CA, Okada RD, et al. Serial thallium-201 myocardial imaging after dipyridamole infusion: diagnostic utility in detecting coronary stenoses and relationship to regional wall motion. Circulation 1982;66:649–57.

37. Gupta N, Mohuiddin S, Siffring PA, et al. Comparative efficacy of adenosine infusion and dipyridamole T1-201 perfusion imaging. J Nucl Med 1989;30:730.

38. Berthe C, Pierard LA, Hiernaux M, et al. Predicting the extent and location of coronary artery disease in acute myocardial infarction by echocardiography during dobutamine infusion. Am J Cardiol 1986;58:1167–72.

39. Tennant R, Wiggers CJ. The effect of coronary occlusion on myocardial contraction. Am J Physiol 1935;112:351–61.

40. Krayenbuehl HP, Schoenbeck M, Rutishauser W, et al. Abnormal segmental contraction velocity in coronary artery disease produced by isometric exercise and atrial pacing. Am J Cardiol 1975;35:785–94.

41. Nesto RW, Kowalchuk GJ. The ischemic cascade: temporal sequence of hemodynamic, electrocardiographic and symptomatic expressions of ischemia. Am J Cardiol 1987;57:23C–30C.

42. Hauser AM, Vellappillil G, Ramos RG, et al. Sequence of mechanical, electrocardiographic and clinical effects of repeated coronary artery occlusion in human beings: echocardiographic observations during coronary angioplasty. J Am Coll Cardiol 1985;5:193–7.

43. Wijns W, Serruys PW, Slager CJ, et al. Effect of coronary occlusion during percutaneous transluminal angioplasty in humans on left ventricular chamber stiffness and regional diastolic pressure-radius relations. J Am Coll Cardiol 1986;7:455–63.

44. Chierchia S, Brunelli C, Simonetti I, et al. A sequence of events in angina at rest: primary reduction in coronary flow. Circulation 1980;61:759–68.

45. Kaul S. A look at 15 years of planar thallium-201 imaging. Am Heart J 1989;118:581–601.

46. Maddahi J, Van Train KF, Wong EC, et al. Comparison of T1-201 single photon emission computer tomography (SPECT) and planar imaging for evaluation of coronary artery disease. J Nucl Med 1986;27:999.

47. Fintel DJ, Links JM, Brinker JA, et al. Improved diagnostic performance of exercise thallium-201 single photon emission computed tomography over planar imaging in the diagnosis of coronary artery disease: a

receiver operations characteristic analysis. J Am Coll Cardiol 1989;13: 600–13.

48. Kahn JK, Pippin JJ, Corbett JR. New radionuclide agents for cardiac imaging: description and application. Cardiol Clin 1989;7:589–605.

49. Okada RD, Glover D, Gaffney T, et al. Myocardial kinetics of technetium-99m-hexakis-2-methoxy-2-methylprophylisonitrile. Circulation 1988;77:491–8.

50. Watson DD, Smith WH, Sinusas AJ, et al. Myocardial defect detection with Tc-99m methoxyisobutyl isonitrile vs T1-201. J Nucl Med 1988;29: 850–6.

51. Kiat H, Maddahi J, Roy LT, et al. Comparison of technetium-99m methoxy isobutyl isonitrile and thallium-201 for evaluation of coronary artery disease by planar and tomographic methods. Am Heart J 1989; 117:1–11.

52. Spirito P, Maron BJ, Bellotti P, et al. Noninvasive assessment of left ventricular diastolic function: comparative analysis of pulsed Doppler ultrasound and digitized M-mode echocardiography. Am J Cardiol 1986;58:837–43.

53. Lavine SJ, Krishnawami V, Shriener DP, et al. Left ventricular diastolic filling in patients with coronary artery disease and normal left ventricular function. Am Heart J 1985;110:318–25.

54. Spirito P, Maron BJ, Bonow RO. Noninvasive assessment of left ventricular diastolic function: comparative analysis of Doppler echocardiographic and radionuclide angiographic techniques. J Am Coll Cardiol 1986;7:518–26.

55. Friedman BJ, Drinkovic N, Miles H, et al. Assessment of left ventricular diastolic function: comparison of Doppler echocardiography and gated blood pool scintigraphy. J Am Coll Cardiol 1986;8:1348–54.

56. Bonow RO, Bacharach SL, Green MV, et al. Impaired left ventricular diastolic filling in patients with coronary artery disease: assessment with radionuclide angiography. Circulation 1981;64:315–23.

57. Rokey R, Kuo LC, Zoghbi WA, et al. Determination of parameters of left ventricular diastolic filling with pulsed Doppler echocardiography: comparison with cineangiography. Circulation 1985;71:543–50.

58. Gill JB, Ruddy TD, Newell JB, et al. Prognostic importance of thallium uptake by the lungs during exercise in coronary artery disease. N Engl J Med 1987;317:1485–9.

59. O'Rourke RA. Post myocardial infarction risk stratification. Circulation (in press).

60. Ryan T, Armstrong WF, O'Donnell JA, et al. Risk stratification after acute myocardial infarction by means of exercise two-dimensional echocardiography. Am Heart J 1987;114:1305–16.

61. Gibson RS, Watson DD, Craddock GB, et al. Prediction of cardiac events after uncomplicated myocardial infarction: a prospective study comparing predischarge exercise thallium-201 scintigraphy and coronary angiography. Circulation 1983;68:321–36.

62. Poliner LR, Buja LM, Parkey RW, et al. Clinic-pathologic findings in 52 patients studied by technetium-99m stannous pyrophosphate myocardial scintigrams. Circulation 1979;59:257–91.

63. Khaw BA, Gold HK, Yasuda T, et al. Scintigraphic quantitation of myocardial necrosis in patients after intravenous injection of myosin-specific antibody. Circulation 1986;74:501–6.

64. Bansal RC, Shah PM. Usefulness of echo-Doppler in management of patients with valvular heart disease. Curr Probl Cardiol 1989;14:283–350.

65. Peller OG, Wallerson DC, Devereux RB. Role of Doppler and imaging echocardiography in selection of patients for cardiac valvular surgery. Am Heart J 1987;114:1445–61.

66. Kleinman JP, Czer LSC, DeRobertis M, et al. A quantitative comparison of transesophageal and epicardial color Doppler echocardiography in the intraoperative assessment of mitral regurgitation. Am J Cardiol 1989;64: 1168–72.

67. Perez JE, Ludbrook PR, Ahumada GG. Usefulness of Doppler echocardiography in detecting tricuspid valve stenosis. Am J Cardiol 1985;55: 601–3.

68. Lima CO, Sahn DJ, Valdes-Cruz LM, et al. Non-invasive prediction of transvalvular pressure gradient in patients with pulmonary stenosis by quantitative two-dimensional echocardiographic Doppler studies. Circulation 1983;67:866–71.

69. Stamm RB, Martin RP. Quantification of pressure gradients across stenotic valves by Doppler ultrasound. J Am Coll Cardiol 1983;2:707–18.

70. Hatle L, Angelsen B, Techn DR, et al. Non-invasive assessment of atrioventricular pressure half-time by Doppler ultrasound. Circulation 1979;60:1096–104.

71. Sahn DJ, Maciel BC. Physiological valvular regurgitation: Doppler echocardiography and the potential for iatrogenic heart disease. Circulation 1988;78:1075–7.

72. Smith MD, Grayburn PA, Spain MG, et al. Observer variability in the quantitation of Doppler color flow jet areas for mitral and aortic regurgitation. J Am Coll Cardiol 1988;11:579–84.

73. Alam M, Rosman HS, Lakier JB, et al. Doppler and echocardiographic features of normal and dysfunctioning bioprosthetic valves. J Am Coll Cardiol 1987;10:851–8.

74. Mugge A, Daniel WG, Frank G, et al. Echocardiography in infective endocarditis: reassessment of prognostic implications of vegetation size determined by the transthoracic and the transesophageal approach. J Am Coll Cardiol 1989;14:631–8.

75. DeBruijn NP, Clements FM, Kisslo J. Transesophageal applications of color flow imaging. Echocardiography 1987;4:557–67.

76. Fyke FE III, Seward JB, Edwards WD, et al. Primary cardiac tumors: experience with 30 consecutive patients since the introduction of two-dimensional echocardiography. J Am Coll Cardiol 1985;5:1465–73.

77. Reeder GS, Tajik AJ, Seward JB. Left ventricular mural thrombus: two-dimensional echocardiographic diagnosis. Mayo Clin Proc 1981;56: 82–6.

78. Bansal RC, Heywood JT, Applegate PM, et al. Detection of left atrial thrombi by two-dimensional echocardiography and surgical correlation in 148 patients with mitral valve disease. Am J Cardiol 1989;64:243–6.

79. Colan SD, Borow KM, Neumann A. Left ventricular end-systolic wall stress-velocity of fiber shortening relation: a load-independent index of myocardial contractility. J Am Coll Cardiol 1984;4:715–24.

80. Toyoka T. A critical review of NMR imaging and spectroscopy for the evaluation of cardiac hypertrophy in humans and experimental animals. J Mol Cell Cardiol 1989;21:141–7.

81. Bittner V, Cranney GB, Lotan CS, et al. Overview of cardiovascular nuclear magnetic resonance imaging. Cardiol Clin 1989;7:631–49.

82. Rakowski H, Sasson Z, Wigle ED. Echocardiographic and Doppler assessment of hypertrophic cardiomyopathy. J Am Soc Echo 1988;1:31–47.

83. Miller JG, Perez JE, Sobel BE. Ultrasonic characterization of myocardium. Prog Cardiovasc Dis 1985;28:85–110.

84. Wickline SA, Thomas LJ, Miller JG, et al. Sensitive detection of the effects of reperfusion on myocardium by ultrasonic tissue characterization with integrated backscatter. Circulation 1986;74:389–400.

85. Chandraratna PAN, Balachandran PK, Shah PM, Hodges M. Echocardiographic observations on ventricular septal rupture complicating myocardial infarction. Circulation 1975;51:506–10.

86. Miyatake K, Okamoto M, Kinoshita N, et al. Doppler echocardiographic features of ventricular septal rupture in myocardial infarction. J Am Coll Cardiol 1985;5:182–7.

87. Eisenberg PR, Barzilai B, Perez JE. Noninvasive detection by Doppler echocardiography of combined ventricular septal rupture and mitral regurgitation in acute myocardial infarction. J Am Coll Cardiol 1984;4: 617–20.

88. Rogers EW, Glassman RD, Feigenbaum H, Weyman AE, Godley RW. Aneurysms of the posterior interventricular septum with postinfarction ventricular septal defect. Echocardiographic identification. Chest 1980; 78:741–6.

89. Feigenbaum H. Echocardiographic diagnosis of pericardial effusion. Am J Cardiol 1970;26:475–9.

90. Hoit B, Shabetai R. Pericardial disease, pp 757–72. In Ref 14.

91. Callahan JA, Seward JB, Nishimura RA, et al. Two-dimensional echocardiographically guided periocardiocentesis: experience in 117 consecutive patients. Am J Cardiol 1985;55:476–9.

92. Singh S, Wann LS, Schuchard GH, et al. Right ventricular and right atrial collapse in patients with cardiac tamponade: a combined echocardiographic and hemodynamic study. Circulation 1984;70:966–71.

93. Appleton CP, Hatle LK, Popp RL. Cardiac tamponade and pericardial effusion: respiratory variation in transvalvular flow resolution studied by Doppler echocardiography. J Am Coll Cardiol 1988;11:1020–30.

94. Hatle LK, Appleton CP, Popp RL. Differentiation of constrictive pericarditis and restrictive cardiomyopathy by Doppler echocardiography. Circulation 1989;79:357–70.

95. Eagle KA, DeSanctis RW. Aortic dissection. Curr Probl Cardiol 1989; 15:225–78.

96. Khanderia BK, Tajik AJ, Taylor CL, et al. Aortic dissection: review of value and limitations of two-dimensional echocardiography in a six-year experience. J Am Soc Echo 1989;2:17–25.

97. Mohr-Kahaly S, Erbel R, Rennollet H, et al. Ambulatory follow-up of aortic dissection by transesophageal two-dimensional and color-coded Doppler echocardiography. Circulation 1989;80:24–33.

98. Kersting-Sommerhoff BA, Higgins CB, White RD, et al. Aortic dissection: sensitivity and specificity of MR imaging. Radiology 1988;166:651–5.

99. Winkle RA. Ambulatory electrocardiography and the diagnosis, evaluation and treatment of chronic ventricular arrhythmias. Prog Cardiovasc Dis 1980;23:99–128.

100. Morganroth J, Michelson EL, Horowitz LN, et al. Limitation of routine long-term electrocardiographic monitoring to assess ventricular ectopic frequency. Circulation 1978;58:408–14.

101. Anderson JL, Mason JW. Testing the efficacy of antiarrhythmic drugs. N Engl J Med 1986;315:391–3.

102. Pratt CM, Therous P, Slymen DJ, et al. Spontaneous variability of ventricular arrhythmias in patients at increased risk of sudden death after acute myocardial infarction: consecutive ambulatory electrocardiographic recordings of 88 patients. Am J Cardiol 1987;59:278–83.

103. Pratt CM, Eaton T, Francis M, et al. Ambulatory electrocardiography recordings: the Holter monitor. Curr Probl Cardiol 1988;13:519–86.

104. Zwicky P, Daniel WG, Mugge A, et al. Imaging of coronary arteries by color-coded transesophageal Doppler echocardiography. Am J Cardiol 1988;62:639–40.

105. O'Rourke RA. Value of Doppler echocardiography for quantitating valvular stenosis or regurgitation. Circulation 1988;78:1–3.

106. Starling MR, Crawford MH, Sorenson SG, et al. Comparative accuracy of apical biplane, cross-sectional echocardiography and gated equilibrium angiography for estimating left ventricular size and performance. Circulation 1981;63:1075–84.

107. Currie PJ, Sweard JB, Chan KL, et al. Continuous wave Doppler determination of right ventricular pressure: a simultaneous Doppler catheterization study in 127 patients. J Am Coll Cardiol 1985;6:750.

108. Bittl JA, Ingwall JS. Intracellular high-energy phosphate transport in normal and hypertrophied myocardium (abstr). Circulation 1987;75(suppl I):I-96.

◆ CHAPTER 4 ◆

The Challenge of Cardiomyopathy

WALTER H. ABELMANN, MD, BEVERLY H. LORELL, MD

"D'où venons nous? Que sommes nous? Où allons nous?"

Thus, Paul Gauguin entitled his monumental canvas of 1897, which addresses the human condition and life cycle. Since then, biomedical science has elucidated much of this cycle, and has prolonged it for many individuals. The same can be said for many diseases of heart muscle. We know a great deal more about their origins and can recognize them earlier and more often. Their life cycle has been extended, and we see their late stages with increasing frequency.

Some afflictions of the heart have decreased in prevalence and importance, at least in the more developed countries, partly because of effective prevention or treatment, or both, and partly for reasons unclear. Among these are syphilis, rheumatic fever, tuberculosis and malignant hypertension. Conversely, diseases of heart muscle appear more prevalent, either having increased in incidence or being recognized more frequently; they have become more prominent as causes of morbidity, disability and mortality. This holds for a wide range of presentations and manifestations, such as decreased tolerance of activity, congestive heart failure, arrhythmias, conduction disturbances, chest pain and sudden death.

This chapter will not review our knowledge and understanding of the cardiomyopathies in detail; many recent comprehensive reviews (1–12) are available. Rather, we emphasize recent contributions, try to present the highlights of our knowledge in perspective, address gaps of knowledge and understanding and raise questions to be addressed in the future.

Historical Perspective

Disease of heart muscle, as distinct from valvular, coronary, pericardial or congenital heart disease, was recognized as early as 1891 by Krehl (13) in Germany and reemphasized in 1901 by Josserand and Gallavardin (14) in France and in 1933 by Christian (15) in the United States. However, it came into prominence and wide recognition only in the second half of this century, thanks largely to the contributions by Mattingly (16), who reintroduced the term "primary myocardial disease," and Harvey et al. (17) in the United States and by Brigden (18), who introduced the term cardiomyopathy, and Goodwin et al. (19) in Great Britain. Originally, the designation "primary" signified that the disease predominantly affected the myocardium. Later, "primary" came to designate idiopathic afflictions of heart muscle as distinguished from diseases of other organ systems that affect the heart secondarily.

Initially, primary myocardial disease was considered a diagnosis of exclusion (that is, a diagnosis to be made after other etiologies had been ruled out). Gradually, it became recognized that there were characteristic albeit nonspecific features that permitted recognition of primary myocardial disease on its own merits. Furthermore, it became evident that there were different groupings of structural and physiologic characteristics, leading to a functional classification first introduced in 1968 by Goodwin et al. (19) and later adopted by the World Health Organization (20). This classification distinguished hypertrophic cardiomyopathy with or without obstruction, initially known in the United States as idiopathic hypertrophic subaortic stenosis or IHSS, congestive cardiomyopathy and restrictive cardiomyopathy. In a later modification, the WHO classification (21) was altered in that "congestive cardiomyopathy" was relabeled "dilated cardiomyopathy," and cases in which a specific etiology or associated systemic disease could be identified were now assigned to the new category of "specific heart muscle disease." Furthermore, two new categories, "obliterative cardiomyopathy" and "indeterminate cardiomyopathy" were added. Although according to the WHO definition (21), heart muscle disease secondary to specific causes or disease entities (for example, thiamine deficiency, hemochromatosis, amyloidosis and muscular dystrophy) is no longer included among the cardiomyopathies, the similar clinical presentations and therapeutic problems have led to widespread continuation of the use of the term cardiomyopathy for such cases, especially the frequently encountered entity of congestive heart failure secondary to chronic ischemic heart disease, generally referred to as "ischemic cardiomyopathy." The pragmatic advantage to the clinician of continuing to include congestive heart failure associated with specific heart muscle disease under the category of dilated cardiomyopathy has been discussed in detail in a previous communication (5).

The original concept that most idiopathic cardiomyopathies were attributable to a specific cause if one just searched long enough and awaited the results of further research has had to be discarded. More than 75 specific heart muscle diseases that may manifest as dilated cardiomyopathy have been described (5,22), but these disorders share common clinical, functional and pathologic manifestations. Moreover, experimental models of heart failure have shown a good deal of communality and overlap in the characteristics of individual forms of cardiomyopathy or specific heart muscle disease. Therefore, the concept of cardiomyopathy as a pluricausal or multifactorial disease has gained increasing acceptance (2,5,23). The principal pathogenetic mechanisms under current consideration include genetic factors, metabolic disturbances, hormonal imbalances, toxins, calcium overload, altered vascular reactivity, hypoxia, free radicals, infection and immune/autoimmune processes.

Incidence and Prevalence of Cardiomyopathy

In developed countries, the annual incidence of cardiomyopathy ranges from 0.7 to 7.5 cases per 100,000 population (24), and the prevalence in England has been reported (25) as 8.317 cases per 100,000 population. At least 0.7% of cardiac deaths in the United States have been attributed to cardiomyopathy (24); the cardiomyopathy mortality rate is in males twice that of females, and blacks have more than twice the mortality rate of whites. It is generally thought that dilated cardiomyopathy accounts for >90% of all cardiomyopathies encountered.

In less developed countries, especially in the tropics, cardiomyopathies are most prevalent and account for a greater if not dominant fraction of all cases of heart disease (24). This greater prevalence is largely in the form of dilated cardiomyopathy and to some extent as restrictive cardiomyopathy; it has been attributed variously to genetic factors, nutritional deficiency, infection including Chagas' disease, physical stress, untreated hypertension, endomyocardial fibrosis and toxins such as ethanol (26).

Hypertrophic Cardiomyopathy

Hypertrophic cardiomyopathy has held the fascination of cardiologists despite its rarity because of its dramatic aberrations of geometry and function and its importance as a cause of disability and death in young, otherwise healthy adults. Over the past three decades, our appreciation of the pleomorphic, geometric and hemodynamic manifestations of hypertrophic cardiomyopathy has greatly increased as a result of an enlarging body of natural history data and technologic advances in cardiac imaging. However, major gaps in knowledge of the etiology and pathophysiology remain.

This discussion first presents the historic perspective of the initial disparate evolution and more recent convergence of concepts regarding pathogenic mechanisms in hypertrophic cardiomyopathy. From this perspective, we highlight major unanswered issues that require attention if further strides are to be made in the treatment of symptomatic patients, prevention of premature sudden death and, ultimately, alteration of natural history and the regression of hypertrophy in this cardiomyopathy.

Historical Perspective

This peculiar disorder has been recognized in clinical practice for only three decades. However, Brigden (27) recently emphasized that isolated cardiac hypertrophy with an element of outflow tract stenosis was identified by pathologists in the 19th century and clearly described by Schminke as "Muskulöse Conusstenosen" in 1907. Both its familial nature and association with sudden death were raised by Evan (28), who described a kindred with unexplained hypertrophy in 1949. However, this disorder first came to widespread international attention as an entity that could mimic valvular stenosis due to functional obstruction by hypertrophied muscle with the publication of a case report by Brock (29) in 1957 and the description of a necropsy finding of unexplained septal hypertrophy in seven young adult victims of sudden death by Teare (30) in 1958. During the 1960s, investigators in the United States, particularly at the National Institutes of Health, focused on the identification and detailed assessment of patients with the obstructive form of the disease. In addition to confirming the familial transmission of this entity, elegant hemodynamic studies elucidated the physiology of this subset of patients whose hallmark was the presence of a dynamic systolic murmur and pressure gradient consistent with the presence of functional obstruction to left ventricular outflow (31,32). The anatomic basis of the dynamic outflow gradient was suggested by angiographic studies and shown by M-mode and later two-dimensional echocardiography to depend on narrowing of the left ventricular outflow tract by asymmetric septal hypertrophy and systolic anterior movement and apposition of the mitral valve leaflet to the septum (33). This concept of hypertrophic cardiomyopathy as a disorder having the fundamental characteristics of the presence of asymmetric septal hypertrophy and dynamic outflow tract obstruction was supported by the clinical improvement of symptomatic patients after interventions aimed at reducing the dynamic outflow gradient, including the use of negative inotropic agents such as propranolol and surgical ablation of the gradient using the myotomy-myectomy procedure pioneered by Morrow et al. (34). Necropsy studies (35) in these patients demonstrated the consistent finding of disorganization and malalignment of the myofibrils (myofibrillar disarray), which is not unique to hypertrophic cardiomyopathy, but is clearly more extensive in this disorder than in secondary hypertrophy from pressure overload or congenital heart disorders. During this exciting period of discovery and description, it was clearly recognized that not all patients had severe outflow tract pressure gradients and that abnormalities of diastolic function were common (36). Nonetheless, the emphasis on regional septal hypertrophy and its relation to the systolic murmur and gradient led to a profusion of terms such as "idiopathic hypertrophic subaortic stenosis" and "muscular subaortic stenosis." Furthermore, particularly in the United States, the widespread interest in the subset of patients with idiopathic hypertrophic subaortic stenosis was accompanied by their ease of recognition by physical examination and office-based echocardiography. It can be argued that this resulted in the widespread perception that hypertrophic cardiomyopathy could only be identified in patients with the clinical signs of rest or provocable outflow tract gradients in whom there was documentation of asymmetric septal hypertrophy and systolic anterior mitral valve motion. As a consequence, during the era of idiopathic hypertrophic subaortic stenosis, patients with other phenotypic manifestations and nonobstructive physiology and older patients with the confounding presence of mild hypertension were outside the mainstream of clinical recognition and study.

In parallel with these lines of investigation, there were the acquisition of natural history data, identification of kindreds and clinical investigation of patients with hypertrophic cardiomyopathy drawn from somewhat different patient referral populations in the United Kingdom. These observations led to the insight that the presence of a systolic murmur indicative of a left ventricular outflow gradient was not an invariable feature of the disease within kinships of patients or in the natural history of an individual followed up from adolescence through adulthood (2,37,38). In individuals who presented with the dramatic signs of outflow obstruction in young adulthood, clinical deterioration in middle age was frequently associated with the disappearance of the dynamic systolic murmur and the development of physiology resembling a restrictive cardiomyopathy. Second, it became apparent that although the extent of septal hypertrophy and duration of mitral leaflet-septal apposition correlate well with the magnitude of the systolic gradient, cardiac morphology does not correlate well with either symptoms or natural history. Severe symptoms of angina, pulmonary congestion and syncope occur in patients with either the obstructive or the nonobstructive forms of the disease, and many but not all investigators (39–41) observed that there appears to be little relation between the magnitude of the systolic gradient and the severity of symptoms or improvement in functional status with pharmacologic agents.

Two-dimensional cineangiographic studies and the ability to look at cardiac geometry in a new way with two-dimensional echocardiography (42–44) revealed that patients with hypertrophic cardiomyopathy can exhibit unexplained hypertrophy in regions other than the upper portion of the ventricular septum, including the mid portion of the left ventricle, the apex and the lower portion of the septum, as well as severe concentric hypertrophy. Furthermore, this variability in cardiac geometry can occur not only in isolated individual patients, but also within kindreds (45). Two morphologic forms of hypertrophic cardiomyopathy merit particular attention: apical hypertrophy and mid-ventricular hypertrophy. These atypical forms of hypertrophic cardiomyopathy are of interest not because of their prevalence, but because they underscore the fact that our perception of hypertrophic cardiomyopathy has been powerfully shaped by the capabilities and limitations of the tools available for the study of patients. Both of these forms of hypertrophic cardiomyopathy are associated with nonspecific physical findings, escape detection by M-mode echocardiography and have come to attention with two-dimensional imaging using either contrast ventriculography or two-dimensional echocardiography. In the late 1970s, Japanese investigators (46) described cohorts of patients with severe apical hypertrophy identified by invasive contrast ventriculography, who lacked signs of outflow tract obstruction and often came to clinical attention because of bizarre electrocardiographic (ECG) findings of severe left ventricular hypertrophy with giant negative T waves. This expression of hypertrophic cardiomyopathy is especially prevalent in Japan, but has now been identified using two-dimensional echocardiography in other genetic and geographic populations and within kindreds with other phenotypic patterns of hypertrophy. A second subset of patients that did not receive attention during the era of the identification of hypertrophic cardiomyopathy with M-mode echocardiography is made up of patients with severe mid-ventricular hypertrophy below the level of the outflow tract at the level of the papillary muscles. At cardiac catheterization, such patients can be shown to have mid-ventricular "obstruction" with a gradient between the left ventricular apical region and the remainder of the chamber due to the generation of markedly elevated levels of left ventricular systolic pressure from an isometric contraction in a discrete apical cavity (42,47). In our experience and that of Wigle et al. (42), some patients show progression to an appearance of a noncontractile apical aneurysm, and apical thrombus formation can occur. In such patients who have documentation of normal epicardial coronary arteries, the responsible mechanism may be the repetitive generation of high levels of isometric pressure, which ultimately results in episodes of ischemic injury and necrosis.

It should be emphasized that the true frequency of these different phenotypes of hypertrophic cardiomyopathy is difficult to ascertain. Referral centers with expertise in the medical and surgical management of the obstructive form of the disease report a predominance of asymmetric septal hypertrophy, whereas this morphologic expression appears to occur in the minority at centers that accrue a different spectrum of patients. Nonetheless, these lines of investigation and observation from different referral populations and different parts of the world have converged to a consensus position that the central morphologic feature of hypertrophic cardiomyopathy is the presence of a nondilated hypertrophied left ventricle detected in the absence of a primary illness that could cause hypertrophy (48,49).

Evolving Concepts and New Questions

Role of ischemia. The importance of ischemia in hypertrophic cardiomyopathy is an area of increasing interest and clinical investigation. Angina pectoris is a cardinal symptom of hypertrophic cardiomyopathy and can occur in all morphologic forms of the disease. There is substantial evidence that the symptom of angina pectoris is related to myocardial ischemia in these patients. Similar to observations in patients with secondary pressure overload hypertrophy (50), interventions such as pacing tachycardia and exercise can provoke chest pain in association with elevation of left ventricular filling pressure, myocardial lactate production and the development of reversible perfusion defects detectable by thallium imaging (51–53). In addition, autopsy studies (49) of patients with hypertrophic cardiomyopathy and patent epicardial coronary arteries have demonstrated the presence of fibrous tissue that varies from a patchy subendocardial distribution to large transmural scars. These observations strongly support a role of repetitive ischemic injury and necrosis in the symptomatology and natural history of the disease. Several mechanisms are likely to be responsible for myocardial ischemia in hypertrophic cardiomyopathy. First, abnormal narrowing of the small intramural coronary arteries as a result of intimal and medial thickening in association with regions of myocardial fibrosis occurs in the majority of patients studied at autopsy (54). The role of this form of small vessel disease as a cause of ischemia is not yet clear. In addition, patients with hypertrophic cardiomyopathy may have impairment of coronary vascular reserve and susceptibility to develop subendocardial ischemia that is characteristic of advanced secondary hypertrophy and related to a reduced capillary density (55). Third, the exacerbation of impaired relaxation and further elevation of left ventricular diastolic pressure during tachycardia or exercise in patients with hypertrophic cardiomyopathy and secondary hypertrophy may itself further limit coronary perfusion, particularly in the subendocardium. This hypothesis is supported by the observation of Cannon et al. (51) that coronary blood flow actually decreases during pacing-induced angina in some patients with hypertrophic cardiomyopathy. Finally, there is experimental evidence (56) in models of pressure overload hypertrophy that myocardial hypoxia is accompanied by an impaired capacity to recruit anaerobic glycolysis. Preliminary studies (57) in patients with hypertrophic cardiomyopathy using positron emission tomography are consistent with a mismatch between impaired myocardial perfusion and utilization of glucose substrate, but further studies are needed to address this issue.

Significance of the systolic pressure gradient. The concept of left ventricular outflow obstruction has been criticized by investigators (58,59) who have argued that intraventricular gradients are related to gradients between rapidly and slowly emptying regions in association with cavity obliteration. Murgo et al. (60) have also challenged this notion on the basis of studies of aortic flow velocity that suggested that patterns of flow were similar in patients with hypertrophic cardiomyopathy with and without outflow gradients and that both groups manifested the very rapid ejection of most of the left ventricular stroke volume very early in systole. However, multiple recent studies using cineangiographic, echocardiographic and Doppler flow methods lend support to the concept of "obstruction," defined as ventricular emptying that occurs in the presence of a pressure gradient across the outflow tract. As recently summarized by Wigle (61) and Maron and Epstein (62), multiple studies indicate that the onset of septal-mitral leaflet contact correlates with both the development of the systolic gradient and the abrupt deceleration of aortic flow, whereas the time of onset and duration of contact predict the magnitude of the gradient, the proportion of ventricular emptying that occurs in the presence of the gradient and the prolongation of left ventricular ejection time. Furthermore, there are substantial data (61) to support the hypothesis that septal-mitral leaflet contact occurs because of a Venturi effect of very rapid velocity of flow across the narrowed outflow tract in early systole. However, we support the concerns of many investigators in the field that the amount of energy that has been expended in the controversy of "proving" or "disproving" the existence of obstruction has not yielded proportionate insight into our understanding of the ways in which the systolic gradient may contribute to symptoms or the natural history of the disease.

A different viewpoint is that the repetitive development of large systolic pressure gradients may be deleterious as a mechanical stimulus for further hypertrophy, as well as being energy-costly in an hypertrophied ventricle with impaired coronary vascular reserve. This concept is supported by the observation that patients with left ventricular outflow obstruction exhibit higher levels of myocardial oxygen consumption at rest and during pacing tachycardia in comparison with patients without outflow obstruction (63). From this perspective, it is possible to have a unifying hypothesis that addresses the fact that symptoms of angina and exertional dyspnea and the development of myocardial fibrosis can occur in patients with classic asymmetric septal hypertrophy and outflow gradients, mid-ventricular obstruction and diffuse hypertrophy with cavity obliteration. In each of these settings, the repetitive development of high levels of left ventricular systolic pressure may trigger a dangerous cycle of increased regional or global systolic wall stress and myocardial oxygen demand, which provokes the development of ischemic injury, necrosis and fibrosis. This hypothesis is consistent with the well-established observation that many patients with large outflow gradients at rest improve symptomatically after myotomy-myectomy. This improvement may be related to the ablation of regional myocardium involved in a vicious cycle of high wall stress and ischemia as opposed to the relief of "obstructed" blood flow. The advent of new technologies that will permit the assessment of global and regional changes in both myocardial perfusion and metabolism provides an exciting opportunity to address this hypothesis.

Diastolic function. The last two decades have seen an explosion of international interest in diastolic function in hypertrophic cardiomyopathy and in secondary pressure overload hypertrophy. In both forms of hypertrophy, clinical congestive heart failure is a major cause of disability despite the preservation of left ventricular systolic function. In both forms of hypertrophy, left ventricular diastolic pressure is usually elevated relative to a normal or diminished diastolic volume consistent with decreased diastolic distensibility of the left ventricular chamber. Similar to secondary pressure overload hypertrophy (64), this is in part due to altered passive diastolic properties of the left ventricle related to both the extent of hypertrophy and changes in composition of the ventricle, including possible alterations in the collagen matrix and deposition of fibrous scars (65). In addition, the elevation of left ventricular filling pressure is in part related to changes in the rate and extent of left ventricular pressure decay (that is, left ventricular relaxation) (66). In some patients, left ventricular relaxation is so aberrant that left ventricular pressure continues to decline sluggishly throughout diastole, instead of showing the usual pattern of rapidly decreasing to its nadir in early diastole at mitral valve opening (67). The responsible mechanisms are as yet incompletely understood and include a slowing of force inactivation at the level of the myofibril related to abnormal calcium handling, abnormal patterns of electromechanical activation, regional dyssynchrony of the time course of contraction and relaxation and impaired relaxation due to ischemia. Many but not all patients also show a slowed rate of left atrial emptying and early left ventricular diastolic filling with an enhanced dependence on left atrial contraction (66–69). These patients usually have an elevation of left atrial pressure, and thus the presence of impaired diastolic filling is striking because increased left atrial pressure and the driving force across the mitral valve would otherwise tend to accelerate left ventricular filling.

The consistent finding of abnormal diastolic function in patients with the obstructive and nonobstructive forms of the disease has led to the hypothesis proposed by Goodwin (48) that diastolic "in-flow obstruction" of the left ventricle is a major defect. The elevation of diastolic pressure and the increased resistance to diastolic filling, which is especially important when the diastolic filling period is shortened by tachycardia, contribute to symptoms of pulmonary venous congestion and easy fatigue and near-syncope during exertion related to inadequate diastolic filling. Because of these abnormalities in diastolic function, the development of atrial fibrillation is a "double whammy" that results in both abbreviation of the time available for diastolic filling and the loss of atrial transport.

Implications for therapy. For this reason, drugs such as beta-adrenergic blockers, which exert a primary myocardial effect of slowing relaxation and do not improve diastolic filling rates, may indirectly improve dyspnea and exercise reserve through improved "diastolic function" by slowing the heart rate, lengthening the diastolic filling period and facilitating a greater extent of diastolic filling. The calcium channel blocking agents such as verapamil, nifedipine and diltiazem have been studied extensively and have been reported (67,69,70) to improve left ventricular relaxation and the rate and extent of left ventricular filling in patients with both the obstructive and nonobstructive forms of the disease. Despite intense clinical study, the mechanisms of action are controversial and may include alteration of loading, induction of increased sympathetic tone, reduction of regional asynchrony and relief of subendocardial ischemia. A controversial issue that has not yet been answered is whether or not these agents exert a direct myocardial effect on cytosolic calcium handling in patients with hypertrophic cardiomyopathy. The benefit tends to be greatest in patients with severe elevation of left ventricular end-diastolic pressure and impairment of relaxation and filling, but the effects of these agents on diastolic function are not uniform and precipitation of pulmonary edema can occur. Although improvement in diastolic function has also been observed with short-term administration of amiodarone, similar to that seen with calcium blockers, long-term therapy has been associated with no improvement in diastolic relaxation and the elevation of left heart filling pressures (73). Although calcium channel blockers have been an important addition to treatment options, these agents must be used with great caution because of their chronotropic side effects (bradycardia and isorhythmic dissociation, with loss of atrial contraction with verapamil and reflex tachycardia with nifedipine) and the risk of excessive vasodilation and hypotension (74,75). Thus, the quest for the ideal lusitropic agent to reliably enhance left ventricular relaxation has not been fulfilled with available agents and merits further investigation by both academic research centers and the pharmaceutical industry.

The dilemma of sudden death. Since the initial case reports, sudden cardiac death has been an ominous feature of hypertrophic cardiomyopathy distinct from its hemodynamic abnormalities. Similar to dilated cardiomyopathy, major unanswered problems are the ability to identify individual patients at high risk of sudden death and define treatment strategies that reduce this risk. Although the overall annual mortality rate for patients studied at referral centers is estimated to be 2% to 3%, the risk of premature death is skewed by a high incidence of sudden cardiac death in children and young adults (39,49,76). In about 50% of patients, death occurs suddenly, is unexpected and can be the index presentation of hypertrophic cardiomyopathy. Ominous prognostic features for an increased risk of sudden death include young age (first three decades of life), documented syncope and a family history of sudden death (39). It is still controversial whether the extent of hypertrophy is an independent predictor of sudden death. Otherwise, it is not predicted by symptoms, functional limitation, hemodynamic abnormalities, including the presence or absence of left ventricular outflow obstruction, or rest ECG abnormalities (40,49). In this disorder, sudden cardiac death can probably occur from multiple mechanisms, including hemodynamic deterioration, complete heart block, bradyarrhythmias and atrial tachycardia with concealed atrioventricular conduction. However, the predominant mechanism is probably the development of sustained ventricular tachyarrhythmia. Although this has been documented only rarely as a cause of witnessed sudden death (77), several centers (78,79) have reported that asymptomatic episodes of ventricular tachycardia detected by ambulatory holter monitoring are predictive of an increased risk of sudden death in adults. In patients referred to the National Institutes of Health (79), a single episode of ventricular tachycardia during ambulatory ECG monitoring was associated with an 8% risk of sudden death per year compared with a 1% risk per year in patients without ventricular tachycardia. The mechanisms responsible for the initiation of ventricular tachycardia in these patients are not known, including the potential contribution of ischemia.

Beta-adrenergic blocking agents have been used widely to reduce the risk of sudden death in symptomatic adults, asymptomatic children and young adults in whom hypertrophic cardiomyopathy is detected incidentally by routine physical examination or screening echocardiography. The rationale for use of these drugs is bolstered by awareness of the potential role of ischemia in this disorder and the striking protective effect of beta-adrenergic blockers in reducing the incidence of death in patients after myocardial infarction and possibly in patients with dilated cardiomyopathy. However, the effect of beta-adrenergic blockers on the risk of sudden death in hypertrophic cardiomyopathy is not established. Propranolol administration does not appear to reduce the frequency of asymptomatic ventricular arrhythmias detected by Holter ECG monitoring, and studies by McKenna et al. (80) in the United Kingdom have failed to demonstrate a protective effect of propranolol against sudden death. However, prospective, controlled, randomized trials have not been done to determine whether or not administration of beta-adrenergic blockers modifies the risk of sudden death in high risk young adults. There is also considerable controversy and few hard data regarding the efficacy of classic type I antiarrhythmic agents (quinidine, procainamide) in suppressing ventricular arrhythmias and preventing sudden death. Preliminary studies using amiodarone are promising. Available clinical trials (81,82) that did not incorporate randomized control subjects suggest that amiodarone reduces the frequency of episodes of ventricular tachycardia detected by ambulatory ECG monitoring and may be more effective than conventional agents, including calcium channel blockers. However, there is great concern about the long-term use of amiodarone in children and young adults because of the difficulty in evaluating its efficacy, proarrhythmic effects, deleterious effects on left heart filling pressure and uncommon but major side effects, including pulmonary fibrosis. The potential role of invasive electrophysiologic testing to identify high risk patients and monitor efficacy of therapy and the use of implantable defibrillators in preventing sudden death also need further study.

Unresolved: the etiologies of hypertrophic cardiomyopathy. There is some uncertainty regarding the true prevalence of familial versus sporadic forms of hypertrophic cardiomyopathy, which is influenced in part by the techniques used to detect occult disease (that is, echocardiographic criteria) and by the fact that morphologic expression of the disease may not be apparent until young adulthood. With these caveats, hypertrophic cardiomyopathy appears to be familial in nearly 60% of cases and sporadic in the remainder (83,84). In about 75% of pedigrees with familial transmission, the pattern of inheritance is consistent with a single or linked gene defect of autosomal dominant transmission with variable penetrance and expression. Within pedigrees with familial transmission, there is marked variability of cardiac morphology, including the site of hypertrophy, and functional limitation. The fact that morphologic evidence of hypertrophy may not be evident until after the pubertal growth spurt suggests that neurohormonal factors, including reproductive hormones, play a poorly understood role in modulating the expression of hypertrophy. The variability of expression also suggests that in genetically susceptible patients, the development of hypertrophy may be modulated by exposure to other stresses, such as mechanical stress imposed by athletic activity or even mild hypertension. The role of pressure overload as a possible stimulus for the development of severe hypertrophy in genetically susceptible individuals has been neglected, in part because of the focus on the "pure" forms of unexplained hypertrophy without contamination by factors such as hypertension. It is noteworthy that hypertension was present in the early case report by Brock (29). In this regard, there is new recognition of the syndrome of hypertensive hypertrophic myopathy, which is defined as the presence of severe left ventricular hypertrophy in older patients with a variable history of hypertension, in which symptoms, cardiac geometry, presence of mitral annular calcification and systolic and diastolic function simulate hypertrophic cardiomyopathy (85). Careful pedigree analysis, histologic studies and ultimately advances in molecular biology are needed to clarify whether this syndrome is completely distinct from hypertrophic cardiomyopathy in the elderly (86) or a phenotypic expression of hypertrophic cardiomyopathy that is triggered by the appearance of systolic hypertension during aging (87).

An important future direction in hypertrophic cardiomyopathy is the confirmation or refutal of the hypothesis that familial hypertrophic cardiomyopathy is a single gene defect with protean manifestations or a combination of several separate genetic defects. Jarcho et al. (88) recently applied the technique of genetic linkage analysis, using multiple polymorphic probes of deoxyribonucleic acid (DNA) that scan large regions of the human genome to study a large kindred in whom there was a pattern of inheritance of hypertrophic cardiomyopathy as an autosomal dominant trait. They identified a DNA locus mapped to chromosome 14 band q1 that was coinherited with the disease in this family; thus, in this kindred, the large "neighborhood" of the genome in which the abnormal gene resides has been identified, although the specific "address" is still elusive. It is intriguing that other genes whose expression is modified during the development of cardiac hypertrophy, such as the genes for myosin heavy chain (89) and heat shock protein, have also been mapped to chromosome 14. Advances in this direction are important not only in developing highly accurate and sensitive markers of this uncommon disease, but also in attempting to identify the location and function of the genetic loci that are critical in the regulation of cardiac hyperplasia and hypertrophy in general.

Just as the specific gene loci and gene products are not yet known, neither are the biologic defects responsible for the expression of hypertrophic cardiomyopathy. It is intriguing that there are case reports of the development of cardiac malformations that mimic the morphology and function of hypertrophic cardiomyopathy in patients with hereditary subcellular defects of skeletal and cardiac muscle, such as hereditary mitochondrial myopathy (90) and myotonic muscular dystrophy (91), and in patients with hereditary storage disorders, such as Fabry's disease (92). These rare experiments of nature suggest that the phenotypic expression of hypertrophy seen in hypertrophic cardiomyopathy can occur as a response to diverse developmental defects in which a common defect is a paucity of normal stress-bearing myocytes.

Two hypotheses to explain the development of hypertrophic cardiomyopathy are currently under scrutiny. Goodwin (2), Perloff (93) and Ferrans and Rodriguez (94) have developed the hypothesis that familial hypertrophic cardiomyopathy is caused by a defective response of developing cardiac cells to sympathetic stimulation, so that there is a failure of regression of the fetal pattern of disproportionate septal thickening and myofiber disarray that results in the fetal "programming" of permanently disturbed numbers and regional distribution of myocytes available to hypertrophy in response to later developmental stimuli. Support for the hypothesis comes from the association of hypertrophy with other congenital disorders of neural crest origin, such as neurofibromatosis, lentiginosis and pheochromocytoma, and from experimental studies in animals and myocyte culture, which have shown that administration of nerve growth factor (a glycoprotein that enhances sympathetic nerve growth) and norepinephrine can stimulate the development of hypertrophy. Support is also drawn from the apparent hyperdynamic contractile state in hypertrophic cardiomyopathy and from the clinical improvement seen with the administration of beta-adrenergic blockers. The perception that the hypertrophied myocyte is a hyperdynamic "superman" that can be tamed by negative inotropic agents has been seriously challenged by recent studies (95,96) of stress-shortening and end-systolic pressure-volume relations in patients with hypertrophic cardiomyopathy, which indicate that myocardial contractility is normal or depressed and not hyperdynamic.

Kawai et al. (97) reported the presence of normal plasma and elevated myocardial catecholamine content in patients with hypertrophic cardiomyopathy, but others (98,99) have failed to substantiate altered levels of myocardial cyclic adenosine monophosphate (AMP), beta-receptor density or adenylate cyclase activity in response to adrenergic agonists in these patients. These observations do not exclude the hypothesis that defective interplay between the cardiac cell and catecholamines may occur in utero and may not be detectable during later development.

A second hypothesis is that the unique biologic defect in hypertrophic cardiomyopathy is the defective regulation of cytosolic calcium (67). This hypothesis is supported by the clinical association of hypercalcemia and hypertrophic cardiomyopathy (100), the apparent hyperdynamic contractile state and the impairment of diastolic relaxation that can be induced by experimental calcium overload (101). Additional support for the notion of defective calcium handling in hypertrophic cardiomyopathy comes from the recent findings (102) of an increased number of calcium antagonist receptors in atrial tissue from patients with this disease. These observations have provided an attractive rationale for the use of calcium channel blockers in hypertrophic cardiomyopathy. Studies (103) of myocardial tissue obtained at surgery from patients with this disorder and from experimental pressure overload hypertrophy have shown a marked prolongation of the cytosolic calcium transient in association with a prolongation of the time course of tension decay. As recently reviewed elsewhere (64), these data and other studies strongly suggest that changes in the regulation of cytosolic calcium by the sarcoplasmic reticulum and sarcolemma pumps are not unique to hypertrophic cardiomyopathy, but appear to be a characteristic adaptation of advanced pressure overload hypertrophy. Thus, impaired regulation of cytosolic calcium is a likely candidate as an important pathogenic mechanism in hypertrophic cardiomyopathy, particularly when the stress of ischemia is superimposed, further impairing calcium handling. However, available evidence does not yet confirm the hypothesis that calcium overload is the primary genetically determined defect in hypertrophic cardiomyopathy.

Restrictive Cardiomyopathy

Of all the forms of cardiomyopathy, this is the one encountered least frequently. In its classic form, restrictive cardiomyopathy manifests as congestive heart failure with a small or only mildly enlarged heart, mimicking constrictive pericarditis. The pathophysiology is that of impaired diastolic function attributable to decreased ventricular distensibility, impairing diastolic filling, secondary to morphologic changes in the endocardium, myocardium or both. In the tropics, the most prevalent form of restrictive cardiomyopathy is endomyocardial fibrosis, which is not really a disease of heart muscle, but primarily a disease of the endocardium, which becomes scarred and thickened, leading to restriction of ventricular filling and diastolic dysfunction (26). However, the subendocardial myocardium is often involved, as are the atrioventricular valves, which become insufficient. Characteristically, the outflow tract is spared. In the Ivory Coast, 20% of deaths due to heart failure in patients <40 years of age are attributed to this disease (26). Tropical endomyocardial fibrosis (now known as EMF) was first reported in 1946 by Bedford and Konstam (104). Ten years earlier, Löffler (105) in Switzerland had described a similar disease associated with eosinophilia, which he named endocarditis parietalis fibroplastica and which has since become known as Löffler's endocardial fibrosis and has been reported from several developed countries. More recently (106), it has been proposed that these are related or identical diseases, the eosinophilia having preceded the clinical manifestations and being observed only rarely in the tropics. The cardiac manifestations have been reported to be associated with degranulation of eosinophils and their severity to be a function of the severity and duration of eosinophilia. Thus, a pathogenetic role has been attributed to degranulated eosinophils, which have been found to bind immunoglobulin-G (IgG) and have an increased peroxidase, which in turn was demonstrated to have direct toxic effects on rat myocytes (107).

In the western nations, myocardial restriction is more common than endocardial restriction. The most frequent forms are idiopathic myocardial fibrosis and amyloid heart disease, the latter by definition really falling into the category of "specific heart muscle disease." Other specific heart muscle diseases, such as hemochromatosis, sarcoid heart disease, myocardial infiltration by tumor, Fabry's disease and radiation fibrosis, may also present as restrictive cardiomyopathy (108). In these instances, the constitutive properties of the ventricular wall are altered: the diffuse increase in fibrous tissue, infiltration by tumor or deposits of foreign substances (for example, amyloid) stiffen ventricular walls and thus prevent normal dilation of ventricular chambers during diastole, eventually reducing stroke volume and cardiac output. However, the syndrome of restrictive cardiomyopathy has also been observed in the absence of histopathologic abnormalities of the endocardium or myocardium (109). Some of these cases are attributable to concentric hypertrophy (110). A neglected potential mechanism is the alteration of collagen and the cytoskeleton, such as described by Caulfield (111).

The diagnosis of restrictive cardiomyopathy, the rarest form of cardiomyopathy, should be considered in patients who present with congestive heart failure in the presence of slight or no cardiomegaly, and the principal differential diagnosis is constrictive pericarditis. Chest pain is not unusual. Elevation of jugular venous pressure is usually prominent. Murmurs of mitral or tricuspid regurgitation, or both, may be heard. Atrial arrhythmias, the brady-tachycardia syndrome or complete heart block may be present (112,113).

In late-presenting cases, the ECG may show low voltage. Noninvasive evaluation and hemodynamic study tend to confirm preservation of normal or near normal systolic function in the presence of elevated but nonequal left and right ventricular filling pressures. The square root sign (diastolic dip and end-diastolic plateau) is often present.

All patients with restrictive pathophysiology should undergo endomyocardial biopsy (114) to rule out specific heart muscle disease such as amyloidosis. If the histology is normal or near normal, constrictive pericarditis should be reconsidered, even if echocardiography did not suggest this. Computed tomography has also been found of value in the differential diagnosis (115).

When one sees the extreme interstitial fibrosis or deposition of amyloid surrounding cardiac myocytes individually or in clusters, it is difficult to think of therapeutic interventions other than nonspecific supportive measures, such as diuretic drugs and vasodilators in cases of congestive heart failure. Even here, caution must be exercised because elevated ventricular filling pressures may be needed to maintain adequate stroke volume and cardiac output. Conversely, as long as idiopathic cases exist without such morphologically evident "restriction," the search must continue for other mechanisms that might lead to specific therapy. For example, vascular lesions and spasm resulting in ischemia have been incriminated in the myocardial fibrosis encountered in scleroderma (116). Contraction band necrosis of myofibers (117) and abnormal thallium scans in the presence of normal coronary angiograms (118) point in this direction. Radiation-induced myocardial fibrosis also appears to involve damage to the myocardial microvasculature. Endocardial fibroelastosis, usually of unknown etiology, has been reported (119) in association with carnitine deficiency. Clinically, the detection of low serum carnitine levels, especially in cases of familial cardiomyopathy or endocardial thickening demonstrated by biopsy, may lead to specific therapy with L-carnitine. Another specific heart muscle disease that may present as restrictive cardiomyopathy and be amenable to specific therapy is hemochromatosis (120); myocardial deposits of iron can be reduced by means of phlebotomy (121) or chelation (122), resulting in functional improvement. Endomyocardial fibrosis may be treated surgically by endocardiectomy and repair or replacement of affected atrioventricular valves (123). Antihypereosinophilic therapy for the hypereosinophilic syndrome with prednisone or hydroxyurea, or both, has been recommended (124). Surprisingly, calcium channel blockers, which are known to improve ventricular diastolic function in hypertrophic cardiomyopathy, have not been studied in restrictive cardiomyopathy.

Dilated Cardiomyopathy

As already discussed, the clinical and pathophysiologic manifestations of dilated cardiomyopathy have been well characterized and are widely known. Its characteristic features are impaired systolic function of both ventricles (although dysfunction of one ventricle may dominate), leading to manifestations of congestive heart failure. In individuals with a sedentary life-style, low sodium intake or on diuretic therapy, even severe systolic dysfunction may not be accompanied by pulmonary or systemic congestion, but rather manifest as easy fatigue and decreased exercise tolerance. Although most clinical cases are recognized when manifestations of heart failure appear, initial presentations as cardiac arrhythmia, conduction disturbance, thromboembolic complication or even sudden death are not uncommon. Such manifestations may even occur before significant ventricular dilation or hemodynamic impairment of myocardial function can be demonstrated.

Although biventricular global hypokinesis in the absence of risk factors and symptoms of coronary artery disease would generally permit a clinical diagnosis of dilated cardiomyopathy, especially in young patients, coronary disease may present in just this manner, and dominance of right or left ventricular dysfunction, regional hypokinesis as well as chest pain may all occur in dilated cardiomyopathy.

Arrhythmogenic Right Ventricular Dysplasia

Cardiomyopathy limited to the right ventricle, associated with arrhythmias and sudden death, especially in young people, has drawn increasing attention (125–127). This rare form of cardiomyopathy is also known as arrhythmogenic right ventricular dysplasia, Uhl's anomaly or parchment heart. Right ventricular myocardium is thinned, partly or completely replaced by fibrous or adipose tissue, and the right ventricle is dilated and hypokinetic. Supraventricular and especially ventricular arrhythmias are characteristically present. Premature death results from early congestive heart failure or sudden, presumably arrhythmic death, which may be the first known manifestation of the disease and is frequently associated with physical exertion. Evidence for familial occurrence of this condition has been reported from Italy (128).

Natural Course and Prognosis

The natural course and prognosis of dilated cardiomyopathy are a function of how early the diagnosis is made. Whereas the annual mortality rate, beginning with the onset of illness, was as low as 5.7% in a series of 258 patients studied by Kuhn et al. (129), a 1 year mortality rate of 23% and a 2 year mortality rate of 48% have been reported (130) in 87 patients with severe congestive heart failure. There is general agreement that significant cardiomegaly, low cardiac output and frank congestive heart failure are associated with a poor prognosis (5,131). In some series (129), the severity of histopathologic abnormalities on myocardial biopsy correlated inversely with life expectancy. Cardiac hypertrophy has a favorable effect on prognosis (132), presumably by limiting systolic wall stress. The presence of etiologic or contributory factors that can be eliminated (for example, ethanol, thiamine deficiency, hypertension, anemia and thyrotoxicosis) may also affect the prognosis favorably.

Pathogenesis

Tabulations of "causes" of dilated cardiomyopathy, namely specific agents, diseases and syndromes associated with the disorder, have been repeatedly published (1–6,8–12). These include, of course, specific heart muscle diseases. Here, we focus on proven and postulated pathogenetic mechanisms that may play a role in dilated cardiomyopathy.

Heredity. The familial occurrence of dilated cardiomyopathy is best known in the specific heart muscle diseases associated with hereditary disorders, such as glycogen storage diseases, Fabry's disease, mucopolysaccharidosis, the muscular dystrophies and Friedreich's ataxia. Specific biochemical and metabolic abnormalities have been identified in many of these disorders, although cardiac tissue itself has only rarely been studied.

The familial incidence of dilated cardiomyopathy has been given less attention. In a retrospective analysis of 169 patients (133), the family history was positive in 6.5% of cases. Recently, X-linked, autosomal dominant and autosomal recessive inheritance of dilated cardiomyopathy has been reported (134–136). The use of echocardiography in systematic surveys of relatives of patients with dilated cardiomyopathy promises to reveal a familial prevalence much more frequently than heretofore suspected (137).

Fatal dilated cardiomyopathy in newborn calves has been attributed to a genetic defect (138). The hereditary cardiomyopathy of the Syrian hamster, transmitted by an autosomal recessive gene, has long been a favorite experimental model of dilated cardiomyopathy (139). Major histocompatibility genes have been shown to play a role in the determination of myocardial damage and the immunologic mechanisms involved in infection with cardiotropic viruses (140–142).

It is not unreasonable to expect that within a few years, it may be possible to identify individuals genetically predisposed to myocardial disease and reduce that risk by control of other risk factors, such as ethanol and viral infections.

Nutritional deficiencies. *Thiamine deficiency.* One of the very few curable as well as preventable forms of dilated cardiomyopathy is wet beriberi due to deficiency of thiamine or vitamin B_1, a coenzyme essential to the decarboxylation of alpha-keto-acids and the utilization of pentose in the hexose-monophosphate shunt. In the absence of thiamine, oxidative phosphorylation and hence myocardial energy production are impaired. Clinically, thiamine deficiency first manifests as a high output state secondary to peripheral vasodilation, at least in part attributable to the accumulation of intermediate carbohydrate metabolites. Eventually, depressed myocardial function in the setting of increased preload and wall stress leads to congestive heart failure, first in the presence of normal to high cardiac output, later in association with a low output state. This sequence is of great interest inasmuch as the peripheral vasodilation undoubtedly acts to delay the onset of left ventricular failure. Indeed, administration of thiamine, resulting in reversal of the peripheral vasodilation, has been reported (143) to precipitate left ventricular failure. A similar protective role of naturally occurring left ventricular unloading by peripheral vasodilation is seen in hyperthyroidism and cirrhosis of the liver.

Selenium deficiency. Another treatable as well as preventable form of dilated cardiomyopathy is that due to selenium deficiency, reported primarily in northeast China, where it is known as Keshan disease (144). The absence of selenium results in decreased activity of glutathione peroxide, an enzyme dependent on selenium, as well as an increase in free radicals that may be toxic to cardiac myocytes. Clinical cardiomyopathy due to a deficiency in selenium has also been reported from the West (145).

Carnitine deficiency. Deficiency of carnitine may present as dilated cardiomyopathy. In this condition, oxidation of fatty acids is impaired, and lipids accumulate in the cytoplasm. The deficiency may be familial, and the cardiac lesions are often associated with endocardial fibroelastosis. Oral therapy with L-carnitine is effective (119). Recent reports of therapeutic benefit of carnitine treatment in the cardiomyopathic hamster (146) and in experimental adriamycin toxicity (147) raise the possibility that carnitine deficiency may also be a contributory factor in human cardiomyopathies. Indeed, Regitz et al. (148) reported reduced myocardial carnitine levels in 30 patients with end-stage heart failure secondary to cardiomyopathy, but also in 22 patients with heart failure secondary to coronary disease.

Toxins and drugs. *Ethanol.* In many populations and series of patients with dilated cardiomyopathy, a history of chronic alcoholism is so prominent that some consider ethanol the major cause of the disorder (149). Although Mackenzie (150) introduced the term "alcoholic heart disease" in 1902, in the first half of this century, congestive heart failure in chronic alcoholic patients was generally attributed to nutritional deficiencies. In 1957, however, Brigden and Robinson (151) reintroduced "alcoholic heart disease." Indeed, depression of myocardial function by chronic intake of ethanol has been well demonstrated in humans as well as in experimental animals (152–155). However, many efforts to produce chronic congestive heart failure by administration of ethanol alone in animal models have failed. Most recently, however, Edes et al. (156) succeeded in producing dilated cardiomyopathy in young turkeys fed ethanol, accounting for 35% of caloric intake, for 16 weeks. Considerable evidence favors the view that other factors may be needed for full expression of the clinical syndrome of dilated cardiomyopathy, including genetic predisposition, malnutrition, infection and other toxins (23,157). There is increasing evidence for a role of altered handling of

calcium, the effects of which may be prevented by verapamil (158).

Clinically, the identification of a history of alcoholism in a patient with dilated cardiomyopathy is important inasmuch as the prognosis may be improved by abstention.

Anthracyclines. Doxorubicin (adriamycin) and daunorubicin, among the most effective agents in the chemotherapy of malignant neoplasms, are highly cardiotoxic. The long-term effects, which include dilated cardiomyopathy, have been studied extensively in humans as well as experimental animals. These studies lead to the conclusion that we may be dealing with a multifactorial pathogenesis, including altered nucleic acid synthesis (159), altered mitochondrial respiration (160), release of vasoactive substances (161), formation of free radicals (162) and calcium overload (163).

Vasoactive agents and microvascular spasm. Studies of cardiac effects of catecholamines have dealt primarily with acute effects, including myocardial necrotic foci resembling ischemic lesions, which have been attributed to microvascular spasm and hypoxia, altered membrane permeability and calcium overload (164). Late effects of acute administration of isoproterenol in rats, however, include cardiomyopathy and congestive heart failure (165). Catecholamine-induced dilated cardiomyopathy in humans is seen most clearly in patients with pheochromocytoma. This form of cardiomyopathy is reversible by removal of the tumor or adrenergic blockade (166,167).

Of wider interest is the evidence that catecholamines play a role in anthracycline cardiotoxicity (161) and diabetic cardiomyopathy (168). Catecholamines also enhance the severity of necrosis seen in the hereditary cardiomyopathy of the Syrian hamster (169).

Recent studies in experimental models of cardiomyopathy have revealed evidence of microvascular spasm in the cardiomyopathic hamster (170), the hypertensive diabetic rat (171) and the mouse infected with *Trypanosoma cruzi* (172). Furthermore, these lesions could be prevented by verapamil, suggesting that calcium overload plays a role in these experimental models, which closely resemble the human disease.

Decreased coronary flow reserve. The not infrequent occurrence of chest pain, often indistinguishable from angina pectoris, in patients with dilated cardiomyopathy has long puzzled clinicians and has led to the postulate of a decrease in maximal coronary blood flow (173). Cannon et al. (174) studied the responses of coronary blood flow in 26 patients with dilated cardiomyopathy and angiographically normal coronary arteries to ergonovine, dipyridamole and rapid atrial pacing. In the subset of patients with a history of angina pectoris, there was a greater response to ergonovine and a significantly decreased coronary flow reserve in response to either dipyridamole or pacing. Recently, DeMarco et al. (175) reported that in patients with chronic heart failure due to either chronic coronary artery disease or dilated cardiomyopathy, both rest coronary blood flow and myocardial oxygen consumption were increased and coronary sinus oxygen content was decreased. Although the mechanism of this decreased coronary flow reserve remains uncertain, myocardial hypoxia not only may explain the anginal pain, but is also implicated as a factor potentially contributing to ongoing myocyte necrosis, replacement fibrosis and deterioration of myocardial function.

Tachyarrhythmia. Reversible heart failure associated with rapid supraventricular arrhythmias has been recognized in patients without evidence of heart disease for some time (176). In a recent report, Packer et al. (177) described eight subjects with long-standing uncontrolled tachycardia associated with depressed left ventricular function, which was at least partly reversed by control of the tachycardia. They thus coined the term "tachycardia-induced cardiomyopathy." It is, of course, possible that they were dealing with subclinical cardiomyopathy enhanced by tachycardia. Conversely, heart failure has been induced by chronic rapid cardiac pacing in healthy dogs, followed by persistence of abnormal cardiac function after return to sinus rhythm (178). Underlying mechanisms may include shortening of diastole, depletion of high energy substrate (179) and ischemia secondary to decreased coronary flow reserve. Evidence that supraventricular tachycardia depresses both systolic and diastolic myocardial reserve in patients with established dilated cardiomyopathy was recently reported by Feldman et al. (180), and studies of isolated cardiac muscle from patients with end-stage heart failure yielded evidence for calcium overload and decreased concentrations of cyclic AMP at high frequencies of stimulation (181).

Calcium overload. The important role of calcium in excitation/contraction coupling and hence in the pump function of the heart has long been recognized (182–184). Increasing evidence derived from studies of both clinical and experimental cardiomyopathy points toward abnormalities in the handling of calcium by heart muscle cells. Thus, there is evidence of impaired calcium regulation in several experimental models of cardiomyopathy. Myocardial calcium is increased in the cardiomyopathic hamster (185,186). Left ventricular function is improved by the calcium channel blocker verapamil (187). Calcium overload has also been demonstrated in experimental adriamycin toxicity (163). In healthy Syrian hamsters fed ethanol until adenosine, high energy phosphates and left ventricular function became depressed, administration of verapamil along with ethanol was shown to have a preventive effect (158). Conversely, streptozotocin-induced diabetes in the rat was associated with depression of the calcium pump, reversible by insulin (188). Recent studies (189) of human heart muscle from patients with end-stage heart failure, including cases of dilated cardiomyopathy, also yielded evidence of abnormal intracellular calcium handling.

Oxygen-free radicals. Oxygen-free radicals have been recognized as toxins that may play a role in several disease processes, of which ischemia/reperfusion injury has been given special attention (190,191). The formation of free radicals has been reported in the cardiomyopathy of the Syrian hamster (192), as well as in adriamycin toxicity (162). In acute but not in chronic experimental adriamycin cardiomyopathy, the free radical scavenger alpha-tocopherol (vitamin E) has been found to be of protective value (193).

Infection. All infectious organisms that are capable of invading the bloodstream may enter the myocardial capillaries and reach the myocardium. Acute necrotic or inflammatory lesions have been associated with many bacterial, spirochetal, rickettsial, viral, mycotic, protozoal and helminthic infections (5,9). Some forms of acute myocarditis have long been recognized as precursors of chronic dilated cardiomyopathy. Thus, both clinical and experimental studies (194–196) have established that the chronic dilated cardiomyopathy so prevalent in Central and South America and known as Chagas' disease is a late sequel of acute myocarditis due to *Trypanosoma cruzi*. Dilated cardiomyopathy has also been recognized as a late sequel of African trypanosomiasis (197) and toxoplasmosis (198).

Increasing evidence also points to dilated cardiomyopathy as a late sequel of acute viral myocarditis (199). This evidence includes clinical follow-up studies (200–206). Support of such a relation has also come from serological surveys of patients with chronic dilated cardiomyopathy (207–209).

Not all viruses, however, are myotropic, and not all patients infected with myotropic viruses develop myocarditis or dilated cardiomyopathy, or both. This should not be surprising in view of the great differences in susceptibility to and expression of cardiac involvement by a given virus seen in different inbred strains of rodents (140,141). Although it has been postulated that the majority of cases of idiopathic dilated cardiomyopathy in countries in which *T. cruzi* is not endemic may be of viral origin (48,210), the fraction of cases for which this holds true is unknown.

Acute as well as chronic dilated cardiomyopathy is encountered with increasing frequency in patients with acquired immunodeficiency syndrome (AIDS) (211), often associated with evidence of myocarditis (212). The majority of cases remained unrecognized before postmortem examination and may have been associated with opportunistic infections. However, human immunodeficiency virus has been cultured for myocardial tissue at least once (213), although it may have originated from perfusing blood. As yet, cardiac involvement has not been reported to occur in experimental models of infection with this or related viruses. It remains an open question whether the human immunodeficiency virus itself is responsible for cardiomyopathy.

Strong support for dilated cardiomyopathy as a sequel of acute myocarditis is also provided by extensive studies of experimental models of myocarditis. The chronic form of Chagas' disease has been reproduced in mice (196), and chronic cardiomyopathy has been demonstrated to develop in mice infected with encephalomyocarditis virus (214,215), herpes simplex virus (216) and especially with coxsackievirus B3 (217) and B4 (218).

Myocarditis may also be subacute and even chronic. In humans, this was first described in 1931 by Boikan (219), who coined the term "myocarditis perniciosa." Additional cases were reported by Kline and Saphir (220). With increasing use of endomyocardial biopsy (221) in patients with chronic dilated cardiomyopathy, the persistence of active inflammation and necrosis has been reported in 3% to 63% of such cases, especially if heart failure was <1 year's duration (223–226). This variability may in part be attributed to variable criteria for the histopathologic diagnosis of myocarditis (227). However, since the establishment of strict criteria for the histopathologic diagnosis of active myocarditis (228), the prevalence of active myocarditis among patients with dilated cardiomyopathy has been reported (229) to be closer to 10%. Chronic myocarditis associated with demonstrably persistent *T. cruzi* infection has also been described (230).

Recent application of in situ hybridization techniques to the study of the pathogenesis of ongoing myocarditis has revealed the presence of encephalomyocarditis viral nucleic acid in cardiac myocytes 2 weeks after isolation of virus was no longer possible (231). Similar results have been obtained in experimental coxsackievirus B3 infection (232) and myocardial biopsy specimens from patients with cardiomyopathy and myocarditis (233,234). Thus, the question of a pathogenetic role of persistent viral infection in subacute and chronic myocarditis must be reconsidered.

Immune/autoimmune mechanisms. Experimental myocarditis has been produced by immunization with myocardial proteins (235–238). The fact that trypanosomes can be demonstrated only rarely in subacute and chronic Chagas' cardiomyopathy has led to the concept of chronic Chagas' disease as an autoimmune disease, as supported by extensive clinical and experimental studies (239). Recent experimental studies (240) suggest that this form of autoimmune myocarditis is attributable to cross-reacting antigens of *T. cruzi* and skeletal muscle (240), presumably mediated by cytotoxic T lymphocytes. Furthermore, experimental myocarditis induced in mice by homologous heart immunization has been shown to resemble chronic murine Chagas' cardiomyopathy (241).

Inasmuch as the isolation of cardiomyotropic viruses from myocardium only rarely is possible >2 weeks after inoculation or infection, subacute and chronic myocarditis as well as later noninflammatory cardiomyopathy have also long been considered of immune or autoimmune etiology. A great deal of evidence has accumulated in favor of immunopathogenesis of myocarditis and its late sequel of cardiomyopathy, derived from studies in humans as well as experimental animals, and several monographs and reviews have been published recently (242–248).

In both humans and experimental animals, there is evidence that either humoral or cellular immunity, or both, may play a role in expression of the short- as well as long-term effects of viral replication in the heart. Evidence to date indicates that many different mechanisms may be operative, that these involve cytotoxic T lymphocytes, suppressor T lymphocytes and natural killer (NK) cells and that the mechanisms as well as the biologic effects may be a function of genetic background, type and strain of virus, age, gender, species, strain and other modifying factors such as stress. The fact that immune processes are involved even in the expression of acute myocarditis was first demonstrated by Woodruff and Woodruff (249), who found that depletion of T lymphocytes in mice infected with coxsackievirus B3 significantly suppressed both cellular infiltration and necrosis in the myocardium. Since then, evidence has accumulated for a cytotoxic role of T helper cells (L3T4) and T cytolytic/suppressor cells (Lyt 2+) and for a myocardial protective role by activated natural killer cells and suppressor T lymphocytes (247,250). Evidence has also been presented for deficient natural killer cell activity in patients with dilated cardiomyopathy (251,252).

Degeneration of cardiac ganglia. The well known dysautonomia associated with degeneration and loss of cardiac ganglia in Chagas' disease led Amorim and Olsen (253) to study seven hearts from patients with dilated cardiomyopathy. They found a significant loss of ganglion cells in the sinoatrial region, whereas collagen tissue was increased. Neither the cause of this neuronal degeneration nor the functional significance is known, nor is it clear whether this is a primary or a secondary phenomenon or even an epiphenomenon.

Alterations in the cardiac cytoskeleton. Noncontractile elements of the myocardium have been relatively neglected in the search for pathogenetic mechanisms in dilated cardiomyopathy. Yet, myocytes are surrounded by a network of bundles of collagen, which are below the limits of resolution of light microscopy and best studied by means of scanning electron microscopy (254). Alterations of the collagen matrix have been observed in experimental cardiac hypertrophy (255) and after a single injection of adriamycin in rats (256).

A correlation study (257) of histopathology and left ventricular function in 24 patients with dilated cardiomyopathy identified a relation of degree of impairment of ventricular function with proliferation of collagen fibers. More recently, studies by Weber et al. (258) of the collagen matrix in three postmortem hearts from patients with dilated cardiomyopathy revealed evidence of pathologic remodeling of collagen, involving a shift from a stronger to a weaker type of collagen. The authors hypothesized that these changes may play a role in cardiac dilation and hence put forward the concept of "interstitial heart disease" and recommend the substitution of "cardiopathy" for "cardiomyopathy."

Diagnosis

In view of the protean manifestations and initial presentations of dilated cardiomyopathy already mentioned, an awareness of its existence and prevalence is paramount for its detection. The failure to diagnose dilated cardiomyopathy is most frequently seen in the early stages of the disease, in association with the custom of limiting cardiac diagnosis to labeling of manifestations such as "cardiac arrhythmia" or "congestive heart failure" and in the mislabeling of dilated cardiomyopathy as ischemic heart disease, attributable in part to the latter's high prevalence. Occasionally, insufficiency of either or both atrioventricular valves may lead to a misdiagnosis of valvular heart disease. In most cases, however, careful clinical evaluation and judicious use of noninvasive methods such as echocardiography and radioventriculography should lead to the correct diagnosis. There remains, however, a group of patients (especially males) with coronary risk factors, whose myocardial dysfunction is regional and who may have a history of typical or atypical anginal chest pain. In these patients, coronary angiography is essential. It must also be kept in mind that three vessel coronary artery disease may be painless and associated with global hypokinesis of the left ventricle. Finally, there are patients with significant coronary atherosclerosis whose myocardial dysfunction appears to be out of proportion to the degree of coronary artery disease. By definition, as long as significant coronary obstruction exists, these patients cannot be classified as having cardiomyopathy. Yet, pathogenetically and pathophysiologically, a cardiomyopathic process may exist, and its recognition and identification of causal factors may be of value for purposes of prognosis, therapy and secondary prevention. Of special importance in this regard is the identification of chronic alcohol abuse.

Therapy

Inasmuch as true dilated cardiomyopathies are of unknown etiology, treatment is symptomatic and nonspecific as contrasted with specific heart muscle diseases, for many of which specific therapy is available (5). Hence, the need to evaluate every patient with dilated cardiomyopathy for the existence of a specific etiology that might identify a specific therapeutic approach. The therapeutic approach to decompensated dilated cardiomyopathy differs little from that to congestive heart failure in general and has been reviewed in depth in recent reports by Parmley (259) and Cohn (260). The discussion here is limited to considerations of special relevance to dilated cardiomyopathy.

In the use of diuretic drugs, it should be kept in mind that loss of electrolytes and water-soluble vitamins may affect the structure and function of myocardium adversely and that excessive volume depletion may result in depression of ventricular filling pressures below the optimal level.

Vasodilators represent the major advance in the therapy of dilated cardiomyopathy in recent years. Unlike ischemic heart disease, an arterial pressure significantly lower than normal may be acceptable in dilated cardiomyopathy, and thus higher doses of vasodilators may be tolerated. However, the physician must be alert to possible deleterious

effects on cerebral and renal function (261). Evidence for prolongation of life has been demonstrated for the combination of hydralazine and isosorbide dinitrate (262) and for converting enzyme inhibitors (263).

Digitalis glycosides, even though recognized as relatively weak positive inotropic agents, are still of value in these patients (264,265). In cases of intractable, advanced congestive heart failure, hospitalization and a course of intravenous amrinone or dobutamine under close supervision may initiate diuresis and result in considerable symptomatic and objective improvement (266,267). Such a course may have to be repeated every few weeks. A sophisticated recent study (268) of the physiologic mechanisms determining the hemodynamic response to dobutamine demonstrated significant differences in responses between a group with appropriate and another with inappropriate hypertrophy, the latter exhibiting a significantly attenuated response.

The considerable evidence for a role of calcium overload and the preventive value of verapamil in several experimental forms of cardiomyopathy, as well as circumstantial evidence for a role of myocardial hypoxia in dilated cardiomyopathy have led to a number of efforts to treat dilated cardiomyopathy with calcium antagonists (269). Evidence for negative inotropic effects of these agents has resulted in their limited clinical use in advanced dilated cardiomyopathy. Most recently, Figulla et al. (270) reported favorable results in a group of patients treated with diltiazem. Controlled trials, especially in early stages of the disease, are needed.

High grade ventricular ectopy is frequent in dilated cardiomyopathy, generally correlating with the severity of systolic dysfunction and often responding to therapeutic improvement of ventricular function. Pharmacologic approaches to the management of arrhythmias in this setting have been discussed recently by Myerburg et al. (271).

Waagstein et al. (272) were the first to report beneficial effects of treatment with beta-adrenergic blockade in patients with dilated cardiomyopathy and a high heart rate at rest. This approach has its conceptual justification inasmuch as it addresses the increased activity of the adrenergic nervous system in congestive heart failure, initially blocks the beta-adrenergic receptors and then permits up-regulation of the beta$_1$-receptors down-regulated by the chronic effects of norepinephrine (273). However, the negative inotropic effects of beta-blockade justifiably have been of concern. A number of studies (274–276), however, have suggested the value of this approach. Until the results of controlled trials now in progress become available, clinical use of this mode of therapy is best restricted to patients with tachycardia and those in relatively early stages of the disease.

Several studies of therapy with coenzyme Q$_{10}$, a redox coenzyme of several mitochondrial enzymes (277,278), which has been thought to be deficient in diseased hearts, have been reported (277,278) in patients with dilated cardiomyopathy. Further study appears warranted.

In view of the high incidence of thromboembolic complications, all patients with dilated cardiomyopathy and chronic heart failure, unless there is a contraindication, should receive therapy with a coumarin derivative. This therapy has been validated (279).

Inasmuch as many patients with dilated cardiomyopathy are young and free of systemic disease and yet carry a guarded prognosis, cardiac transplantation, with its rapidly increasing prognosis, has much to offer and should be considered before secondary changes in the pulmonary and systemic circulation have become irreversible. Indeed, to date, approximately 50% of all patients with cardiac transplantation have suffered from dilated cardiomyopathy. The timing of cardiac transplantation remains a challenge (280–282).

Prevention

At this time, the limited knowledge about the etiology of dilated cardiomyopathy does not permit primary prevention. However, a few words about secondary prevention are in order. The principle is simple: inasmuch as myocardial damage may be pluricausal and cardiac toxins may be additive, a patient with cardiomyopathy must be protected from potential cardiotoxins such as ethanol, anthracyclines, radiation, nutritional deficiency and electrolyte imbalance, as well as excessive preload and afterload such as imposed by anemia and hypertension.

Conclusions

The cardinal clinical and pathophysiologic characteristics, as well as current concepts of pathogenesis and therapy of the principal forms of cardiomyopathy have been reviewed, with emphasis on recent developments and unsolved questions.

In the last 40 years, the understanding of the diseases of heart muscle has advanced from clinical descriptions, first to pathophysiologic understanding and more recently to gradual unveiling of likely pathogenetic mechanisms. The application of techniques of molecular biology and genetics is just beginning to fulfill their early promise. Much of the progress has been facilitated by the development of experimental models of heart muscle disease, and we owe much to the contributions made by experimental animals. The use of isolated and cultured heart muscle cells is still in its infancy, and better techniques for culturing adult myocytes are needed. A major difficulty encountered in the research of human cardiomyopathies and to a lesser extent of experimental cardiomyopathies is the differentiation between primary, causal and secondary abnormalities in structure and function. Thus, greater emphasis must be placed on studying the early (that is, before heart failure) stages of cardiomyopathy.

Dr. Lorell is supported by an Established Investigatorship from the American Heart Association, Inc., Dallas, Texas.

References

1. Wenger NK, Goodwin JF, Roberts WC. Cardiomyopathy and myocardial involvement in systemic disease. In: Hurst JW, ed. The Heart, Arteries and Veins, 6th ed. New York: McGraw-Hill, 1986:1181–248.
2. Goodwin JF. Prospects and predictions for the cardiomyopathies. Circulation 1974;50:210–9.
3. Johnson RA, Palacios I. Dilated cardiomyopathies of the adult. N Engl J Med 1982;307:1050–8, 1119–26.
4. Perloff JK, ed. The Cardiomyopathies. Cardiol Clin 1988;6:185–320.
5. Abelmann WH. Classification and natural history of primary myocardial disease. Prog Cardiovasc Dis 1984;27:73–94.
6. Goodwin JF, ed. Heart Muscle Disease. Lancaster: MTP Press (Kluwer), 1985:291.
7. Unverferth DV, ed. Dilated Cardiomyopathy. Mt. Kisco, NY: Futura, 1985:289.
8. Ten Cate FJ, ed. Hypertrophic Cardiomyopathy: Clinical Recognition and Management. New York: Marcel Dekker, 1985:266.
9. Wenger NK, Abelmann WH, Roberts WC. Myocarditis. In: Hurst JW, ed. The Heart, Arteries and Veins, 6th ed. New York: McGraw-Hill, 1986:1158–80.
10. Giles TD, ed. Cardiomyopathy. Littleton, MA: PSG Publishing, 1988: 501.
11. Engelmeier R, O'Connell JB, eds. Drug Therapy in Dilated Cardiomyopathy and Myocarditis. New York: Marcel Dekker, 1988:288.
12. Wynne J, Braunwald E. The cardiomyopathies and myocarditides. In: Braunwald E, ed. Heart Disease: A Textbook of Cardiovascular Medicine, 3rd ed. Philadelphia: WB Saunders, 1988:1410–69.
13. Krehl L. Beitrag zur Kentniss der idiopathischen Herz-muskelerkrankungen. Dtsch Arch Klin Med 1891;48:414–31.
14. Josserand E, Gallavardin L. De l'asystolie progressive des jeunes sujets par myocardite subaigue primitive. Arch Gen Med 1901;6:684–704.
15. Christian H. Diagnosis of chronic non-valvular heart disease (chronic myocarditis). N Engl J Med 1933;208:574.
16. Mattingly TW. The clinical and hemodynamic features of primary myocardial disease. Trans Am Clin Climatol Assoc 1959;70:132–41.
17. Harvey WP, Segal JP, Gurel T. The clinical spectrum of primary myocardial disease. Prog Cardiovasc Dis 1964;7:17–42.
18. Brigden W. Uncommon myocardial diseases. The non-coronary cardiomyopathies. Lancet 1957;2:1179–243.
19. Goodwin JF, Gordon H, Hollman A, et al. Clinical aspects of cardiomyopathy. Br Med J 1961;1:69–79.
20. Fejfar Z, ed. Accounts of international meetings: idiopathic cardiomegaly. Bull WHO 1968;38:979–92.
21. WHO/ISFC Task Force. Report of the WHO/ISFC Task Force on the Definition and Classification of cardiomyopathies. Br Heart J 1980;44: 672–3.
22. Abelmann WH. The etiology, pathogenesis and pathophysiology of dilated cardiomyopathies. In: Schultheiss H-P, ed. New Concepts in Viral Heart Disease: Virology, Immunology and Clinical Management. Berlin: Springer-Verlag, 1988:3–21.
23. Abelmann WH. The cardiomyopathies. Hosp Pract 1971;6:101–12.
24. Abelmann WH. Incidence of dilated cardiomyopathy. Postgrad Med J 1985;61:1123–4.
25. William DG, Olsen EGJ. Prevalence of overt dilated cardiomyopathy in two regions of England. Br Heart J 1985;54:153–5.
26. World Health Organization. Cardiomyopathies: report of a WHO expert committee. WHO Tech Rep Ser 1984;697:7–68.
27. Brigden W. Hypertrophic cardiomyopathy. Br Heart J 1987;58:299–302.
28. Evans W. Familial cardiomyopathy. Br Heart J 1949;11:68–82.
29. Brock RC. Functional obstruction of the left ventricle (acquired aortic subvalvular stenosis). Guys Hosp Rep 1957;106:221–38.
30. Teare D. Asymmetric hypertrophy of the heart in young adults. Br Heart J 1958;20:1–8.

31. Braunwald E, Morrow AG, Cornell WP, et al. Idiopathic hypertrophic subaortic stenosis: clinical, hemodynamic and angiographic manifestations. Am J Med 1960;29:924–45.

32. Frank S, Braunwald E. Idiopathic hypertrophic subaortic stenosis: clinical analysis of 126 patients with emphasis on the natural history. Circulation 1968;37:759–88.

33. Henry WL, Clark CE, Griffith JM, et al. Mechanism of left ventricular outflow obstruction in patients with obstructive asymmetric septal hypertrophy (idiopathic hypertrophic subaortic stenosis). Am J Cardiol 1975;35:337–45.

34. Morrow AG, Reitz BA, Epstein SE, et al. Operative treatment in hypertrophic subaortic stenosis: techniques, and the results of pre and post operative assessments in 83 patients. Circulation 1975;52:88–102.

35. Maron BJ, Anan TJ, Roberts WC. Quantitative analysis of the distribution of cardiac muscle cell disorganization in the left ventricular wall of patients with hypertrophic cardiomyopathy. Circulation 1981;63:882–94.

36. Steward S, Mason D, Braunwald E. Impaired rate of left ventricular filling in idiopathic hypertrophic subaortic stenosis and valvular aortic stenosis. Circulation 1968;37:8–14.

37. Swan DH, Bell B, Oakley CM, et al. Analysis of symptomatic course and prognosis and treatment of hypertrophic obstructive cardiomyopathy. Br Heart J 1971;33:671–85.

38. Oakley CM. Clinical recognition of the cardiomyopathies. Circ Res 1974;35:II-152–67.

39. McKenna W, Deanfield J, Farugui A, et al. Prognosis in hypertrophic cardiomyopathy: role of age and clinical, electrocardiographic and hemodynamic features. Am J Cardiol 1981;47:532–8.

40. Maron BJ, Roberts WC, Epstein SE. Sudden death in hypertrophic cardiomyopathy: a profile of 78 patients. Circulation 1982;65:1388–94.

41. Spirito P, Maron BJ, Bonow RO, et al. Severe functional limitation in patients with hypertrophic cardiomyopathy and only mild localized left ventricular hypertrophy. J Am Coll Cardiol 1986;8:537–44.

42. Wigle ED, Sasson Z, Henderson MA, et al. Hypertrophic cardiomyopathy: importance of the site and extent of hypertrophy: a review. Prog Cardiovasc Dis 1985;28:1–83.

43. Maron BJ, Gottdiener JS, Epstein SE. Patterns and significance of the distribution of left ventricular hypertrophy in hypertrophic cardiomyopathy: a wide-angle two-dimensional study of 125 patients. Am J Cardiol 1981;48:418–28.

44. Shapiro LM, McKenna WJ. Distribution of left ventricular hypertrophy in hypertrophic cardiomyopathy: a two-dimensional echocardiographic study. J Am Coll Cardiol 1983;2:437–44.

45. Ciro E, Nichols PF, Maron BJ. Heterogeneous morphologic expression of genetically transmitted hypertrophic cardiomyopathy: two dimensional echocardiographic analysis. Circulation 1983;67:1227–33.

46. Yamaguchi H, Ishimura T, Nishiyama S, et al. Hypertrophic nonobstructive cardiomyopathy with giant negative T waves (apical hypertrophy): ventriculographic and echocardiographic features in 30 patients. Am J Cardiol 1979;44:401–12.

47. Falicov RE, Resnekov L, Bharati S, et al. Mid-ventricular obstruction: a variant of hypertrophic obstructive cardiomyopathy. Am J Cardiol 1976;37:432–7.

48. Goodwin JF. The frontiers of cardiomyopathy. Br Heart J 1982;48:1–18.

49. Maron BJ, Bonow RO, Cannon RO, et al. Hypertrophic cardiomyopathy: interrelations of clinical manifestations, pathophysiology and therapy. N Engl J Med 1987;316:780–9.

50. Fifer MA, Bourdillon PD, Lorell BH. Altered left ventricular diastolic properties during pacing-induced angina in patients with aortic stenosis. Circulation 1986;74:675–83.

51. Cannon RO, Rosing DR, Maron BJ, et al. Myocardial ischemia in patients with hypertrophic cardiomyopathy: contribution of inadequate vasodilator reserve and elevated left ventricular filling pressures. Circulation 1985;71:234–43.

52. Ten Cate FJ, Serruys PW. Coronary flow reserve and diastolic function in hypertrophic cardiomyopathy. Int J Cardiol 1987;17:25–36.

53. O'Gara PT, Bonow RO, Maron BJ, et al. Myocardial perfusion abnormalities in patients with hypertrophic cardiomyopathy: assessment with thallium-201 emission computed tomography. Circulation 1987;76:1214–23.

54. Maron BJ, Wolfson JK, Epstein SE, et al. Intramural ("small vessel") coronary artery disease in hypertrophic cardiomyopathy. J Am Coll Cardiol 1986;8:545–57.

55. Marcus ML, Doty DB, Hiratzka LF, et al. Decreased coronary reserve: a mechanism for angina pectoris in patients with aortic stenosis and normal coronary arteries. N Engl J Med 1982;307:1362–6.

56. Cunningham ML, Weinberg CS, Apstein CS, et al. Reversal of exaggerated hypoxic dysfunction in hypertrophied hearts by increased glycolytic substrate (abstr). Circulation 1988;78(suppl II):II-265.

57. Grover-McKay M, Schwaiger M, Krivokapich J, et al. Regional myocardial blood flow and metabolism at rest in mildly symptomatic patients with hypertrophic cardiomyopathy. J Am Coll Cardiol 1989;13:1–8.

58. Criley JM, Lewis KB, White RI Jr, et al. Pressure gradients without obstruction: a new concept of "hypertrophic subaortic stenosis." Circulation 1965;32:881–7.

59. Criley JM, Siegel RJ. Has "obstruction" hindered our understanding of hypertrophic cardiomyopathy? Circulation 1985;72:1148–54.

60. Murgo JP, Alter BR, Dorethy JF, et al. Dynamics of left ventricular ejection in obstructive and nonobstructive hypertrophic cardiomyopathy. J Clin Invest 1980;66:1369–82.

61. Wigle ED. Hypertrophic cardiomyopathy: a 1987 viewpoint. Circulation 1987;75:311–22.

62. Maron BJ, Epstein SE. Clinical significance and therapeutic implications of the left ventricular outflow tract pressure gradient in hypertrophic cardiomyopathy. Am J Cardiol 1986;58:1093–6.

63. Cannon RO, Schenke WH, Maron BJ, et al. Differences in coronary flow and myocardial metabolism at rest and during pacing between patients with obstructive and patients with nonobstructive cardiomyopathy. J Am Coll Cardiol 1987;10:53–62.

64. Lorell BH, Grossman W. Cardiac hypertrophy: the consequences for diastole. J Am Coll Cardiol 1987;9:1189–93.

65. Spirito P, Maron BJ, Chiarella F, et al. Diastolic abnormalities in patients with hypertrophic cardiomyopathy: relation to magnitude of left ventricular hypertrophy. Circulation 1985;72:310–6.

66. Hanrath P, Mathey DG, Siegert R, et al. Left ventricular relaxation and filling pattern in different forms of left ventricular hypertrophy. Am J Cardiol 1980;45:15–23.

67. Lorell BH, Paulus WJ, Grossman W, et al. Modification of abnormal left ventricular diastolic properties by nifedipine in patients with hypertrophic cardiomyopathy. Circulation 1982;65:499–507.

68. St. John Sutton MG, Tajik AJ, Gibson DG, et al. Echocardiographic assessment of left ventricular filling and septal and posterior wall dynamics in idiopathic hypertrophic subaortic stenosis. Circulation 1978;57:512–20.

69. Bonow RO, Rosing DR, Bacharach SL, et al. Effects of verapamil on left ventricular systolic function and diastolic filling in patients with hypertrophic cardiomyopathy. Circulation 1981;64:787–96.

70. Iwase M, Sotobata I, Takagi S, et al. Effects of diltiazem on left ventricular diastolic behavior in patients with hypertrophic cardiomyopathy. J Am Coll Cardiol 1987;9:1099–105.

71. Paulus WJ, Lorell BH, Craig WE, et al. Comparison of the effects of nitroprusside and nifedipine on diastolic properties in patients with hypertrophic cardiomyopathy: altered left ventricular loading or improved muscle activation? J Am Coll Cardiol 1983;2:379–86.

72. Bonow RO, Vitale DF, Maron BJ, et al. Regional left ventricular asynchrony and impaired left ventricular filling in hypertrophic cardiomyopathy: effect of verapamil. J Am Coll Cardiol 1987;9:1108–16.

73. Paulus WJ, Nellens P, Heyndrickx GR, et al. Effects of long-term treatment with amiodarone on exercise hemodynamics and left ventricular relaxation in patients with hypertrophic cardiomyopathy. Circulation 1986;74:544–54.

74. Epstein SE, Rosing DR. Verapamil: its potential for causing serious complications in patients with hypertrophic cardiomyopathy. Circulation 1981;64:437–41.

75. Lorell BH. Use of calcium channel blockers in hypertrophic cardiomyopathy. Am J Med 1985;78(suppl 2B):43–54.

76. Shah PM, Adelman AG, Wigle ED, et al. The natural (and unnatural) history of hypertrophic obstructive cardiomyopathy. Circ Res 1973;34/35(suppl II):II-179–95.

77. Nicod P, Polikar R, Peterson KL. Hypertrophic cardiomyopathy and sudden death. N Engl J Med 1988;318:1255-7.

78. McKenna WJ, England D, Doi YL, et al. Arrhythmia in hypertrophic cardiomyopathy: influence on prognosis. Br Heart J 1981;46:168-72.

79. Maron BJ, Savage DD, Wolfson JK, et al. Prognostic significance of 24 hour ambulatory monitoring in patients with hypertrophic cardiomyopathy: a prospective study. Am J Cardiol 1981;48:252-7.

80. McKenna WJ, Chetty S, Oakley CM, Goodwin JF. Arrhythmia in hypertrophic cardiomyopathy: exercise and 48 hour ambulatory electrocardiographic assessment with and without beta adrenergic blocking therapy. Am J Cardiol 1980;45:1-5.

81. McKenna WJ, Harris L, Perez G, et al. Arrhythmia in hypertrophic cardiomyopathy: comparison of amiodarone and verapamil in treatment. Br Heart J 1981;46:173-8.

82. McKenna WJ, Oakley CM, Krikler DM, et al. Improved survival with amiodarone in patients with hypertrophic cardiomyopathy and ventricular tachycardia. Br Heart J 1985;53:412-6.

83. Maron BJ. The genetics of hypertrophic cardiomyopathy. Ann Intern Med 1986;105:610-3.

84. Greaves SC, Roche AHG, Neutze JM, et al. Inheritance of hypertrophic cardiomyopathy: a cross-sectional and M-mode echocardiographic study of 50 families. Br Heart J 1987;58:259-66.

85. Topol EJ, Traill TA, Fortuin N. Hypertensive hypertrophic cardiomyopathy in the elderly. N Engl J Med 1985;312:277-83.

86. Lewis JF, Maron BJ. Elderly patients with hypertrophic cardiomyopathy: a subset with distinctive left ventricular morphology and progressive clinical course late in life. J Am Coll Cardiol 1989;13:36-45.

87. Petrin TJ, Tavel ME. Idiopathic hypertrophic subaortic stenosis as observed in a large community hospital: relation to age and history of hypertension. J Am Geriatr Soc 1979;27:43-6.

88. Jarcho JA, McKenna W, Pare P, et al. Mapping a gene for familial hypertrophic cardiomyopathy to chromosome 14q1. N Engl J Med 1989;321:1372-8.

89. Saez LJ, Gianola KM, McNally EM, et al. Human cardiac myosin heavy chain genes and their linkage in the genome. Nucleic Acids Res 1987;15:5443-59.

90. van Ekeren GJ, Stadhouders AM, Egberink GJM, et al. Hereditary mitochondrial hypertrophic cardiomyopathy with mitochondrial myopathy of skeletal muscle, congenital cataract and lactic acidosis. Virchows Arch [A] 1987;412:47-52.

91. Pandullo C, Nicolosi GL, Scardi S. Hypertrophic cardiomyopathy associated with myotonic muscular dystrophy. Int J Cardiol 1987;16:205-8.

92. Colucci WS, Lorell BH, Schoen FR, et al. Hypertrophic obstruction cardiomyopathy due to Fabry's disease. N Engl J Med 1982;307:926-8.

93. Perloff JK. Pathogenesis of hypertrophic cardiomyopathy: hypothesis and speculations. Am Heart J 1981;101:219-26.

94. Ferrans VJ, Rodriguez ER. Evidence of myocyte hyperplasia in hypertrophic cardiomyopathy and other disorders with myocardial hypertrophy? Z Kardiol 1987;76(suppl 3):20-5.

95. Pouleur H, Rousseau MF, Eyll CV, et al. Force-velocity-length relations in hypertrophic cardiomyopathy: evidence of normal or depressed myocardial contractility. Am J Cardiol 1983;52:813-7.

96. Saito T, Hirota Y, Kita Y, et al. Evaluation of left ventricular contractility in hypertrophic cardiomyopathy from end-systolic pressure-volume relation. Jpn Circ J 1987;51:511-9.

97. Kawai C, Yui Y, Hoshino T, et al. Myocardial catecholamines in hypertrophic and dilated (congestive) cardiomyopathy: a biopsy study. J Am Coll Cardiol 1983;2:834-40.

98. Golf S, Myhre E, Abdelnoor H, et al. Hypertrophic cardiomyopathy characterized by beta-adrenoceptor density, relative amount of beta-adrenoceptor subtypes and adenylate cyclace activity. Cardiovasc Res 1985;19:693-9.

99. Unverferth DV, Schmidt WR, Fertel RH. Cyclic nucleotide analysis of myocardial biopsies in hypertrophic cardiomyopathy. Am J Cardiol 1987;59:185-6.

100. McFarland KF, Stefadouros MA, Abdulla AM, McFarland DE. Hypercalcemia and idiopathic hypertrophic subaortic stenosis. Ann Intern Med 1978;88:57-8.

101. Lorell BH, Barry WH. Effects of verapamil on contraction and relaxation on cultured chick embryo ventricular cells during calcium overload. J Am Coll Cardiol 1984;3:341-8.

102. Wagner JA, Sax FL, Weisman HF, et al. Calcium-antagonist receptors in the atrial tissue of patients with hypertrophic cardiomyopathy. N Engl J Med 1989;320:755-61.

103. Morgan JP, Morgan KG. Calcium and cardiovascular function: intracellular calcium levels during contraction and relaxation of mammalian and vascular smooth muscle as detected by aequorin. Am J Med 1984;(suppl 5A):33-46.

104. Bedford DE, Konstam GCS. Obscure heart disease in West African troops. Br Heart J 1946;8:236-7.

105. Löffler W. Endocarditis parietalis fibroplastica mit Bluteosinophilie. Schweiz Med Wochenschr 1936;17:817-20.

106. Olsen EGJ, Spry CJF. Relation between eosinophilia and endomyocardial disease. Prog Cardiovasc Dis 1985;27:241-54.

107. Spry CJF, Tai P-C, Davies J. The cardiotoxicity of eosinophils. Postgrad Med J 1983;59:147-53.

108. Abelmann WH. Restrictive and obliterative cardiomyopathy. In: Parmley WW, Chatterjee K, eds. Cardiology. Philadelphia: JB Lippincott, 1987;1-16.

109. McManus BM, Bren GB, Robertson EA, Katz RJ, Ross AM, Roberts WC. Hemodynamic cardiac constriction without anatomic myocardial restriction or pericardial constriction. Am Heart J 1981;102:134-6.

110. Grossman W, McLaurin LP, Moos SP, Stefadoros M, Young DT. Wall thickness and diastolic properties of the left ventricle. Circulation 1974;49:129-35.

111. Caulfield JB. Morphologic alterations of the collagen matrix with cardiac hypertrophy. Perspect Cardiovasc Res 1983;7:167-75.

112. Benotti JR, Grossman W, Cohn PF. Clinical profile of restrictive cardiomyopathy. Circulation 1980;61:1206-12.

113. Siegel RJ, Shah PK, Fishbein MC. Idiopathic restrictive cardiomyopathy. Circulation 1984;70:165-9.

114. Ferriere M, Donnadio D, Gros B, Baissus C, Latour H. Biopsie endoventriculaire droite: indications et resultats: cent seize observations. Presse Med 1985;14:773-6.

115. Isner JM, Carter BL, Blankoff MS, et al. Differentiation of constrictive pericarditis from restrictive cardiomyopathy by computed tomographic imaging. Am Heart J 1983;105:1019-25.

116. Gillette EL, McChesney SL, Hoopes PJ. Isoeffect curves for radiation-induced cardiomyopathy in the dog. Int J Radiat Oncol Biol Phys 1985;11:2091-7.

117. Bulkley BH, Ridolfi RL, Salyer WR, Hutchins GM. Myocardial lesions of progressive systemic sclerosis. A cause of cardiac dysfunction. Circulation 1976;53:483-90.

118. Follansbee WP, Curtiss EI, Medsger TA Jr, et al. Physiologic abnormalities of cardiac function in progressive systemic sclerosis with diffuse scleroderma. N Engl J Med 1984;310:142-8.

119. Tripp ME, Katcher ML, Peters HA, et al. Systemic carnitine deficiency presenting as familial endocardial fibroelastosis: a treatable cardiomyopathy. N Engl J Med 1981;305:385-90.

120. Cutler DJ, Isner JM, Bracey AW, et al. Hemochromatosis heart disease: an unemphasized cause of potentially reversible restrictive cardiomyopathy. Am J Med 1980;69:923-8.

121. Dabestani A, Child JS, Henze E, et al. Primary hemochromatosis: anatomic and physiologic characteristics of the cardiac ventricles and their response to phlebotomy. Am J Cardiol 1984;54:153-9.

122. Ley TJ, Griffith D, Niehuis AW. Transfusion hemosiderosis and chelation therapy. Clin Hematol 1982;11:437-64.

123. Moraes CR, Buffalo E, Lima R, et al. Surgical treatment of endomyocardial fibrosis. J Thorac Cardiovasc Surg 1983;85:738-45.

124. Parillo JE, Borer JS, Henry WC, Wolff SM, Fauci AS. The cardiovascular manifestations of the hypereosinophilic syndrome: prospective study of 26 patients, with review of the literature. Am J Med 1979;67:572-82.

125. Marcus RI, Fontaine GH, Guirauaudon G, et al. Right ventricular dysplasia: a report of 24 adult cases. Circulation 1982;65:384-98.

126. Rossi P, Massumi A, Gillette P, Hall RJ. Arrhythmogenic right ventricular dysplasia: clinical features, diagnostic techniques and current management. Am Heart J 1982;103:415-20.

127. Thiene G, Nava A, Corrado D, Rossi L, Pennelli N. Right ventricular cardiomyopathy and sudden death in young people. N Engl J Med 1988;318:129–33.

128. Nava A, Thiene G, Canciani B, et al. Familial occurrence of right ventricular dysplasia: a study involving nine families. J Am Coll Cardiol 1988;12:1222–8.

129. Kuhn H, Becker R, Fischer J, et al. Studies on the etiology, the clinical course and the prognosis of patients with dilated cardiomyopathy (DCM). Z Kardiol 1982;71:497–508.

130. Franciosa JA, Wilen M, Ziesche S, Cohn JN. Survival in men with severe chronic left ventricular failure due to either coronary heart disease or idiopathic dilated cardiomyopathy. Am J Cardiol 1983;51:831–6.

131. Diaz RA, Obasohan A, Oakley CM. Prediction of outcome in dilated cardiomyopathy. Br Heart J 1987;58:393–9.

132. Benjamin IJ, Schuster EH, Bulkley BH. Cardiac hypertrophy in idiopathic dilated congestive cardiomyopathy: a clinicopathologic study. Circulation 1981;64:442–7.

133. Michels VV, Driscoll IJ, Miller FA Jr. Familial aggregation of idiopathic cardiomyopathy. Am J Cardiol 1985;55:1232–3.

134. Berko BA, Swift M. X-linked dilated cardiomyopathy. N Engl J Med 1987;316:1186–91.

135. Gardner RJM, Hanson WW, Ionasescu HH, et al. Dominantly inherited dilated cardiomyopathy. Am J Med Genet 1987;27:61–73.

136. Goldblatt J, Melmed J, Rose AG. Autosomal recessive inheritance of idiopathic dilated cardiomyopathy in a Madeira Portuguese kindred. Clin Genet 1987;31:249–54.

137. Fragola PV, Auture C, Picelli A, Sommariva L, Cannata D, Sangiorgi M. Familial idiopathic dilated cardiomyopathy. Am Heart J 1988;115:912–4.

138. Morrow CJ, McOrist S. Cardiomyopathy associated with curly hair coat in Poll Hereford calves in Australia. Vet Rec 1985;117:312–3.

139. Bajusz E, Homburger F, Baker JR, Opie LH. The heart muscle in muscular dystrophy with special reference to involvement of the cardiovascular system in the hereditary myopathy of the hamster. Ann NY Acad Sci 1966;138:213–29.

140. Herskowitz A, Wolfgram LJ, Rose NR, Beisel KW. Coxsackievirus B3 murine myocarditis: a pathologic spectrum of myocarditis in genetically defined inbred strains. J Am Coll Cardiol 1987;9:1311–9.

141. Kishimoto C, Kawai C, Abelmann WH. Immuno-genetic aspects of the pathogenesis of experimental viral myocardits. In: Kawai C, Abelmann WH, eds. Pathogenesis of Myocarditis and Cardiomyopathy: Recent Experimental and Clinical Studies. Tokyo: Tokyo University Press, 1987:3–7.

142. Huber SA, Lodge PA. Coxsackievirus B3 myocarditis. Identification of different pathogenetic mechanisms in DBA/2 and BALB/c mice. Am J Pathol 1986;122:284–91.

143. Akbarian M, Yankopoulos NA, Abelmann WH. Hemodynamic studies in beriberi heart disease. Am J Med 1966;41:197–212.

144. Yang GQ, Chen JS, Wen ZM, et al. The role of selenium in Keshan disease. Adv Nutr Res 1984;6:203–31.

145. Johnson RA, Baker SS, Fallon JT, et al. An occidental case of cardiomyopathy and selenium deficiency. N Engl J Med 1981;304:1210–2.

146. Whitmer JT. L-carnitine treatment improves cardiac performance and restores high energy phosphate pools in cardiomyopathic Syrian hamsters. Circ Res 1987;61:396–408.

147. McFalls EO, Paulson DJ, Gilbert EF, Shug AL. Carnitine protection against adriamycin-induced cardiomyopathy in rats. Life Sci 1986;38:497–505.

148. Regitz V, Müller M, Schüler S, et al. Carnitinstoffwechselveränderungen im Endstadium der dilativen Kardiomyopathie und der ischämischen Herzmuskelerkrankung. Z Kardiol 1987;76(suppl 5):1–8.

149. Walsh TK, Vacek JL. Ethanol and heart disease: an underestimated contributory factor. Postgrad Med 1986;79:60–75.

150. Mackenzie J. The study of the pulse. Edinburgh, Y.J. Pentland, 1902:237.

151. Brigden W, Robinson J. Alcoholic heart disease. Br Med J 1964;2:1283–9.

152. Czarnecki CM, Shaffer SW, Evanson OA. Ultrastructural features of ethanol-induced cardiomyopathy in turkey poults. Comp Biochem Physiol 1985;82:939–43.

153. Regan TJ, Levinson GE, Oldewurtel HA, Frank MJ, Weisse AB, Moschos CB. Ventricular function in noncardiacs with alcoholic fatty liver: the role of ethanol in the production of cardiomyopathy. J Clin Invest 1969;48:397–407.

154. Spodick DH, Pigott VM, Chirife R. Preclinical cardiac malfunction in chronic alcoholism: comparison with matched normal controls and with alcoholic cardiomyopathy. N Engl J Med 1972;287:677–80.

155. Kino M, Thorp KA, Bing OHL, Abelmann WH. Impaired myocardial performance and response to calcium in experimental alcoholic cardiomyopathy. J Mol Cell Cardiol 1981;13:981–9.

156. Edes I, Piros G, Forster T, Csandy M. Alcohol-induced congestive cardiomyopathy in adult turkeys: effects of myocardial antioxident defence systems. Basic Res Cardiol 1987;82:551–6.

157. Regan TJ. Alcoholic cardiomyopathy. Prog Cardiovasc Dis 1984;27:141–52.

158. Garrett JS, Wikman-Coffelt J, Sievers R, Finkbeiner WE, Parmley WW. Verapamil prevents the development of alcoholic dysfunction in hamster myocardium. J Am Coll Cardiol 1987;9:1326–31.

159. Rosenoff SH, Brooks E, Bostick F, Young RC. Alterations in DNA synthesis in cardiac tissue induced by adriamycin in vivo—relationship to fetal toxicity. Biochem Pharmacol 1975;14:1898–901.

160. Iwamoto Y, Hansen IL, Porter TH, Folkers K. Inhibition of coenzyme Q_{10}-enzymes, succinoxidase and NADH-oxidase by adriamycin and other quinones having antitumor activity. Biochem Biophys Res Commun 1974;58:633–8.

161. Bristow MR, Minobe WA, Billingham ME, et al. Anthracycline-associated cardiac and renal damage in rabbits: evidence for mediation by vasoactive substances. Lab Invest 1981;45:157–68.

162. Myers CE, McGuire WP, Liss RH, Ifrim I, Grotzinger K, Young RC. Adriamycin: the role of lipid peroxidation in cardiac toxicity and tumor response. Science 1977;197:165–7.

163. Azuma J, Sperelakis N, Hasegawa H, et al. Adriamycin cardiotoxicity: possible pathogenetic mechanisms. J Mol Cell Cardiol 1981;13:381–97.

164. Rona G. Catecholamine cardiotoxicity. J Mol Cell Cardiol 1985;17:291–306.

165. Rona G, Kahn DS, Chappel CI. Studies on infarct-like myocardial necrosis produced by isoproternol: a review. Rev Can Biol 1963;22:241–55.

166. Velasquez G, D'Souza VJ, Hackshaw BJ, Glass TA, Formanek AG. Pheochromocytoma and cardiomyopathy. Br J Radiol 1984;57:89–92.

167. Imperato-McGinley J, Gautier T, Ehlers K, Zullo MA, Goldstein DS, Vaughan ED Jr. Reversibility of catecholamine-induced dilated cardiomyopathy in a child with a pheochromocytoma. N Engl J Med 1987;316:793–7.

168. Ganguly PK, Pierce GN, Dhalla NS. Diabetic cardiomyopathy: membrane dysfunction and therapeutic strategies. J Appl Cardiol 1987;2:323–38.

169. Lossnitzer K. Genetic induction of a cardiomyopathy. In: Schmier J, Eichler O, eds. Experimental Production of Diseases. Part 3: Heart and Circulation. New York: Springer-Verlag, 1975:309.

170. Factor SM, Minase T, Cho S, Dominitz R, Sonnenblick EH. Microvascular spasm in the cardiomyopathic hamster: a preventable cause of focal myocardial necrosis. Circulation 1982;66:342–54.

171. Factor SM, Minase T, Cho S, Fein F, Capasso JM, Sonnenblick EH. Coronary microvascular abnormalities in the hypertensive-diabetic rat: a primary cause of cardiomyopathy? Am J Pathol 1984;116:9–20.

172. Factor SM, Cho S, Wittner M, Tanowitz H. Abnormalities of the coronary microcirculation in the acute murine Chagas' disease. Am J Trop Med Hyg 1985;34:246–53.

173. Pasternac A, Noble J, Streulens Y, Elie R, Henschke C, Bourassa MG. Pathophysiology of chest pain in patients with cardiomyopathies and normal coronary arteries. Circulation 1982;65:88–9.

174. Cannon RO, Cunnion RE, Parrillo JE. Dynamic limitation of coronary vasodilator reserve in patients with dilated cardiomyopathy and chest pain. J Am Coll Cardiol 1987;10:1190–200.

175. DeMarco T, Chatterjee K, Rouleau JL, Parmley WW. Abnormal coronary hemodynamics and myocardial energetics in patients with chronic heart failure caused by ischemic heart disease and dilated cardiomyopathy. Am Heart J 1988;115:809–15.

176. Phillips E, Levine SA. Auricular fibroelastosis without other evidence of heart disease: a case of reversible heart failure. Am J Med 1949;7:479–89.

177. Packer DL, Bardy GH, Worley SJ, et al. Tachycardiainduced cardiomyopathy: a reversible form of left ventricular dysfunction. Am J Cardiol 1986;57:563–70.

178. Moe GW, Stopps TP, Howard RJ, Armstrong PW. Early recovery from heart failure: insights into the pathogenesis of experimental chronic pacing-induced heart failure. J Lab Clin Med 1988;112:426–32.

179. Coleman HN, Taylor RR, Pool PE, et al. Congestive heart failure following chronic tachycardia. Am Heart J 1971;81:790–8.

180. Feldman MD, Alderman JD, Aroesty JM, et al. Depression of systolic and diastolic myocardial reserve during atrial pacing tachycardia in patients with dilated cardiomyopathy. J Clin Invest 1988;82:1661–9.

181. Feldman MD, Gwathmey JK, Phillips PS, Schoen F, Morgan JP. Reversal of the force-frequency relationship in working myocardium from patients with end-stage heart failure. J Appl Cardiol 1988;3:273–83.

182. Fabiato A, Fabiato F. Calcium and cardiac excitation-contraction coupling. Ann Rev Physiol 1979;41:473–84.

183. Katz AM. Regulation of myocardial contractility. 1958-1983: an odyssey. J Am Coll Cardiol 1983;1:42–51.

184. Dhalla NS, Singal PK, Panagia V, Harrow JAC, Anand-Srivastava MB, Beamish RE. Progress and problems in understanding the involvement of calcium in heart failure. Can J Physiol Pharmacol 1984;62:867–73.

185. Lossnitzer K, Bajusz E. Water and electrolyte alterations during the lifecourse of the Bio 14.6 Syrian golden hamster: a disease model of a hereditary cardiomyopathy. J Mol Cell Cardiol 1974;6:163–77.

186. Wrogemann K, Blanchaer M, Thakar JH, Mezon BJ. On the role of mitochondria in the hereditary cardiomyopathy of the Syrian hamster. In: Fleckenstein A, Rona G, eds. Recent Advances in the Studies on Cardiac Structure and Metabolism, Vol 6: Pathophysiology and Morphology Cell Alteration. Baltimore: University Park Press, 1975;231–41.

187. Markiewicz W, Wu S, Parmley WW, et al. Evaluation of the hereditary Syrian hamster cardiomyopathy by ^{31}P nuclear magnetic resonance spectroscopy: improvement after acute verapamil therapy. Circ Res 1986;59:597–604.

188. Makino N, Dhalla KS, Elemban V, Dhalla NS. Sarcolemmal Ca^{2+} transport in streptozotocin-induced diabetic cardiomyopathy in rats. Am J Physiol (Endocrinol Metab 16) 1987;253:E202–E207.

189. Gwathmey JK, Copelas L, MacKinnon R, et al. Abnormal intracellular calcium handling in myocardium from patients with end-stage heart failure. Circ Res 1987;61:70–6.

190. Cross CE, Halliwell B, Borish ET, et al. Davis Conference: oxygen radicals and human disease. Ann Intern Med 1987;107:526–45.

191. Singal PK, ed. Oxygen Radicals in the Pathophysiology of Heart Disease. Boston: Kluwer Academic, 1988;348.

192. Kobayashi A, Yamashita T, Kaneko M, Nishiyama T, Hayashi H, Yamazaki N. Effects of verapamil on experimental cardiomyopathy in the Bio 14.6 Syrian hamster. J Am Coll Cardiol 1987;10:1128–38.

193. Breed JGS, Zimmerman ANE, Dormans JAMA, Pinedo HM. Failure of the antioxidant vitamin E to protect against adriamycin-induced cardiotoxicity in the rabbit. Cancer Res 1980;40:2033–8.

194. Laranja FS, Dias E, Nobrega G, Miranda A. Chagas' disease: a clinical epidemiologic and pathologic study. Circulation 1956;14:1035–60.

195. Köberle F. Chagas' disease and Chagas' syndromes: the pathology of American trypanosomiasis. Adv Parasitol 1968;6:63–116.

196. Abelmann WH. Experimental infection with Trypanosoma cruzi (Chagas' disease): a model of acute and chronic myocardiopathy. Ann NY Acad Sci 1969;156:137–51.

197. Poltera AA, Cox JN, Owor R. Pancarditis affecting the conducting system and all valves in human African trypanosomiasis. Br Heart J 1976;38:827–37.

198. Leak D, Meghji M. Toxoplasmic infection in cardiac disease. Am J Cardiol 1979;43:841–9.

199. Abelmann WH. Myocarditis as a cause of dilated cardiomyopathy. In: Engelmeier RS, O'Connell JB, eds. Therapy of Dilated Cardiomyopathy and Myocarditis. New York: Marcel Dekker, 1988;221–32.

200. Sainani GS, Krompotic E, Slodki SJ. Adult heart disease due to coxsackie virus B infection. Medicine 1968;47:13–23.

201. Smith WG. Coxsackie B myopericarditis in adults. Am Heart J 1970;80:34–46.

202. Miklozek CL, Kingsley EM, Crumpacker CS, et al. Serial cardiac function tests in myocarditis. Postgrad Med J 1986;62:577–9.

203. Obeysekere I, Hermon Y. Arbovirus heart disease: myocarditis and cardiomyopathy following dengue and chikungunya fever-a follow-up study. Am Heart J 1973;85:186–94.

204. Kitaura Y, Morita H. Secondary myocardial disease. Virus myocarditis and cardiomyopathy. Jpn Circ J 1979;43:1017–31.

205. Hasumi M, Sekiguchi M, Morimoto S, Hiroe M, Take M, Hirosawa K. Ventriculographic findings in the convalescent stage in eleven cases with acute myocarditis. Jpn Circ J 1983;47:1310–6.

206. Quigley PJ, Richardson PJ, Meany BT, et al. Long-term follow-up of acute myocarditis. Correlation of ventricular function and outcome. Eur Heart J 1987;8(suppl J):39–42.

207. Kawai C. Idiopathic cardiomyopathy: a study of the infection immune theory as a cause of disease. Jpn Circ J 1971;35:765–70.

208. Ayuthya PSN, Jayavasu VJ, Pongpenich B. Coxsackie group B virus and primary myocardial disease in infants and children. Am Heart J 1974;88:311–4.

209. Cambridge G, MacArthur CGC, Waterson AP, Goodwin JF, Oakley CM. Antibodies to coxsackie B viruses in congestive cardiomyopathy. Br Heart J 1979;41:692–6.

210. Olsen EGJ. Myocarditis—a case of mistaken identity? Br Heart J 1983;50:303–11.

211. Cohen IS, Anderson DW, Virmani R, et al. Congestive cardiomyopathy in association with the acquired immune deficiency syndrome. N Engl J Med 1986;315:628–30.

212. Anderson DW, Virmami R, Reilly JM, et al. Prevalent myocarditis at necropsy in the acquired immunodeficiency syndrome. J Am Coll Cardiol 1988;11:792–9.

213. Calabrese LH, Profitt MR, Yen-Lieberman B, Hobbs RE, Ratliff NB. Congestive cardiomyopathy and illness related to the acquired immunodeficiency syndrome (AIDS) associated with isolation of retrovirus from myocardium. Ann Intern Med 1987;691–2.

214. Matsumori A, Kawai C. An animal model of congestive (dilated) cardiomyopathy: dilatation and hypertrophy of the heart in the chronic stage in DBA/2 mice with myocarditis caused by encephalomyocarditis virus. Circulation 1982;66:355–60.

215. Matsumori A, Kawai C. An experimental model for congestive heart failure after encephalomyocarditis virus myocarditis in mice. Circulation 1982;65:1230–5.

216. Grodums EI, Zbitnew A. Experimental herpes simplex virus carditis in mice. Infect Immun 1976;14:1322–31.

217. Reyes MP, Ho K-L, Smith E, Lerner AM. A mouse model of dilated-type cardiomyopathy due to Coxsackie virus B3. J Infect Dis 1981;155:232–6.

218. Kawai C, Matsumori A, Kumagai N, Tokuda M. Experimental Coxsackievirus B-3 and B-4 myocarditis in mice. Jpn Circ J 1978;42:43–7.

219. Boikan WS. Myocarditis perniciosa. Virchows Arch Pathol Anat Physiol 1931;282:46–66.

220. Kline IK, Saphir O. Chronic pernicious myocarditis. Am Heart J 1960;59:681–97.

221. Mason JW. Techniques for right and left ventricular endomyocardial biopsy. Am J Cardiol 1978;41:887–92.

222. Nippoldt TB, Edwards WD, Holmes DR Jr, Reeder GS, Hartzler GO, Smith HC. Right ventricular endomyocardial biopsy: clinicopathologic correlates in 100 consecutive patients. Mayo Clin Proc 1982;57:407–18.

223. Fenoglio JJ, Ursell PC, Kellogg CF, Drusin RE, Weiss MB. Diagnosis and classification of myocarditis by endomyocardial biopsy. N Engl J Med 1983;308:12–8.

224. Zee-Cheng C, Tsai CC, Palmer DC, Codd JE, Pennington D, William GA. High incidence of myocarditis by endomyocardial biopsy in patients with idiopathic congestive cardiomyopathy. J Am Coll Cardiol 1984;3:63–70.

225. Dec GW Jr, Papacios IF, Fallon JT, et al. Active myocarditis in the spectrum of acute dilated cardiomyopathies: clinical features, histologic correlates, and clinical outcome. N Engl J Med 1985;312:885–90.

226. Cassling RS, Linder J, Sears TD, et al. Quantitative evaluation of inflammation in biopsy specimens from idiopathically failing or irritable hearts: experience in 80 pediatric and adult patients. Am Heart J 1985;110:713–20.

227. Shanes JG, Ghali J, Billingham ME, et al. Interobserver variability in the pathologic interpretation of endomyocardial biopsy results. Circulation 1987;75:401–5.

228. Aretz HT, Billingham ME, Edwards WD, et al. Myocarditis: a histopathologic definition and classification. Am J Cardiovasc Pathol 1986;1:3–14.

229. O'Connell JB, Mason JW. The diagnosis and therapy of active myocarditis. West J Med 1989;150:431–5.

230. Higuchi M de L, de Morais CF, Barreto ACP, et al. The role of active myocarditis in the development of heart failure in chronic Chagas' disease: a study based on endomyocardial biopsies. Clin Cardiol 1987;10:665–70.

231. Cronin ME, Love LA, Miller FW, McClintock PR, Plotz PH. The natural history of encephalomyocarditis virus-induced myositis and myocarditis in mice. Viral persistence demonstrated by *in situ* hybridization. J Exp Med 1988;168:1639–48.

232. Kandolf R, Ameis D, Kirschner P, Canu A, Hofschneider PH: *In situ* detection of enteroviral genomes in myocardial cells by nucleic acid hybridization: an approach to the diagnosis of viral heart disease. Proc Natl Acad Sci USA 1987;84:6272–6.

233. Archard LC, Freeke CA, Richardson PJ, et al. Persistence of enterovirus RNA in dilated cardiomyopathy: a progression from myocarditis. In: Schultheiss H-P, ed. New Concepts in Viral Heart Disease: Virology, Immunology and Clinical Management. Berlin: Springer-Verlag, 1988;349–62.

234. Kandolf R. The impact of recombinant DNA technology on the study of enteroviral heart disease. In: Bendinelli M, Friedman H, eds: Coxsackieviruses: A General Update. New York: Plenum, 1988:293–318.

235. Kaplan MH, Craig JM. Immunologic studies of heart tissue. 4: cardiac lesions in rabbits associated with autoantibodies to heart induced by immunization with heterologous heart. J Immunol 1963;90:725–33.

236. Davies AM, Laufer A, Gery I, Rosenmann E. Organ specificity of the heart. 3: circulating antibodies and immunopathological animals. Arch Pathol 1964;78:369–76.

237. Fukuta S, Kimura Y, Yamakawa K, Iwamoto S, Wada K, Kusukawa R. Experimental myocarditis. 2: cardiac lesions in rats induced by immunization with heterologous heart extracts. Jpn Circ J 1981;45:1399–402.

238. Hosenpud JD, Campbell SM, Niles NR, Lee J, Hart MV. Exercise-induced augmentation of cellular and humoral autoimmunity associated with increased cardiac dilatation in experimental autoimmune myocarditis. Cardiovasc Res 1987;21:217–22.

239. Santos-Buch CA. American trypanosomiasis: Chagas' disease. Int Rev Exp Pathol 1979;19:63–100.

240. Acosta AM, Santos-Buch CA. Autoimmune myocarditis induced by *Trypanosoma cruzi*. Circulation 1985;71:1255–61.

241. Cossio PM, Bustuoabad O, Paterno E, et al. Experimental myocarditis induced in Swiss mice by homologous heart immunization resembles chronic experimental Chagas' heart disease. Clin Immunol Immunopathol 1984;33:165–75.

242. Woodruff JF. Viral myocarditis: a review. Am J Pathol 1980;101:427–83.

243. Robinson JA, O'Connell JB, eds. Myocarditis: Precursor of Cardiomyopathy. Lexington, MA: DC Heath, 1983:167.

244. Bolte H-D. Viral Heart Disease. Berlin: Springer-Verlag, 1984:1–248.

245. Kawai C, Abelmann WH, eds. Pathogenesis of Myocarditis and Cardiomyopathy: Recent Experimental and Clinical Studies. Tokyo: University of Tokyo Press, 1987:1:312.

246. Maisch B, Kochsiek K, Gold R, eds. Inflammatory heart disease. Eur Heart J 1987;8(suppl J):1–465.

247. McManus BM, Gauntt CJ, Cassling RS. Immunopathologic basis of myocardial injury. Cardiovasc Clin 1988;18:163–84.

248. Schultheiss H-P, ed. New Concepts in Viral Heart Disease: Virology, Immunology and Clinical Management. Berlin: Springer-Verlag, 1988:1–504.

249. Woodruff JF, Woodruff JJ. Involvement of T lymphocytes in the pathogenesis of coxsackievirus B3 heart disease. J Immunol 1974;113:1726–34.

250. Lodge PA, Herzum M, Olszewski J, Huber SA. Coxsackie-virus B-3 myocarditis: acute and chronic forms of the disease caused by different immunopathogenic mechanisms. Am J Pathol 1987;128:455–63.

251. Anderson JL, Carlquist JF, Hammond EH. Deficient natural killer cell activity in patients with idiopathic dilated cardiomyopathy. Lancet 1982;2:124–7.

252. Yokoyama A. Natural killer cells in dilated cardiomyopathy. Tohoku J Exp Med 1988;154:335–44.

253. Amorim DS, Olsen EGJ. Assessment of heart neurons in dilated (congestive) cardiomyopathy. Br Heart J 1982;47:11–8.

254. Borg TK, Caulfield JB. The collagen matrix of the heart. Fed Proc 1984;40:2037–41.

255. Abrahams C, Janicki JS, Weber KT. Myocardial hypertrophy in *Macaca fascicularis*: structural remodeling of the collagen matrix. Lab Invest 1987;56:676–83.

256. Caulfield JB, Bittner V. Cardiac matrix alterations induced by adriamycin. Am J Pathol 1988;133:298–305.

257. Nakayama Y, Shimizu G, Hirota Y, et al. Functional and histopathologic correlation in patients with dilated cardiomyopathy: an integrated evaluation by multivariate analysis. J Am Coll Cardiol 1987;10:186–92.

258. Weber KT, Pick R, Janicki JS, Gadodia G, Lakier JB. Inadequate collagen tethers in dilated cardiomyopathy. Am Heart J 1988;116:1641–6.

259. Parmley WW. Pathophysiology and current therapy of congestive heart failure. J Am Coll Cardiol 1989;13:771–85.

260. Cohn JN. Current therapy of the failing heart. Circulation 1988;78:1099–107.

261. Packer M, Lee WH, Yushak M, Medina N. Comparison of captopril and enalapril in patients with severe chronic heart failure. N Engl J Med 1986;315:847–53.

262. Cohn JN, Archibald DG, Francis GS, et al. Veterans Administration Cooperative Study on vasodilator therapy of heart failure: influence of prerandomization variables on the reduction of mortality by treatment with hydralazine and isosorbide dinitrate. Circulation 1987;75(suppl IV):IV-49–54.

263. The Consensus Trial Study Group. Effects of enalapril on mortality in severe congestive heart failure. Results of the cooperative North Scandinavian Enalapril Survival Study (consensus). N Engl J Med 1987;316:1429–35.

264. Smith TW. Digitalis: mechanisms of action and clinical use. N Engl J Med 1988;318:358–65.

265. Captopril-Digoxin Multicenter Research Group. Comparative effects of therapy with captopril and digoxin in patients with mild to moderate heart failure. JAMA 1988;259:539–44.

266. Unverferth DV, Magorien RD, Alyschuld R, Kolibash AJ, Lewis RP, Leier CV. The hemodynamic and metabolic advantages gained by a three-day infusion of dobutamine in patients with congestive cardiomyopathy. Am Heart J 1983;106:29–34.

267. Liang CS, Sherman LG, Doherty JV, Wellington K, Lee VW, Hood WB Jr. Sustained improvement of cardiac function in patients with congestive heart failure after short-term infusion of dobutamine. Circulation 1984;69:113–9.

268. Borow KM, Lang RM, Neumann A, Carroll JD, Rajfer SI. Physiologic mechanisms governing hemodynamic responses to positive inotropic therapy in patients with dilated cardiomyopathy. Circulation 1988;77:625–37.

269. Colucci WS. Usefulness of calcium antagonists for congestive heart failure. Am J Cardiol 1987;59:52B–8B.

270. Figulla HR, Rechenberg JV, Wiegand V, Soballa R, Kreuzer H. Beneficial effects of long-term diltiazem treatment in dilated cardiomyopathy. J Am Coll Cardiol 1989;13:653–8.

271. Myerberg RJ, Kessler KM, Zaman L, Fernandez P, DeMarchena E, Castellanos A. Pharmacologic approaches to management of arrhythmias in patients with cardiomyopathy and heart failure. Am Heart J 1987;114:1273–9.

272. Waagstein F, Hjalmarson A, Varnauskas E, Wallentin I. Effect of chronic β-adrenergic receptor blockade in congestive cardiomyopathy. Br Heart J 1975;37:1022–36.

273. Scarpace BJ, Baresi LA, Sanford DA, Abrass IB. Desensitization and resensitization of β-adrenergic receptors in a smooth muscle cell line. Mol Pharmacol 1985;28:495–501.

274. Anderson JL, Lutz JR, Gilbert EM, et al. A randomized trial of low-dose beta-blockade therapy of idiopathic dilated cardiomyopathy. Am J Cardiol 1985;55:471–5.

275. Engelmeier RS, O'Connell JB, Walsh R, Rad N, Scanlon RJ, Gunnar RM. Improvement in symptoms and exercise tolerance by metoprolol in patients with dilated cardiomyopathy: a double-blind, randomized, placebo-controlled trial. Circulation 1985;72:536–46.

276. Waagstein F, Caidahl K, Wallentin I, Bergh C-H, Hjalmarson A. Long-term β-blockade in dilated cardiomyopathy: effects of short- and long-term metoprolol treatment followed by withdrawal and readministration of metoprolol. Circulation 1989;80:551–63.

277. Langsjoen PH, Vadhanavikit S, Folkers K. Response of patients in classes III and IV of cardiomyopathy to therapy in a blind and crossover trial of coenzyme Q_{10}. Proc Natl Acad Sci USA 1985;82:4240–4.

278. Langsjoen PH, Folkers K, Lyson K, Muratsu K, Lyson T, Langsjoen P. Effective and safe therapy with coenzyme Q_{10} for cardiomyopathy. Klin Wochenschr 1988;66:583–90.

279. Fuster V, Gersh BJ, Giuliani ER, Tajik AJ, Brandenburg RO, Frye RL. The natural history of idiopathic dilated cardiomyopathy. Am J Cardiol 1981;47:525–31.

280. Keogh A, Freund J, Baron DW, Hickie JB. Timing of cardiac transplantation in idiopathic dilated cardiomyopathy. Am J Cardiol 1988;61:418–22.

281. Thompson ME, Zerbe K, Hardesty RL. Patient selection and results of cardiac transplantation in patients with cardiomyopathy. Transplant Proc 1988;20:782–5.

282. Griffin ML, Hernandez A, Martin TC, et al. Dilated cardiomyopathy in infants and children. J Am Coll Cardiol 1988;11:139–44.

CHAPTER 5

Perspective on Valvular Heart Disease: Update II

SHAHBUDIN H. RAHIMTOOLA, MB, FRCP

Many exciting events have occurred in the last 40 years in the field of valvular heart disease. Valve surgery continues to remain the dominant therapeutic technique in the management of patients with severe symptomatic valve lesions; a previous perspective (1) was mainly devoted to that topic. In the last 7 years, new developments (for example, catheter balloon valvuloplasty for stenotic valve lesions [2]) and additional data (for example, randomized trials [3–6] of prosthetic heart valves, better analysis of results of valve surgery and value of various tests) have resulted in a reassessment of some aspects of the management of adult patients with valvular heart disease. This perspective focuses on these and other aspects not covered in the previous perspective (1) and updates an additional recent perspective (7).

Determinants of Results of Valve Surgery (Table 5.1)

About 16 years ago, it was recognized that the preoperative clinical condition of the patient and the intraoperative care influence the results of valve surgery (8,9). Subsequent studies have demonstrated that: 1) the etiology of mitral regurgitation influences the results of mitral valve replacement (10); 2) patients operated on at different periods at the same center by the same surgeons using the same valve replacement device have different outcomes (11,12)—this was called the "time factor" (that is, time as a variable includes differences in the clinical condition, ventricular function and cardiovascular function in patients, in medical treatment, in operative techniques and in pre- and postoperative care) (3,13); 3) valve-related complications are more importantly related to patient-related factors than to the type of prosthesis used (14); and 4) factors other than the type of prosthesis are more important in determining the intermediate results of valve replacement. For example, the Edinburgh and Veterans Administration randomized clinical trials (4–6) compared a mechanical with a bioprosthetic valve and showed that up to 7 to 8 years after surgery, there were no significant differences in the results with regard to survival, reoperation and valve-related complications. The Veterans Administration Cooperative Study also showed that: 1) there is no clinically meaningful or statistically significant difference in the hemodynamics of various commonly used sizes of a tilting disc mechanical and bioprosthetic valves (15); and 2) the effects of valve replacement on hemodynam-

ics and left ventricular function are influenced by patient-related factors (16).

The type of surgery (for example, repair versus replacement) may influence the results of surgery (17). Certain complications (for example, mechanical failure, degeneration, thrombosis and the need for anticoagulation) vary with different prostheses (18), and thus the type of prosthesis also influences the results of valve surgery.

The preoperative clinical condition of the patient may be influenced by health care delivery factors (Table 5.2). The Veterans Administration Cooperative Study (19) showed that the ratio of observed to expected operative deaths varied greatly among the participating centers; it was >1 in 5 of the 13 centers, indicating that the quality of surgical treatment also influences patient outcome. Health care delivery factors are multiple, complex and interrelated (Table 5.2) (3). Some (for example, early diagnosis and treatment of complications of prosthetic valves) are uniquely related to valve disease. Anticoagulant therapy that is inappropriate (20), inadequate or incorrectly discontinued may also have a major impact on the observed results.

Associated Coronary Artery Disease

Coronary bypass surgery plus valve surgery. It was previously emphasized (1) that patients who have associated coronary artery disease should undergo simultaneous coronary bypass surgery and valve replacement because: 1) the combined procedure can be performed at only a slightly higher risk; 2) the 10 year survival rate in patients undergoing the combined procedure was only a little less than that in patients without associated coronary artery disease who underwent isolated valve replacement; 3) large randomized trials of coronary bypass surgery for isolated coronary artery disease had demonstrated an improved survival in several subsets of patients; and 4) there were obvious difficulties in performing an adequate randomized trial of coronary bypass surgery in patients undergoing valve replacement.

Recent data (21) show that the operative mortality rate in patients with associated coronary artery disease who did not undergo bypass surgery with aortic valve replacement was increased and the 10 year survival rate was reduced (Table 5.3). In this study, patients who underwent bypass surgery for associated coronary artery disease had more extensive disease than those who did not have surgery (Table 5.3); therefore, the improvement in the 10 year survival rate in

Table 5.1. Factors That Influence Valve Surgery

Results of valve surgery
  Survival
  Complications
  Valve function
  Cardiac function
  Functional class
Are dependent on:
  Patient-related factors
  Type of surgery
  Type of prosthesis
  Health care delivery factors

Adapted from Rahimtoola (3).

those undergoing bypass surgery would have been greater had the patients in the two groups been comparable.

At the present time, all patients undergoing valve surgery should have myocardial revascularization for associated coronary artery disease, except in special clinical circumstances.

Indications for coronary arteriography. The Joint Task Force of the American College of Cardiology/American Heart Association has issued guidelines for performing coronary arteriography in patients with valvular heart disease (22).

For skilled and experienced coronary arteriographers working in experienced cardiac catheterization laboratories, the recommendations for coronary arteriography can be simplified. In all patients being considered for valve surgery or who are undergoing left heart catheterization for valvular heart disease, coronary arteriography should be performed:

Table 5.2. Health Care Delivery Factors That Influence Surgical Results

Preoperative management
  Time patient seeks medical care
  Patient acceptance of and compliance with diagnostic and
    therapeutic measures
  Expertise of care provided by family practitioners, internists
    and cardiologists
  Timing of referral for specialized cardiac investigation and
    interventional treatment
  Expertise in nonsurgical intervention treatment
Quality of surgical treatment
  Expertise of anesthesiology team
  Expertise of surgical team
  Surgical techniques
  Expertise of perioperative care
Postoperative management
  Expertise in long-term care of patients after interventional
    therapy
  Early diagnosis and treatment of complications
  Specialized care with certain treatments (for example,
    anticoagulant agents)
  Patient cooperation and compliance with long-term care

Adapted from Rahimtoola (3).

1) in those ≥35 years of age; and 2) in those aged <35 years of age if they have left ventricular dysfunction, symptoms or signs suggestive of coronary artery disease or one or more major risk factors for coronary artery disease.

Incidence of associated coronary artery disease. This will vary considerably depending on the prevalence of coronary artery disease in the population being studied. In our studies at the University of Oregon (23,24), the incidence of associated coronary artery disease was about 35% in patients with aortic stenosis, 20% in patients with aortic regurgitation and 45% in patients with aortic stenosis who were ≥60 years of age. In the Veterans Administration Cooperative Study on Valvular Heart Disease, 429 (48%) of 896 patients had ≥50% stenosis of one or more coronary arteries (19); in those with coronary artery disease, the incidence of single, double and triple vessel disease was 36%, 31% and 33%, respectively (16).

Clinical Decision Making

There are usually several steps involved in clinical decision making in patients with valvular heart disease (Table 5.4) (25). The first and most important is a complete clinical evaluation that includes the history, physical examination, electrocardiogram (ECG) and chest X-ray. At the end of this evaluation, the clinician should diagnose and assess the severity of disease of all valves, determine the state of ventricular function, evaluate the hemodynamic effects of the valvular disease and associated ventricular dysfunction, assess the extent and severity of coronary artery disease and diagnose the presence or absence of other cardiovascular disease. Additionally, it is necessary to make an evaluation of the effects of cardiovascular disease on other body organs and obtain a complete evaluation of disease in other organ systems.

The next step is also important: the clinician should list, either in writing or in thought, the questions that need answering for the particular patient and why these questions need to be answered. After this, the critical decision is made about performing the test or tests that are most likely to provide answers to these questions reliably, accurately, at the lowest risk to the patient and at a reasonable cost at *one's own institution*. Depending on the clinical circumstances, the decision to perform the tests may be stepwise, rather than an across the board ordering of several tests. As the results of each test become available, an overall reevaluation and reassessment and a decision about the need for further tests are made. Finally, when all the information from the various tests is available, a complete evaluation of the patient is made and recommendations regarding management are made. Subsequently, these recommendations are discussed with the patient.

The results of a prospective, blinded, clinical decision-making study (25–27) of 98 consecutive patients with valvular heart disease are shown in Table 5.5. The results from

Table 5.3. Effect of Coronary Bypass Surgery (CBS) and Aortic Valve Replacement (AVR) on Operative Mortality (Op Mort) and Late Survival

| | 1982–1983 | 1967–1976 | | | | | |
| | | | 10 Year Survival | | | | |
	Op Mort	Op Mort	All Pts	1VD	2VD	3VD	LM CAD
AVR + No CAD (%)	1.4	4.5	63	—	—	—	—
AVR + CAD + CBS (%)	4.0	6.3	49	38	28	34	11
AVR + CAD + No CBS (%)	9.4	10.3	36	65	22	13	1

Adapted from Mullany et al. (21). CAD = coronary artery disease; LM = left main; Pts = patients; VD = vessel disease.

cardiac catheterization and angiography and the subsequent clinical decision that was made were considered 100% correct. The *most important finding of the study is how commonly the initial clinical evaluation was correct.* Several studies (28,29) have demonstrated the feasibility and practicality of diagnosing the etiology of cardiac murmurs by dynamic auscultation at the bedside. Results of these studies (25–29) emphasize the importance of learning and practicing the cognitive skills and becoming experienced in clinical evaluation.

Rheumatic Fever and Carditis

In recent years, there have been several reports (30–33) of outbreaks of acute rheumatic fever in Salt Lake City, Utah, northeast Ohio and the tristate area of Western Pennsylvania and at a naval training center in San Diego, California. The patients have been predominantly (≥90%)

Table 5.4. Steps in Clinical Decision Making in Patients With Valvular Heart Disease

1) Complete clinical evaluation
   History
   Physical examination
   Electrocardiogram
   Chest X-ray film
2) Diagnose and assess severity of disease
   All valves
   Ventricular function
   Hemodynamic effects
   Coronary artery disease
   Other cardiovascular disease
   Effects on other body organs
   Other organ diseases
3) List questions that need answering
4) Be reasonably certain these questions need to be answered
5) Perform test(s) most likely to provide these answers in one's own institution with the following criteria:
   Reliably
   Accurately
   Lowest risk to patient
   Reasonable (or lowest) cost
6) Review results of test(s)
7) Make an overall assessment of patient
8) Make recommendations regarding management

white, middle class and from nonurban areas. Genetic predisposition and emergence of strains of group A streptococcus more likely to produce rheumatic fever have been suggested as predisposing to the reemergence of this disease (34–36). An increased awareness of the diagnosis and management of rheumatic fever and primary and secondary prevention of recurrence of rheumatic fever and carditis are critical (37–39).

Aortic Stenosis

Natural history. *Severe aortic stenosis.* Ross and Braunwald (40) reviewed seven autopsy studies published before 1955 and concluded that in aortic stenosis, the average life expectancy after the onset of symptoms was 3 years, after the occurrence of angina 5 years, after syncope 3 years and after onset of heart failure <2 years. They documented that 15% to 20% of deaths in patients with aortic stenosis were sudden and that 65% to 80% of sudden deaths occurred in symptomatic patients. Although this was a retrospective postmortem review of patients who died before the use of left heart catheterization, it is interesting how close these estimates may be to the true outcome in these patients. In a prospective study of 35 patients with an aortic valve area <0.8 cm^2 documented by cardiac catheterization and who had refused surgery, Horstkotte and Loogen (41) demonstrated that the average survival period after onset of symptoms was 23 ± 5 months; the mean survival period after occurrence of angina was 45 months, syncope 27 months and left heart failure 11 months.

In the study of Frank et al. (42) in 15 patients (32 to 59 years of age) with an aortic valve area ≤0.7 cm^2/m^2 documented by cardiac catheterization and who had refused surgery, the 3, 5 and 10 year mortality rate was 36%, 52% and 90%, respectively. Another study (43) of severe aortic stenosis (aortic valve area stated to be ≤1 cm^2) showed the 5 and 10 year mortality rate to be 62% and 80%, respectively. Chizner et al. (44) reported on 23 patients (peak to peak catheter gradient 69 ± 33 mm Hg) whose 1, 2, 5 and 11 year mortality rate after the onset of symptoms was 26%, 48%, 64% and 94%, respectively.

Schwarz et al. (45) studied 19 patients (56 ± 8.3 years of age) who were in New York Heart Association functional

Table 5.5. Results of a Prospective, Blinded, Clinical Decision-Making Study of 98 Consecutive Patients With Valvular Heart Disease

Final Diagnosis/Recommendation	After Clinical Evaluation		After Doppler Echo	
	Sensitivity (%)	Specificity (%)	Sensitivity (%)	Specificity (%)
Sensitivity and Specificity of Diagnosis for the Presence of a Valve Lesion				
Aortic stenosis	78	92	100	92
Aortic regurgitation	66	76	79	74
Mitral stenosis	86	87	94	89
Mitral regurgitation	75	88	82	80
Accuracy of Diagnosis Including Severity of the Valve Lesion				
Aortic stenosis	48		65	
Aortic regurgitation	43		57	
Mitral stenosis	44		52	
Mitral regurgitation	50		46	
Accuracy of Diagnosis for Moderate or Severe Valve Lesions				
Aortic stenosis	100		100	
Aortic regurgitation	91		100	
Mitral stenosis	92		97	
Mitral regurgitation	97		100	
Accuracy of Recommendations for Valve Surgery				
Aortic valve replacement	61		58	
No aortic valve replacement	84		90	
Mitral valve replacement	58		50	
No mitral valve replacement or commissurotomy	76		76	

Doppler Echo = Doppler echocardiography.

class III or IV and had refused surgery. Their peak to peak transvalvular gradient was 89.6 ± 17.3 mm Hg, mean left atrial pressure 13.3 ± 11.9 mm Hg, left ventricular end-diastolic volume index 122.8 ± 58.3 ml/m^2 and left ventricular ejection fraction 57.4 ± 12.8%. The 3 year mortality rate in these patients was 79%.

O'Keefe et al. (46) evaluated 50 patients from 1978 through 1985. Twenty-eight of their patients refused surgery and surgery was deferred by the physician in 22 because of "perceived excessive surgical risk." In 30 (60%) of the 50 patients, "precise" (46) quantification of severe aortic stenosis was obtained by Doppler echocardiography, cardiac catheterization or both. In 15 patients, mean maximal Doppler instantaneous gradient was 81 mm Hg; in 20 patients, cardiac catheterization data demonstrated an aortic valve area of 0.3 to 0.8 cm^2. The average age of the patients was 77 years (20 were >80 years), and 65% of those undergoing angiography had coronary artery disease. The 1, 2 and 3 year mortality rate was 43%, 63% and 75%, respectively.

Turina et al. (47) studied 50 patients with severe aortic stenosis (aortic valve area <0.9 cm^2), 39 of whom had aortic stenosis alone and 11 who had aortic stenosis and aortic regurgitation. In their study, patients with aortic stenosis alone and those with aortic stenosis and aortic regurgitation had similar outcomes and are grouped together. The 1 year

mortality rate in these patients was 40%; at 10 years, 91% had had a cardiac event.

In another study, Kelly et al. (48) described 39 symptomatic patients, 26 of whom refused surgery and 13 who did not have surgery because the "supervising physician did not deem symptoms to be of sufficient severity to warrant surgery." Their mean age was 72 ± 11 years (range 59 to 98) and the mean Doppler peak pressure gradient was 68 ± 19 mm Hg (range 50 to 115). Among these patients, the 1 year mortality rate was about 38%.

Horstkotte and Loogen (41) reported on 35 patients with AVA < 0.8 cm^2 at cardiac catheterization who refused surgery. The mean survival was 23 ± 5 months, the 5-year mortality was 82 ± 7%, and all patients were dead within 12 years.

It is clear that symptomatic severe aortic stenosis is associated with a high or very high mortality rate when managed medically; the mortality rate is much higher than that associated with many malignant neoplasms. Therefore, before denying patients interventional therapy for symptomatic severe aortic stenosis, physicians must very carefully weigh the risks and benefits of interventional and noninterventional therapy; these must also be discussed with the patient and family.

Mild aortic stenosis. Horstkotte and Loogen (41) followed 142 patients after cardiac catheterization; these patients had a mean aortic valve area >1.5 cm^2, which they called mild aortic stenosis. At 10 years, aortic stenosis was mild in 88% and moderate in 4%; 8% of these had undergone aortic valve replacement. At 20 years, aortic stenosis was still mild in 63% and moderate in 15%; 22% of these had undergone aortic valve replacement or had severe aortic stenosis. At 25 years, aortic stenosis was mild in 38% and moderate in 25%; 38% of these had undergone aortic valve replacement. Turina et al. (47) followed up 16 patients with mild aortic stenosis or mild aortic stenosis and aortic regurgitation with aortic valve area >1.5 cm^2. At 10 years, no patient had died and 15% had had a cardiac event. In view of this "favorable" natural history, it is clear that patients with an aortic valve area >1.5 cm^2 ("mild" aortic stenosis) should *not* undergo valve surgery or other interventional therapy.

Moderate aortic stenosis. It is difficult to know the natural history of truly moderate aortic stenosis because of varying definitions that have been used to define the term "moderate." Horstkotte and Loogen (41) defined it as aortic valve area of 0.8 to 1.5 cm^2 and aortic valve gradient ≤80 mm Hg; most centers would consider that at least some of the patients in this group had severe aortic stenosis. In this group of patients with mixed moderate and severe aortic stenosis in whom the incidence of moderate and severe aortic stenosis is not known, approximately 5% had progressed to severe aortic stenosis and about 25% had undergone aortic valve replacement at the end of 10 years.

Turina et al. (47) defined moderate aortic stenosis as an aortic valve area of 0.95 to 1.4 cm^2; 30 patients had aortic stenosis alone and 14 had aortic stenosis and regurgitation. The 1 and 10 year mortality rate was 3% and 14.5% respectively, and at 10 years 65% of patients had had a cardiac event.

Chizner et al. (44) defined moderate aortic stenosis as an aortic valve area of 0.71 to 1.09 cm^2 and a peak systolic pressure gradient <70 mm Hg; however, 6 of their 10 patients with "moderate" aortic stenosis died in an average time of 9 months (range 2 days to 22 months). Thus, it may be clinically imprudent to consider all patients with an aortic valve area of 0.71 to 1 cm^2 as having "moderate" aortic stenosis.

Asymptomatic severe aortic stenosis. Ross and Braunwald (40) concluded that 3% to 5% of deaths in acquired aortic stenosis occurred suddenly in asymptomatic patients. In the series of Frank et al. (47), three patients with severe aortic stenosis were asymptomatic; one (33%) died suddenly 19 months after cardiac catheterization. In the study of Horstkotte and Loogen (41), 3 patients died suddenly before onset of symptoms and 10 were asymptomatic at the start of the study (personal communication); thus, 3 (30%) of 10 asymptomatic patients died suddenly before symptom onset. Chizner et al. (44) studied eight asymptomatic patients

(aged 20 to 29 years) with "moderate" and "severe" aortic stenosis. At an average follow-up period of 60 months, five had undergone aortic valve replacement and three had remained asymptomatic. Turina et al. (47) reported on 17 patients with severe aortic stenosis or aortic stenosis and regurgitation who were "asymptomatic" or "mildly symptomatic"; at 5 years, the mortality rate was 6% and 25% had had a cardiac event. Kelly et al. (48) studied 51 asymptomatic patients (aged 63 ± 19 years) with "moderate" and "severe" aortic stenosis. At an average follow-up period of only 17 ± 9 months, 41% of the patients became symptomatic and 16% of the patients had died. Of the eight deaths, two were sudden (both occurred after onset of symptoms), five were from carcinoma and one was from Osler-Weber-Rendu syndrome. Pellikka et al. (49) described 143 asymptomatic patients with "hemodynamically significant" aortic stenosis. Thirty (21%) of the 143 patients underwent a surgical procedure within 3 months. Aortic stenosis was graded only by Doppler gradients; the average of the mean aortic valve gradient in the remaining 113 patients (79%) (mean age 72 years) was 47 mm Hg (range 35 to 90). In 16 patients who underwent cardiac catheterization, the correlation of Doppler and catheterization gradients was only r = 0.76; the standard error (SE) of the regression equation was not given. When compared with the cardiac catheterization gradient, the 95% confidence limit (2 SE) of the Doppler gradient is ±20 mm Hg; thus, the average of the mean aortic valve gradient is likely to be between 27 and 67 mm Hg, indicating that in this study some patients probably had mild stenosis and the majority most likely had moderate stenosis. The mortality rate in the remaining 113 (79%) of the 143 patients was 4% at 6 months, 6% at 1 year and 10% at 2 years. The cardiac event rate was 5% at 6 months, 7% at 1 year and 26% at 2 years. All of these series included patients who had moderate as well as severe stenosis and some with mild stenosis, and five of the eight deaths in one series (48) were from carcinoma, an interesting chance occurrence. The natural history of the asymptomatic patients (asymptomatic status not objectively documented) with a mixture of moderate and severe stenosis is not entirely favorable.

More prospective studies of asymptomatic patients with aortic stenosis are needed where the severity of the stenosis is well documented and results for moderate and severe aortic stenosis are presented separately. From the available data, it seems likely that the outcome of asymptomatic patients with severe aortic stenosis is not necessarily benign.

Grading the degree of aortic stenosis. Many different criteria have been used to define *severe* aortic stenosis: aortic valve area ≤0.5 (50), ≤0.7 (51), ≤0.75 (52–55) and ≤1 cm^2 (43) and ≤0.7 (42,56), ≤0.6 (57) and ≤0.4 cm^2/m^2 (54,55). Another common criterion is a peak systolic gradient ≥50 mm Hg (56). The peak systolic gradient may not have a very good direct relation to orifice size. It is recognized that in most adults, a high peak to peak systolic gradient (for example, >60 mm Hg) will usually signify severe aortic stenosis; however, a gradient between 20 and 59 mm Hg may signify mild, moderate or severe aortic stenosis. For any size of stenotic aortic valve, the systolic gradient is determined by the stroke volume and systolic ejection period (58), both of which are dependent on the loading conditions of the left ventricle, resistance in the arterial system and the contractile state of the left ventricle (59). Moreover, the stenotic valve area is inversely related not to the mean systolic gradient, but to the square root of the mean systolic gradient (58). Thus, it seems best to define severe aortic stenosis in terms of valve area. Also, people of different body size of necessity have different values for aortic valve area and therefore it is best to correct the valve area for body surface area (60). Although calculation of valve area by the method of Gorlin and Gorlin (58) was criticized 37 years ago (61), it is still widely used, is clinically useful and has withstood the test of time.

Braunwald and Morrow (56) defined severe aortic stenosis as an aortic valve area index ≤ 0.7 cm^2/m^2. The subsequent natural history study of Frank et al. (42) used this criterion; however, all the patients in their study had an aortic valve area index ≤ 0.63 cm^2/m^2; thus, this criterion (≤ 0.63 to 0.7 cm^2/m^2) now has the backing of a natural history study. Tobin et al. (57), on the basis of left ventricular stroke work loss $\geq 30\%$ and knowledge that an orifice must be reduced to $\leq 25\%$ of its natural size before serious consequences occur (62,63), showed that aortic stenosis was severe when the valve area was ≤ 0.7 to 1 cm^2 or ≤ 0.4 to 0.6 cm^2/m^2. The valve area values from these two studies are very close (≤ 0.63 and ≤ 0.6 cm^2/m^2); the value of ≤ 0.6 cm^2/m^2 is equal to ≤ 1 cm^2, assuming an average body size of 1.75 m^2.

Rapaport (43) assumed severe aortic stenosis as a valve area ≤ 1 cm^2; however, in that natural history study, it is not clear how this value was obtained in his patients. The other authors provide no rationale for the criteria they used in assessing severe aortic stenosis.

The natural history study reported by Horstkotte, Turina and their coworkers (41,47) provides a reasonable basis for considering a calculated aortic valve area >1.5 cm^2 as being *mild* aortic stenosis.

Authors who consider an aortic valve area ≤ 0.8, ≤ 0.75 or ≤ 0.7 cm^2 as severe aortic stenosis would have to include patients with a valve area >0.8, >0.75 or >0.7 cm^2 up to 1 or 1.1 cm^2 as having moderate aortic stenosis. The study of Chizner et al. (44) shows that asymptomatic patients with an aortic valve area of 0.71 to 1.09 cm^2 had a very poor outcome—60% died in an average time of 9 months (range 2 days to 22 months) and another 20% underwent aortic valve replacement. This outcome can hardly be considered as consonant with moderate aortic stenosis, and most of these patients should be considered as having severe aortic stenosis. The study of Turina et al. (47) shows that patients with a valve area of 0.95 to 1.4 cm^2 had an outcome that would be more compatible with moderate aortic stenosis.

Table 5.6. Suggested Grading of the Degree of Aortic Stenosis

Aortic Stenosis	AVA (cm^2)	AVA Index (cm^2/m^2)
Mild	>1.5	>0.9
Moderate	1.1–1.5	$\geq$0.6–0.9
Severe*	$\leq$0.8–1.0	$\leq$0.4–0.6

*Patients with aortic valve area (AVA) that is at a borderline value between the moderate and severe grades (0.9 to 1.1 cm^2; 0.55 to 0.65 cm^2/m^2) should be individually considered for reasons discussed in the text.

A suggested schema for grading the severity of aortic stenosis in adults is shown in Table 5.6. Values of aortic valve area, particularly those borderline between the moderate and severe grades (0.9 to 1.1 cm^2; 0.55 to 0.65 cm^2/m^2), should be interpreted in association with other clinical features for several reasons: 1) the accuracy of the calculated valve area is dependent on the care with which the gradient and flow measurements are made and the values calculated; 2) in an individual patient, the normal value for aortic valve area is unknown; 3) body size is an important variable; and 4) the constant in the Gorlin formula may not be accurate in an individual clinical circumstance.

Doppler echocardiography versus cardiac catheterization for assessing severity of aortic stenosis. A number of studies have examined the relation of aortic valve gradient and area obtained by Doppler echocardiography to that obtained by cardiac catheterization and have shown that the r value of the relationship is ≥ 0.8. Importantly, one needs to know the precision (or the confidence limit) of a value obtained by the noninvasive method, which is obtained from the standard error (SE) of the regression equation (Fig. 5.1). Thus, even if

Figure 5.1. Hypothetic relation of Doppler-derived mean systolic aortic valve gradient to that obtained by cardiac catheterization. Even though the gradients by Doppler and cardiac catheterization are identical at 50 mm Hg by regression equation, 2SE shows that when the Doppler gradient is 50 mm Hg, the 95% confidence limit predicts that the gradient by cardiac catheterization is likely to be between 30 and 70 mm Hg.

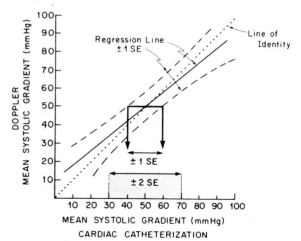

Table 5.7. Relation of Doppler to Cardiac Catheterization Determined Gradient and Valve Area in Aortic Stenosis

Reference	No. of Pts	2 SE of Regression Equation Estimate	
		Mean Aortic Valve Gradient (mm Hg)	Aortic Valve Area (cm^2)
Currie et al.* (64)	100	20	—
Skjaerpe et al. (65)	30	18	—
	16–30	—	0.20 to 0.42
Krafchek et al. (66)	39	18	—
Currie et al.* (67)	62	16	—
Smith et al. (68)	40	12	—
Yeager et al. (69)	58	22	—
Zoghbi et al. (70)	39	—	0.22 to 0.30
Otto et al. (71)	48	24	0.80
Teirstein et al. (72)	30	16	0.34
Come et al.† (73)	31	—	0.32
Oh et al.* (74)	100	20	0.38
Nishimura et al.* (75)	55	—	0.20 to 0.34
Come et al.† (76)	30	—	0.36
Davidson et al. (77)	20	22	—
Range		±12 to ±24	±0.20 to ±0.80

*Same medical center; † same medical center. Pts = patients.

the Doppler gradient of 50 mm Hg is equal to 50 mm Hg on cardiac catheterization from the regression equation and 1 SE is 10 mm Hg, then the 95% confidence limit (2 SE) would estimate that when the Doppler gradient is 50 mm Hg, the gradient obtained by cardiac catheterization is likely to be between 30 and 70 mm Hg (Fig. 5.1). The range of 95% confidence limits of the regression equation (2 SE) for aortic valve gradient and area from several studies is shown in Table 5.7. Ideally, one should know the relation of Doppler gradient and valve area to cardiac catheterization findings at one's own institution. These measurements should be simultaneously obtained prospectively in a blinded study of a significant number of consecutive patients; in one such study (64), 2 SE of the regression equation was 20 mm Hg. Some conservative general guidelines for estimating severe aortic stenosis from Doppler gradients are shown in Table 5.8.

Doppler estimates of the pressure drops across a stenotic valve depend on the application of Bernoulli's law for the calculation of valve area. Energy losses, nonuniform velocity profiles, pressure recovery, unsteady flow and omission of the upstream velocity affect the accuracy of Doppler

Table 5.8. Suggested Conservative Guidelines for Relating Doppler-Determined Gradient to Severity of Aortic Stenosis (AS) in Adults with Normal Cardiac Output

Peak Gradient (mm Hg)	Mean Gradient (mm Hg)	Severe AS
≥80	≥70	Highly likely
60–79	50–69	Probable
<60	<50	Uncertain

measurements of pressure drop (78). The simplified Bernoulli equation used in Doppler estimates does not completely describe the relation between the pressure drop at the inlet of the obstruction and the Doppler velocity measurement (78); these are some other reasons for the discrepancy between the measurements obtained by Doppler and those obtained at cardiac catheterization. Another reason for the discrepancy between Doppler- and catheterization-derived measurements is that the quality of the Doppler signal is clearly operator-dependent (68,79) and even at a single experienced medical center the regression equation can vary at different times (Fig. 5.2). Similarly, the care with which gradient and flow measurements are made during cardiac catheterization and the values calculated also affect the results.

Catheter balloon valvuloplasty. Since November 1986 (2), there has been a great increase in the number of patients who have undergone catheter balloon valvuloplasty. We do not yet know the full extent of the results that can be achieved, the complications, late survival and the clear definition of those who will be benefited and those who will not. Nevertheless, a few observations are worth emphasizing at this time.

Aortic valve area. 1) The average aortic valve area achieved after catheter balloon valvuloplasty (Table 5.9) is not different now from that which was reported earlier (0.8 to 0.9 cm^2) (2); 2) the increase in average valve area after valvuloplasty is 0.2 to 0.4 cm^2 (Table 5.9), although most centers have cases where the increase has been greater (0.5 cm^2; at times, 0.6 cm^2) (Fig. 3); 3) those patients with a larger aortic valve area after valvuloplasty frequently have a larger valve area before valvuloplasty (Table 5.10); and 4)

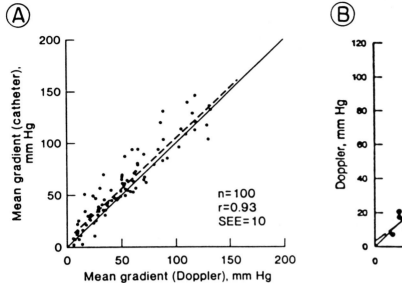
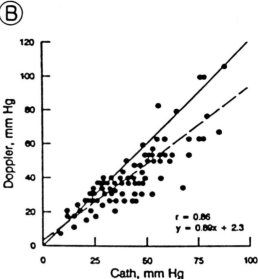

Figure 5.2. Relation of mean systolic aortic valve gradient to that obtained by cardiac catheterization at the same experienced medical center at two different times. Note the different regression equations. In **panel B**, a Doppler-derived gradient of approximately 35 to 40 mm Hg is associated with a catheterization-derived gradient of approximately 25 to 70 mm Hg. **Panel A** from Currie et al. (64) reproduced with permission of the American Heart Association Inc. **Panel B** Oh et al. (74) reproduced with permission from the American College of Cardiology.

there may be a learning curve or advances in technology that have contributed to an improvement in results (Table 5.11) (80).

Restenosis may occur quite rapidly (75,81). At an average follow-up period of 6 months, it may be as high as 65% or 77% (83,92). The restenosis rate currently ranges from 42% to 83% at an average follow-up period of 5 to 9 months (93). The restenosis rate is higher when the final valve area after valvuloplasty was <0.7 cm² and when the increase in area as a result of valvuloplasty was small (83,94).

The hospital mortality rate has ranged from 7% to 13% (75,95,96); the "procedure mortality" rate may be 3% to 5% (75). Currently, the hospital mortality rate ranges from 3% to 9% (93).

Complications, including death, may occur in 25% of patients (95). The incidence of aortic regurgitation is 1% to 2%, vascular complications requiring surgery 4% to 10%, cardiac tamponade 1% to 4%, cerebrovascular accident 0 to 3% and myocardial infarction 0 to 0.5% (93). However, the

Table 5.9. Aortic Valve Area (AVA) Before and After Catheter Balloon Valvuloplasty (CBV)

Reference	No. of Pts	AVA (cm²)		Increase in Average AVA by CBV
		Pre-CBV	Post-CBV	
Nishimura et al.* (75)	55	0.54 ± 0.15	0.85 ± 0.23	0.31
Safian et al. (81)	170	0.6 ± 0.2	0.9 ± 0.3	0.3
Cribier et al. (82)	350	0.47 ± 0.14	0.9 ± 0.02	0.43
Block and Palacios (83)	162	0.5 ± 0.01	0.9 ± 0.02	0.4
†M-Heart Group (84)	166	0.5 ± 0.17	0.77 ± 0.24	0.27
‡MSAVR Registry (85)				
Before July 1987	285	0.5 ± 0.18	0.8 ± 0.3	0.3
July–Dec 1987	231	0.49 ± 0.17	0.82 ± 0.31	0.33
Desnoyers et al. (86)	47	0.5 ± 0.06	0.9 ± 0.07	0.4
Litvac et al. (87)	24	0.5 ± 0.17	0.7 ± 0.26	0.2
Brady et al. (88)	26	0.45 ± 0.03	0.67 ± 0.04	0.22
Holmes et al.* (89)	88	0.48 ± 0.20	0.74 ± 0.26	0.26
Sherman et al. (90)	36	0.5 ± 0.2	0.9 ± 0.3	0.4

*Same medical center; †Multi-Hospital Eastern Atlantic Restenosis Trial; ‡Mansfield Scientific Aortic Valve Registry (many patients in this Registry are probably also included in the other series). Data are mean ± SD. Post = after; Pre = before; Pts = patients.

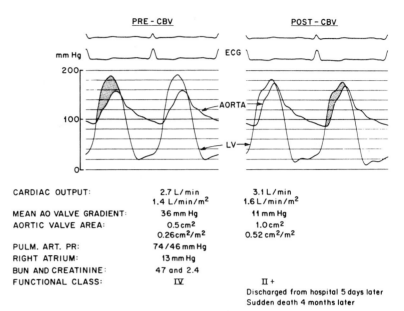

Figure 5.3. Catheter balloon valvuloplasty (CBV) for severe aortic stenosis in a patient with carcinoma of the lung. The procedure resulted in an increase in aortic valve area from 0.5 to 1 cm^2, with rapid relief of symptoms. The patient was discharged from hospital and died suddenly (? cause of death) 4 months later. Catheter balloon valvuloplasty played an important palliative, supportive therapeutic role in this patient. Reproduced with permission from Daniel L. Kulick, MD, Veterans Administration Medical Center, Albuquerque, New Mexico.

incidence of "clinically silent" cerebrovascular embolism is quite high (97).

At an average follow-up period of 6 months, the mortality rate ranges from 15% to 22% (75,81). At 1 year, the actuarial mortality rate has been reported to be 24% (98), 43% (99) and 60% (100); about 25% of patients have undergone repeat valvuloplasty or valve replacement. Currently, the late mortality rate ranges from 17% to 40% at an average follow-up period of 6 to 18 months (93). Late mortality (average of 16 months) appears to be related to a small valve area after valvuloplasty, particularly if it is <0.7 cm^2 and a low left ventricular ejection fraction (90,94,99,100).

In patients with impaired left ventricular function, the results have been mixed. Desnoyers et al. (102) described two patients with "cardiogenic shock" from severe aortic stenosis (aortic valve area 0.2 cm^2); valvuloplasty that resulted in a final valve area of 0.6 and 0.5 cm^2 had a dramatic impact on the patients' immediate clinical condition (both patients rapidly came out of shock). Of 28 patients described by Safian et al. (103), 13 (46%) had a major improvement in left ventricular ejection fraction, whereas the remainder had no change. Among 55 patients studied by

Berland et al. (104), the 1 year actuarial mortality rate was 40%.

Catheter balloon valvuloplasty for aortic stenosis has been shown to be an effective palliative procedure to partially relieve severe aortic stenosis as preoperative preparation for emergent noncardiac surgery (104–106).

These results must be kept in perspective. The average age of the patients in these series ranged from 73 to 86 years, most patients were stated to be inoperable or at very high risk for surgery, the majority were in clinical class III or IV and many had associated coronary artery disease. It is uncertain as to which group of patients (that is, those treated medically or surgically) the results from this cohort of patients can be compared; it is important to avoid making inappropriate comparisons and conclusions (3).

These results are not surprising. It was pointed out very early in the experience with catheter balloon valvuloplasty that in view of the limited and modest increase in valve area after the procedure, valve replacement may be more beneficial in terms of symptomatic status, hemodynamics, left ventricular function and survival (2). The average aortic valve area after valvuloplasty (Table 5.9) (that is, 0.8 to 0.9

Table 5.10. Range of Aortic Valve Area Values Before and After Catheter Balloon Valvuloplasty

| Reference | AVA (cm^2) | | Patients | |
	Pre-CBV	Post-CBV	No.	(%)
Cribier et al. (91)	0.5 ± 0.1	0.8 ± 0.1	139	(68)
	0.7 ± 0.2	1.3 ± 0.3	69	(32)
Block and Palacios (83)	*	No change from pre-CBV	6	(4)
	*	<0.7	62	(39)
	*	0.8, 0.9	51	(32)
	*	≥1.0	40	(25)

*Not given in abstract. Abbreviations as in Table 5.9.

Table 5.11. Experience Curve for Aortic Valve Catheter Balloon Valvuloplasty

Patient Nos.*	AVA (cm²)		Final AVA (cm²)			
	Pre-CBV	Post-CBV	<0.7	0.7–0.99	1.0–1.19	≥1.2
51–135	0.53	0.84	30%	45%	10%	15%
136–218	0.54	0.99	15%	41%	21%	23%

*In this series, results in Patients 1 to 50 were not reported. Abbreviations as in Table 5.9. Modified from Letac et al. (80).

cm²) is still in the range of severe aortic stenosis. After catheter balloon valvuloplasty, >40% of patients have an aortic valve area <0.7 cm², which represents very severe aortic stenosis known to be associated with a high mortality rate. The improvement in severe heart failure with a small increase in valve area was also predicted (2) and subsequently proven by the two patients with cardiogenic shock studied by Desnoyers et al. (102); however, in the latter report, both patients had a poor "late" outcome probably because valve area after valvuloplasty was only 0.5 and 0.6 cm², respectively. Thus, to achieve better late results, it is important that once such patients are improved, they should undergo another intervention (preferably aortic valve replacement) if it is not otherwise clinically contraindicated.

Catheter balloon valvuloplasty for aortic stenosis has been successfully performed in combination with valvuloplasty for mitral stenosis (108,109) and percutaneous transluminal coronary angioplasty (110).

Catheter balloon valvuloplasty for aortic stenosis is still in an evolving phase; improvements in equipment and technique could have a major impact. A suggested list of indications for the procedure in patients ≥70 to 75 years of age with aortic stenosis is given in Table 5.12. Although it is clear that the procedure has an important clinical role in the management of some of these patients (Fig. 5.3) (102), there

Table 5.12. Suggested Indications for Catheter Balloon Valvuloplasty

Severe aortic stenosis in patients >70–75 years*

Patient at high risk for cardiac surgery
  Cardiac reasons
  Noncardiac reasons
Patient with limited life-span
  Cardiac reasons nonvalve related
  Noncardiac reasons
Patient in urgent need for noncardiac surgical procedures
Cardiac surgery undesirable for noncardiac reasons
Patient with moderate to severe CHF and LV dysfunction
Patient with severe CHF of uncertain etiology but aortic stenosis of uncertain severity
Patient refuses surgery
Mitral stenosis*
In experienced and skilled centers, procedure of first choice in most patients, particularly in patients with mobile, nonthickened valves

*The techniques, results and, therefore, indications and contraindications are still evolving. CHF = congestive heart failure; LV = left ventricular.

are insufficient data in younger patients to provide any guidelines at present.

At present, the Food and Drug Administration has approved the clinical use of the Mansfield catheter for catheter balloon valvuloplasty in the treatment of aortic stenosis.

Mitral Stenosis

Atrial fibrillation. Digoxin remains the drug of choice for the control of ventricular rate in patients with atrial fibrillation (111). However, digoxin is much less effective during exercise (112), which is of particular importance in patients with mitral stenosis. The combination of digitalis with beta-adrenergic blocking agents is effective in controlling ventricular rate; however, beta-adrenergic blocking agents are not ideal for long-term control because they may reduce exercise capacity (113) and their negative inotropic effect may pose a problem in patients with impaired left ventricular function. Verapamil, a calcium channel blocking agent, controls ventricular rate, but also poses problems because of its negative inotropic effect and its interaction with digoxin, which leads to a decrease in digoxin renal clearance and, at times, to a marked elevation of serum digoxin concentration and digoxin toxicity (114).

Diltiazem, another calcium channel blocking agent, has similar electrophysiologic properties as those of verapamil, resulting in a depression of conduction and prolongation of refractory period in the atrioventricular node. In contrast, there is no significant interaction between digoxin and diltiazem (115). Combination therapy with diltiazem (240 mg/day) and digoxin (0.25 mg/day) provides good control of ventricular rate at rest and during exercise (116) and results in no change in exercise capacity (117).

Doppler echocardiography versus cardiac catheterization for assessing severity of mitral stenosis. The range of 95% confidence limits of the regression equation for mitral valve gradient and area obtained from Doppler echocardiography compared with that obtained from cardiac catheterization is shown in Table 5.13.

Catheter balloon commissurotomy for mitral stenosis. We do not yet have long-term results, but several facts have rapidly emerged.

The average mitral valve area is doubled after catheter balloon commissurotomy, an increase that averages 1 cm² (Table 5.14, Fig. 5.4). The increase in mitral valve area is

Table 5.13. Relation of Doppler to Cardiac Catheterization Determined Gradient and Valve Areas in Mitral Stenosis

| | | 2 SE of Regression Equation Estimate | |
| | | Mean Mitral Valve Gradient (mm Hg) | MVA (cm²) |
Reference	No. of Pts.		
Hatle et al. (118)	25	4	—
Stamm and Martin (79)	26,27	4.8	0.36
Smith et al. (119)*	45	—	0.40
Grayburn et al. (120)*	38 without AR	—	0.38
	17 with AR	—	0.42
	55 with or without AR	—	0.38
Nakatani et al. (121)	21 without AR	—	0.56
	41 with or without AR	—	0.88
Reid et al. (122)	46	8	—
	53	—	0.70
	27 with Doppler MVA <1.5 cm²	—	0.30
	Range	±4 to ±8	±0.30 to ±0.88

*Same medical center. AR = aortic regurgitation; MVA = mitral valve area; Pts = patients.

similar to that observed after surgical mitral commissurotomy (137) and may be larger than that seen with valve replacement.

There is a marked improvement in the functional class of the patient, which has been objectively documented by exercise testing (Fig. 5.5) (138).

The improvement in mitral valve area and functional class is maintained for up to 1 year of follow-up (Table 5.14) (124–126).

There is a reduction in left atrial pressure, pulmonary artery pressure and pulmonary vascular resistance (Fig. 5.6)

(138–140). These reductions can be dramatically rapid, with equally rapid improvement in the patient's clinical condition (Table 5.15).

During exercise, the left atrial and pulmonary artery pressures and mitral valve gradient are lower after than before catheter balloon commissurotomy (Fig. 5.6) (138).

Left ventricular size and function show no significant change (138).

The magnitude of the increase in mitral valve area is dependent on several factors, including the experience of the

Table 5.14. Mitral Valve Area Before and After Catheter Balloon Commissurotomy (CBC)

| Reference | No. of Pts | Mitral Valve Area (cm²) (mean ± SD) | | | | Immediate Increase in Average MVA by CBC (cm²) |
		Pre-CBC	Immediate Post-CBC	3–6 Mos Post-CBC	1 Yr Post-CBC	
Reid et al. (123,124)	33	1.0 ± 0.3	2.0 ± 0.6	1.8 ± 0.7 (3 mos)	1.8 ± 0.4	1.0
Palacios and Block (125)*	172	0.9 ± 0.1	2.0 ± 0.1	—	—	1.1
Abascal et al. (126)*	20		1.90 ± 0.59	1.62 ± 0.55 (6 mos)	—	
NHLBI Registry (127)†	72	0.9 ± 0.5	2.0 ± 1.0	—	—	1.1
Cequier et al. (128)	48	1.0 ± 0.4	2.5 ± 1.0	2.1 ± 0.6 (6 mos)	—	1.5
Tamai et al. (129)	19	0.8 ± 0.2	1.4 ± 0.4	—	—	0.6
Chen et al. (130)	54	0.8 ± 0.2	2.0 ± 0.5	—	—	1.2
Nakatani et al. (131)	12	1.0 ± 0.2	1.9 ± 0.6	—	—	0.9
Inoue et al. (132)	515	1.2 ± 0.37	1.9 ± 0.46	—	—	0.7
Babic et al. (133)	72	1.2 ± 0.2	2.3 ± 0.6	—	—	1.1
Vahanian et al. (134)	200	1.1 ± 0.3	2.2 ± 0.5	—	—	1.1
Nobuyoshi et al. (135)	106	1.4 ± 0.4	2.0 ± 0.5	—	—	0.6
Herrmann et al. (136)‡	74	1.0 ± 0.04	2.0 ± 0.1	—	—	1.0

*Data from the same center; †It is likely patients in this series are also included in other series; ‡M-Heart Valvuloplasty Registry. Abbreviations as in Tables 5.9 and 5.13.

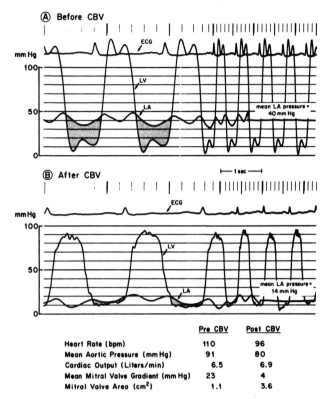

	Pre CBV	Post CBV
Heart Rate (bpm)	110	96
Mean Aortic Pressure (mm Hg)	91	80
Cardiac Output (Liters/min)	6.5	6.9
Mean Mitral Valve Gradient (mm Hg)	23	4
Mitral Valve Area (cm²)	1.1	3.6

Figure 5.4. Catheter balloon valvuloplasty (CBV) for severe mitral stenosis, showing major reductions in mitral valve gradient and left atrial pressure. Reproduced with permission from the American Medical Association (137).

operator, use of double balloon technique, size of the mitral valve anulus diameter, effective balloon dilating diameter and, importantly, the morphologic characteristics of the

Figure 5.5. Treadmill exercise test demonstrating significant improvement in exercise capacity within 1 month of catheter balloon valvuloplasty (CBV). The first exercise test after the procedure was done at 1 month; the improvement persisted for 3 months. Adapted from McKay et al. (137).

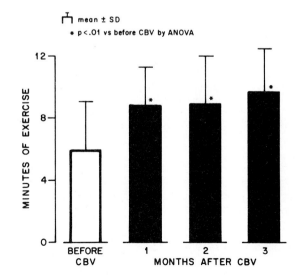

Figure 5.6. Mean mitral valve gradient (**top panel**), mean pulmonary artery wedge pressure (**center panel**) and mean pulmonary artery pressure (**lower panel**) at rest and during exercise before and after catheter balloon valvuloplasty (CBV) for mitral stenosis. After the procedure, there is reduction in all pressures measurements at rest and during exercise [pre-CBV Ex 1-Symptom limited (SxLTD) vs post-CBV Ex 1]. Three months after catheter balloon valvuloplasty at a higher level of exercise (post-CBV, Ex 2, SxLTD), pressures are lower than those present before the procedure (Ex 1 SxLTD).

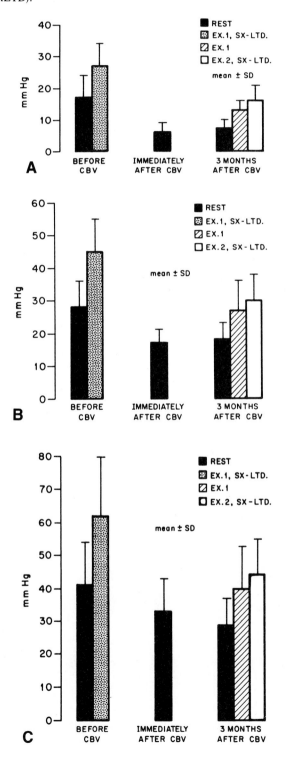

Table 5.15. Hemodynamic Findings After Catheter Balloon Commissurotomy (CBV) in a 23 Year Old Man With Severe Mitral Stenosis, Mitral Regurgitation and a Calcified and Moderately Mobile Mitral Valve*

	Pre-CBC	Post-CBC (2/14/89)	Next Day (2/15/89)
Pressure (mm Hg)			
Mean right atrial	8	8	4
Pulmonary artery	84/45 ($\overline{61}$)	51/29 ($\overline{39}$)	28/19 ($\overline{22}$)
Mean pulmonary artery wedge	43	26	15
Left ventricular	122/1–12	116/6–20	—
Heart rate (beats/min)	88	77	85
Cardiac output (liters/min)	4.9	6.3	6.3
Pulmonary vascular resistance (dynes·s·cm^{-5})	294	160	89
Mean mitral valve gradient (mm Hg)	22	9	—
Mitral valve area (cm^2)	0.8	1.5	—
Functional class	III	—	—*

*Left ventricular volume and ejection fraction were normal both before (Pre) and immediately after (Post) catheter balloon valvuloplasty (CBV). On the day after valvuloplasty, he had spontaneous 3.5 liter diuresis. Two days after valvuloplasty, the patient was "asymptomatic," wanted to walk home, and was discharged from hospital. Reproduced by permission of Drs. D.T. Kawanishi, D.L. Kulick and C.L. Reid, LAC/USC Medical Center, Los Angeles, California.

mitral valve (Tables 5.16 and 5.17, Figs. 5.7 and 5.8) (123,126,139,141,142).

Doppler estimates of mitral valve area immediately after commissurotomy are frequently inaccurate (122,141) because of their dependence on transmitral gradients and atrial and ventricular compliance (142).

The 30 day mortality rate is ≤3%. The incidence of moderate to severe mitral regurgitation is ≤4% and thromboembolism ≤4% (143). A number of complications, including tamponade, heart block and vascular injury, have been reported (144).

The incidence of atrial septal defect after the procedure is as high as 53% (122,140,144), but many of the defects close by 3 to 12 months, at which time most are small with a pulmonary to systemic flow ratio <1.5 (122,123,144–146). The incidence of atrial septal defect may be as high as 40%, but some series have reported a much lower incidence (≤20%). The reasons for these differences are complex and

Table 5.16. Two-Dimensional Echocardiographic Assessment of Mitral Valve Morphology

Morphologic Feature	Definition	Grade	Score
Leaflet motion			
H/L ratio			
≥0.45		Mild	0
0.26–0.44		Moderate	1
<0.25		Severe	2
Leaflet thickness			
MV/PWAo ratio			
1.5–2.0		Mild	0
2.1–4.9		Moderate	1
Subvalvular disease	Thin, faintly visible chordae tendineae	Absent-mild	0
	Areas of increased density equal to endocardium	Moderate	1
	Areas denser than endocardium with thickened chordae tendineae	Severe	2
Commissural calcium	Homogeneous density of MV orifice	Absent	0
	Increased density of anterior/posterior commissure	One commissure	1
	Increased density of both commissures	Two commissures	2

H = height of doming of mitral valve; L = length of dome of mitral valve; MV = mitral valve; PWAo = posterior wall of aorta. From Reid et al. (123).

Table 5.17. Stepwise Analysis of Predictors of Mitral Valve Area Immediately After Catheter Balloon Commissurotomy

Variables Selected	Regression Coefficient	R^2	p Value
All		0.65	0.0001
Leaflet motion	3.96		0.0001
EBDA	0.04		0.03
Cardiac output	0.20		0.002
Only mitral valve morphology		0.49	0.0001
Leaflet motion score	0.62		0.0001
All nonhemodynamic		0.56	0.0001
Leaflet motion score	0.58		0.0001
EBDA	0.05		0.04

EBDA = effective balloon-dilating area; from Reid et al. (122).

may include differences in patient characteristics, technique and diagnostic criteria. In some studies (141,146), atrial septal defect has been diagnosed on the basis of a ≥7% increase in oxygen saturation; others (132) disregarded a pulmonary to systemic blood flow ratio (Qp/Qs) <1.4. These criteria result in a lowered incidence of atrial septal defect and a greater mitral valve area after commissurotomy (because of use of pulmonary blood flow as a measure of cardiac output); possibly, Qp/Qs may be lower in those in whom it

Figure 5.7. Relation of mitral valve leaflet motion (**panel A**) and thickness (**panel B**) as a continuous variable by two-dimensional echocardiography with mitral valve area determined immediately after catheter balloon valvuloplasty (POST-CBV). As the leaflet motion decreases and leaflet thickness increases, the mitral valve area immediately after the procedure is smaller.

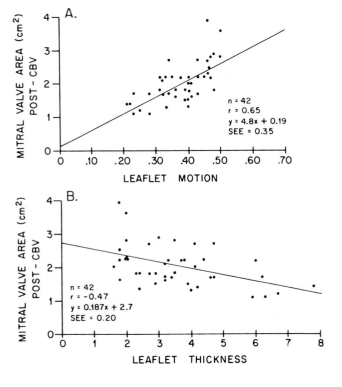

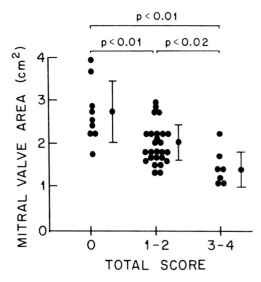

Figure 5.8. Total score for mitral valve leaflet motion and thickness plotted against mitral valve area immediately after catheter balloon valvuloplasty. Among the patients with a score of 0, 89% had a mitral valve area >2 cm². Of those with a score of 1 or 2, 65% had a mitral valve area ≥1.5 cm², whereas among those with a score of 3 or 4, only 29% had a mitral valve area ≥1.5 cm².

was actually calculated. Using transesophageal Doppler color flow mapping, Yoshida et al. (148) demonstrated left to right shunting with the single balloon Inoue catheter in 87% of patients immediately after catheter balloon commissurotomy; the incidence of a left to right shunt was reduced to 20% 6 months later (148).

Atrial septal defect is more likely to occur with smaller increases in valve area, absence of previous surgical commissurotomy, small left atria and mitral valve calcification (124,145,146). The size of the defect can be reduced by use of a single as opposed to two separate atrial punctures and withdrawal of completely deflated balloon catheters in tandem fashion (149).

There is a rapid reduction in plasma atrial natriuretic peptide levels (150,151).

The immediate results of catheter balloon and closed mitral commissurotomy are similar, as indicated by results from a prospective randomized clinical trial of 40 patients (136).

Catheter balloon commissurotomy for mitral stenosis is somewhat similar to closed surgical mitral commissurotomy. The results of closed mitral commissurotomy are excellent in appropriate patients and in experienced, skilled centers (151). However, closed mitral commissurotomy is "rarely" performed in the United States today, one major reason being the lack of skill and experience, another being the low frequency of suitable patients. Open mitral commissurotomy is considered by many to be the preferred operation in those not undergoing valve replacement. However, there is no well-documented superiority of open over closed commissurotomy in centers with the necessary skill and experience; a recent study from the University of Alabama (153) showed that the technique of the surgical commissurotomy (closed versus open) was *not* a risk factor for time-related death, mitral valve reintervention, subsequent mitral valve replacement, thromboembolism or poor functional status. Results with catheter balloon commissurotomy and closed mitral commissurotomy for mitral stenosis are excellent in patients with mobile, pliable and nonthickened valves, which occur more frequently in young patients; results in these patients are also likely to be more durable. In patients with nonmobile, rigid and thickened valves, which occur more frequently in older patients, results are less satisfactory and less durable. However, it needs to be recognized that if the latter group of patients were to have surgery at the present time, many would be more likely to undergo valve replacement rather than commissurotomy or valvuloplasty. Thus, even if catheter balloon commissurotomy delays surgery for ≥2 to 5 years in the latter group of patients, it may not be an undesirable palliative option. Moreover, the hemodynamic results may be better than or at least as good as those seen with valve replacement.

These findings are encouraging and indicate that in experienced, skilled centers, double balloon commissurotomy is the procedure of choice in most patients with mitral stenosis, particularly those in whom the valve is mobile and pliable (Table 5.12).

Valvular Regurgitation

Left ventricular ejection fraction during exercise. Radionuclide angiography has been used to study left ventricular ejection fraction at rest and during exercise in patients with severe chronic aortic regurgitation. In symptomatic patients, left ventricular ejection fraction at rest is below normal in up to 50% of patients and decreases with exercise in virtually all patients; in asymptomatic patients, rest left ventricular ejection fraction is normal in most patients, and the response to exercise is mixed, with about 50% of the patients showing a normal increase in left ventricular ejection fraction (154). As a result, it was hoped that the response of left ventricular ejection fraction to exercise would: 1) detect latent abnormalities of left ventricular function; 2) have prognostic value; 3) help determine the timing of aortic valve replacement in asymptomatic patients; and 4) predict the results of valve replacement.

Left ventricular ejection fraction during exercise in valve regurgitation is dependent on at least two factors: 1) state of myocardial function at rest (155), and 2) change in systemic vascular resistance during exercise (156). If systemic vascular resistance declines sufficiently, the left ventricle can meet the requirements of increased blood flow during exercise

without a change in left ventricular ejection fraction (156). Thus, no reasonable conclusion can be made about myocardial or ventricular function from the change in left ventricular ejection fraction during exercise without knowledge of the change in systemic vascular resistance. Therefore, an "abnormal" left ventricular ejection fraction during exercise without knowledge of any change in systemic vascular resistance is of little prognostic value. For example, in one study (157), two-thirds of patients with an "abnormal" left ventricular ejection fraction during exercise (asymptomatic + normal ejection fraction at rest) did well for the 4 year follow-up period (that is, they continued to remain asymptomatic and have normal left ventricular function at rest); the remaining one-third underwent aortic valve replacement because they became symptomatic. Moreover, there is no correlation between this variable and death or left ventricular dysfunction after aortic valve replacement (158).

Vasodilators. Previously (1), it was summarized that: 1) in aortic and mitral regurgitation, vasodilators improve cardiac hemodynamics and left ventricular function at rest and during exercise and improve functional class; 2) in symptomatic patients with mitral regurgitation, long-term therapy with hydralazine, an arteriolar dilator, is disappointing because of a high incidence of side effects and an unsatisfactory result in the majority of patients; 3) in a single symptomatic patient with chronic aortic regurgitation, left ventricular function and symptomatic state improved with 12 months of treatment with hydralazine; and 4) additional long-term studies of *symptomatic* and *asymptomatic* patients are needed.

In a trial of 19 hydralazine-treated patients with *symptomatic*, chronic, severe aortic regurgitation demonstrated by cardiac catheterization and angiography, we (159) were able to demonstrate an improvement in exercise capacity and cardiac output and a reduction in systemic vascular resistance. None of the other hemodynamic or left ventricular size and function variables (on echocardiography and radionuclide and contrast angiography) changed significantly (Table 5.18). Further review of the data showed that in the hydralazine-treated group, only 37% had an increase in cardiac output and exercise capacity, with a major reduction in left ventricular end-diastolic volume index and an increase in left ventricular ejection fraction occurring in 21%. However, the latter subgroups of patients could not be predicted from baseline clinical, exercise, hemodynamic or left ventricular function data. These data combined with the known beneficial effects of aortic valve replacement indicate that hydralazine is of limited clinical value in *symptomatic* patients with severe aortic regurgitation.

In a randomized trial (160), 2 years of therapy with hydralazine in patients with chronic aortic regurgitation who were *asymptomatic* or *"minimally"* symptomatic resulted in an average reduction of 24 ± 6 ml/m^2 in left ventricular end-diastolic volume index and 12 ± 3 ml/m^2 in left ventricular end-systolic volume index and an increase of 0.02 ±

Table 5.18. Long-Term Response to Hydralazine in 19 Symptomatic Patients with Chronic Severe Aortic Regurgitation

	Hydralazine		
	Initial	Late	p Value
Follow-up (mon)		11 ± 3	
Treadmill time			
(min; Bruce protocol)	6.3 ± 2.6	7.8 ± 2.8	0.04
Echocardiography			
LV end-diastolic dimension (mm)	64 ± 12	61 ± 11	
LV end-systolic dimension (mm)	44 ± 9	42 ± 9	
Fractional shortening (%)	31 ± 6	30 ± 7	
Radionuclide ventriculography			
Rest LVEF	0.54 ± 0.12	0.52 ± 0.13	
Exercise LVEF	0.52 ± 0.10	0.49 ± 0.14	
Main aortic pressure (mm Hg)	95 ± 10	86 ± 10	0.006
Cardiac output (liters/min)	4.8 ± 1.1	5.9 ± 1.2	0.0006
Systemic resistance (dynes·s·cm^{-5})	1511 ± 334	1124 ± 218	0.00007
LV function at angiography			
EDVI (ml/m^2)	161 ± 64	174 ± 60	
ESVI (ml/m^2)	76 ± 45	78 ± 48	
Ejection fraction	0.55 ± 0.13	0.59 ± 0.17	

Values are mean ± standard deviation. EDVI = end-diastolic volume index; EF = ejection fraction; ESVI = end-systolic volume index; LV = left ventricular.

0.01 in left ventricular ejection fraction; all these changes were statistically significant compared with the changes seen in the placebo-treated group. The reduction in left ventricular end-diastolic volume index at 1 year was not significant. Although these are interesting and helpful data (160), certain issues need to be recognized. 1) Of the hydralazine-treated patients, 13 (29%) of 45 discontinued the drug, and at 3 months 76% experienced side effects, indicating that this is not a satisfactory drug for long-term treatment. Interestingly, 44% of the placebo-treated patients also had side effects (the content of the placebo tablets was not given). Only 37 (46%) of 80 patients completed the 2 year follow-up study. 2) Both asymptomatic and "minimally" symptomatic patients as well as patients with moderate and severe aortic regurgitation were studied, and thus there is uncertainty about to which of the four subgroups the results apply. The findings in subgroups of asymptomatic and symptomatic patients with *severe* aortic regurgitation are of considerable interest. 3) Individual data are not presented, and thus there is uncertainty regarding the percent of patients who responded favorably. 4) Some of the improvement was minimal. 5) There was no significant reduction in either systolic or diastolic blood pressure. 6) The definition of "minimally" symptomatic was not given and objective testing of exercise capacity was not performed. Thus, there is uncertainty about the make-up of this subset of patients, and the effect on exercise capacity was not studied. 7) This small trial was not designed to study the improvement in survival or the delay in the need for aortic valve replacement.

In a randomized 12 month trial of a calcium channel blocking agent, nifedipine, in 72 *asymptomatic* patients with severe aortic regurgitation, Scognamiglio et al. (161) demonstrated a significant reduction in left ventricular end-diastolic volume index by 26 ml/m^2 and mass by 27 g/m^2 and an increase in ejection fraction by 0.12 units. At 3 months, the incidence of side effects in the nifedipine and placebo groups was 60% and 26% and at 12 months was 11% and 9%, respectively; 92% of patients completed the trial and only one nifedipine-treated patient discontinued therapy.

The studies of Greenberg, Scognamiglio and their co-workers (160,161) demonstrated a small reduction in left ventricular ejection fraction in placebo-treated patients. In one study (162) of 1 month duration, digitalis therapy was demonstrated to improve ejection fraction (from 0.47 ± 0.08 to 0.54 ± 0.08, p < 0.05), an effect not seen with hydralazine or nifedipine. Thus, digitalis therapy may be of benefit in asymptomatic patients with severe aortic regurgitation.

Venodilation with intravenous nitroglycerin has been shown to reduce left ventricular filling pressure, end-diastolic volume and regurgitant volume in patients with chronic mitral regurgitation (163), suggesting that venodilators may also have a role in the treatment of patients with valve regurgitation.

Thus, studies to date have failed to demonstrate a clear-cut role for hydralazine in the long-term treatment of patients with chronic *severe* valve regurgitation. The results with nifedipine are most encouraging. Additional studies using angiotensin converting enzyme inhibitors (which are arterial and venous dilators), nifedipine and digitalis are needed to determine the best therapeutic option, particularly for the *asymptomatic* patient (164).

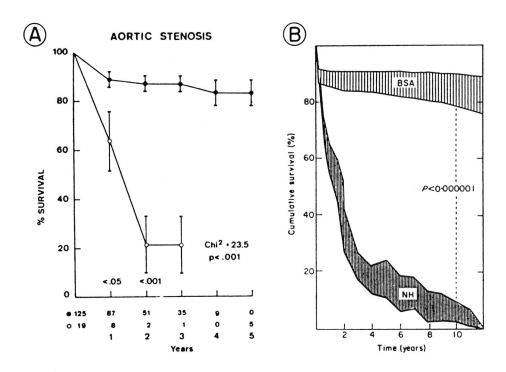

Valve Replacement/Repair

Improved survival. There are no prospective randomized clinical trials that have compared valve replacement and medical treatment. Two concurrent series (41,45) compared aortic valve replacement and medical treatment in patients with severe aortic stenosis and demonstrated increased survival after aortic valve replacement (Fig. 5.9). Similar data from Roy and Gopinath (165) suggested improved survival with closed mitral commissurotomy in symptomatic patients with severe mitral stenosis who were in functional class II, III or IV (Fig. 5.10). However, data from Schwarz et al. (45) suggested no benefit from valve replacement for up to 4 years of follow-up study in patients with aortic regurgitation.

Left ventricular function and hemodynamics. *Aortic valve disease.* Patients with severe aortic stenosis who undergo valve replacement have significant early (up to 6 months)

Figure 5.9. Survival curves in patients with severe aortic stenosis. **Panel A,** Patients who had valve replacement (closed circles) had a better survival rate than those treated medically (open circles). In **Panel B,** those treated with valve replacement (BSA) also had a better survival rate than those treated medically (NH). **Panel A** Schwartz et al. (45) reproduced with permission from the American Heart Association. **Panel B** Horstkotte and Loogen (41) reproduced with permission from the European Society of Cardiology.

Figure 5.10. Survival curves in patients with severe mitral stenosis. Patients in New York Heart Association functional class II (**left panel**) and class III or IV (**right panel**) who underwent closed surgical commissurotomy had a better survival than those treated medically. Roy and Gopinath (164) reproduced with permission from the American Heart Association.

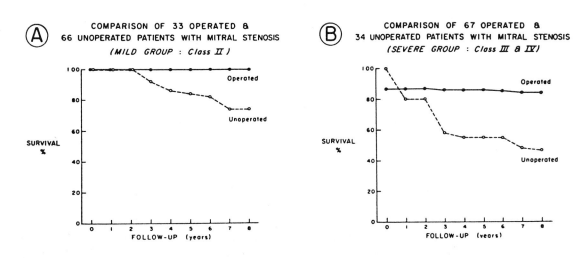

Table 5.19. Effect of Aortic Valve Replacement (AVR) on Left Ventricular Function in Patients With Aortic Stenosis

	Control Valve	Before AVR	After AVR (yr)	
			1.6 ± 0.5	8.1 ± 2.9
LV EDVI (ml/m²)	93 ± 14	108 ± 35	89 ± 26	82 ± 20
LV ESVI (ml/m²)	31 ± 9	43 ± 33	32 ± 22	29 ± 24
LVEF*	67 ± 7	64 ± 15	66 ± 11	67 ± 16
LV muscle mass index (g/m²)	85 ± 9	158 ± 33	114 ± 27	97 ± 28

*Change not statistically significant. Abbreviations as in Table 5.18. From Monrad et al. (167).

and intermediate (0.5 to 2 years) improvement in hemodynamics, left ventricular function and regression of left ventricular hypertrophy (1). Left ventricular ejection fraction improves in most patients, the most dramatic improvement being seen in patients with impaired left ventricular function who are in clinical heart failure (1,166). Recent data from Monrad et al. (167) indicate further "late" improvement (to 8.1 ± 2.9 years) after aortic valve replacement (Table 5.19). At that time, further small but significant reductions had occurred in left ventricular systolic and diastolic pressures and end-diastolic and end-systolic volumes, and there was an increase in cardiac index. Importantly, hypertrophy regressed, left ventricular mass decreased from 158 ± 33 g·m² preoperatively to 114 ± 27 g·m² at 1.6 ± 0.5 years (p < 0.01) and to 97 ± 28 g·m² at 8.1 ± 2.9 years (p < 0.01) after aortic valve replacement (167).

Patients with severe aortic regurgitation who undergo valve replacement also have significant early and intermediate improvement in hemodynamics and regression of left ventricular hypertrophy; impaired left ventricular ejection fraction improves in many patients (1). Data from Monrad et al. (167) indicate that late (8.1 ± 2.9 years) after aortic valve replacement, there are further reductions in left ventricular mass and end-diastolic and end-systolic volumes (Table 5.20). Recent data from Bonow et al. (168) show that late (3 to 7 years, mean 5) after aortic valve replacement, left ventricular dimensions decrease further and ejection fraction increases in patients with a normal left ventricular ejection fraction before operation, but not in those with an abnormal

left ventricular ejection fraction (Table 5.21). It was felt that late improvement in left ventricular ejection fraction was more likely to occur in those who had an improvement early after aortic valve replacement (168) but apparently without accompanying late changes in left ventricular dimensions or mass (169). However, late improvement in left ventricular ejection fraction occurred only in patients with a normal left ventricular ejection fraction before operation and these patients did indeed have a further reduction in left ventricular end-diastolic dimension (Table 5.21) (168). Earlier data from Bonow et al. (170) had shown that an abnormal preoperative left ventricular ejection fraction in aortic regurgitation usually normalized if the preoperative abnormality had been present for ≤14 months; if the preoperative ejection fraction had been abnormal for ≥18 months, it usually did not improve after valve replacement.

Data from the Veterans Administration Cooperative Study indicate that severely depressed preoperative left ventricular ejection fraction (≤0.35) improves after valve replacement in patients with mixed aortic stenosis/regurgitation (left ventricular ejection fraction 0.31 ± 0.05 preoperatively, 0.52 ± 0.10 postoperatively; p < 0.001). In this regard, these patients appear to have a response more like that in patients with aortic stenosis (166) than in those with aortic regurgitation (171).

The Veterans Administration Cooperative Study also identified preoperative predictors of postoperative left ventricular dysfunction (172). In patients with aortic stenosis, the predictors of postoperative left ventricular dysfunction were preoperative left ventricular ejection fraction, myocardial infarction, aortic valve gradient and incomplete revascularization. In patients with aortic regurgitation, the predictors were preoperative left ventricular ejection fraction, left ventricular systolic pressure and arteriovenous oxygen difference. For patients with combined aortic stenosis/regurgitation, the predictors were preoperative left ventricular systolic pressure and myocardial infarction. In this study, postoperative left ventricular dysfunction was defined as a left ventricular ejection fraction ≤0.50 or left ventricular end-diastolic volume index >101 ml/m², or both, which is an uncommon definition of left ventricular dysfunction; a left ventricular end-diastolic volume index >101 ml/m² is 1.5 standard deviations greater than normal, which seems an

Table 5.20. Effect of Aortic Valve Replacement (AVR) on Left Ventricular Function in Patients With Aortic Regurgitation

	Control Valve	Before AVR	After AVR (yr)	
			1.6 ± 0.5	8.1 ± 2.9
LV EDVI (ml/m²)	93 ± 14	225 ± 49	123 ± 36	111 ± 53
LV ESVI (ml/m²)	31 ± 9	99 ± 35	51 ± 30	46 ± 47
LVEF (%)*	67 ± 7	57 ± 11	61 ± 9	64 ± 14
LV muscle mass index (g/m²)	85 ± 9	191 ± 36	128 ± 29	113 ± 35

*Changes not statistically significant. Abbreviations as in Table 5.18. From Monrad et al. (167).

Table 5.21. Effects of Aortic Valve Replacement (AVR) on Left Ventricular Function in Patients With Aortic Regurgitation

	Before AVR	p Value	6–8 Months After AVR	p Value	5 Years (range 3–7) After AVR
Normal LVEF Before AVR (n = 22)					
LV end-diastolic dimension (mm)	75 ± 6	<0.001	53 ± 6	<0.05	51 ± 5
LV muscle cross-sectional area (cm²)	36 ± 4	<0.001	26 ± 5	NS	26 ± 5
LVEF (%)	52 ± 8	<0.001	61 ± 11	<0.01	68 ± 11
Abnormal LVEF Before AVR (n = 39)					
LV end-diastolic dimension (mm)	75 ± 7	<0.001	57 ± 9	NS	57 ± 11
LV muscle cross-sectional area (cm²)	34 ± 7	<0.001	27 ± 8	NS	26 ± 8
LVEF (%)	39 ± 6	<0.005	46 ± 15	NS	49 ± 19

Abbreviations as in Table 5.18. From Bonow et al. (168).

arbitrary cutoff value. Predictors of abnormal left ventricular systolic pump function were not presented (172), which limits the clinical value of the data at the present time.

Mitral valve disease. Data from the Veterans Administration Cooperative Study (16) show that patients with mitral stenosis have significant improvement in hemodynamics after valve replacement; left ventricular function does not change (Table 5.22). Mitral valve area increased from 1.2 ± 0.4 to 1.8 ± 0.6 cm², an average increase of only 0.6 cm². In patients with mitral stenosis/regurgitation, regurgitant volume was reduced and the calculated mitral valve area remained unchanged. Patients with mitral regurgitation had significant improvement in hemodynamics and reductions in left ventricular end-diastolic and regurgitant volumes after valve replacement; left ventricular ejection fraction de-

creased from 0.56 to 0.45 (Table 5.22). The most powerful predictor of abnormal postoperative left ventricular ejection fraction was an abnormal preoperative ejection fraction, followed by total cardiopulmonary bypass time and left ventricular systolic pressure (16). There were no significant multivariate determinants of postoperative ejection fraction in the mitral stenosis and mitral stenosis/regurgitation groups (16). Nine (90%) of 10 patients with mitral regurgitation who had an abnormal ejection fraction preoperatively had an abnormal ejection fraction postoperatively; 12 (50%) of 24 patients with mitral regurgitation who had a normal ejection fraction preoperatively had an abnormal ejection fraction postoperatively and the other 50% continued to have a normal ejection fraction postoperatively. A postoperative left ventricular end-diastolic volume index >101 ml/m² in patients with

Table 5.22. Hemodynamics and Left Ventricular Function Before and After Mitral Valve Replacement (MVR) in the Veterans Administration Cooperative Study (16)

	Mitral Stenosis		Mitral Stenosis/Regurgitation		Mitral Regurgitation	
	Pre-MVR	Post-MVR	Pre-MVR	Post-MVR	Pre-MVR	Post-MVR
No. of patients	33		23		48	
LV end-diastolic pressure (mm Hg)	11 ± 5	12 ± 6	14 ± 6	13 ± 7	18 ± 8	12 ± 6*
Mean PA wedge pressure (mm Hg)	36 ± 15	28 ± 14*	30 ± 12	25 ± 11	29 ± 11	22 ± 9*
Mean systolic PA pressure (mm Hg)	54 ± 24	42 ± 22†	47 ± 18	36 ± 15†	43 ± 16	33 ± 13*
Cardiac index (liters/min per m²)	2.1 ± 1.5	2.3 ± 0.6	2.3 ± 0.6	2.3 ± 0.5	2.5 ± 1.0	2.7 ± 0.7
LV EDVI (ml/m²)	79 ± 18	72 ± 24	109 ± 55	85 ± 25	117 ± 51	89 ± 27*
LV ESVI (ml/m²)	41 ± 13	39 ± 21	54 ± 30	45 ± 22	54 ± 42	50 ± 25
LVEF	0.48 ± 0.10	0.47 ± 0.14	0.51 ± 0.13	0.49 ± 0.13	0.56 ± 0.15	0.45 ± 0.13*
Mitral regurgitant volume (ml)	—	—	53 ± 68	18 ± 22‡	59 ± 45	11 ± 17*
Regurgitant volume/end-diastolic volume	—	—	0.37 ± 0.34	0.19 ± 0.20‡	0.49 ± 0.31	0.12 ± 0.17*
Mitral valve gradient (mm Hg)	15 ± 7	8 ± 3*	12 ± 5	7 ± 4†	—	—
Mitral valve area (cm²)	1.2 ± 0.4	1.8 ± 0.6*	1.8 ± 1.2	1.9 ± 0.5	—	—

*p < 0.001, †p < 0.01 comparing before and after mitral valve replacement; ‡p < 0.05. LV = left ventricle; MVR = mitral valve replacement; PA = pulmonary artery.

Table 5.23. Aortic Homograft Primary Valve Failure

Reference	Valve Characteristics	No. of Pts.	Valve Failure (yr)		
			5	10	15
Barrat-Boyes et al. (181)	Antibiotic sterilized valve*				
	All patients	252	4%	19%	54%
	Low risk	144	2%	13%	38%
	High risk	108	10%	35%	60%
O'Brien et al. (182)	Allograft aortic valve†				
	Preservation				
	Fresh 4°C	124	—	11%	41%
	Viable cryopreserved	192	—	0%	0%
Matsuki et al. (183)	Aortic homografts‡				
	Several preservation techniques	555	—	43.2 ± 10%	87.6 ± 4.8% at 20 years

*Failure = incidence of aortic incompetence; High risk = donor age >55 years/recipient's age <15 years/recipient's aortic root size >30 mm. †There were many statistically significant patient-related factors that were different between the two groups; failure = reoperation for valve degeneration. ‡Failure = reoperation or death.

mitral regurgitation was best predicted by a preoperative left ventricular end-systolic volume index >50 ml/m^2 and mean pulmonary artery pressure >20 mm Hg (16).

Mechanical versus bioprosthetic valves. Two prospective randomized clinical trials (the Edinburgh and Veterans Administration Cooperative Studies [4–6]) compared a mechanical prosthetic valve with a bioprosthetic valve. Up to 7 years after surgery, there were no significant differences in the results in terms of survival, reoperation and valve-related complications. Thus, factors other than the type of prosthesis were more important in determining the intermediate (5 to 7 years) results of valve replacement.

Both trials failed to confirm that thromboembolism was a greater hazard with mechanical valves than with bioprosthetic valves, probably because the risks of thromboembolism in valvular heart disease are multifactorial (3). The major difference between the two trials was the incidence of anticoagulation-related bleeding. In the Veterans Administration Cooperative Study, the incidence of anticoagulation-related bleeding was 4% to 5%/year (4); conversely, the Edinburgh Study reported that bleeding complications were rare (1% to 1.5%/year) (6). In the Veterans Administration Cooperative Study, the recommended level of anticoagulant therapy was a prothrombin time of 2 to 2.5 times the control value, which is much higher than is usually recommended in patients with prosthetic heart valves (prothrombin time of 1.6 to 1.9 times control value) (3). A prothrombin time >2 times the control value increases the incidence of bleeding without a further reduction in the incidence of thromboembolism. Other differences between the studies, such as patient-related and health care delivery factors (Table 5.2), probably account for most of the observed differences between the two trials.

It needs to be reemphasized that *all* mechanical valves in patients who are not on anticoagulant therapy or receive only aspirin or dipyridamole, or both, are associated with a high or very high incidence of thromboembolism (1,9,20, 173–179). Therefore, patients with any type of mechanical prosthetic heart valve must receive long-term anticoagulant therapy with sodium warfarin unless there is a specific contraindication to its use.

Mitral valve repair. Galloway et al. (17) recently presented an extensive review of mitral valve reconstruction for mitral regurgitation. The operative mortality rate ranged from 2.3% to 8%; the mortality rate at 5 years ranged from 8% to 40% and at 9 to 10 years from 18% to 27%. The late valve replacement rate at 5 years ranged from 3% to 16%. The incidence of thromboembolism ranged from 0.2% to 1.8%/year; the incidence at 5 years was 3% to 6%. The incidence of late endocarditis was very low (17).

Cosgrove and Stewart from the Cleveland Clinic (180) also reviewed the topic of mitral valve repair and presented the results in patients with all types of mitral lesions. Between 1985 and 1988, valve repair was performed in 69% of patients with pure mitral regurgitation, 54% of patients with mitral stenosis and 42% of those with mitral stenosis/regurgitation. Valve repair was performed in 75% of patients with degenerative disease, 68% of those with "ischemic" disease and 49% of those with rheumatic valve disease. The operative mortality rate was 2.4% in degenerative disease and 13% in ischemic disease. The rate of thromboembolism and reoperation was 2.6% and 2% per patient-year, respectively (179). Clearly, in selected patients, mitral valve repair yields very good results and should be performed whenever it can be done and a good result obtained.

Durability of valve replacement material. *Aortic homografts (Table 5.23).* Barrat-Boyes et al. (181) described 248 patients followed up for 9 to 16.5 years (mean 10.8) and showed that the homograft failure rate was 19% at 10 years and 54% at 15 years; it was lower in the low risk group (Table 5.24), but at 15 years, it was still 38%. O'Brien et al. (182) presented data on homografts preserved by two different

Table 5.24. Porcine Bioprosthetic Failure Rate*

Valve Characteristics	Reference	No. of Pts.	10 Years (%)	12–12.5 Years (%)	15 Years (%)
Mitral	Foster et al. (184)	111	25 ± 6	42 ± 8	60 ± 12
	Gallo et al. (185)	193	35 ± 5	48 ± 5	—
	Jamieson et al. (186)	509	27.9 ± 4.9	—	—
	Gallucci et al. (187)	502	—	—	59 ± 5.5
	Magilligan et al. (188)	562	29 ± 1.6	—	70 ± 13
Aortic	Gallo et al. (185)	126	30 ± 7	42 ± 6	—
	Jamieson et al. (186)	572	16.9 ± 3.7	—	—
	Gallucci et al. (187)	196	—	—	63 ± 10
	Magilligan et al. (188)	479	24 ± 3.4	—	63 ± 18
Multiple valves	Jamieson et al. (186)	111	34.5 ± 7.8	—	—
	Gallucci et al. (187)	71	—	51 ± 13	—
Single and multiple valves	Spampinato et al. (189)	1.098	14.9 ± 2.0	39.4 ± 9.6	—
	Approximate average incidence (%)		25	45	65

*Based on diagnosis at valve replacement or by pathologic examination, or both.

techniques; viable allografts cryopreserved in liquid nitrogen at −196°C did not degenerate during up to 15 years of follow-up study. Matsuki et al. (183) presented data on homografts inserted between 1964 and 1986. The linearized failure rate was 4.8 ± 0.4%/year for 20 years; the failure rate was very low up to 4 to 5 years and then was steep and steady up to 18 years. The incidence of homograft endocarditis was probably low in the first year (180,181) and was 8% to 11% at 15 years and 17.3% at 20 years (180–182), which may not be significantly different from that with other valve replacement devices. However, a most interesting finding in these studies is the very low thromboembolic rate (≤4% up to 15 years).

Porcine bioprosthetic valves (Table 5.24). The primary tissue failure rate of bioprosthetic valves ranged from 24% to 35% at 10 years (in one study [186], it was 17% for aortic valve replacement), 42% to 48% at 12 years and 60% to 70% at 15 years (184–188). The primary tissue failure rate was very low in the first 5 years (2% to 3% at 5 years), with a steady increase during years 6 to 10 and a marked increase after year 11. The higher failure rate was statistically signif-

icant for mitral valves in only one series (186). Patients aged ≤30 to 35 years were at higher risk for bioprosthetic valve failure (156); those aged ≥50 to 60 years were at lower risk for bioprosthetic valve failure (186,187).

The incidence of thromboembolism is very low with mitral valve repair and aortic homografts. Likewise, the

Figure 5.11. Eighteen to 20 year survival curves after mitral (**top panel**) and aortic (**bottom panel**) valve replacement using the silastic ball Starr-Edwards prosthetic heart valve. Reproduced by permission of A. Starr, MD, Heart Institute at St. Vincent Hospital and Medical Center, Portland, Oregon.

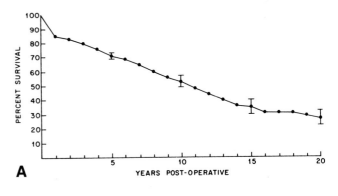

A

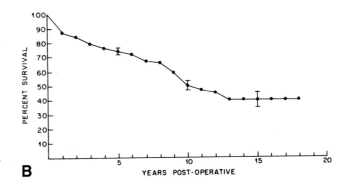

B

Table 5.25. Long-Term Results With Silastic Ball Starr-Edwards Prosthetic Heart Valve

	Mitral 6120 at 20 Years	Aortic 1260 at 15 Years
Total no. of patients	458	660
Survival (%)	27 ± 4.7	40 ± 4.5
Valve-related deaths (%)	22 ± 7	9 ± 3
Thromboembolism (%)	55 ± 8	16 ± 2
Bleeding (%)	33 ± 7	44 ± 14
Prosthetic endocarditis (%)	3 ± 2	4 ± 1
Thrombotic stenosis (%)	7 ± 3	1 ± 1
Reoperation (%)	25 ± 6	5 ± 2

Reproduced by permission from Starr (unpublished observations).

incidence of "late" endocarditis is very low with mitral valve repair. Porcine bioprostheses do not share these advantages. One reason for this may be related to the fact that metallic and other materials are incorporated in the fabrication of porcine prosthetic heart valves.

However, both porcine bioprostheses and homografts have a *significant* and *major problem of valve degeneration*, which for porcine bioprostheses averages approximately ≤5% at 5 years, 25% at 10 years, 45% at 12 years and 65% at 15 years (Table 5.25). Additional studies of cryopreserved viable allografts that confirm the findings of O'Brien et al. (182) are needed. The reported incidence rates of degeneration refer to those confirmed at operation, pathologic examination or autopsy; thus, the actual clinical incidence of valve degeneration may be higher. These data mandate a careful reevaluation of the indications for and use of biological material as valve replacement substitutes.

Mechanical valves. It is clear that at least some of the currently available mechanical valves are durable. The one with the longest proven record is the silastic ball Starr-Edwards valve (Fig. 5.11). Structural failure has been virtually nonexistent in the 20 to 23 years of use with the silastic ball Starr-Edwards valve, during which time the device has not undergone any significant change. There are no good data to show that any valve replacement device is superior to the silastic ball Starr-Edwards valve in overall performance; the long-term results of its use are shown in Table 5.25. It needs to be reemphasized that results from valve surgery are dependent on many factors (Tables 5.1 and 5.2) (3); one should avoid making inappropriate comparisons and thereby arriving at inappropriate conclusions.

References

1. Rahimtoola SH. Valvular heart disease: a perspective. J Am Coll Cardiol 1983;1:199–215.
2. Rahimtoola SH. Catheter balloon valvuloplasty in adults with aortic and mitral stenosis: 1987. Circulation 1987;75:895–901.
3. Rahimtoola SH. Lessons learned about the determinants of the result of valve surgery. Circulation 1988;78:1503–7.
4. Hammermeister KE, Henderson WG, Burchfiel CM, et al. Comparison of outcome after valve replacement with a bioprosthesis versus a mechanical prosthesis: initial 5 year results of a randomized trial. J Am Coll Cardiol 1987;10:719–32.
5. Sethi G, Hammermeister K, Henderson W, et al. Comparison of outcome at an average of 7+ years between a mechanical valve and a bioprosthesis: results of a VA cooperative study on valvular heart disease. In: Bodnar E, ed. Surgery for Heart Valve Disease. London: ICR Publishers, 1990:253–61.
6. Bloomfield P, Kitchin AH, Wheatley DJ, Walbaum PR, Lutz W, Miller HC. A prospective evaluation of the Bjork-Shiley, Hancock and Carpentier-Edwards heart valve prostheses. Circulation 1986;73:1213–22.
7. Rahimtoola SH. Perspective on valvular heart disease: an update. J Am Coll Cardiol 1989;14:1–23.
8. McGoon D. On evaluating valves (editorial). Mayo Clin Proc 1974;49:233–5.
9. Rahimtoola SH. Valve replacement—a perspective. Am J Cardiol 1975;35:711–5.
10. Salomon NW, Stinson EB, Griepp RB, Shumway NE. Patient-related risk factors as predictors of results following isolated mitral valve replacement. Ann Thorac Surg 1977;24:519–30.
11. Macmanus Q, Grunkemeier GL, Lambert LE, Teply JF, Harlan BJ, Starr A. Year of operation as a risk factor in the late results of valve replacements. J Thorac Cardiovasc Surg 1980;80:834–41.
12. Turina J, Turina M, Rothlin M, Krayenbuehl HP. Improved late survival in patients with chronic aortic regurgitation by earlier operation. Circulation 1984;70(suppl I):I-147–52.
13. Bonow RO, Picone AL, McIntosh CL, et al. Survival and functional results after valve replacement for aortic regurgitation for 1976 to 1983: impact of preoperative left ventricular function. Circulation 1985;72:1244–56.
14. Mitchell RS, Miller DC, Stinson EB, et al. Significant patient-related determinants of prosthetic valve performance. J Thorac Cardiovasc Surg 1986;91:807–17.
15. Khuri SF, Folland ED, Sethi GK, et al. Six month postoperative hemodynamics of the Hancock heterograft and the Bjork-Shiley prosthesis: results of the Veterans Administration cooperative prospective randomized trial. J Am Coll Cardiol 1988;12:8–18.
16. Crawford MH, Souchek J, Oprian CA, et al. Determinants of survival and left ventricular performance after mitral valve replacement. Circulation 1990;81:1173–81.
17. Galloway AC, Clvin SB, Baumann FG, Spencer FC. Current concepts of mitral valve reconstruction for mitral regurgitation. Circulation 1988;78:1087–98.
18. Starr A, Grunkemeier GL. Selection of a prosthetic heart valve. JAMA 1984;251:1739–42.
19. Sethi GK, Miller DC, Souchek J, et al. Clinical, hemodynamic and angiographic predictors of operative mortality in patients undergoing single valve replacement. J Thorac Cardiovasc Surg 1987;93:884–7.
20. Myers ML, Lawrie GM, Crawford ES, et al. The St. Jude valve prosthesis: analysis of the clinical results in 815 implants and the need for systemic anticoagulation. J Am Coll Cardiol 1989;13:57–62.
21. Mullany CJ, Elveback ER, Frye RL, et al. Coronary artery disease and its management: influence on survival in patients undergoing aortic valve replacement. J Am Coll Cardiol 1987;10:66–72.
22. ACC/AHA Task Force on Assessment of Diagnostic and Therapeutic Cardiovascular Procedures, Subcommittee on Coronary Angiography. Guidelines for coronary angiography. J Am Coll Cardiol 1987;10:935–50.
23. Greves J, Rahimtoola SH, McAnulty JH, et al. Preoperative criteria predictive of late survival following valve replacement for severe aortic regurgitation. Am Heart J 1981;101:300–8.
24. Murphy ES, Lawson RM, Starr A, Rahimtoola SH. Severe aortic stenosis in the elderly: state of left ventricular function and result of valve replacement on ten-year survival. Circulation 1981;64(suppl II):II-184–8.
25. Kotlewski A, Rahimtoola SH. Imaging and clinical decision-making in patients with acquired valvular heart disease. In: Pohost GM, O'Rourke RA, eds. Cardiac Imaging. Boston: Little, Brown, 1991.
26. Kotlewski A, Kawanishi DT, McKay CR, et al. The relative value of clinical examination, echocardiography with Doppler, and cardiac catheterization with angiography in the evaluation of aortic valve disease. In Ref 5:66–72.
27. Kawanishi DT, Kotlewski A, McKay CR, et al. Incremental value of clinical examination, echocardiography with Doppler, and cardiac catheterization with angiography in the evaluation of mitral valve disease. In Ref 5:73–8.
28. Lembo NJ, Dell'Italia LJ, Crawford MH, O'Rourke RA. Bedside diagnosis of systolic murmurs. N Engl J Med 1988;318:1572–8.
29. Crewe K, Crawford MH, O'Rourke RA. Differentiation of cardiac murmurs by dynamic auscultation. Curr Probl Cardiol 1988;13:675–721.
30. Veasy LG, Wiedmeier SE, Orsmond GS, et al. Resurgence of acute rheumatic fever in the intermountain area of the United States. N Engl J Med 1987;316:421–7.
31. Congeni B, Rizzo C, Congeni J, Sreenivassan VV. Outbreak of acute rheumatic fever in northeastern Ohio. J Pediatr 1987;111:176–9.
32. Wald ER, Dashefsky B, Feidt C, Chiponis D, Byers C. Acute rheumatic fever in western Pennsylvania and the tristate area. Pediatrics 1987;80:371–4.
33. Papadimos T, Escamilla J, Garst P, et al. Acute rheumatic fever at a navy training center—San Diego, California. JAMA 1988;259:1782–7.

34. Zabriske JB. Rheumatic fever: the interplay between host, genetics, and microbe. Circulation 1985;71:1077–86.

35. Kaplan AL. Return of rheumatic fever: consequences, implications and needs. J Pediatr 1987;111:244–6.

36. Bisno AL, Shulman ST, Dajani AS. The rise and fall (rise ?) of rheumatic fever. JAMA 1988;259:728–9.

37. Denny FW. T Duckett Jones and rheumatic fever in 1986. Circulation 1987;76:963–70.

38. Bland EF. Rheumatic fever: the way it was. Circulation 1987;76:1190–5.

39. Dajani AS, Bisno AL, Chung KJ, et al. Prevention of rheumatic fever. Circulation 1988;78:1083–6.

40. Ross J Jr, Braunwald E. Aortic stenosis. Circulation 1968;36(suppl IV):IV-61–7.

41. Horstkotte D, Loogen F. The natural history of aortic valve stenosis. Eur Heart J 1988;9(suppl E):57–64.

42. Frank S, Johnson A, Ross J Jr. Natural history of valvular aortic stenosis. Br Heart J 1973;35:41–6.

43. Rapaport E. Natural history of aortic and mitral valve disease. Am J Cardiol 1975;35:221–7.

44. Chizner MA, Pearle DL, deLeon AC. The natural history of aortic stenosis in adults. Am Heart J 1980;99:419–24.

45. Schwarz F, Banmann P, Manthey J, et al. The effect of aortic valve replacement on survival. Circulation 1982;66:1105–10.

46. O'Keefe JH Jr, Vlietstra RE, Bailey KR, Holmes DR Jr. Natural history of candidates for balloon aortic valvuloplasty. Mayo Clin Proc 1987;62: 986–91.

47. Turina J, Hess O, Sepulcri F, Krayenbuehl HP. Spontaneous course of aortic valve disease. Eur Heart J 1987;8:471–83.

48. Kelly TA, Rothbart RM, Cooper M, Kaiser DL, Smucker ML, Gibson RS. Comparison of outcome of asymptomatic to symptomatic patients older than 20 years of age with valvular aortic stenosis. Am J Cardiol 1988;61:123–30.

49. Pellikka PA, Nishimura PA, Bailey KR, Tajik AJ. The natural history of adults with asymptomatic, hemodynamically significant aortic stenosis. J Am Coll Cardiol 1990;15:1012–27.

50. Conn HL Jr, Horwitz O. Cardiac and Vascular Diseases. Philadelphia: Lea & Febiger, 1971:812.

51. Hancock EW, Fleming PR. Aortic stenosis. Quart J Med 1960;29:209–34.

52. Wood P. Aortic stenosis. Am J Cardiol 1958;1:553–71.

53. Ross J Jr. Left ventricular function and the timing of surgical treatment in valvular heart disease. Ann Intern Med 1981;84:498–504.

54. Ross J Jr. Afterload mismatch in aortic and mitral valve disease: implications for surgical therapy. J Am Coll Cardiol 1985;5:811–26.

55. Braunwald E. Valvular heart disease. In: Braunwald E, ed. Heart Disease. Philadelphia: WB Saunders, 1984:1103.

56. Braunwald E, Morrow AG. Obstruction to left ventricular outflow: current criteria for the selection of patients for operation. Am J Cardiol 1963;12:53–9.

57. Tobin JR Jr, Rahimtoola SH, Blundell PE, Swan HJC. Percentage of left ventricular stroke work loss: a simple hemodynamic concept for estimation of severity in valvular aortic stenosis. Circulation 1967;35:868–79.

58. Gorlin R, Gorlin SG. Hydraulic formula for calculation of the area of the stenotic mitral valve, other cardiac valves, and central circulatory shunts. Am Heart J 1951;41:1–29.

59. Braunwald E, Sarnoff SJ, Stainsby WN. Determinants of duration and mean rate of ventricular ejection. Circ Res 1958;6:319–25.

60. Rahimtoola SH. The problem of valve prosthesis-patient mismatch. Circulation 1978;58:20–4.

61. Rodrigo FA, Snellen HA. Estimation of valve and "valvular resistance": a critical study of the physical basis of the methods employed. Am Heart J 1953;45:1–12.

62. Allan GO. A schema of the circulation with experiments to determine the additional load on the apparatus produced by conditions representing valvular lesions. Heart 1925;12:181.

63. DeHeer. Cited by: Wiggens CJ. Physiology in Health and Disease, 5th ed. Philadelphia: Lea & Febiger, 1949:786.

64. Currie PJ, Seward JB, Reeder GS, et al. Continuous-wave Doppler echocardiographic assessment of severity of calcific aortic stenosis: a simultaneous Doppler-catheter correlative study in 100 adult patients. Circulation 1985;71:1162–9.

65. Skjaerpe T, Hegrenaes L, Hatle L. Noninvasive estimation of valve area in patients with aortic stenosis by Doppler ultrasound and two-dimensional echocardiography. Circulation 1985;72:810–5.

66. Krafchek J, Robertson JH, Radford M, Adams D, Kisslo J. A reconsideration of Doppler assessed gradients in suspected aortic stenosis. Am Heart J 1985;110:765–73.

67. Currie PJ, Hagler DJ, Seward JB, et al. Instantaneous pressure gradient: a simultaneous Doppler and dual catheter correlative study. J Am Coll Cardiol 1986;7:800–6.

68. Smith MD, Dawson PL, Elion DL, et al. Systematic correlation of continuous wave Doppler and hemodynamic measurements in patients with aortic stenosis. Br Heart J 1986;111:245–52.

69. Yeager M, Yock PG, Popp RL. Comparison of Doppler derived pressure gradient to that determined at cardiac catheterization in adults with aortic valve stenosis: implications for management. Am J Cardiol 1986;57:644–8.

70. Zoghbi WA, Farmer KL, Soto JG, Nelson JG, Quinones MA. Accurate noninvasive quantification of stenotic aortic valve area by Doppler echocardiography. Circulation 1986;73:452–9.

71. Otto CM, Pearlman AS, Comess RA, Reamer RP, Janko CL, Huntsman LL. Determination of the stenotic aortic valve area in adults using Doppler echocardiography. J Am Coll Cardiol 1986;7:509–17.

72. Teirstein P, Yaeger M, Yock PG, Popp RL. Doppler echocardiographic measurement of aortic valve area in aortic stenosis: a noninvasive application of the Gorlin formula. J Am Coll Cardiol 1986;8:1059–65.

73. Come PC, Riley MF, McKay RG, Safian R. Echocardiographic assessment of aortic valve area in elderly patients with aortic stenosis and of changes in valve area after percutaneous balloon valvuloplasty. J Am Coll Cardiol 1987;10:115–24.

74. Oh JK, Taliercio CP, Holmes DR Jr, et al. Prediction of the severity of aortic stenosis by Doppler aortic valve area determination: prospective Doppler-catheterization correlation in 100 patients. J Am Coll Cardiol 1988;11:1227–34.

75. Nishimura RA, Holmes DR Jr, Reeder GS, et al. Doppler evaluation of results of percutaneous aortic balloon valvuloplasty in calcific aortic stenosis. Circulation 1988;78:791–9.

76. Come PC, Riley MF, Safian RD, Ferguson JF, Diver DD, McKay RG. Usefulness of noninvasive assessment of aortic stenosis before and after percutaneous aortic valvuloplasty. Am J Cardiol 1988;61:1300–6.

77. Davidson CJ, Harpole DA, Kisslo K, et al. Analysis of the early rise in aortic transvalvular gradient after aortic valvuloplasty. Am Heart J 1989;117:411–7.

78. Rijsterborgh H, Roelandt J. Doppler assessment of aortic stenosis: Bernoulli revisited. Ultrasound Med Biol 1987;13:241–84.

79. Stamm RB, Martin RP. Quantification of pressure gradients across stenotic valves by Doppler ultrasound. J Am Coll Cardiol 1983;2:707–18.

80. Letac B, Cribier A, Konnig B, Bellefleur JP. Results of percutaneous transluminal valvuloplasty in 218 adults with valvular aortic stenosis. Am J Cardiol 1988;62:598–605.

81. Safian RD, Berman AD, Diver DJ, et al. Balloon aortic valvuloplasty in 170 consecutive patients. N Engl J Med 1988;319:125–31.

82. Cribier A, Koning R, Eltchaninoff H, Joannides R, Berland J, Letac B. Results of aortic balloon valvuloplasty in patients with aortic stenosis nonsuitable for valve replacement (abstr). Circulation 1988;78(suppl II):II-592.

83. Block PC, Palacios IF. Percutaneous aortic balloon valvuloplasty (PAV) in the elderly: update of immediate results and follow-up (abstr). Circulation 1988;78(suppl II):II-593.

84. Kleaveland JP, Hill J, Margolis J, et al. M-Heart Registry for percutaneous transluminal aortic valvuloplasty: follow-up report (abstr). Circulation 1988;78(suppl II):II-533.

85. Block PC, for the MSAVR Investigators. The "experience curve" for percutaneous aortic valvuloplasty: report from the Mansfield Scientific Aortic Valvuloplasty Registry (MSAVR) (abstr). Circulation 1988; 78(suppl II):II-531.

86. Desnoyers MR, Isner JM, Pandian NG, et al. Clinical and noninvasive hemodynamic results after aortic balloon valvuloplasty for aortic stenosis. Am J Cardiol 1988;62:1078–84.

87. Litvack F, Jakubowski AT, Buchbinder NA, Eigler N. Lack of sustained clinical improvement in an elderly population after percutaneous aortic valvuloplasty. Am J Cardiol 1988;62:270–5.

88. Brady ST, Davis CA, Kussmaul WG, Laskey WK, Hirshfield JW, Herrmann HC. Percutaneous aortic balloon valvuloplasty in octogenarians: morbidity and mortality. Ann Intern Med 1989;110:761–6.

89. Holmes DR, Nishimura RA, Reeder GS, Wagner PJ, Ilstrup DM. Clinical follow-up after percutaneous aortic balloon valvuloplasty. Arch Intern Med 1989;149:1405–9.

90. Sherman W, Hershman R, Lazzam C, Cohen M, Ambrose J, Gorlin R. Balloon valvuloplasty in adult aortic stenosis: determinants of clinical outcome. Ann Intern Med 1989;110:421–5.

91. Cribier A, Berland J, Konig R, Bellefleur JP, Letac B. Determinant of best results of balloon aortic valvuloplasty in adults (abstr). J Am Coll Cardiol 1988;11:14A.

92. Leonard BM, Berman AD, Kuntz RE, et al. Follow-up of balloon aortic valvuloplasty: results in 170 cases (abstr). Circulation 1988;78(suppl II):II-593.

93. Kulick DL, Kawanishi DT, Reid CL, Rahimtoola SH. Catheter balloon valvuloplasty in adults, Part 1: aortic stenosis. Curr Probl Cardiol 1990;15:359–95.

94. Leonard BM, Harvey JR, Berman AD, et al. Predictors of initial success and long-term survival for balloon aortic valvuloplasty (abstr). Circulation 1988;78(suppl II):II-533.

95. McKay RG, for the Mansfield Scientific Aortic Valvuloplasty Registry. Balloon aortic valvuloplasty in 285 patients: initial results and complications (abstr). Circulation 1988;78(suppl II):II-594.

96. Desnoyers M, Fields C, Lucas A, et al. Extended clinical and noninvasive hemodynamic follow-up of patients treated with balloon valvuloplasty for aortic stenosis (abstr). Circulation 1988;78(suppl II):II-593.

97. Davidson CJ, Skelton TN, Kisslo KB, et al. The risk for systemic embolization associated with percutaneous balloon valvuloplasty in adults. Ann Intern Med 1988;108:557–60.

98. Holland K, Brown K, Kirsh M, et al. One year clinical follow-up of balloon aortic valvuloplasty vs aortic valve replacement in elderly operative candidates (abstr). Circulation 1988;78(suppl II):II-593.

99. Letac B, Cribier A, Berland J, Eltchaninoff H, Joannides R. Clinical follow-up in adult aortic stenosis treated by balloon valvuloplasty (abstr). Circulation 1988;78(suppl II):II-532.

100. O'Neill WW, for Mansfield Registry. Long-term survival after percutaneous balloon valvuloplasty: preliminary report of the Mansfield Scientific Registry (abstr). Circulation 1988;78(suppl II):II-594.

101. Sherman W, Hershman R, Lazzam C, Cohen M, Ambrose J, Govlin R. Balloon valvuloplasty in adult aortic stenosis: determinants of clinical outcome. Ann Int Med 189;110:421–5.

102. Desnoyers MR, Salan DN, Rosenfield K, MacKay W, O'Donnell T, Isner JM. Treatment of cardiogenic shock by emergency aortic balloon valvuloplasty. Ann Intern Med 1988;108:833–5.

103. Safian RD, Warren SE, Berman AD, et al. Improvement in symptoms and left ventricular performance after balloon aortic valvuloplasty in patients with aortic stenosis and depressed left ventricular ejection fraction. Circulation 1988;78:1181–91.

104. Berland J, Cribier A, Savin T, Lefebvre E, Koning, Letac B. Percutaneous balloon valvuloplasty in patients with severe aortic stenosis and low ejection fraction. Circulation 1989;79:1189–96.

105. Roth RB, Palacios IF, Block PC. Percutaneous aortic balloon valvuloplasty: its role in the management of patients with aortic stenosis requiring major noncardiac surgery. J Am Coll Cardiol 1989;13:1039–41.

106. Levine MJ, Berman AD, Safian RD, Diver DJ, McKay RG. Palliation of valvular aortic stenosis by balloon valvuloplasty as preoperative preparation for noncardiac surgery. Am J Cardiol 1988;62:1309–10.

107. Hayes SN, Holmes DR, Nishimura RA, Reeder GS. Palliative percutaneous aortic balloon valvuloplasty before noncardiac operations and invasive diagnostic procedures. Mayo Clin Proc 1989;64:753–7.

108. McKay CR, Kawanishi DT, Chatterjee S, Reid CL, Rahimtoola SH. Stenotic aortic and mitral valves treated with catheter balloon valvuloplasty in a patient with small valve annuli. Ann Intern Med 1988;108:568–9.

109. Berman AD, Weinstein JS, Safian RD, Diver DJ, Grossman W, McKay RG. Combined aortic and mitral balloon valvuloplasty in patients with

critical aortic and mitral valve stenosis: results in six cases. J Am Coll Cardiol 1988;11:1213–8.

110. McKay RG, Safian RD, Berman AD, et al. Combined percutaneous aortic valvuloplasty and transluminal coronary angioplasty in adult patients with calcific aortic stenosis and coronary artery disease. Circulation 1987;76:1298–306.

111. Mackenzie J. Diseases of the Heart, ed. 3, London: Oxford Medical Publications, 1914:211.

112. Goldman S, Probst P, Selzer A, Cohn K. Inefficacy of "therapeutic" serum levels of digoxin in controlling the ventricular rate in atrial fibrillation. Am J Cardiol 1975;35:651–5.

113. DiBianco R, Morganroth J, Freitag JA, et al. Effects of uadolol on the spontaneous and exercise-provoked heart rate of patients with chronic atrial fibrillation on receiving stable doses of digoxin. Am Heart J 1984;108:1121–7.

114. Schwartz JB, Keefe D, Kates RF, Kirsten E, Harrison DC. Acute and chronic pharmacodynamic interaction of verapamil and digoxin in atrial fibrillation. Circulation 1982;65:1163–70.

115. Elkayam U, Parikh H, Torkan B, Weber L, Cohen JL, Rahimtoola SH. Effect of diltiazem on renal clearance and serum concentration of digoxin in patients with cardiac disease. Am J Cardiol 1985;55:1393–5.

116. Roth A, Harrison E, Mitani G, Cohen J, Rahimtoola SH, Elkayam U. Efficacy and safety of medium- and high-dose diltiazem alone and in combination with digoxin for control of heart rate at rest and during exercise in patients with chronic atrial fibrillation. Circulation 1986;73:316–24.

117. Atwood JE, Myers JN, Sullivan MJ, Forbes SM, Pewen WF, Froelicher VF. Diltiazem and exercise performance in patients with chronic atrial fibrillation. Chest 1988;93:1–25.

118. Hatle L, Angelsen B, Tromsdal A. Noninvasive assessment of atrioventricular pressure half-time by Doppler ultrasound. Circulation 1979;60:1096–104.

119. Smith MD, Handshoe R, Handshoe S, Kwan OL, DeMaria AN. Comparative accuracy of two-dimensional echocardiography and Doppler pressure half-time methods in assessing severity of mitral stenosis in patients with and without prior commissurotomy. Circulation 1986;73:100–7.

120. Grayburn PA, Smith MD, Gurley JC, Booth DC, DeMaria AN. Effect of aortic regurgitation on the assessment of mitral valve orifice area by Doppler pressure half-time in mitral stenosis. Am J Cardiol 1987;60:322–6.

121. Nakatani S, Masuyama T, Kodama K, Kitabatake A, Fujii K, Kamada T. Value and limitations of Doppler echocardiography in the quantification of stenotic mitral valve area: comparison of the pressure half-time and the continuity equation methods. Circulation 1988;77:78–85.

122. Reid CL, Kawanishi DT, Chandraratna PA, Kotlewski A, Rahimtoola SH. Doppler/two-dimensional echocardiographic assessment of catheter balloon valvuloplasty for mitral stenosis: changes in correlation with cardiac catheterization. In Ref 5:136–44.

123. Reid CL, Chandraratna PAN, Kawanishi DT, Kotlewski A, Rahimtoola SH. Influence of mitral valve morphology upon double-balloon catheter balloon valvuloplasty in patients with mitral stenosis: analysis of factors predicting immediate and 3 month results. Circulation 1989;80:515–24.

124. Reid CL, Kawanishi DT, Rahimtoola SH. One year clinical and echocardiographic follow-up of patients having double balloon catheter balloon valvuloplasty for mitral stenosis (abstr). J Am Coll Cardiol 1989;13:115A.

125. Palacios IF, Block PC. Percutaneous mitral balloon valvotomy (PMV): update of immediate results and follow-up (abstr). Circulation 1988;78(suppl II):II-489.

126. Abascal VM, Wilkins GT, Choong CY, et al. Echocardiographic evaluation of mitral valve structure and function in patients followed up for at least 6 months after percutaneous balloon mitral valvuloplasty. J Am Coll Cardiol 1988;12:606–15.

127. Block PC, for the NHLBI Balloon Valvuloplasty Registry (BVR). Early results of mitral balloon valvuloplasty (MBV) for mitral stenosis: report from the NHLBI Registry (abstr). Circulation 1988;78(suppl II):II-489.

128. Cequier A, Bonan R, Dyrda I, Crepeau J, Dethy M, Petitclerc R. Percutaneous mitral valvuloplasty: long-term clinical and hemodynamic follow-up (abstr). Circulation 1988;78(suppl II):II-529.

129. Tami J, Nagata S, Akaike M, Ishikura F, Yamagishi M, Miyatake K.

Improvement in exercise hemodynamics after balloon mitral valvulo-plasty: noninvasive examination using continuous wave Doppler (abstr). Circulation 1988;78(suppl II):II-530.

130. Chen C, Wang Y, Duan Q, Lin Y, Lan Y. Comparative results of percutaneous mitral balloon dilatation by various techniques (abstr). Circulation 1988;78(suppl II):II-530.

131. Nakatani S, Nagata S, Beppu S, Kimura K, Takamiya M, Nimura Y. Time related changes in mitral valve area after balloon mitral valvulo-plasty assessed by Doppler continuity equation method (abstr). Circulation 1988;78(suppl II):II-487.

132. Inoue K, Nobuyoshi M, Chen C, Hung JS. Advantage of inoue-balloon (self-positioning balloon) in percutaneous transvenous mitral commissurotomy (abstr). Circulation 1988;78(suppl II):II-490.

133. Babic UU, Dorros G, Pejcic P, et al. Percutaneous mitral valvuloplasty: retrograde, transarterial double-balloon technique utilizing the transseptal approach. Cathet Cardiovasc Diagn 1988;14:229–37.

134. Vahanian A, Michel PL, Cormier B, et al. Results of percutaneous mitral commissurotomy in 200 patients. Am J Cardiol 1989;63:847–52.

135. Nobuyoshi M, Hamasaki N, Kimura T, et al. Indications, complications, and short-term clinical outcome of percutaneous transvenous mitral commissurotomy. Circulation 1989;80:782–92.

136. Herrmann HC, Kleaveland JP, Hill JA, et al. The M-Heart Percutaneous Balloon Mitral Valvuloplasty Registry: initial results and early follow-up. J Am Coll Cardiol 1990;15:1221–6.

137. Reyes VP, Raju BS, Raju ARG, Turi ZG, for the WSU-Nizam's Institute Valvuloplasty Study Group. Percutaneous balloon mitral valvuloplasty vs surgery: results of a randomized clinical trial (abstr). Circulation 1988;78(suppl II):II-489.

138. McKay CR, Kawanishi DT, Kotlewski A, et al. Improvement in exercise capacity and exercise hemodynamics 3 months after double balloon catheter balloon valvuloplasty in the treatment of patients with symptomatic mitral stenosis. Circulation 1988;77:1013–21.

139. McKay CR, Kawanishi DT, Rahimtoola SH. Catheter balloon valvuloplasty (CBV) of the mitral valve in adults using a double balloon technique: early hemodynamic results. JAMA 1987;257:1753–61.

140. Block PC, Palacios IF. Pulmonary vascular dynamics after percutaneous mitral valvotomy. J Thorac Cardiovasc Surg 1988;66:39–43.

141. Reid CL, McKay CR, Chandraratna PAN, Kawanishi DT, Rahimtoola SH. Mechanisms of increase in mitral valve area and influence of anatomic features in double balloon, catheter balloon valvuloplasty in adults with rheumatic mitral stenosis: an echocardiographic-Doppler study. Circulation 1987;76:628–36.

142. Pallacios IF, Block PC, Wilkins GT, Weyman AE. Follow-up of patients undergoing percutaneous mitral balloon valvotomy: analysis of factors determining restenosis. Circulation 1989;79:573–9.

143. Thomas JD, Wilkins GT, Choony CYP, et al. Inaccuracy of mitral pressure half-time immediately after percutaneous mitral valvotomy: dependence on transmitral gradient and left atrial and ventricular compliance. Circulation 1988;78:980–93.

144. Kulick DL, Kawanishi DT, Reid CL, Rahimtoola SH. Catheter balloon commissurotomy in adults, Part II: mitral and other stenosis. Curr Probl Cardiol 1990;15:403–70.

145. Cequier A, Bonan R, Serra A, et al. Left-to-right atrial shunting after percutaneous mitral valvuloplasty: incidence and long-term hemodynamic follow-up. Circulation 1990;81:1190–7.

146. Palacios IF, Block PC. Atrial septal defect during percutaneous mitral balloon valvotomy (PMV): immediate results and follow-up (abstr). Circulation 1988;78(suppl II):II-529.

147. Casale P, Block PC, O'Shea JP, Palacios IF. Atrial septal defect after percutaneous mitral balloon valvuloplasty: immediate results and follow-up. J Am Coll Cardiol 1990;15:1300–4.

148. Yoshida K, Yoshikawa J, Akasaka T, et al. Assessment of left-to-right shunting after percutaneous mitral valvuloplasty by transesophageal color Doppler flow-mapping. Circulation 1989;80:1521–6.

149. Fields CD, Isner JM. Size of atrial septostomy resulting from transseptal delivery of balloon catheters used for mitral valvuloplasty (abstr). Circulation 1988;78(suppl II):II-488.

150. Waldman HM, Palacios IF, Block PC, et al. Responsiveness of plasma atrial natriuretic factor to short-term changes in left atrial hemodynamics

after percutaneous balloon mitral valvuloplasty. J Am Coll Cardiol 1988;12:649–55.

151. Ishikura F, Nagata S, Hirata Y, et al. Rapid reduction of plasma atrial natriuretic peptide levels during percutaneous transvenous mitral commissurotomy in patients with mitral stenosis. Circulation 1989;79:47–50.

152. John S, Bashi VV, Jairaj PS, et al. Closed mitral valvotomy: early results and long-term follow-up of 3,742 consecutive patients. Circulation 1983;68:891–6.

153. Hickey MSJ, Blackstone EH, Kirklin JW, Dean LS. Outcome probabilities after surgical commissurotomy: implications for balloon commissurotomy. J Am Coll Cardiol (in press).

154. Borer JS, Bacharach SL, Green MV, et al. Exercise-induced left ventricular dysfunction in symptomatic and asymptomatic patients with aortic regurgitations: assessment with radionuclide cineangiography. Am J Cardiol 1978;42:351–7.

155. Shen WR, Roubin GS, Choong CYP, et al. Evaluation of relationship between myocardial contractile state and left ventricular function in patients with aortic regurgitation. Circulation 1985;71:31–8.

156. Kawanishi DT, McKay CR, Chandraratna PAN, et al. Cardiovascular response to dynamic exercise in patients with chronic symptomatic mild-to-moderate and severe aortic regurgitation. Circulation 1986;73:62–72.

157. Bonow RO, Rosing DR, McIntosh CL, et al. The natural history of asymptomatic patients with aortic regurgitation and normal left ventricular function. Circulation 1983;68:509–17.

158. Bonow RO, Picone AL, McIntosh CL, et al. Survival and functional results after valve replacement for aortic regurgitation from 1976 to 1983: impact of preoperative left ventricular function. Circulation 1985;72:1244–56.

159. McKay CR, Nanna M, Kawanishi DT, et al. Long-term hydralazine treatment in patients with symptomatic chronic aortic regurgitation: results of a prospective clinical trial (in preparation).

160. Greenberg B, Massie B, Bristow JD, et al. Long-term vasodilator therapy of chronic aortic insufficiency: a randomized double-blinded, placebo-controlled clinical trial. Circulation 1988;78:92–103.

161. Scognamiglio R, Fasoli G, Pouchia A, Dalla-Volta S. Long-term nifedipine unloading therapy in asymptomatic patients with chronic, severe aortic regurgitation. J Am Coll Cardiol 1990;16:430–2.

162. Crawford MH, Wilson RS, O'Rourke RA, Vittitoe JA. Effect of digoxin and vasodilators on left ventricular function in aortic regurgitation. Int J Cardiol 1989;23:385–93.

163. Elkayam U, Roth A, Kumar A, et al. Hemodynamic and volumetric effects of venodilation with nitroglycerin in chronic mitral regurgitation. Am J Cardiol 1987;60:1106–11.

164. Rahimtoola SH. Vasodilator therapy in chronic, severe aortic regurgitation. J Am Coll Cardiol 1990;16:430–2.

165. Roy SB, Gopinath N. Mitral stenosis. Circulation 1968;38(suppl V):V-68–76.

166. Smith N, McAnulty JH, Rahimtoola SH. Severe aortic stenosis with impaired left ventricular function and clinical heart failure: results of valve replacement. Circulation 1978;58:255–64.

167. Monrad ES, Hess OM, Murakami T, Nonogi H, Corin WJ, Krayenbuehl HP. Time course of regression of left ventricular hypertrophy after aortic valve replacement. Circulation 1988;77:1345–55.

168. Bonow RO, Dodd JT, Maron BJ, et al. Long-term serial changes in left ventricular function and reversal of ventricular dilatation after valve replacement for chronic aortic regurgitation. Circulation 1988;78:1108–20.

169. Levine HJ. Left ventricular function after correction of chronic aortic regurgitation. Circulation 1988;78:1319–21.

170. Bonow RO, Rosing DR, Maron BJ, et al. Reversal of left ventricular dysfunction after aortic valve replacement for chronic aortic regurgitation: influence of duration of preoperative left ventricular dysfunction. Circulation 1984;70:570–9.

171. Clark DG, McAnulty JH, Rahimtoola SH. Valve replacement in aortic insufficiency with left ventricular dysfunction. Circulation 1980;61:411–21.

172. Hwang MH, Hammermeister KE, Oprian C, et al. Preoperative identification of patients likely to have left ventricular dysfunction after aortic

valve replacement: participants in VA cooperative study on valvular heart disease. Circulation 1989;80(suppl I):I-65-76.

173. Bjork VO, Henze A. Management of thromboembolism after valve replacement with the Bjork-Shiley tilting disc valve. Scand J Thorac Cardiovasc Surg 1975;9:183-91.

174. Limet L, Lepage E, Grondin CM. Thromboembolic complications with the cloth covered Starr-Edwards aortic prosthesis in patients not receiving anticoagulants. Ann Thorac Surg 1977;23:529-33.

175. St. John Sutton MG, Miller GAH, Oldershaw PJ. Anticoagulants and the Bjork-Shiley prosthesis: experience of 390 patients. Br Heart J 1978;40:558-62.

176. Chaux A, Czer LSC, Matloff JM, et al. The St. Jude medical bileaflet valve prosthesis: a 5 year experience. J Thorac Cardiovasc Surg 1984;88:706-17.

177. Rahimtoola SH. Anticoagulant treatment and cardiac valvular surgery: coumadin and other alternatives. In: Matloff JM, Cardiac Valve Replacement: Current Status. The Hague: Martinus Nijhoff, 1985:25-28.

178. Baudet EM, Oca CC, Roques XF, et al. A 5½ year experience with St. Jude medical cardiac valve prosthesis: early and late results of 737 valve replacements in 671 patients. J Thorac Cardiovasc Surg 1985;90:137-44.

179. Chesbro JH, Adams PC, Fuster V. Antithrombotic therapy in patients with valvular heart disease and prosthetic heart valves. J Am Coll Cardiol 1986;8:41B-56B.

180. Cosgrove DM, Stewart WJ. Mitral valvuloplasty. Curr Probl Cardiol 1989;14:359-415.

181. Barrat-Boyes BG, Roche AHG, Subramanyan R, Pemberton JR, Whitlock RML. Long-term follow-up of patients with the antibiotic-sterilized aortic homograft inserted freehand in the aortic position. Circulation 1987;75:768-77.

182. O'Brien MF, Stafford EG, Gardner MAH, Pohlner PG, McGiffin DC. A comparison of aortic valve replacement with viable cryopreserved and fresh allograft valves, with a note on chromosomal studies. J Thorac Cardiovasc Surg 1987;94:812-23.

183. Matsuki O, Robles A, Gibb S, Bodnar E, Ross DN. Long-term performance of 555 aortic homografts in the aortic position. Ann Thorac Surg 1988;46:187-91.

184. Foster AH, Greenberg GJ, Underhill DJ, McIntosh CL, Clark RE. Intrinsic failure of Hancock mitral bioprosthesis: 10-15 year experience. Ann Thorac Surg 1987;44:568-77.

185. Gallo I, Nistal F, Blasquez R, Arbe E, Artinano E. Incidence of primary tissue valve failure in porcine bioprosthetic heart valves. Ann Thorac Surg 1988;45:66-70.

186. Jameison WRE, Rosado LJ, Muriro AI, et al. Carpentier-Edwards standard porcine bioprosthesis: primary tissue failure (structural valve deterioration) by age groups. Ann Thorac Surg 1988;46:155-62.

187. Gallucci V, Mazzucco A, Bortolotti U, Milano A, Guerra F, Thieuke G. The standard Hancock porcine bioprosthesis: overall experience at the University of Padova. J Cardiovasc Surg 1988;3(suppl):337-45.

188. Magilligan DJ Jr, Lewis JW Jr, Stein P, Alam M. The porcine bioprosthetic heart valve: experience at fifteen years. Ann Thorac Surg 1989;48:324-9.

189. Spampinato N, Stassano P, Cammarota A, et al. Bioprostheses at twelve years. J Cardiovasc Surg 1988;(suppl)3:383-90.

◆ CHAPTER 6 ◆

The Evolution of Antihypertensive Therapy: An Overview of Four Decades of Experience

GEORGE L. BAKRIS, MD,* EDWARD D. FROHLICH, MD†

Hypertension is a major public health problem amenable to treatment. Numerous large-scale clinical trials have demonstrated that effective sustained control of elevated arterial pressure to a level <140/90 mm Hg results in reduced cardiovascular morbidity and mortality. Over the past four decades, antihypertensive drug therapy has evolved from a stepwise but physiologically rational selection of agents to specific programs tailored to individualized therapy for specific clinical situations. This evolution has occurred because of a greater understanding of the pathophysiology of hypertensive diseases, the development of new classes of antihypertensive agents that attack specific pressor mechanisms and the ability to wed these concepts into a rational and specific therapeutic program. Thus, with the currently available spectrum of antihypertensive therapy, it is now possible to select treatment for special groups of patients utilizing a single agent, thus protecting the heart, brain and kidneys and maintaining organ function without exacerbating associated diseases. This transfer of careful, painstaking and purposeful investigative experiences into clinical practice has resulted in clear-cut benefits for millions of patients.

The introduction of indirect blood pressure measurement in the mid 19th century permitted the later correlation with hypertensive diseases (1). Thus, over the past 150 years, a number of fundamental and clinical concepts have been elucidated that have permitted a greater understanding of the pathophysiology of hypertensive diseases. These include a clearer understanding of pressor and depressor mechanisms involving neurohumoral, hormonal, cardiovascular and renal responses that serve to control arterial pressure (2–6). Hence, a better comprehension of these mechanisms has enabled the purposeful development and application of several different classes of therapeutic agents that intercede in the responses of these systems and ultimately correct abnormally elevated arterial pressure.

Over these past 40 years, the emergence of numerous therapeutic innovations and drug discoveries resulted in better control of hypertensive disease (Table 6.1). With greater understanding of these new classes of agents, it was possible to regulate arterial pressure and develop therapeutic regimens that have progressed from direct-acting smooth muscle-relaxing vasodilators, which require diuretic drugs to protect against intravascular fluid expansion, to more specific agents, which act on cardiovascular function through specific mechanisms that control vascular smooth muscle

tone and cardiac responses (for example, alpha- and beta-adrenoreceptor inhibition, calcium antagonism and angiotensin converting enzyme inhibition).

The evolution of these major classes of antihypertensive agents, their mechanisms of action and hemodynamic effects and their relations to specific cardiovascular risk factors are reviewed. Our discussion emphasizes their relation to specific cardiovascular problems that are associated with hypertension and suggests an evolved approach for tailoring antihypertensive therapy.

Agents That Inhibit the Sympathetic Nervous System

A number of neural mechanisms serve to modulate circulatory control of arterial pressure (6,7). These include neural afferents in baroreceptors (or mechanoreceptors) located in arteries, veins and the heart (7). Signals from these receptors travel centrally to the medullary vasomotor centers of the brain and result in efferent reflexive cardiovascular responses. These efferent impulses are conducted to the periphery by means of sympathetic and parasympathetic nerve fibers to affect changes in vessel caliber, heart rate and myocardial contractility through the release of various neurohumoral substances (namely, catecholamines, indoles and peptide hormones). The responses elicited by these impulses modulate cardiovascular and renal homeostatic regulation of arterial pressure (6–9).

Therapeutic agents that modify neural input to the cardiovascular and renal systems were among the first introduced for the management of hypertensive diseases (9). Over the years, this array of compounds has permitted the possibility of virtual pharmacologic dissection of the entire autonomic nervous system. Thus, it is possible to select agents that inhibit the outflow of impulses from various cardiovascular control centers in the brain (ganglionic neurotransmission and the release of neurohumoral substances from nerve endings) and alpha- or beta-adrenoreceptors, or both, on presynaptic nerve endings or at postsynaptic sites on cardiac and vascular smooth muscle cells (10,11).

Ganglionic Blockers

This potent group of antihypertensive agents (for example, hexamethonium and trimethaphan) was synthesized in the late 1940s and was the first group used to treat hyper-

Table 6.1. Evolutionary Use of Antihypertensive Drugs

Drugs or Drug Classes	Year
Ganglionic Blocking Agents (hexamethonium, tetraethylammonium chloride, pentdinium tartarate)	late 1940s
Rauwolfa and Veratrum Alkaloids (reserpine, cryptenamine tannate)	1931 (India) 1952 (U.S.)
Vasodilator (hydralazine)	1951
Alpha-adrenergic Receptor Blockers (phentolamine phenoxybenzamine)	1954
Thiazide Diuretics (chlorothiazide, hydrochlorothiazide, etc.)	1957
Post-Ganglionic Blocker (guanethedine)	1959
Potassium-Sparing Diuretics (spironolaetone, amiloride, triameterine)	1958–1964
Central Alpha-2 Receptor Agonist (methyldopa, clonidine)	1963 and 1974
Beta Adrenergic Receptor Blockers (propranolol)	1964 (Europe) 1974 (U.S.)
Vasodilator (minoxidil)	1968
Peripheral Alpha-1 Adrenergic Receptor Blocker (prazosin)	1976
*Calcium Channel Antagonist (verapamil)	1980
Angiotensin Converting Enzyme Inhibitor (captopril)	1981
Alpha-Beta-Adrenergic Receptor Blocker (labetalol)	1984
New Investigational Classes of Drugs: Serotonergic Receptor Antagonists (ketanserin) Selective Dopamine-1 Antagonists (fenoldopam) Renin Inhibitors	1990s

#Year approved for use as antihypertensive in U.S. unless otherwise noted. *Verapamil was synthesized and used for investigation as early as 1962 in Europe.

tension (12,13). They inhibit the neurotransmission at the thoracolumbar ganglia by blocking the action of released acetylcholine to interfere with postganglionic neuronal propagation of the impulse (13). This results in reduced sympathetic tone and arterial and venodilation. The pressure decrease is most pronounced with upright posture as a result of peripheral blood pooling and reduced venous return to the heart (13). Declines in arterial pressure, therefore, result from diminished cardiac output as well as reduced total peripheral resistance (13,14). Although these agents are less used today, they were responsible for the dramatic reversal of morbidity from malignant hypertension and other severe hypertensive complications in the early years of therapy (15). However, trimethaphan continues to be used for the management of certain hypertensive crises (for example, for dissecting aortic aneurysm and intraoperative control of arterial pressure) (15,16).

Postganglionic Adrenergic Inhibitors

Reserpine. This agent was introduced in the mid-1950s and is still widely used throughout the world. It acts by depleting neurotransmitters (for example, norepinephrine, epinephrine and serotonin) from postganglionic nerve endings as well as in the brain (11,17). As a result, arterial pressure and total peripheral resistance are reduced, heart

rate is slowed and cardiac output and renal blood flow are maintained (18,19).

The Veterans Administration Cooperative Studies (20,21) supplied some of the first evidence that low doses of reserpine (0.1 to 0.5 mg/day) in combination with a diuretic drug effectively lower arterial pressure with relatively few side effects. Shortly thereafter, these landmark multicenter studies by the Veterans Administration (22,23) demonstrated a dramatic reduction in cardiovascular morbidity and mortality and diminished progression of diseases associated with hypertension. Furthermore, studies (24–29) with a number of adrenergic inhibitors (for example, the centrally acting agents and beta-adrenoreceptor blockers, angiotensin converting enzyme inhibitors and calcium antagonists) have shown reversal of left ventricular hypertrophy, a known risk factor for myocardial infarction. In the United States, reserpine is used less often today because of the availability of other agents with fewer side effects.

Guanethidine. This agent became available for the management of hypertension in the late 1950s and remains one of the most potent sympatholytic drugs (30). It acts by depleting norepinephrine from the postganglionic nerve endings, but unlike reserpine, it has no central action (30–32). This results in reduced total peripheral resistance and venous tone, which permits a decrease in arterial pressure, particularly with assumption of upright posture. When this drug is given intravenously, it produces a transient increase in arterial pressure secondary to catecholamine release (32,33). This increase in pressure may be attenuated by pretreatment with beta-adrenergic receptor blocking drugs (11,32).

Prolonged therapy with guanethidine results in a negative cardiac chronotropic and inotropic effect secondary to myocardial catecholamine depletion (34). The reduced venous return results from peripheral venous pooling, accounting for the reduction in cardiac output and the possible decrease in blood flow to major circulatory beds, including the kidney (35). Furthermore, intravascular volume expansion attenuates its hypotensive effect, a problem that is resolved by the addition of a diuretic drug (36,37).

Guanethidine has been used less frequently in recent years, even when hypertension is severe, primarily because of the availability of other potent and specific agents having fewer side effects. However, a congener of guanethidine, guanadrel, is used for the treatment of mild to moderate hypertension in less potent dosages. Nevertheless, its mechanism of action is similar to guanethidine.

Peripheral Alpha-Adrenergic Inhibitors

The first alpha-adrenoreceptor blocking agents used to treat hypertension were phentolamine and phenoxybenzamine (38). These agents inhibit norepinephrine stimulation of both postsynaptic (alpha$_1$) and presynaptic (alpha$_2$) adrenergic receptor sites. The major clinical indications for phentolamine (an intravenous compound) or phenoxybenzamine (for oral use) are hypertensive states associated with catecholamine excess (for example, pheochromocytoma and clonidine withdrawal) (38,39). These agents, like the adrenolytic agents, also reexpand intravascular (plasma) volume associated with pressure reduction. This action has been exploited clinically in the preoperative preparation of patients with pheochromocytoma. These agents prevent intraoperative hypotension associated with tumor removal in these catecholamine-induced volume-contracted patients (39). These agents do not prevent cardiac arrhythmias associated with catecholamine excess, a problem that may be alleviated with beta-adrenoreceptor blockers (40).

The more selective alpha$_1$-receptor antagonists directly inhibit norepinephrine stimulation of these receptor sites on vascular smooth muscle without altering myocardial contractility and cardiac output or reflexively stimulating an increase in heart rate (41). This lack of reflex increase in heart rate, even with rapid pressure reduction after the first dose, has been attributed to direct alpha$_1$-receptor inhibition at the cardiac myocyte (41–43). The clinical manifestations of the "first dose phenomenon" (for example, orthostatic hypotension) may be minimized by the initial administration of prazosin at bedtime.

The alpha$_1$-adrenoreceptor inhibitors now include a number of agents (namely, prazosin, terazosin, doxazosin and indoramin), each of which dilate the arterioles and hence reduce arterial pressure (41,42). In addition to arterial pressure reduction, these agents have been used to treat patients with congestive heart failure. By virtue of their potential vasodilating effect on constricted peripheral venules, alpha$_1$-adrenoreceptor blockers reduce cardiac preload and afterload, an effect not observed in patients with uncomplicated hypertension (44). However, this beneficial effect on systemic hemodynamics, noted in early studies with prazosin, was not substantiated. Furthermore, long-term studies (44) in patients with heart failure demonstrated a tachyphylactic response with prolonged use of the drug. This response presumably is secondary to maximal alpha$_1$-adrenoreceptor blockade. Thus, the use of prazosin in patients with heart failure has diminished, although this may reflect the more recent introduction of angiotensin converting enzyme inhibitors.

Centrally Active Alpha$_2$-Receptor Agonists

Clonidine. This drug, an imidazoline derivative, is a prototype of agents that stimulate central alpha$_2$-receptors (45,46). It is chemically related to tolazoline and phentolamine, although it has little direct peripheral vasodilating effects in therapeutic dosages (46). Clonidine acts by stimulating alpha$_2$-receptors in the nucleus tractus solitarii of the brain, which in turn decrease central adrenergic outflow to the heart, vessels and kidney (47). Thus, the resultant decrease in arterial pressure is not accompanied by reflex tachycardia (46,48). Interestingly, the hypotensive effect of

central alpha$_2$-receptor agonists, is attenuated in the presence of tricyclic antidepressant medications, a response that is apparently independent of the alpha$_2$-receptor (49).

With long-term treatment, clonidine decreases total peripheral resistance in both supine and standing positions. Furthermore, in response to exercise, cardiac output and oxygen consumption remain unchanged compared with pretreatment values (49). In addition, clonidine does not alter renal blood flow, glomerular filtration rate or renal sodium handling; however, renin release is suppressed (50).

Clonidine acts promptly and, when administered at hourly intervals, may be useful in treating hypertensive urgencies and emergencies (15). If clonidine is abruptly withdrawn, rebound hypertension may ensue and may be associated with a hypertensive crisis (51). However, the newer and longer-acting agents (for example, guanabenz and guanfacine) may not be associated with this adverse effect (52). Other side effects produced by clonidine and shared by all central alpha$_2$-receptor agonists include drowsiness, dry mouth and impaired sexual function (19,46). These problems may limit their clinical usefulness.

Methyldopa. This agent is the other prototype of a centrally active alpha$_2$-receptor agonist. It was synthesized in the early 1950s and described as a dopa-decarboxylase inhibitor (53). Later, false neurohumoral transmission (54) and other antihypertensive mechanisms, including direct inhibition of central vasomotor centers (55) and renal suppression of renin release (56), were suggested. At present, it appears to act similar to clonidine, although it must be initially metabolized in the nuclei tractus solitarii neurons to alpha-methyl-norepinephrine, the direct central alpha$_2$-receptor agonist (57).

Hemodynamically, methyldopa acts promptly (within a few hours) to reduce arterial pressure through a slight decrease in cardiac output that is associated with a diminished total peripheral resistance (58,59). This decline in output is transient and does not affect renal blood flow or glomerular filtration rate. Thus, renal function is preserved even in patients with renal insufficiency (10,60). In addition to the side effects detailed for clonidine, hepatocellular dysfunction and a Coombs-positive hemolytic anemia have been described with methyldopa administration (10,11,19).

Beta-Adrenergic Receptor Antagonists

Pronethalol was the first beta-adrenoreceptor blocker synthesized (61), but it was not used clinically because of adverse effects. Shortly thereafter, propranolol, a beta$_1$- and beta$_2$-adrenoreceptor blocker, was introduced for the treatment of angina pectoris and hypertension (62). Since then, many other compounds have been introduced, including agents that are more water-soluble (naldolol and atenolol) (63,64), agents with intrinsic sympathomimetic activity (oxyprenolol, pindolol and acebutolol) (65,66) and those with some degree of cardioselectivity (atenolol, metoprolol and acebutolol) (64,66–68). Notwithstanding these varied characteristics, in the dosages employed for the treatment of hypertension and angina pectoris, their more receptor-specific actions appear to have little variance. Despite their widespread use over the past 25 years, their antihypertensive action remains unresolved. However, a number of mechanisms have been postulated, including decreased cardiac output (69), resetting of arterial baroreceptors (70), reduced circulating plasma renin activity (71), central adrenoreceptor stimulation (19,72) and peripheral alteration of catecholamine release (73).

Hemodynamically, the beta-adrenoreceptor inhibitors decrease heart rate, cardiac output and myocardial oxygen consumption and increase total peripheral resistance (66,69). Conversely, renal blood flow and glomerular filtration rate are maintained despite a reduction in cardiac output in the supine position (66). However, studies (74) examining the renal effects of propranolol demonstrate that quiet standing significantly decreases renal blood flow and results in avid sodium retention in normal and hypertensive subjects. Whereas these agents are useful in patients with uncomplicated essential hypertension and ischemic heart disease, their cardiac and renal hemodynamic effects and other metabolic effects may preclude their use in other groups of patients (for example, diabetes mellitus, congestive heart failure, pulmonary disease and peripheral arterial insufficiency).

These agents may also have adverse effects on lipid profiles (75,76), and some studies (76) have shown that nonspecific beta-blockers increase triglycerides and decrease the high density lipoprotein (HDL)/low density lipoprotein (LDL) cholesterol ratio; no such adverse effects on the HDL/LDL cholesterol ratio have been shown with agents having intrinsic sympathomimetic activity. Nevertheless a number of large-scale, double-blind, prospective trials (77–84) with beta-adrenoreceptor blockers clearly demonstrate a reduction in cardiovascular morbidity and mortality and improved myocardial preservation. Thus, these agents serve to protect patients with prior myocardial infarction from increased myocardial oxygen demands and high circulating catecholamine levels, factors that contribute to cardiac arrhythmias in this setting. Furthermore, these agents diminish the mass of the hypertrophied left ventricle (85) and improve symptoms from angina pectoris (86).

Several studies (77,80,82,84) have compared the effects of the thiazide diuretic drugs with beta-blockers (most notably, propranolol). Two trials conducted by the Medical Research Council and the Australian Mild Hypertension Group (77,79) demonstrated that thiazide diuretic drugs protected hypertensive patients who were smokers from subsequent stroke better than propranolol, even though they were equally efficacious in controlling arterial pressure. At present, however, there is no available explanation for this finding.

Combined Alpha- and Beta-Blocker

Labetalol combines (within the same molecule) nonselective beta-adrenoreceptor as well as alpha$_1$-receptor inhibitory properties. This agent lowers arterial pressure by reducing total peripheral resistance without changing rest heart rate or cardiac output (87,88). Thus, when administered intravenously, arterial pressure promptly decreases without the reflex stimulation of the heart (88). Hence, this agent is useful in patients with hypertension and other concomitant problems (namely, symptomatic coronary arterial disease, congestive heart failure or hypertensive emergencies with and without dissecting aneurysm) (89).

Diuretic Drugs

Repeated studies (90) have demonstrated that the prevalence of hypertension in any particular culture is directly related to the dietary sodium intake of its population. Moreover, in those cultures that consume <60 mEq of sodium daily, arterial pressure does not increase with aging and hypertension is virtually nonexistent. In contrast, hypertension is highly prevalent in those industrialized societies in which sodium intake is higher (90,91). Diuretic drugs seem to offset these effects by their natriuretic action and, when employed as single agents for the management of hypertension, have been effective for >30 years (92). Several mechanisms have been proposed for their antihypertensive action, including intravascular volume contraction, reduced vascular responsiveness to naturally occurring vasoconstrictor substances, enhanced responsiveness to depressor substances, decreased sodium content of the arterial wall, altered transmembrane ionic exchange, diminished baroreceptor activity, induction of local tissue dilators (for example, kinins and prostacylins) in the arterial wall and a direct vasodilating action on the arteriole (92,93).

The initial hemodynamic effect of diuretic drugs relates to decreased cardiac output in response to intravascular volume contraction produced by diuresis (92). However, within several weeks, plasma volume and cardiac output return toward pretreatment levels and total peripheral resistance decreases. Thus, the net long-term hemodynamic effect of diuretic therapy is reduced total peripheral resistance with minimal decreases in plasma and extracellular fluid volumes. Diuretic drugs also induce a sustained increase in plasma renin activity; when therapy is stopped (even after several years), plasma volume expands and plasma renin activity decreases (92,93). This effect has been employed in treating patients with low renin essential hypertension to optimize conditions for angiotensin converting enzyme inhibitors (94).

Most of the major clinical trials have employed diuretic drugs for initial monotherapy of essential hypertension and, more recently, the Systolic Hypertension in the Elderly Program (SHEP) (95) has used them for the treatment of isolated systolic hypertension. Moreover, the European Working Party Trial for Hypertension in the Elderly and the

Medical Research Council Trial (77,80) have reaffirmed the safety and efficacy of these agents for the treatment of diastolic hypertension in elderly patients. Thus, diuretic drugs continue to be recommended as one of four major classes of therapeutic agents for first time antihypertensive therapy (96).

Diuretic drugs have important metabolic side effects that may bear on their use in other clinical conditions (for example, hypokalemia, diabetes mellitus, hyperlipidemia, renal diseases and gout) (11,81). Hypokalemia has been implicated in the Multiple Risk Factor Intervention Trial (MRFIT) (81) as a possible factor accounting for sudden death in patients with cardiac involvement. As a result, the Joint National Committee on the Detection, Evaluation and Treatment of High Blood Pressure (96) recommended reduced dosages of diuretic drugs for pressure control because they are equally effective and induce less disturbing hypokalemia. Moreover, sodium restriction in patients treated with diuretic drugs diminishes potassium wastage abetted by the induced hyperaldosteronism. Therefore, it seems reasonable to administer lower doses of the thiazide diuretic drugs (for example, 12.5 to 25 mg of hydrochlorothiazide) and, if necessary, to prescribe a potassium-sparing agent (for example, spironolactone, triameterene or amiloride) to protect patients with left ventricular hypertrophy, cardiac failure, digitalis therapy or long-term diarrhea from further ventricular irritability resulting from hypokalemia (96).

Angiotensin Converting Enzyme Inhibitors

The finding of Yang et al. (97) that snake venom contains an enzyme that converts angiotensin I to angiotensin II, a potent vasoconstrictor, supplied a critical link in the understanding of the renin-angiotensin system. With this knowledge, Ondetti et al. (98) were the first to describe a group of angiotensin converting enzyme inhibitors and illustrate their importance as agents for lowering arterial pressure. This work then led to human investigations (99–102) on the role of the renin-angiotensin system in both hypertensive and heart failure states.

The first angiotensin converting enzyme inhibitor was developed in the 1970s and introduced in the early 1980s for the treatment of hypertension (Table 6.1). These agents have emerged over the past 10 years as a major therapeutic option for the initial treatment of hypertension (102,103). They inhibit the conversion of angiotensin I to angiotensin II and inactivate circulating bradykinin, a potent naturally occurring vasodilating agent. Furthermore, they interfere with the interaction of angiotensin II with norepinephrine and with local tissue prostacyclin. They also reduce the formation of the heptapetide, angiotensin III, that ultimately stimulates the adrenal cortical synthesis of aldosterone, thus decreasing a known sodium-retaining hormone (102). Hemodynamically, these agents lower arterial pressure by reducing total peripheral resistance without increasing heart rate, cardiac output or myocardial contractility. Renal blood flow may increase without altering glomerular filtration rate, thereby reducing the glomerular filtration rate (104,105).

In the mid-1970s studies utilized angiotensin converting enzyme inhibitors to demonstrate a marked reduction in arterial pressure among hypertensive patients, as well as significant improvement in patients with congestive heart failure (99,106,107). Other investigators followed up with similar results. In a multicenter study, captopril (50 to 75 mg/day) controlled arterial pressure in patients with mild to moderate hypertension (105) and was as effective as hydrochlorothiazide (50 mg/day) (105,108,109). Captopril, enalapril and lisinopril are equally effective in reducing arterial pressure in patients with hypertension and have a low side effect profile. Nevertheless, they should be used with extreme caution in patients with functional renal impairment and those receiving potassium supplements or potassium-sparing agents, which may lead to hyperkalemia either by exacerbating renal insufficiency or inhibiting aldosterone production (110,111). Likewise, they should not be administered to patients with bilateral renal arterial disease or arterial disease of solitary kidneys because renal failure and malignant hypertension may be produced (112–114).

Angiotensin converting enzyme inhibitors are particularly effective in hypertensive patients with high plasma renin activity states, including congestive heart failure (107). These agents are also effective in patients with normal or low plasma renin activity and in anephric individuals presumably because of the pressure of the renin-angiotensin system in vascular smooth muscle, myocardial and other extra-renal cells (102,103). Because of their beneficial renal hemodynamic effects, angiotensin converting enzyme inhibitors are useful in patients with diabetes mellitus and collagen vascular diseases (105,110).

Calcium Antagonists

These agents represent another new class of antihypertensive compounds. Verapamil was the first to be synthesized (in the late 1950s), but was not made available for treatment of hypertension in the United States for almost 30 years. At present, a large number of such compounds have been approved for the treatment of hypertension and heart disease, including nifedipine, diltiazem, nicardipine, isradipine, nitrendipine and others (96). Although all these agents are classified as calcium antagonists, they differ greatly with respect to chemical structure, physiologic action and related cardiovascular and renal hemodynamic problems.

Vasoconstriction, myocardial contractility and cardiac automaticity all depend on transmembrane calcium fluxes, and altered permeability of the calcium ion in these cells results in changes in vessel caliber and cardiac function (115–119). As a result, calcium antagonists reduce intracellular influx of calcium, which results in reduced binding to the calmodulin and thus reduced contraction.

The calcium antagonists all produce arteriolar dilation and reduce arterial pressure, with variable effects on cardiac output and myocardial contractility. Verapamil alters heart rate conduction, whereas nifedipine reflexively increases heart rate. Diltiazem has little effect on heart rate and depresses myocardial contractility less than does verapamil.

In general, most studies have revealed that the calcium antagonists are as effective as the other classes of agents for reducing arterial pressure. They do so while maintaining cardiac output and renal blood flow as total peripheral and organ vascular resistances decrease (119–121). Diltiazem, however, increases renal blood flow, while maintaining glomerular filtration rate by lowering efferent glomerular arteriolar resistance and hence glomerular capillary pressure (122). Furthermore, in preliminary studies (123) involving diabetic hypertensive subjects, diltiazem was shown to reduce urinary protein excretion to a similar degree as angiotensin converting enzyme inhibitors. Verapamil has been shown to reduce proteinuria in a renal ablation model of nephropathy (124). Conversely, nifedipine actually increases urinary protein excretion in patients with preexisting renal insufficiency (125,126). Thus, these studies should help guide the choice of calcium antagonists in this group of patients.

The side effects of calcium antagonists are minimal. The most frequent side effect of verapamil is constipation; diltiazem and nifedipine produce edema, and nifedipine produces headache, flushing and dizziness (119,120).

Direct-Acting Vasodilators

Hydralazine. This drug was one of the first antihypertensive agents to produce arteriolar dilation and decreased total peripheral resistance through direct action on arteriolar smooth muscle (127,128). Many studies have attested to the efficacy of hydralazine in lowering arterial pressure (129,130), but its principal clinical usefulness has been as an adjunct to other therapies (131,132). In the Veterans Administration Cooperative Study (22), hydralazine produced an additional decrease in mean arterial pressure of 7 mm Hg after the addition of hydrochlorothiazide. Several other studies (133,134) showed that the combination of thiazide and hydralazine produced an additional mean decrease of 11 mm Hg in patients with mild to moderate hypertension.

The usefulness of hydralazine is limited by several side effects, including reflex sympathetic stimulation and tachycardia (135). This increase in heart rate that generally accompanies hydralazine has been associated with precipitation of myocardial infarction in high risk patients (134). It does not adversely affect plasma lipids or glucose; however, it may increase the antinuclear antibody titer consistent with a diagnosis of lupus erythematosus, hepatitis or peripheral neuropathy in a dose-related fashion (134,136,137).

Minoxidil. This agent was initially synthesized in 1965; however, it was not approved for use as an antihypertensive

agent until 1980. It is a potent vasodilator that acts directly on arteriolar smooth muscle cells, thus, reducing total peripheral resistance without modifying sympathetic nervous system responses or increasing venous capacitance (138). Early studies (138,139) demonstrated its effectiveness in combination with propranolol in patients with refractory hypertension, and it has been particularly useful in severely hypertensive patients with chronic renal failure receiving hemodialysis. Its limitations include marked sodium and water retention, edema, pulmonary hypertension and hirsutism (140,141). Pericardial effusion, angina pectoris and lupus reactions have been associated with minoxidil (11,141,142). Thus, minoxidil should not be used as a single agent and should be reserved for patients with refractory hypertension who have failed triple drug therapy.

Miscellaneous New Compounds

Several new and unique compounds have been synthesized to evaluate the pathophysiologic alterations in hypertension. They include agents that antagonize serotonin, the statine-substituted peptides that inhibit renin and selective dopamine$_1$-receptor antagonists (143–148).

Ketanserin is a selective (S$_2$) serotonergic antagonist with additional alpha$_1$-adrenoreceptor blocking properties. The interaction between the two receptors seems to be necessary for its antihypertensive action (143,144). After its intravenous administration, arterial pressure decreases, with minimal associated cardiovascular reflexive changes. Several studies (143,144) have shown that ketanserin is more effective in elderly rather than younger patients. Its major side effects include dizziness, somnolence and dry mouth, similar to those commonly observed with the centrally acting alpha$_2$-agonists.

The renin inhibitors are peptides with an unusual amino acid, statine, in their structures. These agents inhibit human renin and have promise in the management of hypertension and as a physiologic probe. Although most studies (145,146) have been performed in primates and animals with experimental hypertension, renin inhibitors have been given to human patients. Oral administration to conscious sodium-depleted marmosets resulted in a significant blood pressure reduction secondary to complete inhibition of plasma renin activity (145).

Dopamine infusion increases arterial pressure, but infusion of the selective dopamine$_1$-agonist, fenoldopam, reduces arterial pressure, while increasing renal blood flow and sodium excretion (147,148). Studies in human patients (147,148) have documented that arterial pressure is lowered by selective dopamine$_1$-receptor stimulation through a decrease in total peripheral resistance with associated reflex cardiovascular stimulation.

A Perspective on the Treatment of Arterial Hypertension

The Veterans Administration Cooperative Studies (96) over the past 30 years have clearly demonstrated reduced morbidity and mortality with adequate control of arterial pressure. These initial multicenter studies were followed by numerous large-scale clinical trials (149,150) involving >50,000 patients, all of which confirm this observation. In the earlier studies, a diuretic agent was prescribed initially and, if necessary, an antiadrenergic agent (for example, reserpine, methyldopa or a beta-blocker) was added, followed by a direct-acting smooth muscle vasodilator (that is, hydralazine). This stepped-care approach was both physiologically rational and empirically sound. The diuretic agent was added first to prevent pseudotolerance of the expansion of intravascular volume with the second- and third-step agents (36,37). However, more recently (36,37,63,66,101, 119–121), other classes of antihypertensive agents were introduced and found to be as effective as "first-step" therapy; these include the beta-adrenoreceptor inhibitors, calcium antagonists and the angiotensin converting enzyme inhibitors. Thus, all four classes of compound reduce pressure without intravascular volume expansion. Moreover, continued use of these agents has provided considerable insight into their efficacy in the treatment of concomitant diseases frequently encountered in patients with hypertension. With this additional information, it is now possible to tailor a therapeutic regimen for individual patients, especially those with multiple diseases in which one agent may serve the purpose of treating more than one disease.

Coronary Artery Disease

Ischemic heart disease is usually associated with arterial spasm or atherosclerotic occlusive disease of the coronary arteries. Patients with hypertension and coronary artery disease have increased myocardial tension and oxygen demands on the basis of the elevated pressure and increased cardiac size; this may be aggravated by the restricted blood flow resulting from coronary artery disease (86). Thus, an ideal therapeutic agent in these patients would be one that improves coronary circulation, decreases pressure overload imposed on the left ventricle and reduces myocardial oxygen demand.

Coronary artery disease is a major cause of death in the United States, and hypertension is among its leading treatable risk factors (151). Many studies (20–23,77–84,149,150) investigating the interrelation between hypertension and other risk factors associated with the development of coronary artery disease utilized a variety of antihypertensive agents to demonstrate that a reduction in arterial pressure reduced the overall morbidity and mortality. Beta-adrenoreceptor blocking agents were used in many of these studies (78–84) because they have the advantage of reducing the "double product" (that is, the product of systolic pressure and heart rate), which is a major determinant of myocardial tension. Thus, these agents reduce myocardial oxygen demand and improve myocardial performance (25). Because of their peripheral vasoconstrictive effects, beta-adrenoreceptor blockers should be used with caution in patients with diffuse peripheral vascular disease. However, naldolol and atenolol have been shown to improve the renal circulation in patients with hypertension (63,64).

Most beta-adrenoreceptor blockers tend to adversely affect lipid profiles (for example, decrease the HDL/LDL cholesterol ratio). However, this ratio is not affected by beta-adrenoreceptor antagonists with intrinsic sympathomimetic activity (75,76). These agents primarily increase the LDL component in the blood, whereas others may have effects on triglycerides (76).

Most large-scale clinical trials (78–84) have also utilized diuretic drugs alone or in combination with other agents for control of arterial hypertension in patients with coronary artery disease. Because these agents may produce various electrolyte and metabolic side effects (for example, hypokalemia, hyperglycemia, increased cholesterol levels and hyperuricemia) (10,11), it is possible that they might have attenuated their overall effectiveness in preventing myocardial infarction and sudden death (81,152). Hypokalemia associated with an abnormal electrocardiogram or left ventricular hypertrophy may increase the incidence of death in patients with coronary heart disease independent of their effect on blood pressure (81,153). Thus, patients using diuretic drugs should have their serum potassium levels monitored carefully (and corrected if necessary) to prevent these problems. Moreover, if single agent therapy is desired and hypercholesterolemia is of concern, it might be prudent to use an alternative single agent (for example, a calcium antagonist or an angiotensin converting enzyme inhibitor). These latter agents usually do not significantly alter serum potassium, glucose, uric acid or lipids, each of which contribute to the risk of coronary artery disease (98,154).

Angiotensin converting enzyme inhibitors reduce total peripheral resistance without increasing heart rate and therefore serve to reduce myocardial oxygen demand while maintaining renal blood flow (104,155). Likewise, calcium antagonists also attenuate the peripheral vasoconstrictor response to catecholamines and alter calcium influx into vascular smooth muscle, thereby reducing coronary arterial spasm and myocardial oxygen demand while improving coronary blood flow (116–118,156). Furthermore, calcium antagonists have been shown in experimental studies (157) to reduce atherogenesis, a major factor in the pathogenesis of coronary artery disease. Therefore, the optimal agents for the treatment of hypertension in patients with coronary artery disease would be those groups of drugs that control arterial pressure without adversely effecting electrolytes, plasma lipids or other metabolic processes, thereby improving myocardial oxygen demand and left ventricular afterload. It follows that the calcium channel antagonists, angiotensin converting enzyme inhibitors and some beta-adrenoreceptor blockers would be optimal for this group of patients.

Myocardial Infarction

Hypertension has a profound deleterious effect on the clinical course of patients with acute myocardial infarction or unstable angina pectoris (158). The elevated arterial pressure that results in increased ventricular afterload and outflow tract impedance also increases myocardial oxygen demand, further limiting ventricular function (86). Many studies (159,160,162) have shown that a reduction in pressure, especially with agents that reduce myocardial oxygen consumption, preserves or improves myocardial function and reserve. Such agents reduce the incidence of death after a myocardial infarction and include the beta-adrenoreceptor blockers without intrinsic sympathomimetic activity and the calcium antagonist, diltiazem, in patients with non Q wave infarction (161,162). However, none of the calcium antagonists and only the beta-adrenoreceptor antagonist, timolol, have been shown to limit infarct size or prevent myocardial infarction (159,163). Likewise, angiotensin converting enzyme inhibitors have not prevented reinfarction of myocardium, although in preliminary trials, (163–168), captopril has been shown to protect the heart from developing cardiac failure after myocardial infarction. This has been attributed to "remodeling" of the myocardium; however, the mechanism is unclear. As a group, angiotensin converting enzyme inhibitors are beneficial in these patients because they reduce total peripheral resistance and myocardial oxygen demand, but do not increase heart rate in the postmyocardial infarction period (164).

Clearly, arterial pressure control through venodilation with nitrates and other antihypertensive agents has been shown to relieve symptoms of coronary ischemia. However, in contrast to the aforementioned drugs, agents such as nitroprusside and nitroglycerin, while reducing pressure and improving coronary blood flow, increase heart rate and myocardial oxygen demand (159). Thus, drugs that reduce myocardial oxygen demand, improve pump function and diminish end-diastolic volume and myocardial tension are preferred in this clinical setting.

Finally, recent reports (84,169) have suggested that patients with hypertension who are treated vigorously with antihypertensive agents and whose diastolic arterial pressure is reduced to <90 mm Hg may demonstrate a greater predisposition to myocardial infarction and an increased incidence of death. This so-called "J-shaped" curve of cardiovascular morbidity and mortality has been explained variously by an excessive reduction in pressure and too vigorous use of antihypertensive agents (170,171). A further possibility is that these patients with greater pressure reduction had more severe hypertension and vascular disease that required the greater decrement in diastolic pressure. Clearly, this is an area of current controversy that demands clarification.

Congestive Heart Failure

Approximately 500,000 people develop congestive heart failure each year in the United States, and hypertension is the major causative factor (172). In those patients with hypertension-induced left ventricular failure, the primary goal of therapy is to control pressure and ultimately reduce left ventricular pressure overload. This involves the use of agents that diminish left ventricular preload and afterload, as well as those that reestablish normal electrolyte balance by attenuating the effects of secondary hyperaldosteronism (165–168). Angiotensin converting enzyme inhibitors, alone or in conjunction with diuretic drugs or digitalis, are particularly useful in this setting.

One factor that has correlated with the incidence of death in patients with congestive heart failure is elevated plasma catecholamine levels (173). However, other humoral pressor substances, such as vasopressin and angiotensin II, are also elevated in cardiac failure (174). Pharmacologic agents that modify these hormonal actions would improve myocardial function.

Several studies (99,106,107,158,161,165,175,176) have evaluated the role of calcium antagonists, angiotensin converting enzyme inhibitors, beta-adrenoreceptor blockers, diuretic drugs and vasodilators in the improvement of ventricular function in patients with congestive heart failure with or without hypertension. These studies have shown that the mortality rate is reduced by ≥50% in patients with New York Heart Association class IV congestive heart failure. Furthermore, they demonstrate that beta-adrenoreceptor blockers and calcium antagonists are relatively contraindicated in patients with severe cardiac failure.

The advent of angiotensin converting enzyme inhibitors provided an important new tool in the armentarium for treating congestive heart failure. Although vasodilators improve myocardial function, they are known to increase myocardial oxygen demand and heart rate. Gavras et al. showed that ACE inhibitors improve myocardial performance by decreasing afterload and preload; a process that was independent of baseline arterial pressure on plasma renin activity. As previously mentioned, these agents also decrease myocardial oxygen demand and do not cause tachycardia. They also preferentially dilate vital organs (heart, kidney, brain) which probably enables patients to tolerate lower arterial pressures (155,177). Furthermore, ACE inhibitors, in part, attenuate aldosterone synthesis, thereby alleviating sodium retention seen with congestive heart failure. Thus, these agents attenuate the pathophysiologic consequence of low perfusion states.

Diuretic therapy in cardiac failure is fraught with the intrinsic danger of electrolyte problems, specifically, hypokalemia, hypomagnesemia, and alkalosis (81,151). The ACE inhibitors will help circumvent this problem by permitting lower doses of diuretics to be used (94). Recent studies have suggested that the shorter acting ACE inhibitors might have an advantage over the more long-acting agents, possibly due to their effects on renal function in patients with heart failure (178). Thus, in patients with congestive heart failure the ACT inhibitors, and perhaps cautiously administered calcium blockers, are indicated for the control of arterial pressure. These agents would serve to complement the therapeutic armamentarium of diuretics, digitalis, and nitrates.

Mitral Valve Prolapse

This problem has been related to a variety of causes ranging from myxomatous generation of the mitral valve leaflets to the functional creation of prolapse by enhanced myocardial contractility on the posterior valve leaflet (179). Hemodynamically, this may result in mitral regurgitation, as well as cardiac dysrhythmias and chest discomfort. When hypertension is present, left ventricular hypertrophy may also occur.

Agents that have been beneficial to relieve the symptoms associated with mitral valve prolapse—the altered function as well as the elevated arterial pressure—include the β-adrenoreceptor blocking agents or calcium antagonists (179).

Hyperkinetic Heart Syndrome

Many patients with hypertension, particularly young patients with a milder degree of disease severity, have a hyperdynamic circulation that is manifested by a higher cardiac output, faster heart rate, increased myocardial contractility, and oxygen consumption, and (in some) increased responsiveness to circulating catecholamines (180–181). The mechanism for the increase in cardiac output has been shown to be increased adrenergic function or enhanced β-adrenoreceptor responsiveness. Clinically, these patients complain of palpitations, extra heart beats, and tachycardia; sometimes their symptoms are reproducible or aggravated by isoproterenol infusion (182). The β-adrenoreceptor blocking agents appear to be best for this population. However, if they are contraindicated secondary to other preexisting medical conditions, other adrenergic inhibitors, or the calcium antagonists, may serve as an alternative therapy.

Left Ventricular Hypertrophy

Several studies have shown that left ventricular hypertrophy, as assessed by echocardiography, is common in patients with hypertension (183–185). This hypertrophy is an independent risk factor for cardiovascular morbidity and mortality (153,184–186). Since the increased geometry of the left ventricle is a major determinant of ventricular tension, this (and the increased intraventricular systolic pressure) may explain some of this risk (86). Left ventricular hypertrophy impairs coronary arterial blood flow. This impairment leads to a relative coronary ischemia in the presence of atherosclerotic occlusive coronary disease, a process further exacerbated by hypertension (85–86). Thus, control of arterial pressure will reduce myocardial oxygen consumption and help potentiate regression of left ventricular hypertrophy (24–25).

Most agents that reduce arterial pressure, and maintain that reduction over a long period of time, will decrease left ventricular mass, although minoxidil may actually increase left ventricular mass further in spite of arterial pressure regulation (186). Of the agents that diminish left ventricular mass, some have been shown experimentally as well as clinically to work faster than others (187–188). Thus, within three weeks experimentally, and from four to 12 weeks clinically, the centrally active adrenergic inhibitors, the ACE inhibitors, and calcium antagonists reduce left ventricular mass (25–29).

The mechanisms whereby these drugs seem to diminish left ventricular mass is unknown; however, they seem to involve nonhemodynamic as well as hemodynamic factors (188). Methyldopa is the prototype of the centrally acting agents (27–29). Clonidine does not reduce mass unless the dose providing equivalent hemodynamic effects as methyldopa is tripled; then it acts as a peripheral α-adrenergic receptor agonist to increase pressure and total peripheral resistance (28). Further adding to this intriguing hemodynamic/nonhemodynamic dissociation is the finding that methyldopa reduces the mass of the nonhypertrophied left ventricles of normotensive rats as well as of nonhypertrophied right ventricles (28,189). The ACE inhibitors and calcium antagonists also reduce left ventricular mass in experimental as well as clinical hypertension (97,118–121,187–188,190–191). It is of interest that they do not decrease right ventricular mass, although some ACE inhibitors may also diminish the mass of nonhypertrophied normotensive rat left ventricles (190).

Clinical studies have yet to demonstrate the record of risk from regression of left ventricular hypertrophy, although a preliminary report from the Framingham Heart Study supplies some data (192). Still to be demonstrated is the improvement of risk with reversal of ventricular hypertrophy independent of arterial pressure control. Moreover, there are no clinical studies showing improved function of the left ventricle with pharmacologically reduced mass. Methyldopa (189) and captopril (193), in fact, showed no improvement or even deterioration of left ventricular pumping ability at normal or elevated arterial pressures. Clearly, this is an active area of study and new and exciting information will, no doubt, be forthcoming in the near future.

Peripheral Vascular Disease

The most common diseases of the aorta and peripheral vessels are aneurysms and occlusive arterial disease (194). They are more commonly seen in patients with diabetes mellitus, hyperlipidemia, and/or hypertension (194–195). Cigarette smoking significantly increases the probability of occlusive arterial disease in this population (195). It would seem that agents that control elevated arterial pressure should improve peripheral vascular disease; however, until recently, this had not been demonstrated. Agents such as calcium antagonists, angiotensin converting enzyme inhibitors and alpha$_1$-adrenoreceptor blockers, which do not exacerbate symptoms of peripheral arterial insufficiency, have been useful in controlling arterial pressure in these patients. Conversely, beta-adrenoreceptor blockers would be expected to exacerbate symptoms of claudication by their peripheral vasoconstricting effect (66).

Antihypertensive drugs that should be selected to manage patients with dissecting aortic aneurysms should decrease arterial pressure without reflexively increasing the shearing forces on the aortic wall (11,15). The ganglionic blocker trimethaphan, the combined and alpha/beta-adrenoreceptor blocking agent, labetalol, possibly the angiotensin converting enzyme inhibitor, enalaprilat and sodium nitroprusside satisfy these criteria. The vasodilators, hydralazine and diazoxide, are contraindicated unless there is pre-existing protection with a beta-adrenoreceptor blocking drug (11,15).

Conclusions

In light of these advances in our understanding of the pathophysiology and pharmacology of hypertension, its management should no longer be considered empiric. The clinician now has the opportunity to prescribe therapy that will control arterial pressure and provide benefit to the heart, kidneys and other organs without exacerbating concomitant diseases (for example, gout, diabetes and hyperlipidemia) or create new problems. Moreover, with continuing advances, and new focus on the molecular mechanisms of disease and the design of new therapy (for example, renin inhibitors), enlightened insights into the pathophysiology of hypertension and more specific therapy will no doubt ensue. These past four decades have been exciting and satisfying. Those ahead will be astounding.

We extend our gratitude and appreciation to Peggy Bourque for excellent secretarial assistance in typing the manuscript.

References

1. Major RH, ed. A History of Medicine. Springfield, IL: Charles C. Thomas, 1954:610–1.
2. Goldblatt H, Lynch J, Hanzal RF, Summerville WW. Studies on experimental hypertension: production of persistent elevation of systolic blood pressure by means of renal ischemia. J Exp Med 1934;59:347–79.
3. Page IH. On the nature of the pressor action of renin. J Exp Med 1939;70:521–9.
4. Von Euler US. A specific sympathomimetic ergone in adrenergic nerve fibers and its relation to adrenalin and noradrenalin. Acta Physiol Scand 1946;12:73–97.
5. Cuche JL, Kuchel O, Barbeau A, Langlois Y, Boucher R, Genest J. Autonomic nervous system and benign essential hypertension in man. I. Usual blood pressure, catecholamines, renin and their interrelationships. Circ Res 1974;35:281–9.
6. Frohlich ED, Messerli FH, Re RE, Dunn FG. Mechanisms controlling arterial pressure. In: Frohlich ED, ed. Pathophysiology: Altered Regulatory Mechanisms in Disease. 3rd ed. Philadelphia: Lippincott, 1984: 45–81.
7. Eckstein JW, Abboud FM. Circulatory effects of sympathomimetic amines. Am Heart J 1962;63:119–35.
8. Alquist R. A study of the adrenotropic receptor. Am J Physiol 1948;153: 586–600.
9. Nickerson M. The pharmacology of adrenergic blockade. Pharmacol Rev 1949;1:27–101.
10. Blaschke TF, Melmon KL. Antihypertensive agents and drug therapy in hypertension. In: Goodman AG, Goodman LS, Gilman A, eds. The Pharmacological Basis of Therapeutics. 6th ed. New York: Macmillan, 1980:793–810.
11. Gerber JG, Nies AS. Pharmacology of antihypertensive drugs. In: Genest J, Kuchel O, Hamet P, Cautin M, eds. Hypertension: Physiopathology and Treatment. 2nd ed. New York: McGraw-Hill, 1983;1093–127.
12. Paton WD, Zaimis EJ. The methonium compounds. Pharmacol Rev 1952;4:219–53.
13. Freis ED, Rose JC, Partenope EA, et al. The hemodynamic effects of hypotensive drugs in man: III. hexamethonium. J Clin Invest 1953;32:1285–98.
14. Wang HH, Liu LM, Katz RL. A comparison of the cardiovascular effects of sodium nitroprusside and trimethaphan. Anesthesiology 1977;46:40–8.
15. Vidt DG. Current concepts in treatment of hypertensive emergencies. Am Heart J 1986;111:220–5.
16. Bhatia S, Frohlich ED. Hemodynamic comparisons of agents useful in hypertensive emergencies. Am Heart J 1973;85:367–73.
17. Iggo A, Vogt M. Preganglionic sympathetic activity in normal and in reserpine treated cats. J Physiol 1960;150:114–20.
18. Moyer JG. Cardiovascular and renal hemodynamic response to reserpine and clinical results of using this agent for treatment of hypertension. Ann NY Acad Sci 1954;59:82–94.
19. Frohlich ED. Inhibition of adrenergic function in the treatment of hypertension. Arch Intern Med 1974;133:1033–48.
20. Veterans Administration Multi-Clinic Cooperative Study on Antihypertensive Agents. A double blind control study of antihypertensive agents. Arch Intern Med 1960;106:133–42.
21. Veterans Administration Cooperative Study on Antihypertensive Agents. Double-blind control study on the comparative effectiveness of reserpine, reserpine and hydralazine and three ganglionic blocking agents, chlorisondamine, mecamylamune and pentolinium tartrate. Arch Intern Med 1962;110:222–9.
22. Veterans Administration Cooperative Study Group on Antihypertensive Agents. Effects of treatment in morbidity in hypertension: results in patients with diastolic blood pressure averaging 115 through 120 mm Hg. JAMA 1967;202:116–22.
23. Veterans Administration Cooperative Study Group on Antihypertensive Agents. Effects of treatment in morbidity in hypertension: II. Results in patients with diastolic blood pressures averaging 90 through 114 mm Hg. JAMA 1970;213:1143–52.
24. Frohlich ED. The heart in hypertension. In Ref 11:791–810.
25. Frohlich ED. The heart in hypertension. In: Rosenthal J, Chobanian AV, eds. Arterial Hypertension. 2nd ed. New York: Springer-Verlag (in press).
26. Dunn FG, Chandraratna P, de Carvalho JG, Basta LL, Frohlich ED. Pathophysiologic assessment of hypertensive heart disease with echocardiology. Am J Cardiol 1977;39:789–95.

27. Ishise S, Pegram BL, Frohlich ED. Disparate effects of methyldopa and clonidine on cardiac mass and haemodynamics in rats. Clin Sci 1980;59:449–52.

28. Pegram BL, Ishise S, Frohlich ED. Effect of methyldopa, clonidine and hydralazine on cardiac mass and hemodynamics in Wistar Kyoto and spontaneously hypertensive rats. Cardiovasc Res 1982;16:40–6.

29. Kuwajima I, Kardon MB, Pegram BL, Sesoko S, Frohlich ED. Regression of left ventricular hypertrophy in two-kidney, one-clip Goldblatt hypertension. Hypertension 1982;4:113–8.

30. Maxwell RA, Plummer AJ, Schneider F, Povalski H, Daniel AI. Pharmacology of [2(octahydro-1-azocinyl)-ethyl]-guanidine sulfate (SU 5864). J Pharmacol Exp Ther 1960;128:22–9.

31. Baura ALA, Green AF. Adrenergic neurone blocking agents. Ann Rev Pharmacol 1965;5:183–212.

32. Mull RP, Maxwell RA. Guanethidine and related adrenergic neuronal blocking agents. In: Schlittler E, ed. Antihypertensive Agents. New York: Academic, 1967:115–49.

33. Harrison DC, Chidsey CA, Goldman R, Braunwald E. Relationships between the release and tissue depletion of norepinephrine from the heart by guanethidine and reserpine. Circ Res 1963;12:256–68.

34. Gaffney TE, Braunwald E, Cooper T. Analysis of the acute circulatory effects of guanethidine and bretylium. Circ Res 1962;10:83–8.

35. Richardson DW, Wyso EM, Magee JH, Cavell GC. Circulatory effects of guanethidine: clinical, renal and cardiac responses to treatment with a novel antihypertensive drug. Circulation 1960;22:184–90.

36. Weil JV, Chidsey CA. Plasma volume expansion resulting from interference with adrenergic function in normal man. Circulation 1968;37:54–61.

37. Dustan HP, Tarazi RC, Bravo EL. Dependence of arterial pressure on intravascular volume in treated hypertensive patients. N Engl J Med 1972;286:861–6.

38. Weiner N. Drugs that inhibit adrenergic nerves and block adrenergic receptors. In Ref 10:176–84.

39. Ram EVS, Engelman R. Pheochromocytoma: recognition and management. In: Harvey WI, DeLeon AC Jr, Leonard JJ, et al, eds. Current Problems in Cardiology. Vol 4. Chicago: Year Book Medical, 1979.

40. Kuchel O. Adrenal medulla: pheochromocytoma. In Ref 11:947–63.

41. Graham RM, Pettinger WA. Prazosin. N Engl J Med 1979;399:232–6.

42. Bolli P, Wood AJ, Simspon FO. Effects of prazosin in patients with hypertension. Clin Pharmacol Ther 1976;20:138–218.

43. Graham RM, Thomell IR, Gain JM, et al. Prazosin: the first dose phenomena. Br Med J 1976;2:1293–4.

44. Colluci WS. Alpha-adrenergic receptor blockade with prazosin. Ann Intern Med 1982;97:67–77.

45. Schmitt H, Bossier JR, Giudicelli JF. Centrally mediated decrease in sympathetic tone induced by 2-(2,6-dichlorophenylamine)-2-imidazoline (ST 155, Catapressan). Eur J Pharmacol 1967;2:147–8.

46. Onesti G, Bock KD, Heimsoth V, Kim KE, Merguet P. Clonidine: a new antihypertensive agent. Am J Cardiol 1971;28:74–83.

47. Katic F, Lavery H, Lowe RD. The central action of clonidine and its antagonism. Br J Pharmacol 1972;44:779–87.

48. Vorbuger C, Butikofer E, Renbi F. Dieakute Wirkung on St-155 anf de corvdiale und renale themodinamik. In: Heilmeyer L, Hohmeier JH, Pfeiffer EF, eds. Hochdrucktherapie: Symposion uber 2(2,6-dichlorophenyl-amino)-2-imidazolin-hydrochloride. Stuttgart: Georg Thieme Verlag, 1986:86.

49. Van Zweiten PA. Reduction of the hypotensive effect of clonidine and alpha methyldopa by various psychotropic drugs. Clin Sci 1976;51:4115–55.

50. Green S, Zawada ET, Musakkassa W, et al. Effect of clonidine therapy on renal hemodynamics in renal transplant hypertension. Arch Intern Med 1984;144:1205–8.

51. Hansson L, Hunyor SN, Julius S, Hoobler SW. Blood pressure crisis following withdrawal of clonidine (Catapres, Catapresan) with special reference to arterial and urinary catecholamine levels, and suggestions for acute management. Am Heart J 1973;85:605–10.

52. Motulsky H, O'Connor DT, Insel PA. Platelet alpha-2-adrenergic receptors are normal in untreated and treated hypertensive man. Clin Sci 1983;64:265–72.

53. Oates JA, Gillespie L, Udenfriend S, Sjoerdsma A. Decarboxylase inhibition and blood pressure reduction by alpha methyl-3,4,dihydroxy DL-phenylalmine. Science 1960;131:1890–1.

54. Kopin IJ. False adrenergic transmitters. Ann Rev Pharmacol 1968;8:377–94.

55. Henning M, Van Zwieten PA. Central hypotensive effect alpha-methyldopa. J Pharm Pharmacol 1969;20:409–17.

56. Mohammed S, Fasola AF, Privitera PJ, Lipicky RJ, Martz BL, Gaffney TE. Effect of methyldopa on plasma renin activity in man. Circ Res 1969;25:543–8.

57. Henning M, Rubenson A. Evidence that the hypotensive action of methyldopa is mediated by central actions of methylnoradrenaline. J Pharm Pharmacol 1971;23:1–5.

58. Wilson WR, Fisher FD, Kirkendall WM. The acute hemodynamic effects of alpha-methyldopa. J Chronic Dis 1962;15:907–13.

59. Sannerstedt R, Varnauskas F, Werko L. Hemodynamic effects of methyldopa (Aldomet) at rest and during exercise in patients with arterial hypertension. Acta Med Scand 1962;171:75–82.

60. Mohammed S, Hanenson IB, Magenheim AG, Gaffney TE. The effects of alpha-methyldopa on renal function in hypertensive patients. Am Heart J 1968;76:21–7.

61. Powell CE, Slater IH. Blocking of inhibitory adrenergic receptors by a dichloro analog of isoproterenol. J Pharmacol Exp Ther 1958;122:480–8.

62. Prichard BNC, Gillam PMS. The use of propranolol in the treatment of hypertension. Br Med J 1965;2:725–8.

63. Waal-Manning JG, Hobson CH. Renal function in patients with essential hypertension receiving nadolol. Br Med J 1980;2:423–4.

64. Dreslinski GR, Messerli FH, Dunn FH, Suarez DH, Reisin E, Frohlich ED. Hemodynamics, biochemical and reflexive changes produced by atenolol in hypertension. Circulation 1982;65:1365–8.

65. Frishman W. Pindolol: a new beta-adrenoreceptor antagonist with partial agonist activity. N Engl J Med 1983;308:940–5.

66. Frishman WH. Beta-adrenoreceptor antagonists: new drugs and new indications. N Engl J Med 1981;305:500–4.

67. Brogden RN, Heel RC, Speight TM, Avery GS. Metoprolol: a review of its pharmacological properties and therapeutic efficacy in hypertension. Drugs 1977;14:321–48.

68. Karow AM Jr, Riley MW, Ahlquist RP. Pharmacology and clinically useful beta-adrenergic blocking drugs. Fortschr Arneimittforsch 1971;15:103–22.

69. Frohlich ED, Tarazi RC, Dustan HP, Page IH. The paradox of beta-adrenergic blockade in hypertension. Circulation 1968;37:417–23.

70. Prichard BNC, Gillam PMS. Treatment of hypertension with propranolol. Br Med J 1969;1:7–11.

71. Buhler FR, Laragh JH, Baer L, Vaughn ED, Brunner HR. Propranolol inhibition and renin secretion: a specific approach to diagnosis and treatment of renin dependant hypertensive diseases. N Engl J Med 1972;287:1209–16.

72. Murmann W, Almirante L, Saccani-Guelfi M. Central nervous system effects of four adrenergic blocking agents. J Pharm Pharmacol 1966;18:317–9.

73. Frohlich ED, Tarazi RC, Dustan HP. Beta adrenergic blocking therapy in hypertension: selection of patients. Int J Pharmacol Ther Toxicol 1970;4:151–6.

74. Bakris GL, Wilson DM, Burnett JC Jr. The renal, forearm and hormonal responses to standing in the presence and absence of propranolol. Circulation 1986;74:1061–5.

75. Eliasson K, Lin LE, Rossner S. Serum lipoprotein changes during atenolol treatment of essential hypertension. Eur J Clin Pharmacol 1981;20:335–9.

76. Lucas CP. The effects of antihypertensive agents on serum lipids and lipoproteins. Pract Cardiol 1986;12:55–63.

77. Medical Research Council Working Party. MCR trial of treatment of mild hypertension. Br Med J 1985;291:97–104.

78. Hypertension Detection and Follow-Up Program Cooperative Group. Reduction in mortality of persons with high blood pressure, including mild hypertension. JAMA 1979;242:2562–72.

79. Report by the Management Committee. The Australian therapeutic trial in mild hypertension. Lancet 1980;1:1261–7.

80. Amery A, Birkenhager W, Brixko P, et al. Mortality and morbidity results from the European Working Party on high blood pressure in the elderly trial. Lancet 1985;1:1349–54.

81. Multiple Risk Factor Intervention Trial Research Group. Coronary heart disease death, nonfatal acute myocardial infarction and other clinical outcomes in the Multiple Risk Factor Intervention Trial. Am J Cardiol 1986;58:1–13.

82. Furberg CD, Cutler JA. Diuretic agents versus beta-blockers: comparison of effects on mortality, stroke, and coronary heart disease. Hypertension 1989;13(suppl I):I-57–61.

83. IPPPSH Collaborative Group. Cardiovascular risk and risk factors in a randomized trial of treatment based on the beta-blocker oxprenolol: the International Prospective Primary Prevention Study in Hypertension. J Hypertens 1985;3:379–92.

84. Urlhelmsen L, Berglund G, Emlfeddt D, et al. Beta-blockers versus diuretics in hypertensive men: main results from the HAPPHY trial. J Hypertens 1987;5:561–72.

85. Dunn FG, Ventura HO, Messerli FH, Kobrin I, Frohlich ED. Time course of regression of left ventricular hypertrophy in hypertensive patients treated with atenolol. Circulation 1987;76:254–8.

86. Dunn FH, Frohlich ED. Hypertension and angina pectoris. In: Yu PN, Goodwin JF, eds. Progress in Cardiology. Vol. 7. Philadelphia: Lea & Febiger, 1978:163–96.

87. Mehta J, Cohn JH. Hemodynamic effects of labetalol and alpha and beta-adrenergic blocking agents in hypertensive subjects. Circulation 1977;55:370–5.

88. Dunn FG, Oigman W, Messerli FH, Dreslinski GR, Reisin E, Frohlich ED. Hemodynamic effects of intravenous labetalol in essential hypertension. Clin Pharmacol Ther 1983;33:139–43.

89. Cressman MD, Vidt DG, Gifford RW Jr, Moore WS, Wilson DJ. Intravenous labetalol in the management of severe hypertension and hypertensive emergencies. Am Heart J 1984;107:980–5.

90. Page LH. Hypertension and atherosclerosis in primitive and accultorating societies. In: Hunt JC, Cooper I, Frohlich ED, et al, eds. Hypertension Update: Mechanisms, Epidemiology, Evaluation, Management. Bloomfield, NJ: HLS Press, 1980:1–12.

91. Freis ED. Salt volume and prevention of hypertension. Circulation 1976;53:589–94.

92. Frohlich ED. Diuretics in hypertension. J Hypertens 1987;5:43–9.

93. Guedon J, Chaignon M, Lucsko M. Diuretics as antihypertensive drugs. Kidney Int 1988;34:S177–80.

94. Weinberger MH. Comparison of captopril and hydrochlorothiazide alone and in combination in mild to moderate essential hypertension. Br J Clin Pharmacol 1982;14:5127–31.

95. Perry HM Jr, McDonald RH, Hulley SB, et al. Systolic Hypertension in the Elderly Program Pilot Study (SHEP-PS): morbidity and mortality experience. J Hypertens 1986;4:21–3.

96. The Joint National Committee on the Detection, Evaluation, and Treatment of High Blood Pressure. The 1988 Report of the Joint National Committee on the Detection, Evaluation, and Treatment of High Blood Pressure. Arch Intern Med 1988;148:1023–38.

97. Yang HYT, Erdos EG, Levin Y. A dipeptidyl carboxypeptidase that converts angiotensin I and inactivates bradykinin. Biochem Biophys Acta 1970;214:374–6.

98. Ondetti MA, Rubin B, Cushman DW. Design of specific inhibitors of angiotensin-converting enzyme: new class of orally active antihypertensive agents. Science 1977;196:441–4.

99. Gavras H, Faxon DP, Berkoben J, Brunner HR, Ryan TJ. Angiotensin-converting enzyme inhibition in patients with congestive heart failure. Circulation 1978;58:770–6.

100. Gavras H, Brunner HR, Turini GA, et al. Antihypertensive effect of the oral angiotensin converting-enzyme inhibitor SQ 14225 in man. N Engl J Med 1978;298:991–5.

101. Gavras H, Brunner HR, Laragh JH, Gavras I, Vukovich RA. The use of angiotensin-converting enzyme inhibitor in the diagnosis and treatment of hypertension. Clin Sci 1975;48:575–605.

102. Frohlich ED. Angiotensin converting enzyme inhibitors: present and future. Hypertension 1989;13:125–30.

103. Williams GH. Converting enzyme inhibitors in the treatment of hypertension. N Engl J Med 1988;319:1517–25.

104. Ram CV. Captopril. Arch Intern Med 1982;142:914–6.

105. Fusita T, Ando K, Noda H, et al. Hemodynamic and endocrine changes associated with captopril in diuretic resistant patients. Am J Med 1982;73:341–7.

106. Turini GA, Gribic M, Brunner HR, Waeber B, Gavras H. Improvement of chronic congestive heart failure by oral captopril. Lancet 1979;1:1213–5.

107. Gavras H, Flessas A, Ryan TJ, Brunner HR, Faxon DP, Gavras I. Angiotensin II inhibition: treatment of congestive heart failure in a high renin hypertension. JAMA 1977;237:880–2.

108. Vlasses PH, Rotmensch HH, Swanson BN, et al. Low-dose captopril: its use in mild to moderate hypertension unresponsive to diuretic treatment. Arch Intern Med 1982;142:1098–101.

109. Ferguson R, Blasses P, Swanson BN, McJarerian P, Koplin JR. Comparison of the effects of captopril, diuretic and their combination in low and normal renin essential hypertension. Life Sci 1982;30:59–65.

110. Valvo E, Bedogna V, Casagrande P, et al. Captopril in patients with type II diabetes and renal insufficiency: systemic renal hemodynamic alterations. Am J Med 1988;85:344–8.

111. Textor SC, Bravo EL, Fouad FM, Tarazi RC. Hyperkalemia in azotemic patients during angiotensin converting enzyme inhibition and aldosterone reduction with captopril. Am J Med 1982;73:719–25.

112. Schreiber MJ Jr, Fang LST. Renal failure associated with captopril. JAMA 1983;250:31–34.

113. Re R, Novelline R, Escourrou MT, Athanasoulis C, Burton J, Haber E. Inhibition of angiotensin-converting enzyme for diagnosis of renal artery stenosis. N Engl J Med 1978;298:582–6.

114. Hollenberg NK. Renal response to angiotensin-converting enzyme inhibition. Am J Cardiol 1983;49:1425–9.

115. Almers W. Gating currents and charge movements in excitable membranes. Rev Physiol Biochem Pharmacol 1978;82:96–190.

116. Bers DM, Langer GA. Uncoupling cation effects on cardiac contractility and sarcolemmal Ca^{2+} binding. Am J Physiol 1979;237:H332–41.

117. McAllister RG. Clinical pharmacology of slow channel blocking agents. Prog Cardiovasc Dis 1982;25:83–102.

118. Henry PD. Comparative pharmacology of calcium antagonists: nifedipine, verapamil and diltiazem. Am J Cardiol 1980;46:1047–58.

119. Amodeo C, Kobrin I, Ventura HO, Messerli FH, Frohlich ED. Immediate and short-term hemodynamic effects of diltiazem in patients with hypertension. Circulation 1986;73:108–13.

120. Schmieder RE, Messerli FH, Gararaglia GE, Nunez BD. Cardiovascular effects of verapamil in patients with essential hypertension. Circulation 1987;75:1030–6.

121. Grossman E, Oren S, Gararaglia GE, Messerli FH, Frohlich ED. Systemic and regional hemodynamic and humoral effects of nitrendipine in essential hypertension. Circulation 1988;78:1394–400.

122. Isshiki T, Amodeo C, Messerli FH, Pegram B, Frohlich ED. Diltiazem maintains renal vasodilation without hyperfiltration in hypertension: studies in essential hypertensive man and spontaneously hypertensive rat. Cardiovasc Drugs Ther 1987;1:359–66.

123. Bakris GL. Effects of diltiazem or lisinopril on massive proteinuria in diabetic subjects. Ann Intern Med 1990;112:707–708.

124. Yoshioka T, Shiraga H, Hoshida Y, et al. "Intact nephrons" as the primary origin of proteinuria in chronic renal disease. J Clin Invest 1988;82:1614–23.

125. Mimran A, Insua A, Ribstein J, Monnier L, Bringer J, Mirouze J. Contrasting effects of captopril and nifedipine in normotensive patients with incipient diabetic nephropathy. J Hypertens 1988;6:919–23.

126. Diamond JR, Cheung JY, Fang LS. Nifedipine-induced renal dysfunction. Am J Med 1984;77:905–8.

127. Moyer J, Handley C, Huggins R. Some pharmacodynic effects of 1-hydrazinophthalazine (C-5968) with particular reference to renal function and cardiovascular response. J Pharmacol 1951;103:368–72.

128. Mackinnon J. Effect of hypotension-producing drugs in the renal circulation. Lancet 1952;2:12–5.

129. Ueda H, Yagi S, Kaneko Y. Hydralazine and plasma renin activity. Arch Intern Med 1968;122:387–91.

130. Zacest R, Gilmore E, Koch-Weser J. Treatment of essential hypertension with combined vasodilation and beta-adrenergic blockage. N Engl J Med 1972;286:617–22.

131. Stein DH, Hecht HH. Cardiovascular and renal responses to the combination of hexamethonium and 1-hydrazinophthalazine (Apresoline) in hypertensive subjects. J Clin Invest 1955;34:867–74.

132. Gottlief TB, Kata FH, Chidsey CA III. Combined therapy with vasodilatory drugs and beta-adrenergic blockage in hypertension: a comparative study of minoxidil and hydralazine. Circulation 1972;45:571–8.

133. Zacest R, Gilmore E, Koch-Weser J. Treatment of essential hypertension with combined vasodilation and beta-adrenergic blockage. N Engl J Med 1972;286:617–22.

134. Koch-Weser J. Vasodilatory drugs in the treatment of hypertension. Arch Intern Med 1974;133:1017–22.

135. Morrow JD, Schroeder HA, Perry HM Jr. Studies in the control of hypertension by hydralazine. II. Toxic reactions and side effects. Circulation 1953;8:829–33.

136. Comens P, Schroeder HA. The "LE" cell as a manifestation of delayed hydralazine intoxication. JAMA 1956;160:1134–5.

137. Baer AN, Pincus T. Occult systemic lupus erythematosus in elderly men. JAMA 1983;249:3350–1.

138. Pettinger WA, Mitchell HC. Minoxidil: an alternative to nephrectomy for refractory hypertension. N Engl J Med 1973;289:167–71.

139. Wiburn R, Blaufuss A, Bennett C. Long term treatment of severe hypertension with minoxidil, propranolol and furosemide. Circulation 1975;52:706–13.

140. Earhart RN, Ball J, Nuss DC, Aeling JL. Minoxidil induced hypertrichosis: treatment with calcium thiologycolate depilatory. South Med J 1977;70:442–3.

141. Campese VM, Stein D, DeQuattro V. Treatment of severe hypertension with minoxidil: advantages and limitations. J Clin Pharmacol 1979;19:231–41.

142. Tunkel AR, Shuman M, Popken M, Seth R, Hoffman B. Minoxidil-induced systemic lupus erythematosus. Arch Intern Med 1987;147:599–600.

143. Vanhoutte P, Amery A, Birkenhager W, et al. Serotoninergic mechanisms in hypertension. Hypertension 1988;11:111–33.

144. Van Neuter JM, Janssen PAJ, Van Beck J, et al. Vascular effects of ketanserion (R41468), a novel antagonist of 5-HT$_2$ serotonergic receptors. J Pharmacol Exp Ther 1981;218:217–30.

145. Hiwada K, Kokubu T, Murakami E, et al. A highly potent and long acting oral inhibitor of human renin. Hypertension 1988;11:708–11.

146. Szelke M, Leckie B, Hallet A, et al. Potent new inhibitors of human renin. Nature 1982;299:555–7.

147. Murphy MB, McCoy CE, Weber RR, et al. Augmentation of renal blood flow and sodium excretion in hypertensive patients during blood pressure reduction by intravenous administration of the dopamine-1 agonist, fenoldopam. Circulation 1987;76:1312–8.

148. Ventura HO, Messerli FH, Frohlich ED, et al. Immediate hemodynamic effects of a dopamine receptor agonist (fenoldopam) in patients with essential hypertension. Circulation 1984;69:1142–6.

149. Moser M. Treating hypertension: a review of clinical trials. Am J Med 1986;81(suppl 6C):25–32.

150. Hypertension Detection and Follow-up Program Cooperative Group. Persistence of reduction in blood pressure and mortality of participants in the Hypertension Detection and Follow-Up Program. JAMA 1988;259:2112–22.

151. Castelli WP. The epidemiology of coronary heart disease: the Framingham Study. Am J Med 1984;76(suppl 2A):4–12.

152. Messerli FH, Nunez BD, Nunez MM, Garavaolia GE, Schmeider RG, Ventura HO. Hypertension and sudden death: disparate effects of calcium entry-blockers and diuretic therapy on cardiac dysrhythmias. Arch Intern Med 1989;149:1263–7.

153. Kannel WB, Gordon T, Offutt D. Left ventricular hypertrophy by electrocardiogram: prevalence, incidence and mortality in the Framingham Study. Ann Intern Med 1969;71:89–105.

154. Pool PE, Seagren SC, Salel AF. Effects of diltiazem on serum lipids, exercise performance and blood pressure: randomized, double blind, placebo controlled evaluation for systemic hypertension. Am J Cardiol 1985;56:86H–91H.

155. Ventura HO, Frohlich ED, Messerli FH, Korbin I, Kardon MB. Cardiovascular effects and regional blood flow distribution associated with angiotensin converting enzyme inhibition in essential hypertension. Am J Cardiol 1985;55:1023–6.

156. Winniford MD, Hillis LD. Calcium antagonists in patients with cardiovascular disease. Medicine 1985;64:61–73.

157. Weinstein DB, Heider JG. Protective action of calcium channel antagonists in atherogenesis and experimental vascular injury. Am J Hypertens 1989;2:205–12.

158. Kannel WB, Dannenberg AL, Abbott RD. Unrecognized myocardial infarction and hypertension: the Framingham Study. Am Heart J 1985;109:581–5.

159. Roberts R. Acute myocardial infarction. In: Kelley WN, DeVita VD, DuPont HL, et al, eds. Internal Medicine. Philadelphia: Lippincott, 1989:152–69.

160. Hillis LD, Braunwald E. Myocardial ischemia. N Engl J Med 1977;296:1093–6.

161. Pederson TR. Six year follow-up of the Norwegian Multicenter Study on Timolol After Acute Myocardial Infarction. N Engl J Med 1985;313:1055–9.

162. Gibson RS, Boden WE, Theroux P, et al. Diltiazem and reinfarction in patients with non-Q wave myocardial infarction: results of a double blind multicenter trial. N Engl J Med 1986;315:423–9.

163. Yusuf S, Wittes J, Friedman L. Overview of results of randomized clinical trials in heart disease: treatments following myocardial infarction. JAMA 1988;260:2088–94.

164. Pfeffer MA, Pfeffer JM, Steinbert C, Finn P. Survival after an experimental infarction: beneficial effects of long-term therapy with captopril. Circulation 1985;72:406–10.

165. The Consensus Trial Study Group. Effects of enalapril on mortality in severe congestive heart failure. N Engl J Med 1987;316:1429–34.

166. Captopril Multicenter Research Group. A placebo-controlled trial of captopril in refractory congestive heart failure. J Am Coll Cardiol 1983;2:755–63.

167. Dzau VJ, Colucci WS, Williams GH, et al. Sustained effectiveness of converting enzyme inhibition in patients with severe congestive heart failure. N Engl J Med 1980;302:1373–9.

168. Kramer BL, Massie BM, Topic N. Controlled trial of captopril in chronic heart failure: a rest and exercise hemodynamic study. Circulation 1983;67:801–16.

169. Berglund G. Goals of antihypertensive therapy: Is there a point beyond which pressure reduction is dangerous? Am J Hypertens 1989;2:586–93.

170. Cruickshank JM, Thorp JM, Zacharias FJ. Benefits and potential harm of lowering high blood pressure. Lancet 1987;1:581–4.

171. Samuelsson O, Wilhelmsen L, Andersson OK, et al. Cardiovascular morbidity in relation to change in blood pressure and serum cholesterol levels in treated hypertension. JAMA 1987;258:1768–76.

172. McKee PA, Castelli WP, McNamara PM, Kannel WB. The natural history of congestive heart failure: the Framingham Study. N Engl J Med 1971;285:1441–5.

173. Cohn JN, Levine TB, Olivari MT, et al. Plasma norepinephrine as a guide to prognosis in patients with chronic congestive heart failure. N Engl J Med 1984;311:819–23.

174. Cohn JN. New concepts in the mechanisms and treatment of congestive heart failure. Am J Cardiol 1985;55:1A–10A.

175. MacMahon SM, Cutler JA, Furberg CD, et al. The effects of drug treatment for hypertension on morbidity and mortality from cardiovascular disease. Prog Cardiovasc Dis 1986;29:99–118.

176. Furberg CD, Yusuf S. Effects of vasodilators on survival in chronic congestive heart failure. Am J Cardiol 1988;62:41–5.

177. Gavras H, Liang CS, Brunner HR. Redistribution of regional blood flow after inhibition of the angiotensin converting enzyme. Circ Res 1978;26(suppl I):59–63.

178. Suki WN. Renal hemodynamic consequences of angiotensin converting enzyme inhibition in congestive heart failure. Arch Intern Med 1989;149:669–73.

179. Rahimtoola SH. Valvular heart disease. In Ref 159:217–9.

180. Frohlich ED, Tarazi RC, Dustan HP. Hyperdynamic beta-adrenergic circulatory state: increased beta-receptor responsiveness. Arch Intern Med 1969;123:1–7.

181. Frohlich ED, Dustan HP, Tarazi RC. Hyperdynamic beta-adrenergic circulatory state: an overview. Arch Intern Med 1970;126:1068–9.

182. Frohlich ED. Hemodynamic factors in the pathogenesis and maintenance of hypertension. Fed Proc 1982;41:2400–8.

183. Savage DD, Garrison RJ, Kannel WB, et al. The spectrum of left ventricular hypertrophy in a general population sample: the Framingham Study. Circulation 1987;75:16–23.

184. Pringle SD, MacFarlane PW, McKillop JH, Lorimer AR, Dunn FG. Pathophysiologic assessment of left ventricular hypertrophy and study in asymptomatic patients with essential hypertension. J Am Coll Cardiol 1989;13:1377–81.

185. Devereaux RB. Importance of left ventricular mass as a predictor of cardiovascular morbidity in hypertension. Am J Hypertens 1989;2:650–4.

186. Tsoporis J, Yuan B, Leenen FH. Arterial vasodilators, cardiac volume load, and cardiac hypertrophy in normotensive rats. Am J Physiol 1989;256:H876–80.

187. Frohlich ED. The heart in hypertension: unresolved conceptual challenges. Hypertension 1988;11:19–24.

188. Frohlich ED. The first Irvine H. Page lecture: the mosaic in hypertension: past, present and future. J Hypertens 1988;6:2–11.

189. Sasaki O, Kardon MB, Pegram BL, Frohlich ED. Aortic distensibility and left ventricular pumping ability after methyldopa in Wistar Kyoto and spontaneous hypertensive rats. J Vasc Med Biol 1989;1:59–66.

190. Frohlich ED, Sasaki O. Dissociation of changes in cardiovascular mass and performance with angiotensin converting enzyme inhibitors. Hypertension 1989;14:341(abstract).

191. Frohlich ED, Sasaki O. Calcium antagonists variably change cardiovascular mass and improve function in rats. J Am Coll Cardiol (in press).

192. Kannel WB, D'Agostino RB, Levy KD, Belanger AJ. Prognostic significance of regression of left ventricular hypertrophy (abstr). Circulation 1988;78(suppl II):II-89.

193. Natsume T, Kardon MB, Pegram BL, Frohlich ED. Ventricular performance in spontaneously hypertensive rats with reduced cardiac mass. Cardiovasc Drugs Ther 1989;3:433–9.

194. Juergens JL, Barker NW, Hines EA Jr. Arteriosclerosis obliterans: review of 570 cases with special reference to pathogenic and prognostic factors. Circulation 1960;21:188–96.

195. Imparato AM, Kim GE, Davidson T, Crowley JG. Intermittent claudication: its natural course. Surgery 1975;78:795–812.

CHAPTER 7

Left Ventricular Hypertrophy, Cardiac Diseases and Hypertension: Recent Experiences

EDWARD D. FROHLICH, MD

Heart disease in the patient with hypertension is many-faceted (1–4). It may be an adaptive response to sustained and protracted pressure overload or it may coexist with an associated disease. It may vary according to the severity of the hypertensive vascular disease, the complexity of the pathophysiologic mechanisms involved or the coexisting problems offered by one or more associated diseases. As a result, the management of cardiac disease in the patient with hypertension is dependent on the nature and extent of cardiac involvement and the pathophysiologic mechanisms involved.

This report provides a review of the variability and extent of the functional involvement of the heart in hypertension. It is written with a plea to the student, practitioner and investigator of this major clinical problem to consider it apart from other diseases associated with pressure overload of the left ventricle. The pathogenesis, the involved pathophysiologic mechanisms, the rate of development of cardiac involvement and other aspects of hypertensive heart disease are different from those of other conditions associated with pressure overload (4–6).

Hyperdynamic Heart

Early in the development of hypertensive heart disease, cardiac involvement may be manifested by findings associated with a hyperdynamic circulation (4,7–9). These may include a faster heart rate, greater cardiac output than normal, an increased myocardial contractility with increased oxygen consumption and, perhaps, increased circulating catecholamines or responsiveness of the myocardial and vascular beta-adrenergic receptor sites (6–10).

Borderline or mild essential hypertension. This hyperdynamic circulation associated with hypertensive disease may have various expressions. One common manifestation is frequently found in patients with borderline (labile) or mild essential hypertension. In these patients, an elevated cardiac output, faster heart rate and increased myocardial contractility may be the pathophysiologic manifestations of early disease that involve the same pressor mechanism. In the early stage of the disease this may appear to be the result of increased adrenergic input to the heart, arterioles and venules, but these changes may also reflect interactions with the renopressor or other pressor or modulating systems (1,2). Moreover, the elevated cardiac output is not secondary to an expanded intravascular (plasma) volume; in fact,

plasma volume is usually normal or contracted (7,11,12). However, the increased output results from peripheral venoconstriction that redistributes the circulating intravascular volume centrally to the cardiopulmonary area, thereby increasing venous return (13). Furthermore if autonomic input to the heart is inhibited pharmacologically with parasympathetic (i.e., atropine) and beta-adrenergic receptor (i.e., propranolol) blocking agents, the elevated cardiac output is equilibrated with that of normotensive individuals who are similarly treated (14,15), thereby demonstrating that the so-called normal total peripheral resistance in the untreated individual was "inappropriately normal" and actually increased (7–9).

Thus, this hyperdynamic state is one of a net increase in adrenergic input to the cardiovascular system, and it still is not known whether this results from increased sympathetic outflow from the brain, hyperresponsiveness of beta-adrenergic receptor sites, increases in circulating levels of catecholamines, adrenergic "drive" mediated by the peripherally circulating or centrally active renopressure system or other mechanisms (16).

"Hyper-beta state." Another segment of patients with hyperdynamic circulation comprises those patients with a hyperdynamic beta-adrenergic circulatory state (17,18). These patients present clinically with variable cardiovascular manifestations that reflect increased adrenergic input to the heart and vessels. Thus, in contrast to the foregoing group of asymptomatic patients with borderline (labile) or mild to moderate essential hypertension, these patients have complaints related to excess stimulation of myocardial or vascular smooth muscle beta-adrenergic receptor sites. These symptoms include a more forceful or rapid heart rate, ectopic cardiac (atrial or ventricular) beats, palpitation in the rest or reflexively stimulated (e.g., upright posture or exercise) state or feelings of flushing, hot flashes, weakness or faintness. Physically, the findings may be manifested by systolic or systolic and diastolic pressure elevation, faster heart rate, systolic ejection type murmur, cardiac dysrhythmias and flushing (often in the facial or neck and upper thoracic areas). The findings in earlier years prompted such diagnoses as irritable heart, soldier's heart, effort syndrome, hyperkinetic heart syndrome or neurocirculatory asthma (19,20).

Physiologic findings include a hyperkinetic circulation, as outlined previously, slight elevation of circulating catecholamines (not as high as levels associated with those in patients having pheochromocytoma) and increased responsiveness of myocardial beta-adrenergic receptor sites to infusion of the synthetic beta-adrenergic receptor agonist isoproterenol. In fact, intravenous infusion of isoproterenol will provoke the symptoms experienced by these patients when they are active or assume upright posture (17,18). These symptoms may include anxiety attack, hysteric outbursts and accentuation of milder symptoms that would ordinarily be associated with beta-adrenergic receptor stimulation. Moreover, after intravenous administration of a beta-adrenergic blocking agent (e.g., propranolol) these physiologic and clinical findings will be normalized or prevented.

Mitral valve prolapse. A third manifestation of a hyperdynamic circulation may be seen in patients with idiopathic mitral valve prolapse syndrome. These findings are not unlike those of the previously defined group of patients with a "hyper-beta state" except that these patients will also demonstrate the physical, clinical and echocardiographic findings of mitral valve prolapse (21,22). In addition, they may demonstrate the physiologic findings of a hyperkinetic circulation, elevated levels of circulating catecholamines (not as high as those levels associated with pheochromocytoma), increased responsiveness of myocardial beta-adrenergic receptor sites and aggravation of the mitral valve prolapse during isoproterenol infusion (21,22). Reversal of the findings and improvement of the prolapsed valve may be expected with beta-blocker therapy.

Thus, these alterations constitute a hyperdynamic heart syndrome and patients with these changes may be treated best with beta-adrenergic receptor blocking drugs. However, if a beta-blocker cannot be prescribed, calcium antagonists, adrenergic inhibitors and angiotensin-converting enzyme (ACE) inhibitors may be used, although clinical improvement may not be as clear-cut as with the beta-blocking agents.

Left Ventricular Hypertrophy

Hemodynamic factors. As hypertension becomes well established in patients with essential hypertension, arterial pressure rises pari passu with the increasing total peripheral resistance, the classic hemodynamic hallmark of hypertension (8,9,23). This increased pressure overload imposed on the left ventricle results in a structural hypertrophic adaptation that is generally concentric in nature (24,25). The development of left ventricular hypertrophy, however, may not be totally explained by hemodynamic pressure overload (1–4,26,27). Some patients with hypertension may also have a component of volume overload imposed on the left ventricle by various factors including physiologic volume overload associated with prolonged exercise; pathologically induced volume overload associated with either volume-dependent essential hypertension or other forms of volume-dependent

secondary forms of hypertension (e.g., renal parenchymal disease, steroidal hypertension, primary aldosteronism or congestive heart failure) or exogenous obesity (3,4,28–30).

Nonhemodynamic factors. Still another very important and exciting new aspect of the development of left ventricular hypertrophy relates to specific "nonhemodynamic" factors that have been clinically and experimentally associated with the development of left ventricular hypertrophy (26,27). These findings are supported by clinical observations that indicate that height of arterial pressure in itself may not be correlated totally with developed left ventricular mass or wall thickness. In part, this may be because the pressures obtained to relate with mass and wall thickness do not reflect the integrated arterial pressures actually occurring throughout the 24 h period and over a longer term that are "seen" hemodynamically by the left ventricle. However, there also is increasing evidence (31) to show that patient groups matched for level of arterial pressure, systemic hemodynamics and clinical and demographic features have better (or worse) correlations of hemodynamics with structural changes associated with left ventricular hypertrophy. Moreover, hemodynamic indexes are more directly related to structural changes in black rather than white (32) or male rather than female (33) patients. Experimentally, the lack of correlation between arterial pressure and left ventricular mass has been shown in the laboratory model of essential hypertension, the spontaneously hypertensive rat, but not in the Goldblatt (two-kidney, one-clip renal) hypertensive rat (34); and this same dissociation has been shown in the male and female spontaneously hypertensive rat treated from conception with beta-adrenergic blocking drugs (35).

More compelling evidence relating development of left ventricular hypertrophy to "nonhemodynamic" factors may be offered by in vitro tissue culture studies (1–5,36,37) that demonstrate development of hypertrophy and myocardial protein synthesis when norepinephrine, isoproterenol or angiotensin II is added to tissue culture. Molecular and cellular biologic support for this thesis was offered recently (1,37) by the demonstration of the "on switch" for cellular events that mediate call growth by proto-oncogenes. (This latter subject will be discussed more extensively later.) Thus, increasing clinical, physiologic and experimental evidence is being amassed to alter the long-standing belief that hemodynamic events alone are sufficient to explain the long-standing structural adaptation of the left ventricle to the pressure overload in systemic arterial hypertension (and, perhaps in other pressure overload diseases) (38,39). Therefore, factors are being identified that stimulate myocardial (and probably vascular smooth muscle) mechanisms that serve as the biologic "transducers" that translate the hemodynamic and other pathophysiologic mechanisms of hypertensive disease into structural manifestations of left ventricular and arteriolar wall thickening and hypertrophy (1,38,40,41).

Clinical correlates. Left ventricular hypertrophy in hypertensive disease may be identified initially by electrocardiographic (ECG) means using the criteria of left atrial enlargement (e.g., increased P wave amplitude or duration or the relation of atrial contraction to its depolarization and polarization processes) (23,42,43). This involvement does not reflect atrial disease primarily but the adaptation of the atria to the reduced compliance or distensibility of the hypertrophying chamber of the left ventricle as diastolic filling becomes impaired (44). Left ventricular hypertrophy may also be demonstrated by the more classic chest roentgenogram and the many ECG criteria that are associated with hypertrophy (23).

The echocardiogram, however, is a far more sensitive means for detecting this hypertrophic process. Not only is it able to demonstrate increased left ventricular mass and wall thicknesses before these are evident by ECG, but also it demonstrates the structural analog for atrial enlargement and the structural and functional evidence of that hypertrophy as well as of hypertrophy of the right ventricle (25,45). Moreover, echocardiography has related altered diastolic function to these structurally and systolic functional changes associated with hypertrophy (25). Furthermore, impaired diastolic filling of the left ventricle has also been demonstrated functionally by a reduced filling rate of the left ventricle with use of echocardiographic (46) and nuclear scintigraphic (47) techniques.

Left Ventricular Hypertrophy: An Independent Risk

Risk factors in hypertensive disease. Patients with left ventricular hypertrophy are at increased risk of cardiovascular morbidity and mortality (48–51). This risk has been shown by prospective clinical and population-based as well as clinical investigative studies to be independent of that increased risk associated with the systolic and diastolic pressure elevations observed in the patient with systemic arterial hypertension. Although the precise mechanism or mechanisms responsible for the increased risk are not known, patients with left ventricular hypertrophy demonstrate premature sudden and ischemic heart-related death (48–50), an increased number of premature ventricular contractions throughout a 24 h period (52), more runs of ventricular tachycardia during a 24 h period (53) and insufficiency of absolute and "reserve" arterial blood supply to the myocardium (54). This latter coronary artery insufficiency may solely reflect the increased myocardial oxygen demand offered by the two determinants of left ventricular wall tension: the increased (intraventricular) systolic pressure and the greater left ventricular radius that is produced by the elevated arterial pressure and the hypertrophy process necessary to overcome more efficiently the increased pressure overload imposed on the chamber (55). Alternatively, the coronary insufficiency may be produced by an inadequate reserve of the coronary blood supply of the hypertrophied muscle (56) or by coexisting coronary artery disease because the occlusive arterial atherosclerotic process is enhanced by arterial hypertension (57,58). Of course, with coexisting hypertension and coronary artery disease, both increased oxygen demand and diminished oxygen supply are at least additive in the ischemic effects on the myocardium in these patients. Other factors that may also be related to the increased risk associated with left ventricular hypertrophy include fibrous tissue deposition or fatty amyloid infiltration, diabetic vascular disease or other, as yet undescribed, possibilities (4,5,59).

Therapy to reduce risks. Therapy of patients with left ventricular hypertrophy is based on effective and strict control of the elevated arterial pressure with consequent reduction of the pressure overload (and its attendant increased oxygen demands) imposed on the hypertrophied left ventricle. Physiologically, this may be achieved by the beta-adrenergic receptor blocking drugs, calcium antagonists or angiotensin-converting enzyme inhibitors. However, any therapeutic program designed to provide sustained reduction and control of arterial pressure associated with sustained essential hypertension will reverse left ventricular hypertrophy if the therapeutic program is maintained for a sufficient time period. A recent report (60) from the Framingham study has shown that treated patients will have improved morbidity and mortality associated with the reversal of this hypertrophy. If one agent does not provide effective control of pressure, a second agent (including the addition of a diuretic) may achieve this goal (61).

Reversal of Hypertrophy

It is important to reemphasize that all agents that control arterial pressure, if used for a long enough period of time, may be expected to reduce left ventricular mass and, hence, hypertrophy (1,2). However, certain agents may reverse this process more rapidly (within 4 to 12 weeks) in animals with experimental hypertension or in patients (1,2,62,63). The rapid response has suggested that certain antihypertensive agents possess specific nonhemodynamic qualities that may also participate in the reversal of the development of hypertrophy and "regression" process (1–6,26,27).

Hemodynamic versus structural effects of antihypertensive agents. Several experimental findings support the thesis that nonhemodynamic as well as hemodynamic factors participate in the development of as well as the process that reduces cardiac mass. These findings have whetted the broad clinical and experimental interest in certain groups of pharmacologic agents that rapidly reduce cardiac mass. Indeed, the clinical studies have led to inferred (but not implied) thinking that centrally active adrenergic inhibiting agents, angiotensin-converting enzyme inhibitors and calcium antagonists best "reverse" left ventricular hypertrophy. It is true, as already indicated, that these agents reverse the increased mass more rapidly than do certain other agents. But, at present, we do not know whether associated with the reduced cardiac and vascular wall thickness and mass there is a resulting improvement in cardiac and vascular function (1). Recent experimental findings have failed to confirm the inference and, in fact, show varying findings among these pharmacologic agents that reflect a dissociation between their hemodynamic and structural effects (64,65).

Methyldopa and clonidine. The classic agent that has reversed the increased mass of left ventricular hypertrophy is methyldopa (34,66,67). However, when another centrally acting adrenolytic compound (i.e., clonidine) was used to produce the identical hemodynamic effects, left ventricular mass was not reduced (67). Nevertheless, when the dose of clonidine was tripled, producing an agonist effect on peripheral $alpha_1$-adrenergic receptors, which in turn *increased* total peripheral resistance, cardiac mass then became reduced.

Moreover, recently, similar hemodynamic effects were achieved when we employed the same doses of methyldopa that were used previously. In these studies (64) we demonstrated that the left ventricular mass of both the spontaneously hypertensive rat and the Wistar-Kyoto normotensive control rats (without left ventricular hypertrophy) was also diminished significantly. Coincident with these reductions in left ventricular mass were significant decreases in the mass of the nonhypertrophied right ventricle of both rat groups; however, aortic mass failed to change.

Angiotensin-converting enzyme inhibitors. In contrast to the changes associated with methyldopa were distinctly different findings with two angiotensin-converting enzyme inhibitors (68). These agents (cilazapril and CGS-16617) reduced the mass of both the hypertrophied left ventricle of the spontaneously hypertensive rat and nonhypertrophied left ventricle of the Wistar-Kyoto rat but had no effect on right ventricular mass. Aortic mass was reduced with both agents in the spontaneously hypertensive rat although CGS-16617 did not reduce aortic mass in the normotensive Wistar-Kyoto rat. Other studies (69) with calcium antagonists revealed findings that were still different. In these later studies, both nifedipine and nitrendipine reduced the mass of the hypertrophied left ventricle of the spontaneously hypertensive rat but not that of the nonhypertrophied left ventricle of the Wistar-Kyoto rat. And, more perplexing, right ventricular mass *increased* in the Wistar-Kyoto rat but not in the spontaneously hypertensive rat.

Thus, it seems premature to ascribe changes of reduced left ventricular or total cardiac mass to certain classes of antihypertensive agents. More precise studies demonstrating changes of all cardiac chambers are necessary; and it is also important to know the effect of reduced mass on cardiac performance and contractility, irritability, and overall risk and on whether the reduced mass is simply a reduction in muscle mass or a reversal of true hypertrophy. None of these answers is available today. Those clinical studies that have been reported either show physiologic changes while the patients are still receiving therapy or fail to demonstrate performance under a pressure or exercise load.

Effect of reducing left ventricular mass on pumping performance. We recently reported our experiences of assessing left ventricular pumping ability before inducing reductions in cardiac mass after pharmacologic reduction of mass both at the reduced pressures and when pressure was increased abruptly by placing a snare around the ascending aorta (64,65). Those studies reported with methyldopa (64) showed that pumping ability was impaired after mass was reduced and this impairment was aggravated by increasing pressure. Pumping performance was changed little by captopril but, when pressure was elevated, performance deteriorated (65). In contrast to these findings with captopril, performance actually increased with cilozapril in both Wistar-Kyoto and spontaneously hypertensive rats whose left ventricular mass did not change or was reduced (68); an improvement in pumping ability was not observed with the angiotensin-converting enzyme inhibitor CGS-16617, although function did not deteriorate. The findings with the two calcium antagonists were likewise challenging to reason; thus, pumping ability improved whether left ventricular mass was reduced in spontaneously hypertensive rats or was not reduced in Wistar-Kyoto rats. However, there was no improvement or impairment in performance when aortic pressure was increased in the spontaneously hypertensive rats with reduced left ventricular mass, but performance improved in the Wistar-Kyoto rats without reduced mass.

These findings demonstrated a definite dissociation between the structural and hemodynamic effects of certain antihypertensive agents in this experimental setting. The differences (even in studies using similar pharmacologic classes of agents) suggest differences among drugs in their action, penetrance into the cardiac myocyte, or on local myositic systems affected by these agents (e.g., proto-oncogenes, local renin-angiotensin systems, available calcium ion-protein synthesis interaction or other as yet undefined effects) (1,2).

Implications. At this time, it is not known with certainty whether pharmacologically this reduction in left ventricular mass actually reduces the increased cardiovascular risk imparted by the left ventricular hypertrophy. Moreover, we also do not know with certainty whether the reduction in left ventricular mass or wall thickness represents a true "reversal" of the process of cellular hypertrophy and of the increased risk that is associated with left ventricular hypertrophy.

Nevertheless, one extremely important factor that should be stressed is the importance of careful monitoring of serum electrolyte levels (particularly potassium) in predisposed patients with hypertension, particularly those with left ventricular hypertrophy. The hypertrophied left ventricle is more predisposed to ventricular dysrhythmias (49,52,53), and this irritability may be exacerbated if the patient is receiving diuretics or digitalis. This consideration is of particular relevance if the patient already has congestive heart failure (with secondary aldosteronism and hypokalemia or cardiac dysrhythmias).

Cardiac Failure

Predisposing factors to cardiac failure. Left ventricular failure is the end-stage of hypertensive heart disease, and it results from inability of the heart to adapt further to the ever increasing pressure overload (3–5). Alternatively, this complication may be precipitated earlier in the natural history of hypertensive heart disease if there is a second, coexisting disease that involves the heart (such as atherosclerotic coronary artery disease, exogenous obesity or diabetes mellitus). Thus, for example, in patients with atherosclerotic coronary artery disease, the myocardial ischemia further aggravates the performance of the pressure-overloaded left ventricle (55). Under these circumstances there is insufficient blood supply to satisfy the myocardial oxygen demands associated with pressure overload and hypertrophy. And, in hypertensive patients with exogenous obesity, the left ventricle adapts structurally to the pressure overload by concentric chamber hypertrophy; and the volume overload associated with obesity provokes an eccentric form of hypertrophy (30). This "dimorphic" structural adaptation of the left ventricle to the dual overload predisposes the obese hypertensive patient to premature cardiac failure.

As with other problems that are associated with diabetes mellitus, careful metabolic control of the diabetes as well as control of arterial pressure will assure a better overall cardiovascular prognosis. Early clinical studies (70) have suggested that angiotensin-converting enzyme inhibitors not only provide pressure control, but also may reduce renal glomerular hydrostatic pressure and consequent hyperfiltration with the postulated resultant glomerulosclerosis associated with diabetes. These observations remain to be confirmed in ongoing multicenter trials; and, certain calcium antagonists (i.e., diltiazem and nitrendipine) may also have similar renal effects (71–73).

Therapy. In those patients with hypertension-induced left ventricular failure, the primary goals of therapy are 1) control of arterial pressure and the reduction of the left ventricular pressure overload; 2) contraction of the volume overload associated with congestive heart failure; and 3) reestablishment of normal electrolyte balance resulting from the secondary hyperaldosteronism. Digitalis and diuretics may help to augment the cardiac pumping ability as they reduce the left ventricular preload. The newer angiotensin-converting enzyme inhibitors are of particular value in this situation by their ability to reduce the increased preload and impedance imposed on the left ventricle; and, in doing so, they improve cardiac output and the performance of the failing heart (70). Should hypokalemia exist before the use of the angiotensin-converting enzyme inhibitor (as a result of

the secondary hyperaldosteronism), and should its correction have been attempted by prescribing potassium-retaining agents or supplemental potassium compounds, particular care and biochemical monitoring must be exercised to assure that the angiotensin-converting enzyme inhibitor does not provoke a seemingly paradoxical, life-threatening hyperkalemia. If the angiotensin-converting enzyme inhibitor is not prescribed (e.g., because of insensitivity to or side effects of these agents in the past), other vasodilating drugs that reduce arterial pressure may be employed. However, the beta-adrenergic receptor blocking agents are contraindicated in patients with cardiac failure, and certain calcium antagonists must be used with caution in these patients because of their potential negative inotropic effects on the myocardium.

One final word is in order concerning cardiac failure in patients with hypertension. Occasionally, pressure overload may not appear to be severe enough clinically to produce cardiac failure. In these patients, the physician should consider the coexistence of a second disease—particularly "silent" myocardial ischemia or infarction, extensive coronary artery disease or cardiac dysrhythmias.

Coronary Artery Disease

Therapy. As already indicated, insufficiency (i.e., inadequacy) of oxygen delivery to the hypertension-hypertrophied myocardium is produced by the increased tension of the left ventricle (55). More often than not, however, this insufficiency may be associated with coexisting ischemic coronary artery disease, which may be on the basis of coronary artery spasm or occlusive atherosclerotic disease. In any event, when coronary artery disease is associated with systemic arterial hypertension, the goal of therapy should be control of arterial pressure to reduce the pressure overload and thereby diminish the associated oxygen demand of the myocardium (55).

Calcium channel antagonists and beta-adrenergic blockers. In those patients with coronary artery spasm, this control of arterial pressure may be best achieved with the calcium channel antagonists. Under this circumstance, arterial pressure is controlled through a reduction in total peripheral resistance, and the calcium antagonists are also effective in relieving the coronary artery spasm (74). This effect may also be achieved with the beta-adrenergic receptor blocking agents or the angiotensin-converting enzyme inhibitors. By reducing pressure and heart rate (and, hence, the so-called double product, the product of systolic pressure and heart rate), the beta-blockers reduce the oxygen demand of the myocardium and, as a result, angina pectoris may be relieved. Simply because the beta-blockers reduce cardiac output and therefore increase the calculated total peripheral resistance, there is no reason to exclude these agents from the treatment of patients with coronary artery disease. The beta-blockers do not increase vascular resistance in every regional organ circulation; in fact, they may be associated with an unchanged (or even slightly higher) renal blood flow and a reduced renal vascular resistance in patients with hypertension (75,76). However, should these agents fail to control arterial pressure adequately, a calcium antagonist may be substituted or added to the overall treatment program (61).

Frequently, the physician may wish to maintain therapy with the beta-adrenergic receptor blocking drug because of its myocardial protective effect. Beta-adrenergic blocking agents (exclusive of those with intrinsic sympathomimetic activity) have been shown to protect the patient with a previous myocardial infarction from developing a subsequent infarction and to have an antiarrhythmic effect (77,78). In general, the calcium antagonists have not been demonstrated to protect the patient with a previous myocardial infarction; however, the calcium antagonist diltiazem (79) may protect patients with a prior "non-Q wave" myocardial infarction from a subsequent similar event.

Angiotensin-converting enzyme inhibitors. Administration of an angiotensin-converting enzyme inhibitor may also control arterial pressure and the attendant increased oxygen demands of the hypertrophied myocardium by reducing total peripheral resistance and by maintaining blood flow to the kidney (73). This class of antihypertensive agents has not been shown to protect the myocardium from a second myocardial infarction; however, they have been reported (80) to protect the heart of a patient with a recent myocardial infarction from subsequent potentially complicating cardiac failure. The mechanism for this protection has been explained on the basis of so-called remodeling of the infarcted left ventricle, perhaps through mechanisms similar to those offered for "regression" of left ventricular mass with angiotensin-converting enzyme inhibitors.

Conclusion

Any patient with hypertension has hypertensive heart disease. By virtue of the elevated pressure, there is a greater oxygen demand of the left ventricle and the heart must have adapted structurally and functionally to the increased work load. Effective control of arterial pressure not only assures improved overall morbidity and mortality from hypertension but may even prevent further development of the disease and its associated complications.

Whether reversal of left ventricular hypertrophy reduces its independent risk of cardiovascular morbidity and mortality is not yet known, but experience and common sense dictate that early and vigorous blood pressure control is indicated in all patients with hypertension whether or not hypertrophy is present. Moreover, this aggressive antihypertensive therapeutic approach is also indicated with other associated cardiac diseases that complicate hypertension.

References

1. Frohlich ED. The first Irvine H. Page lecture: the mosaic of hypertension: past, present, and future. J Hypertens 1988;6(suppl 4):S2–11.
2. Frohlich ED. The heart in hypertension: unresolved conceptual challenges. Hypertension 1988;11(suppl I):I-19–I-24.
3. Frohlich ED. The heart in hypertension. In: Genest J, Kuchel O, Hamet P, Cantin M, eds. Hypertension: Physiopathology and Treatment. 2nd ed. New York: McGraw-Hill, 1983:791–810.
4. Frohlich ED. The heart in hypertension. In: Rosenthal J, Chobanian AV, eds. Arterial Hypertension. 2nd ed. Springer-Verlag (in press).
5. Frohlich ED. Cardiac hypertrophy: stimuli and mechanisms. In: Sleight P, ed. Scientific Foundations of Cardiology. London: William Heinemann Medical Books, 1983:182–90.
6. Frohlich ED. Hemodynamics and other determinants in development of left ventricular hypertrophy: conflicting factors in its regression. Fed Proc 1983;42:2709–15.
7. Frohlich ED, Kozul VJ, Tarazi RC, Dustan HP. Physiological comparison of labile and essential hypertension. Circ Res 1970;27:55–69.
8. Frohlich ED. Hemodynamic factors in the pathogenesis and maintenance of hypertension. Fed Proc 1982;41:2400–8.
9. Frohlich ED. Hemodynamics of hypertension. In: Genest J, Koiw E, Kuchel O, eds. Hypertension: Physiopathology and Treatment. New York: McGraw-Hill, 1977:15–49.
10. Messerli FH, de Carvalho JG, Mills NL, Frohlich ED. Renal artery stenosis and polycystic kidney disease. Arch Intern Med 1978;138:1282–3.
11. Tarazi RC, Frohlich ED, Dustan HP. Plasma volume in men with essential hypertension. N Engl J Med 1968;278:762–5.
12. Julius S, Pascual AV, Reilly K, London R. Abnormalities of plasma volume in borderline hypertension. Arch Intern Med 1971;127:116–9.
13. Ulrych M, Frohlich ED, Dustan HP, Page IH. Cardiac output and distribution of blood volume in central and peripheral circulations in hypertensive and normotensive man. Br Heart J 1969;31:570–4.
14. Julius S, Pascual AV, London R. Role of parasympathetic inhibition in the hyperkinetic type of borderline hypertension. Circulation 1971;44:413–8.
15. Frohlich ED, Pfeffer MA. Adrenergic mechanisms in human and SHR hypertension. Clin Sci Mol Med 1975;48:25s–38s.
16. Julius S, Weder AB. Brain and the regulation of blood pressure: a hemodynamic perspective. Clin Hypertens 1989;A11(suppl 1):1–19.
17. Frohlich ED, Dustan HP, Page IH. Hyperdynamic beta-adrenergic circulatory state. Arch Intern Med 1966;117:614–9.
18. Frohlich ED, Tarazi RC, Dustan HP. Hyperdynamic beta-adrenergic circulatory state: increased beta receptor responsiveness. Arch Intern Med 1969;123:1–7.
19. Frohlich ED. Beta-adrenergic receptor blockage in the treatment of essential hypertension. In: Strauer BC, ed. The Heart in Hypertension. New York: Springer-Verlag, 1981:53–71.
20. Boudoulas H, Reynolds JC, Mazzaferri E, Wooley CF. Mitral valve prolapse syndrome: the effect of adrenergic stimulation. J Am Coll Cardiol 1983;2:638–44.
21. De Carvalho JG, Messerli FH, Frohlich ED. Mitral valve prolapse and borderline hypertension. Hypertension 1979;1:518–22.
22. Boudoulas H, Reynolds JC, Mazzaferri E, Wooley CF. Metabolic studies in mitral valve prolapse syndrome: aneuroendocrine-cardiovascular process. Circulation 1980;61:1200–5.
23. Frohlich ED, Tarazi RC, Dustan HP. Clinical-physiological correlations in the development of hypertensive heart disease. Circulation 1971;44:446–55.
24. Linzbach AJ. Heart failure from the point of view of quantitative anatomy. Am J Cardiol 1960;5:370–82.
25. Dunn FG, Chardrartna P, de Carvalho JG, Basta LL, Frohlich ED. Pathophysiologic assessment of hypertensive heart disease with echocardiography. Am J Cardiol 1977;39:789–95.
26. Frohlich ED, Tarazi RC. Is arterial pressure the sole factor responsible for hypertensive cardiac hypertrophy? Am J Cardiol 1979;44:959–63.
27. Tarazi RC, Frohlich ED. Is reversal of cardiac hypertrophy a desirable goal of antihypertensive therapy? Circulation 1987;75:113–7.
28. Tarazi RC. Hemodynamic role of extracellular fluid in hypertension. Circ Res 1976;38(suppl 2):73–83.

29. Tarazi RC, Dustan HP, Frohlich ED, Gifford RW Jr, Hoffman GC. Plasma volume and chronic hypertension: relationship to arterial pressure levels in different hypertensive diseases. Arch Intern Med 1970;125:835–42.

30. Frohlich ED, Messerli FH, Reisin E, Dunn FG. The problem of obesity and hypertension. Hypertension 1983;5:71–8.

31. Messerli FH, Sundgaard-Riise K, Ventura HO, Dunn FG, Oigman W, Frohlich ED. Clinical and hemodynamic determinants of left ventricular dimensions. Arch Intern Med 1984;144:477–81.

32. Dunn FG, Oigman W, Sundgaard-Riise K, et al. Racial differences in cardiac adaptation to essential hypertension determined by echocardiographic indexes. J Am Coll Cardiol 1983;1:1348–51.

33. Messerli FH, Garavaglia GE, Schmieder RE, Sundgaard-Riise K, Nunez BD, Amodeo C. Disparate cardiovascular findings in men and women with essential hypertension. Ann Intern Med 1987;107:158–61.

34. Kuwajima I, Kardon MB, Pegram BL, Sesoko S, Frohlich ED. Regression of left ventricular hypertrophy in two-kidney, one clip Goldblatt hypertension. Hypertension 1982;4:113–8.

35. Messerli FH, Ventura HO, Reisin E, et al. Borderline hypertension and obesity: two prehypertensive states with elevated cardiac output. Circulation 1982;66:55–60.

36. Khairrallah PA, Robertson AL, Davilla D. Effects of angiotensin II on DNA, RNA and protein synthesis. In: Genest J, Koiw E, eds. Hypertension. New York: Springer-Verlag, 1972:212–20.

37. Starksen NF, Simpson PC, Bishopric N, et al. Cardiac myocyte hypertrophy is associated with c-myc proto-oncogene expression. Proc Natl Acad Sci USA 1986;83:8348–50.

38. Frohlich ED. An epilogue: on target-organ involvement in essential hypertension based on presented concepts and discussions. Am J Cardiol 1987;60:1271–321.

39. Schmieder RE, Frohlich ED, Messerli FH. Pathophysiology of hypertension in the elderly. In: Abrams WB, Frohlich ED, eds. Cardiology Clinics, Vol 4. Philadelphia: WB Saunders, 1986:235–43.

40. Dzau VJ, Gibbons GH. Autocrine-paracine mechanisms of vascular myocytes in systemic hypertension. Am J Cardiol 1987;60:99–103.

41. Re RN. Cellular mechanisms of growth in cardiovascular tissue. Am J Cardiol 1987;60(suppl 1):156–61.

42. Dustan HP, Frohlich ED, Geller RG, et al. Current research and recommendations from the task force subgroups on therapeutics, pregnancy, obesity, Vol. 9. Report of the Hypertensive Task Force. Washington, D.C.: NIH publication no. 79-1631, 1979.

43. Messerli FH, Aristimuño GG, Dreslinski GR, et al. Effect of acute alpha-adrenergic blockage on systemic hemodynamics, circulating catecholamine levels, and reflexive cardiovascular changes. In: Les Alpha-Bloquants: Pharmacologie Experimentale et Clinique. Paris: Masson, 1981:259–62.

44. Braunwald E, Frahm CF. Studies on Starling's law of the heart. IV. Observations in the hemodynamic functions of the left atrium in man. Circulation 1961;244:633–42.

45. Nunez BD, Messerli FH, Garavaglia GE, Schmieder RE, Amodeo C, Frohlich ED. Right ventricular adaptation in obese hypertensive patients (abstr). J Am Coll Cardiol 1987;9:244A.

46. Dreslinski GR, Frohlich ED, Dunn FG, Messerli FH, Suarez DH, Reisin E. Echocardiographic diastolic ventricular abnormality in hypertensive heart disease: atrial emptying index. Am J Cardiol 1981;47:1087–90.

47. Inouye I, Massie B, Loge D, et al. Abnormal left ventricular filling: an early finding in mild to moderate systemic hypertension. Am J Cardiol 1984;53:120–6.

48. Kannel WB, Gordon T, Offutt D. Left ventricular hypertrophy by electrocardiogram: prevalence, incidence and mortality in the Framingham study. Ann Intern Med 1969;71:89–105.

49. Frohlich ED. Potential mechanisms explaining the risk of left ventricular hypertrophy. Am J Cardiol 1987;59:91A–7A.

50. Savage DD, Garrison RJ, Kannel WB, et al. The spectrum of left ventricular hypertrophy in a general population sample: the Framingham study. Circulation 1987;25:16–23.

51. Levy D, Garrison RJ, Savage DD, Kannel WB, Castelli WP. Left ventricular mass and incidence of coronary heart disease in an elderly cohort: the Framingham heart study. Ann Intern Med 1989;110:101–7.

52. Messerli FH, Ventura HO, Elizardi DJ, Dunn FG, Frohlich ED. Hypertension and sudden death: increased ventricular ectopic activity in left ventricular hypertrophy. Am J Med 1984;77:18–22.

53. McLenachan JM, Henderson E, Morris KL, Dargie HJ. Ventricular arrhythmias in hypertensive left ventricular hypertrophy. N Engl J Med 1987;317:787–92.

54. Pringle SD, Macfarlane PW, McKillop JH, Lorimer AR, Dunn FG. Pathophysiologic assessment of left ventricular hypertrophy and strain in asymptomatic patients with essential hypertension. J Am Coll Cardiol 1989;13:1377–81.

55. Dunn FG, Frohlich ED. Hypertension and angina pectoris. In: Yu PN, Goodwin JF, eds. Progress in Cardiology, Vol 7. Philadelphia: Lea & Febiger, 1978:163–96.

56. Harrison DG, Barnes DH, Hiratzka LF, Eastham CL, Kerber RE, Marcus ML. The effect of cardiac hypertrophy on the coronary collateral circulation. Circulation 1985;71:1135–45.

57. Wittels EW, Gotto AM Jr. Atherogenic mechanisms. In: Frohlich ED, ed. Pathophysiology: Altered Regulatory Mechanisms in Disease. 3rd ed. Philadelphia: JB Lippincott, 1984:107–18.

58. Dustan HP. George Lyman Duff Lecture. Atherosclerosis complicating chronic hypertension. Circulation 1974;50:871–9.

59. Sen S, Bumpus FM. Collagen synthesis in development and reversal of cardiac hypertrophy in spontaneously hypertensive rats. Am J Cardiol 1979;44:954–8.

60. Kannel WB, D'Agostino RB, Levy D, Belanger AJ. Prognostic significance of regression of left ventricular hypertrophy (abstr). Circulation 1988;78(suppl II):II-89.

61. The Joint National Committee on the Detection, Evaluation, and Treatment of High Blood Pressure: The 1988 Report of the Joint National Committee on Detection, Evaluation, and Treatment of High Blood Pressure. Arch Intern Med 1988;148:1023–38.

62. Frohlich ED. Changes in hypertrophy by treatment in hypertension: results of experimental research. In: Kaufmann W, Bonner G, Lang I, Meurer KA, eds. Primary Hypertension. Berlin: Springer-Verlag, 1986:105–14.

63. Frohlich ED. Reversal of target-organ involvement in systemic hypertension: a pharmacologic experience. Am J Cardiol 1987;60:1I–2I.

64. Sasaki O, Kardon MG, Pegram BL, Frohlich ED. Aortic distensibility and left ventricular pumping ability after methyldopa in Wistar-Kyoto and spontaneously hypertensive rats. J Vascular Med Biol 1989;1:59–66.

65. Natsume T, Kardon MB, Pegram BL, Frohlich ED. Ventricular performance in spontaneously hypertensive rats with reduced cardiac mass. Cardiovasc Drugs Ther 1989;3:433–9.

66. Sen S, Tarazi RC, Bumpus FM. Reversal of cardiac hypertrophy in renal hypertensive rats: medical versus surgical therapy. Am J Physiol 1981;240:H408–H12.

67. Pegram BL, Ishise S, Frohlich ED. Effect of methyldopa, clonidine, and hydralazine on cardiac mass and haemodynamics in Wistar-Kyoto and spontaneously hypertensive rats. Cardiovasc Res 1982;16:40–6.

68. Frohlich ED, Sasaki O. Dissociation of changes in cardiovascular mass and performance in converting enzyme inhibitors (abstr). Hypertension 1989;14:341.

69. Frohlich ED, Sasaki O. Calcium antagonists variably change cardiovascular mass and improve function in rats (abstr). J Am Coll Cardiol (in press).

70. Frohlich ED. Angiotensin converting enzyme inhibitors: present and future. Hypertension 1989;13(suppl I):I-125–I-30.

71. Amodeo C, Kobrin I, Ventura HO, Messerli FH, Frohlich ED. Immediate and short-term hemodynamic effects of diltiazem in patients with hypertension. Circulation 1986;73:108–13.

72. Isshiki T, Amodeo C, Messerli FH, Pegram BL, Frohlich ED. Diltiazem maintains renal vasodilation without hyperfiltration in hypertension: studies in essential hypertensive man and the spontaneously hypertensive rat. Cardiovasc Drugs Ther 1987;1:359–66.

73. Grossman E, Oren S, Garavaglia GE, Messerli FH, Frohlich ED. Systemic and regional hemodynamic and humoral effects of nitrendipine in essential hypertension. Circulation 1988;78:1394–400.

74. McCall D, Walsh RA, Frohlich ED, O'Rourke RA. Calcium entry blocking drugs: mechanisms of action, experimental studies, and clinical uses. Curr Probl Cardiol 1985;10:7–80.

75. Nishiyama K, Nishiyama A, Pfeffer MA, Frohlich ED. Systemic and regional blood flow distribution in normotensive and spontaneously hypertensive young rats subjected to lifetime beta-adrenergic receptor blockage. Blood Vessels 1978;15:333–47.

76. Frohlich ED, Messerli FH, Dreslinski GR, Kobrin I. Long-term renal hemodynamic effects of nadolol in patients with essential hypertension. Am Heart J 1984;108:1141–3.

77. Beta-Blocker Heart Attack Trial Research Group. A randomized trial of propranolol in patients with acute myocardial infarction. I. Mortality results. JAMA 1982;247:1707–914.

78. The Norwegian Multicenter Study Group. Timolol-induced reduction in mortality and reinfarction in patients surviving acute myocardial infarction. N Engl J Med 1981;304:801–7.

79. Perryman B, Roberts R. Diltiazem Reinfarction Study Group: Diltiazem and reinfarction in patients with non-Q-wave myocardial infarction: results of a double-blind randomized, multicenter trial. N Engl J Med 1986;315:423–9.

80. Pfeffer MA, Pfeffer JM, Steinbert C, Finn P. Survival after an experimental infarction: beneficial effects of long-term therapy with captopril. Circulation 1985;72:406–12.

◆ CHAPTER 8 ◆

Pathophysiology and Current Therapy of Congestive Heart Failure

WILLIAM W. PARMLEY, MD

Congestive heart failure is a common clinical syndrome and, in its advanced stages, has a grave prognosis. Much has been learned about this syndrome, especially through a better understanding of its pathophysiology. The purpose of this review is to update our knowledge of congestive heart failure, and especially relate our current therapy to an understanding of its pathophysiology.

Epidemiology (1)

It is estimated that about 3 million Americans have congestive heart failure. This represents about 1% of the population. For those aged >75 years, the prevalence of congestive heart failure is about 10%. Congestive heart failure is now the most common hospital discharge diagnosis for those over the age of 65. Approximately 400,000 individuals develop heart failure each year.

Age dependence of congestive heart failure (Fig. 8.1). As expected, there is a significant increase in the incidence of congestive heart failure at advanced ages (2). This seems to correspond somewhat with the increase in left ventricular hypertrophy seen with age, as determined by echocardiography (3).

Mortality (Fig. 8.2). The mortality from congestive heart failure has been detailed in several studies. It appears that women have a lesser mortality after the diagnosis of congestive heart failure than do men. The 5 year mortality in men is about 60%, whereas in women it is about 45%. When symptoms of heart failure occur at rest (New York Heart Association functional class IV), however, the 1 year mortality rate approaches 50% (4). About 40% of the time, the mode of death is sudden, implicating serious arrhythmias as the underlying cause (5).

Although the mortality from cardiovascular disease has been steadily declining since 1968 (6), the incidence and prevalence of congestive heart failure have been increasing. These trends may be due, in part, to the aging population, and in part to the improvements in therapy that have allowed patients with cardiovascular disease to live longer, so that congestive heart failure becomes a more common clinical problem.

Definition

A traditional definition of congestive heart failure is "the inability of the heart to deliver enough blood to peripheral tissues to meet metabolic demands." This definition, however, does not fully describe the syndrome of congestive heart failure as we see it in clinical practice. The two major symptom complexes of congestive heart failure are dyspnea (particularly dyspnea with exercise) and fatigue. It is presumed that these two major symptoms relate to the two major hemodynamic abnormalities of congestive heart failure—namely, an increase in left atrial pressure and a decrease in cardiac output. Thus, from a functional viewpoint, it is clear that congestive heart failure also includes the symptoms of dyspnea and fatigue and a decrease in exercise tolerance. Therefore, there is not only a decrease in peripheral blood flow to meet metabolic demands, but also an increase in atrial pressures leading to the signs and symptoms of either right or left heart failure, or both.

Etiology

In the Framingham study (7), which prospectively examined the development of heart failure in a cohort of the population of Framingham, Massachusetts, it appeared that hypertension was one of the major factors leading to heart failure. Over the past 2 decades, however, better recognition and treatment of high blood pressure have reduced the relative importance of this factor. Certainly, better treatment of hypertension has dramatically reduced the incidence of stroke. In current series in the United States, it appears that in about 50 to 75% of patients with heart failure, coronary artery disease is the underlying cause (8). Hypertension may be a contributing factor in some patients, but is clearly less important than myocardial infarction and ischemia. The next most common cause appears to be cardiomyopathy. Rheumatic heart disease is declining significantly in the United States, although valvular heart disease due to mitral regurgitation or aortic stenosis is still reasonably common in the population at large. Congenital heart disease represents only a small portion of adult patients presenting with congestive heart failure.

General Principles

When a patient presents with the signs and symptoms of congestive heart failure it is important that the etiology of this syndrome be carefully identified. In addition to history and physical examination, echocardiography and other noninvasive and invasive tests can be very helpful in assessing the precise cause of the congestive heart failure. It is also important to determine whether the signs and symptoms are due primarily to ventricular systolic dysfunction, diastolic dysfunction or a combination of the two. In most cases

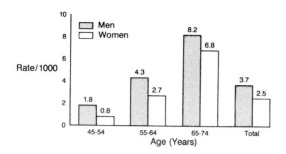

Figure 8.1. The average annual incidence of congestive heart failure for men and women at different ages. In all age groups there is a reduced incidence of the development of heart failure in women as compared with men. Reprinted with permission from McFate-Smith (2).

systolic dysfunction, as manifested by a decreased ejection fraction, will be the most common cause of congestive heart failure. In a minority of cases, diastolic dysfunction will be the predominant cause (9). The latter circumstances would include patients with hypertrophic cardiomyopathy, hypertrophy from any cause, restrictive cardiomyopathy, pericardial disease, certain infiltrative diseases such as amyloid or any process that impedes filling of the ventricle and thus leads to an increase in atrial pressures when cardiac output is increased. It is likely that almost all patients who have systolic dysfunction have some element of diastolic dysfunction as a contributing cause. Our inability to effectively treat diastolic dysfunction, however, limits our ability to provide major therapeutic benefit to patients with this disorder. Certainly if patients have constrictive pericarditis, removal of the pericardium can be quite dramatic in improving function. Similarly, valvotomy in patients with mitral stenosis can also produce a dramatic benefit in what is primarily a filling problem of the left ventricle. Some patients with severe hypertrophic cardiomyopathy may benefit from calcium channel blocker therapy, which can increase left ventricular volume at the same end-diastolic pressure (10). Similarly, in patients with severe hypertensive hypertrophy, which may restrict ventricular filling, control of hypertension with antiadrenergic drugs, the angiotensin-converting enzyme inhibitors or calcium channel blockers can cause regression of the hypertrophy (11) and thus reduce diastolic dysfunction. It is clear, however, that we need to learn much more about diastolic dysfunction and ways to alter it to effectively treat this component of congestive heart failure.

Our current understanding of congestive heart failure is based on our understanding of changes that occur in the myocardium as well as peripheral changes, including neurohumoral alterations, that affect the circulation. These changes will be described in the next sections.

Decrease in Myocardial Contractility

A fundamental problem for patients with systolic dysfunction is a decline in myocardial contractility. This can be

the result of prolonged pressure or volume overload or an intrinsic decline associated with cardiomyopathy. In patients with ischemic heart disease, loss of muscle with myocardial infarction imposes an additional volume and wall stress overload on the remaining normal myocardium. These changes lead to remodeling of the ventricle over time and, eventually, to a similar intrinsic decline in contractility. In general, therefore, therapy has been directed toward earlier recognition and treatment of increased loading conditions of the ventricle. For example, angiotensin-converting enzyme inhibitors may prevent remodeling and delay or attenuate the irreversible decline in contractility that occurs with increased loading after myocardial infarction (12).

Indexes of reduced muscle contraction. A reduction in myocardial contractility is manifested by decreased force development, decreased rate of force development and decreased velocity of shortening at given loading conditions. These changes are frequently accompanied by a delay in relaxation (Table 8.1). These indexes of muscle contraction (13) are reflected in the intact heart by a decrease in ejection fraction and stroke volume and by a shift downward in the ventricular function curve with an increase in atrial pressure.

Biochemical changes. A number of biochemical changes have been noted to accompany the process of congestive heart failure. Although it is outside the scope of this review to examine all of these, a few are listed in Table 8.1. A reduction in contractility is frequently accompanied by a shift in myosin isozymes, such that rapidly contracting V_1 forms with high adenosine triphosphatase (ATPase) activity are converted into slower contracting V_3 forms with slower ATPase activity (14). The relation between maximal velocity of shortening and myosin ATPase activity seen over a wide variety of species (15) also occurs in animal models of congestive heart failure and in patients. A reduction in velocity of shortening and actomysin ATPase activity has the potential benefit of reducing oxygen consumption and thus conserving energy in circumstances where it may be limited. Clearly, however, this compensatory aspect does

Figure 8.2. Survival curves of men and women after the onset of congestive heart failure (CHF) in the Framingham study. The data are compared with the total population sample at the top of each graph. The survival of women is higher than that of men throughout the follow-up. Reprinted with permission from Stamler (6).

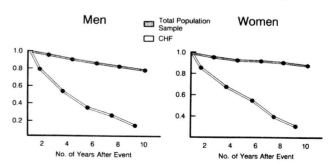

not make up for the dramatic reduction in function that leads to reduced cardiovascular performance.

Hypertrophy is one of the most important compensatory mechanisms available to heart muscle as function decreases, and it is accompanied by an increase in connective tissue that may stiffen the diastolic properties of the heart (16). In animal models of heart failure, calcium overload may play an important role in the development of congestive heart failure (17). This may occur through damage of the sarcolemma or perhaps through increased calcium entry due to increased sympathetic tone or increased sodium-calcium exchange. Certainly, the sarcoplasmic reticulum exhibits decreased function (18). An excess of myoplasmic calcium can reduce mitochondrial function and decrease the production of high energy phosphates. At least in animal models of congestive heart failure, such as the hereditary cardiomyopathy of the Syrian hamster, calcium overload plays a major role (19). The calcium channel blocker, verapamil, is effective in attenuating or treating this form of experimental heart failure. Microvascular spasm (20) has also been implicated in some experimental models of congestive heart failure and has responded to a vasodilator, such as prazosin (21). It is not clear, however, whether these specific biochemical changes in experimental models of heart failure have any application to the clinical syndrome of congestive heart failure.

Sympathetic nervous system and neuroendocrine activity. The activity of the sympathetic nervous system is increased in congestive heart failure (22). A reflex increase in sympathetic tone is presumably designed to maintain cardiovascular compensation by increasing heart rate and contractility. This increased tone leads to a decline in stores of norepinephrine in the myocardium (23) that spill over into the circulation. In some animal species there is also a decline in the production of norepinephrine (24). Increased catecholamines lead to a decline in beta$_1$-receptors (25), although beta$_2$-receptors may be little affected. These latter changes reduce the responsiveness of the myocardium to catecholamines, but the marked increase in plasma catecholamines in congestive heart failure is still sufficient to produce important sympathetic support of the circulation. Some studies in dilated cardiomyopathy suggest that this increased sympathetic drive may actually be deleterious. Some patients with dilated cardiomyopathy have responded beneficially to low dose metoprolol (26); this finding suggests that excess sympathetic drive may be directly harmful to the heart. Certainly high dose catecholamine infusions can directly cause myocardial necrosis in experimental animals (27). The combination of tachycardia and prolonged sympathetic stimulation may be deleterious in some patients with congestive cardiomyopathy. Tachycardia in and of itself not only increases myocardial oxygen demand, but also, by reducing diastolic time, can reduce coronary blood flow to the myocardium and contribute to an imbalance between supply and demand.

Although beta-blocker therapy may be beneficial for

Table 8.1. Myocardial Changes in Congestive Heart Failure

Mechanical
1. Decreased force development
2. Decreased rate of force development
3. Decreased velocity of shortening
4. Delayed relaxation

Biochemical
1. Shift in myosin isozymes
2. Hypertrophy and increase in connective tissue
3. Calcium overload
4. Decreased function of sarcoplasmic reticulum
5. Decreased stores of myocardial norepinephrine
6. Decreased production of norepinephrine
7. Decreased beta-receptors

some patients with cardiomyopathy, it is clear that it does not have widespread application to all forms of heart failure. In fact, beta-blockade can suddenly and dramatically worsen function in some patients who have severe congestive heart failure. The precise role, therefore, of the sympathetic nervous system and its potential benefit and harm have yet to be firmly elucidated in different patient subsets.

Pressure and volume overloading. If increased loading factors are deleterious to heart muscle, it is clear that unloading therapy may be one of the most beneficial ways to attenuate the adverse effects of prolonged pressure or volume overloading. In general, the decline in contractility that accompanies severe heart failure appears to be mostly irreversible and to continue in a downward spiral. Relief of pressure or volume overload in circumstances of valvular disease, however, has shown that there can be some restitution of function (28). This emphasizes the importance of earlier intervention before these irreversible changes produced by pressure and volume overloading cause an irreversible decline in cardiac contractility.

Neurohormonal and Other Peripheral Factors in Congestive Heart Failure

Increased sympathetic nerve reflexes and plasma catecholamines. A number of neurohormonal factors contribute to the syndrome of congestive heart failure. Three hormonal systems that are activated in congestive heart failure include the renin-angiotensin-aldosterone system (29), the sympathetic nervous system (22) and arginine vasopressin (antidiuretic hormone) (30). The marked increased in catecholamines is probably a reflection of the overall severity of the heart failure state (31), because it is presumed that this increase in sympathetic tone is intended to be compensatory. For example, the decrease in stroke volume and cardiac output that accompanies heart failure leads to a decrease in arterial pressure. The baroreceptor-mediated reflex increase in systemic vascular resistance produced by an increase in sympathetic tone would initially be helpful in maintaining arterial pressure during a decrease in cardiac output. Similarly, the decline in contractility that occurs in heart failure would be supported by the increased activity of the sympathetic nervous system, which could thus help to maintain stroke volume and cardiac output. Not only is there an increase in plasma catecholamines, but also there is an abnormal response of the sympathetic nervous system to physiologic interventions. Some examples are listed below. When patients with heart failure are subjected to upright tilt, there may be no change in plasma norepinephrine, although in normal subjects there would be an increase in plasma norepinephrine levels (32). This blunting of baroreceptor responses appears to form a component of the heart failure syndrome (33). Whether this is due to a smaller reduction in atrial pressures, changes in afferent stimulation or changes in central integration is not clear. Increasing or decreasing arterial pressures also does not produce the same responsiveness in patients with congestive heart failure. During exercise there may be a more abrupt increase of plasma norepinephrine at lower work loads in patients with failure, although the relative change in plasma norepinephrine may be less appropriate to the maximal achievable exercise response (34). Thus, overall there may be some blunting of the catecholamine response to exercise.

The arginine vasopressin system. This system is also increased in most patients with congestive heart failure (30). Because this antidiuretic hormone is such a potent vasoconstrictor, it could contribute to the peripheral vasoconstriction which can be so deleterious to patients with severe heart failure. Studies (35) suggest that osmoreceptor function is essentially intact in patients with congestive heart failure. In a few patients, arginine vasopressin may directly contribute to adverse sympathetic tone.

Atrial natriuretic hormones. Patients with heart failure generally have higher levels of atrial natriuretic factor than do normal persons (36). Data suggest that the effects of atrial natriuretic factor on diuresis are diminished in patients with congestive heart failure. Although infusion of this hormone has produced increases in cardiac output and increased renal excretion (37), it is unclear that this will be a major therapeutic intervention in relation to all of the other drugs available in patients with congestive heart failure.

The renin-angiotensin-aldosterone system. This system is also activated in patients with congestive heart failure (29). The three primary mechanisms whereby renin increase is promoted include reduced serum sodium, an increase in sympathetic tone and decreased blood pressure perfusing the macula densa. All three of these factors are frequently present in patients with congestive heart failure. Furthermore, diuretic usage is extremely common in such patients and may contribute directly to the observed rise in renin activity in this group. Renin, in turn, converts an angiotensinogen made in the liver to angiotensin I, which is an inactive decapeptide. Angiotensin I is then converted to angiotensin II by converting enzyme. Converting enzyme is

Table 8.2. Neurohormonal and Peripheral Changes in Congestive Heart Failure

Neurohormonal
1. Increased plasma catecholamines
2. Activation of renin-angiotensin-aldosterone system
3. Increased arginine vasopressin (antidiuretic hormone)
4. Increased atrial natriuretic factors

Peripheral factors
1. Increased systemic vascular resistance
2. Blunting of baroreceptor reflexes
3. Decreased vasodilatory response of peripheral vasculature
4. Altered regional flows
5. Venoconstriction

located everywhere in the body but appears to predominate in pulmonary capillary endothelial cells.

Angiotensin II has three effects that may be deleterious to patients with congestive heart failure. First, it is a potent vasoconstrictor that may contribute to excess systemic vascular resistance. Second, it tends to facilitate sympathetic outflow that may contribute to the already elevated levels of plasma catecholamines. Third, it feeds back on the adrenal gland to release aldosterone and thus further contributes to the increased salt retention seen in patients with heart failure. Patients with a low serum sodium level appear to have the highest renin levels (38). They are also the patients who have the highest mortality rate (39), and may be the most responsive to the angiotensin-converting enzyme inhibitors.

Antagonists to the three neurohormonal systems. The relative importance of the three vasoconstrictor hormone systems was evaluated in a study by Creager et al. (40) (Fig. 8.3). In that study, patients were given antagonists to the three neurohormonal systems to counteract their vasoconstriction. The resultant hemodynamic response, therefore, represents the ability to reverse the adverse hemodynamic effects of these systems. On average, the antagonist to arginine vasopressin produced only minimal hemodynamic changes. Captopril, which interferes with the renin-angiotensin system, produced moderate beneficial hemodynamic effects, including an increase in cardiac output and a reduction in filling pressures. The greatest changes in hemodynamics were produced by an alpha-adrenergic blocker (phentolamine), which antagonized the peripheral vasoconstrictive effects of increased catecholamines. This produced the greatest change in forward cardiac output and the greatest reduction in filling pressures. These findings suggest that the relative effects of vasoconstriction are produced in order by 1) excess sympathetic stimulation and catecholamines, 2) the renin-angiotensin-aldosterone system, and 3) the arginine vasopressin system.

Peripheral vascular changes: alterations in regional flow. Several peripheral vascular changes accompany the heart failure state. In addition to the increase in systemic vascular resistance, some studies (41) have suggested that there is an inability of the peripheral vasculature to dilate normally in response to stimuli such as hyperemia after transient vascular occlusion. A blunting of the baroreceptor mechanism has also been found and may explain why some vasodilator drugs do not result in an increase in heart rate in the same way that they do in patients with normal ventricular function. A limitation of cardiac output requires that regional flows be preserved for vital organs such as the heart and brain, whereas there may be a substantial reduction of the circulation in the skin, splanchnic bed, skeletal muscle and kidney (42). These alterations in regional flow may contribute greatly to some of the associated signs and symptoms accompanying severe congestive heart failure. In addition to arteriolar vasoconstriction, there is also venoconstriction especially due to increased catecholamines.

Compensatory Mechanisms

The four primary determinants of cardiac function are preload, afterload, contractility and heart rate. There is evidence that each of these mechanisms may provide some compensation for the failing circulatory system, especially early in its course. An important concept, however, developed over the past decade, is that these compensatory mechanisms can overshoot and become deleterious (43).

Overshoot of compensatory mechanisms. The increase in extracellular volume that occurs through retention of sodium and water is initially helpful in augmenting preload and thus increasing stroke volume by the Frank-Starling mechanism. Clearly, this mechanism overshoots when increased atrial pressures produce pulmonary or systemic congestion, or both. This overshoot then must be appropriately treated with diuretics or venodilators, or both. An increase in systemic vascular resistance, as an index of afterload, is initially helpful in maintaining blood pressure despite a decrease in cardiac output. It is clear, however, that this increase in systemic vascular resistance may eventually become harmful as shown by the beneficial effects of arteriolar vasodilators that can dramatically increase forward cardiac output. It is also clear that an increase in contractility can be beneficial in maintaining cardiac function. The increase in catecholamines that is required to produce this increase in contractility, however, may be too great and produce damage to heart muscle and result in arrhythmias. Heart rate is one of the most important compensatory mechanisms available to the circulation. With a decline in stroke volume, an increase in heart rate is essential to maintain a reasonably normal cardiac output. As heart rate increases, however, not only does it increase myocardial oxygen demand but also it impinges on diastolic time during which coronary flow can occur. Excess tachycardia, therefore, may contribute directly to continuing cardiac damage, by causing an imbalance between myocardial oxygen supply and demand.

Deleterious vicious cycles contributing to heart failure. This overshoot in compensatory mechanisms can produce vicious cycles such as those illustrated in Figure 8.4. The

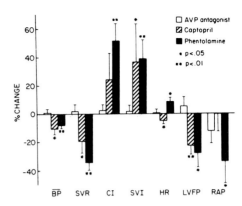

Figure 8.3. Effects of antagonists to three neurohormonal systems in patients with congestive heart failure. The percent change in hemodynamic values is shown with the administration of the three antagonists. The percent change was least with the arginine vasopressin (AVP) antagonist and greatest with the alpha-adrenergic blocker, phentolamine. Changes with captopril were intermediate. See text for discussion. Reprinted with permission from Creager et al. (40). BP = blood pressure; CI = cardiac index; HR = heart rate; LVFP = left ventricular filling pressure; RAP = right atrial pressure; SVI = stroke volume index; SVR = systemic vascular resistance.

decline in cardiac contractility leads, by potent neurohumoral mechanisms, to an increase in systemic vascular resistance. This increased resistance can act as an increased afterload and impedance to ejection, and thus further reduce cardiac output. The downward spiral continues until a new low steady state level is reached at which cardiac output is lower and systemic resistance higher than is optimal for the circulation. Similarly, a reduction in cardiac output contributes to decreased renal perfusion, which also leads to an increase in salt and water retention. In excess, this can also worsen the heart failure state and contribute to a further downward spiral. It is clear that a complex interaction of a number of factors contributes to the development of heart failure. It is therefore possible for a variety of interventions to counteract the overshoot and thus beneficially affect cardiac function.

Therapeutic Approach to Congestive Heart Failure (Table 8.3)

After one has identified the syndrome of congestive heart failure, it is mandatory to determine its cause and to assess the relative contribution of diastolic dysfunction. These steps may indicate the need for therapeutic interventions apart from the pharmacologic treatment to be described later. For example, patients with severe aortic stenosis need replacement of the aortic valve. Similarly, patients with other types of valvular disease may be benefited by appropriate valve replacement or repair. In patients in whom ischemia is an important factor, revascularization procedures or antiischemic therapy may be of great benefit in

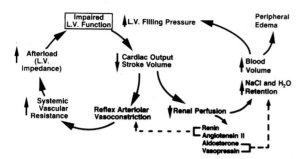

Figure 8.4. Two interrelated vicious cycles in congestive heart failure. **Left panel,** The impairment of left ventricular (LV) function leads to a decrease in cardiac output. In turn, this leads to a reflex increase in systemic vascular resistance by the neurohormonal mechanisms that were described in Figure 8.3. This, in turn, increases the effective afterload of the left ventricle and further reduces stroke volume. **Right panel,** A reduction in cardiac output and arterial pressure leads to a decrease in renal perfusion. This activates the renin-angiotensin-aldosterone system. Overall, there is retention of salt (NaCl) and water (H_2O) leading to a further increase in filling pressure and to peripheral edema. These vicious cycles therefore can feed back on each other to worsen the heart failure state. Reprinted with permission from McCall et al. (43).

alleviating some of the signs and symptoms of congestive heart failure, especially those that are transient and due to intermittent myocardial ischemia.

Nonsurgical, nonpharmacologic approaches. In some patients who do not need (or cannot undergo) surgical correction, a variety of nonpharmacologic approaches should be considered. Reduction of the work load of the heart by reducing overall activity, including both emotional and physical stress, can be of great benefit to some patients. Salt restriction and avoidance of salt overload can be useful in patients who are prone to retention of fluid and whose symptoms appear to be closely linked to an increase in extracellular volume. A number of specific, although rare, circumstances must also be addressed. For example, hyperthyroidism can contribute dramatically to deterioration in patients who have an underlying cause for heart failure. Similarly, anemia and other causes of high cardiac output (44) may contribute to the borderline compensation seen in some patients. When attention has been paid to these nonpharmacologic approaches to therapy, one can then consider the use of drugs from the three major classes of antifailure drugs now available—the diuretics, inotropic agents and vasodilator drugs. These will be discussed in the sections that follow.

Diuretics

Under normal circumstances, renal plasma flow is approximately 10% of the cardiac output and thus is about 500 ml/min (45). When mean arterial pressure ranges from about 80 to 200 mm Hg, glomerular filtration rate is kept approximately constant by autoregulation. Below these lev-

els, however, renal blood flow is decreased as arterial pressure is decreased and glomerular filtration may stop at an arterial pressure of about 40 mm Hg. In general, about 20% of the plasma that enters the glomerulus is filtered and, as an end result, about 1% of the filtrate is excreted in the urine. In patients with congestive heart failure, there is a reduction in cardiac output and arterial pressure. The renal response to this hemodynamic change is retention of salt and water. This has led to the use of diuretics as the most practical way of improving diuresis. Not only can diuretics be effective in increasing salt and water excretion, but, for example, when given intravenously, furosemide directly increases venous capacitance and can acutely reduce left ventricular filling pressure by redistributing blood away from the chest (46).

Choice of diuretic. It is reasonable to begin treatment of congestive heart failure with a thiazide diuretic. Usually, however, a more potent loop diuretic will eventually be needed by patients who have at least moderate heart failure. Attention must be paid to electrolyte imbalance in patients with congestive heart failure because hypokalemia and hypomagnesemia can lead to serious arrhythmias, especially in patients who are taking digitalis. Potassium supplementation is frequently required in patients with congestive heart failure who are taking potent diuretics. Alternatively, a potassium-retaining diuretic might be considered. It should be remembered, however, that the angiotensin-converting enzyme inhibitors retain potassium. Therefore, it is important to discontinue potassium-retaining diuretics and potassium supplementation in patients receiving angiotensin-converting enzyme inhibitors. In patients who become refractory to loop diuretics, one may get additional benefit by adding a thiazide such as metolazone (47). The fact that the two classes of diuretics work at different places in the nephron appears to explain their synergistic effect, which may be quite dramatic in some patients.

Table 8.3. Therapeutic Approach to Congestive Heart Failure

1. Determine the etiology
2. Evaluate relative importance of diastolic dysfunction
3. Surgical correction where possible
4. Nonpharmacologic treatment
   A) Reduce salt intake; avoid salt excess
   B) Reduce physical and emotional stress
5. Pharmacologic approach
   A) Either diuretic, digoxin or vasodilator as first line therapy
   B) Add second and third drugs as necessary
   C) Vasodilators are generally used because they can prolong life
      1) ACE inhibitors
      2) Combination of hydralazine and isosorbide dinitrate
   D) Add potent inotropic agents if the above is ineffective
      1) Intermittent dobutamine
      2) Phosphodiesterase inhibitors
   E) For dilated cardiomyopathy consider low dose metoprolol
6. Consider heart transplant for appropriate patients with end-stage heart failure

ACE = angiotensin-converting enzyme.

Clinical effect. Long-term experience has shown that diuretics can be extremely effective in some patients with congestive heart failure. They certainly are required in patients whose peripheral edema and excess fluid retention become major components of the syndrome of heart failure. Although we have no firm data suggesting that diuretics can prolong life in patients with heart failure, it is intuitive that these agents have been beneficial in alleviating symptoms and, in some circumstances, had the appropriate studies been done, they might have been found to have contributed to longevity.

Inotropic Agents

Digitalis

The most commonly used inotropic agent is digitalis. Numerous questions have arisen over the past few years about the potential benefit of digitalis and have probably led to a decline in its use, particularly in the United Kingdom. In the United States, however, digitalis is still a commonly used agent. It is effective in patients who have atrial fibrillation and a rapid ventricular response. A reduction in the ventricular rate, together with a positive inotropic effect, are generally quite beneficial in these patients. The greatest controversy, however, has arisen about the use of digitalis in patients with congestive heart failure and sinus rhythm. In some studies of such patients discontinuation of digitalis produced no detrimental effects (48,49). In other studies of such patients (50) the patients' heart failure clearly deteriorated (50) after withdrawal of digitalis. In a double blind placebo-controlled crossover study, Lee et al. (51) compared the effects of digoxin and placebo in 25 outpatients with sinus rhythm. In general, there was benefit in patients with a dilated heart, a reduced ejection fraction and a third sound gallop. Other studies with digitalis have also suggested that this drug may be more beneficial in sicker patients as compared with patients with mild heart failure. Dobbs et al. (52) reported a double blind crossover comparison of digitalis versus placebo in 46 patients with sinus rhythm. Approximately 33% of the patients receiving placebo showed deterioration that was followed by improvement after the reintroduction of digitalis therapy.

Clinical application. Overall, the data suggest that digitalis has modest beneficial effects in patients with congestive heart failure (53) and that these effects are probably of greater benefit as the heart failure becomes worse. Certainly, it has no benefit in patients with diastolic dysfunction when ejection fraction is preserved. It must also be used with caution in elderly patients, in whom toxicity may be a greater problem. Dose-response relations must be carefully considered as renal function becomes impaired because digoxin is cleared primarily by the kidney. Within these constraints, however, it appears that digoxin still has value in patients with sinus rhythm and congestive heart failure.

Toxicity and mortality. Some studies (54,55), however, have suggested that patient mortality may be increased by the administration of digoxin, especially after myocardial infarction. Other studies (56) in patients with coronary artery disease have not confirmed this finding. Nevertheless, the known toxicity of this agent raises important questions about its long-term effects. A proposed multicenter study to assess the effect of digoxin on mortality in congestive heart failure will soon be underway to provide a more definitive answer to this question. Until that time, however, it appears reasonable to consider digoxin for its modest inotropic support to the heart in an appropriate clinical setting.

Combination therapy. More recent studies have raised the question as to whether or not vasodilator therapy might be appropriately started before digoxin therapy. In the recent captopril-digoxin study (57), captopril was more effective in increasing exercise tolerance than was digoxin, whereas digoxin was more effective in increasing ejection fraction than was captopril. This study suggests that one can consider all three classes of drugs as initial therapy for heart failure. Thus, depending on the individual patient, one might want to begin treatment with a diuretic, an inotropic agent like digitalis or a vasodilator drug. Combination therapy may be more effective than either class alone.

Phosphodiesterase Inhibitors

There has been considerable interest in the phosphodiesterase inhibitors, which are potent inotropic agents and vasodilators (58). Inhibition of phosphodiesterase leads to an increase in cyclic adenosine monophosphate (AMP), which enhances calcium entry and thus improves contractility. These agents are also potent peripheral vasodilators, and produce significant hemodynamic effects in patients with heart failure. When given on a short-term basis to patients with heart failure, they result in an increase in cardiac output and a reduction in atrial pressures (59). Similarly, exercise tolerance is increased acutely in most studies (60). Despite these short-term beneficial effects, however, these drugs (amrinone and milrinone) are not yet available for oral use in the United States. Part of the uncertainty regarding their use relates to the long-term effects of these agents, both on exercise tolerance and on mortality (61). Until appropriate studies can clearly define a long-term clinical benefit or a reduction in mortality, these agents are best reserved for patients who have not responded in a beneficial fashion to usual therapy but continue to require some pharmacologic support to maintain an appropriate quality of life or to remain outside of the hospital.

Oral Catecholamines

A number of oral catecholamines have been used in patients with heart failure; these include L-dopa, pirbuterol, prenalterol and salbutamol (62–65). It appears that these agents can produce short-term beneficial hemodynamic effects. However, a high side effect profile and problems with arrhythmias and potential sudden death have raised serious questions about the use of such agents in patients with congestive heart failure. Intermittent dobutamine in some controlled studies (66) has shown prolonged benefit in such patients. Short-term infusions for 24 to 72 h have been shown to improve both exercise time and ejection fraction over a subsequent period up to 4 weeks. Although the mechanism of this benefit is unclear, a potential training effect has been implicated as has an improvement in mitochondrial function. A recent multicenter study of patients with heart failure treated at home with dobutamine was stopped because of an increase in serious arrhythmias in the treated group. It appears, therefore, that this form of therapy is best administered in a controlled hospital setting.

Overall, it is clear that inotropic agents are much like a double-edged sword; although they can increase hemodynamics and exercise tolerance, their other effects may be potentially harmful to the patient. These include an increase in oxygen consumption, the generation of arrhythmias and the potential for more rapid deterioration of muscle function. It is less certain, therefore, about the long-term role of potent inotropic agents in the management of severe heart failure.

Vasodilator Drugs

Arteriolar Vasodilators

Hydralazine. As illustrated in Figure 8.4, a major component of the vicious cycle in congestive heart failure is an excess increase in systemic vascular resistance. This increase sets the stage for arteriolar vasodilators, which can decrease systemic resistance and increase cardiac output. Hydralazine is the prototypic agent that has been used in this regard. When administered to patients with severe congestive heart failure, hydralazine increases cardiac output approximately 50% in association with a concomitant reduction in systemic vascular resistance (67). In general, there is little change or a slight decrease in atrial pressures with hydralazine therapy. This pharmacologic result underscores the reality of the vicious cycle in congestive heart failure, where neurohumoral mechanisms have overshot in their compensatory response and set systemic vascular resistance too high. On the other hand, it is clear that this increase in cardiac output may not necessarily be directed to organs that need it. For example, in a placebo-controlled trial (68) examining the effects of hydralazine on exercise tolerance, hydralazine or placebo was given to patients with moderate heart failure already receiving digitalis and diuretics. Over several weeks there was a slight improvement in the exercise tolerance of the hydralazine-treated patients, but it was no greater than the improvement in exercise tolerance seen in the patients receiving placebo. Thus, this arteriolar vasodilator was effective in increasing cardiac output but ineffective in improving exercise tolerance.

Hydralazine has been used with some effectiveness, however, in unloading the ventricle in patients with volume overload due to valvular regurgitation (69). Hydralazine is effective in both mitral and aortic regurgitation in this regard. In patients who are still asymptomatic but with moderate volume overload due to valvular regurgitation, it seems intuitive that, if one could unload the ventricle, one might delay the rate at which the ventricle dilates and therefore delay the onset of irreversible changes in ventricular function.

In patients with aortic regurgitation it appears that hydralazine may be of some benefit in this regard (70). It should be emphasized, however, that unloading therapy should never act as a substitute for surgical replacement of the valve. When severe changes in contractility occur, they appear to be mostly irreversible.

The effective dose of hydralazine is generally between 200 to 300 mg/day given in divided doses. Hydralazine is metabolized by acetylation. Approximately 50% of the United States population are rapid acetylators and half are slow acetylators. In rapid acetylators, higher doses of hydralazine may be required. Similarly, the lupus syndrome tends to occur primarily in patients who are slow acetylators. The primary side effects of hydralazine are related to the gastrointestinal tract and require discontinuation of this drug in a fair proportion of patients.

Minoxidil. Another potent arteriolar vasodilator that has been evaluated in congestive heart failure is minoxidil, which is approved for the treatment of resistant hypertension. The hemodynamic effects of minoxidil are similar to those of hydralazine (71). The drug produces a substantial increase in cardiac output, together with a minor decrease in atrial pressures. In a placebo-controlled trial (72), however, minoxidil did not increase exercise tolerance as compared with placebo. Side effects included sodium retention and hair growth, the latter being quite troublesome to female patients. Results with these two arteriolar vasodilators suggest a simple but important principle, namely, that arteriolar vasodilators do not increase exercise tolerance, although they are effective in increasing cardiac output.

Venodilators

Nitrates. Nitrates are the prototypic venodilators (73); they are available in many preparations, including sublingual, oral and transdermal. If given in effective doses, they can reduce atrial pressures, presumably by dilating peripheral veins and redistributing blood so that more is in the peripheral veins and less is in the chest. When nitrates are given to individuals with normal filling pressures, filling pressures frequently become too low and hypotension and tachycardia result. In patients with congestive heart failure, however, this is not a problem. Nitrates generally do not produce tachycardia in patients with congestive heart failure.

The nitrates have produced an improvement in exercise tolerance in patients with congestive heart failure, as compared with those receiving placebo (74,75). This appears to be true of virtually all agents that lower atrial pressures. Thus, venodilators that lower atrial pressures not only are effective in relieving dyspnea, but also are effective in improving exercise tolerance in patients with congestive heart failure.

Combination therapy. The fact that arteriolar vasodilators can increase cardiac output and that venodilators can reduce filling pressures has led to their combined use in patients with congestive heart failure (76). This combination was able to prolong life in patients with moderate heart failure in the V-HEFT trial (77). This trial was the first trial to demonstrate that vasodilator therapy could prolong life in patients with congestive heart failure and therefore becomes a landmark trial in encouraging physicians to use vasodilators relatively commonly in the management of patients with congestive heart failure.

Nitrate dosage and administration. The usual doses of isosorbide dinitrate range from 20 to 80 mg four times daily. Patches are generally ineffective at usual doses (78) and, even when they are given at high doses, one must employ a nitrate free interval to retain responsiveness to the drug. Shorter-acting forms of nitrates such as sublingual nitroglycerin can be effective for short-term episodes of dyspnea or ischemia. Nitroglycerin ointment can be effective in some patients whose dyspnea occurs primarily during the sleeping hours.

Drugs With Combined Arteriolar and Venodilating Effects

Prazosin. The prototypic drug in this category is prazosin, which is an alpha$_1$ receptor blocker and can produce both arteriolar and venous dilation (79). Studies with prazosin have shown that it can reduce filling pressures and increase cardiac output, and thus produce the same hemodynamic effects as those of combined hydralazine and isosorbide dinitrate. Unfortunately, there appears to be a hemodynamic tachyphylaxis with prazosin, such that there are no sustained long-term effects (80). This may explain why prazosin was ineffective in the V-HEFT trial in prolonging life compared with placebo (77). Because of this hemodynamic tachyphylaxis and inability to prolong life, prazosin does not appear to have a role in the management of congestive heart failure as compared with the combination of hydralazine plus isosorbide dinitrate, and the angiotensin-converting enzyme inhibitors.

Angiotensin-Converting Enzyme Inhibitors

Captopril, enalapril and lisinopril. These agents have been extremely effective in managing congestive heart failure and appear to represent the vasodilators of choice at present (81). They currently are the three angiotensin-converting enzyme inhibitors available in the United States. The benefit produced by these drugs underscores the concept that the renin-angiotensin-aldosterone system has overshot in patients with congestive heart failure and can produce adverse hemodynamic effects. It should be remembered that diuretics and arteriolar vasodilators activate this system and thus help to set the stage for the use of angiotensin-converting enzyme inhibitors. The short-term administration of these agents to patients with congestive heart failure produces a reduction in blood pressure and systemic vascular resistance and a striking reduction in left and right atrial pressures. This is accompanied by a modest increase in cardiac output (82). Of some importance is the ability of angiotensin-converting enzyme inhibitors to increase exercise tolerance in patients with congestive heart failure (83). This improvement in exercise tolerance occurs over a period of several weeks, which is different, for example, from the short-term improvement in exercise tolerance that occurs with the potent inotropic agents such as dobutamine or the phosphodiesterase inhibitors (84). More important, this improvement in exercise tolerance appears to be accompanied by an improvement in patient well-being and quality of life. The angiotensin-converting enzyme inhibitors have especially become popular because of their demonstrated effect in prolonging life in the CONSENSUS trial (85). In this trial, patients with severe heart failure (mostly functional class IV) had either an angiotensin-converting enzyme inhibitor (enalapril) or placebo added to their regimen; there was a reduction in mortality in the enalapril-treated group (Fig. 8.5). A review of some of the captopril data (86) suggests a similar beneficial effect on mortality. It is likely that all of the angiotensin-converting enzyme inhibitors will have generally similar effects, although their short-term effects may be slightly different, in part related to the time course of their action (87).

Dosage. An important aspect of the angiotensin-converting enzyme inhibitors is their dose response relation (81). When one has achieved inhibition of converting enzyme, one has reached the appropriate therapeutic dose. This makes it relatively easy to titrate the angiotensin-converting enzyme inhibitors to an appropriate level. One starts with a low dose to avoid or minimize hypotensive effects and then gradually works up to a standard dose. This would be approximately 25 mg three times daily of captopril, 5 to 10 mg twice daily of enalapril and 10 to 20 mg once daily of lisinopril. The newest of these agents, lisinopril, is a long-acting angiotensin-converting enzyme inhibitor and will

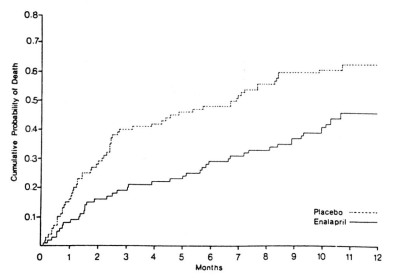

Figure 8.5. Cumulative total mortality in the CONSENSUS trial. The enalapril-treated patients showed a statistically significant reduction in mortality as compared with placebo-treated patients. This was most marked in the first 3 months, with the curves remaining relatively parallel thereafter. Reprinted with permission from the CONSENSUS Trial Study Group (85).

thus have the advantage of being given only once daily, which may well improve patient compliance (88).

Combination Therapy

Selection of drugs for new onset congestive failure. In the past a step-care approach to the management of heart failure has been suggested. This step-care approach generally included starting with a diuretic and then adding digoxin if necessary. This was followed by the addition of vasodilators if digoxin and diuretics were ineffective together. Recent studies (57), however, have suggested that the vasodilators may be appropriate alternatives to digoxin for first-line therapy. The following approach, therefore, is suggested for patients with new onset congestive heart failure (Table 8.3). If the patient has evidence of volume excess or systemic or pulmonary edema, it is likely that diuretics will be required as a permanent part of the therapy of these patients. It makes sense, therefore, to start with the diuretics as first-line therapy and then to add other drugs as appropriate. In patients with left ventricular dysfunction or early signs of congestive heart failure, there is important evidence that unloading therapy with the angiotensin-converting enzyme inhibitors may alter remodeling and slow the intrinsic decline in cardiac contractility (12). Thus, vasodilator therapy can be considered much earlier than in the past, and may prove useful in the earliest forms of heart failure to unload the ventricle. On the other hand, digoxin appears to be most effective in patients who have more severe heart failure (51). The benefit of its use in mild heart failure is less certain.

Thus, this approach would consider any of the three classes of drugs as potential first-line therapy in patients with heart failure. Additional classes would be added as needed because of their demonstrated additive effects. For example,

digoxin added to captopril has been shown to improve hemodynamics in patients with congestive heart failure (89). Similarly, hydralazine as an arteriolar vasodilator when added to captopril has been shown to be beneficial in further improving cardiac output (90).

Effect on survival. In selecting drugs one must remember that only the vasodilators have shown a prolongation of life in placebo-controlled trials (91). In the V-HEFT trial, the combination of hydralazine plus isosorbide dinitrate was effective in prolonging life in the treatment group as compared with the patients receiving placebo or prazosin (77). All had moderate heart failure and baseline therapy of digitalis and diuretics. In the CONSENSUS trial (85) enalapril was effective in prolonging life in patients with severe heart failure (Fig. 8.5). Thus, vasodilators have been shown to prolong life in patients with both moderate and severe heart failure. Because of their potential benefit in mild heart failure, or even in left ventricular dysfunction, it appears that a vasodilator regimen may emerge as core therapy for patients with all stages of congestive heart failure. Because of their potential beneficial effects they should be used in patients with severe heart failure unless there are contraindications such as renal insufficiency.

Hemodynamic effects. In virtually all studies in which combination therapy with different classes of drugs has been used, it appears that their hemodynamic effects are generally additive. Thus, in patients with severe heart failure it makes good sense to consider the combination of diuretics, inotropic agents and vasodilators to maximize beneficial hemodynamic effects. This is conceptually shown in Figure 8.6. In general, therefore, one can start with any of the classes of drugs as suggested above and then gradually add other classes as the heart failure worsens so that patients are eventually receiving all three types of antifailure therapy.

Antiarrhythmic Drugs

The mode of death in patients with severe heart failure is sudden approximately 40% of the time (5). Studies (92) with Holter electrocardiographic (ECG) monitors in patients with congestive heart failure have demonstrated that arrhythmias occur in approximately 90% of patients and that nonsustained ventricular tachycardia or multifocal premature ventricular complexes are relatively common. The data suggest that arrhythmias add independently to an adverse prognosis in patients with congestive heart failure (93), although the level of left ventricular dysfunction remains the most important adverse prognostic factor. It has therefore been reasonable to consider some form of antiarrhythmic therapy in patients with severe heart failure and associated serious arrhythmias. The value of this therapy is uncertain at present. The following discussion represents potential directions that one might take until more definitive data are available.

Reduction of proarrhythmic factors. It seems prudent initially to reduce or eliminate all proarrhythmic factors (94) that can be recognized (Table 8.4). These might include adverse effects of inotropic agents, such as digitalis in the presence of hypokalemia. Electrolyte imbalance should be corrected wherever possible. Ischemia can be an important contributory factor to prognosis, and can be treated with appropriate anti-ischemic agents such as nitrates. High catecholamine levels may also contribute to arrhythmias. In patients with severe heart failure it would be difficult to consider using beta-blockers or calcium channel blockers as antianginal agents, although such therapy could be used in patients with less severe congestive heart failure. Because of the evidence that increased stretch might play a role in producing arrhythmias in heart failure, vasodilator therapy may be helpful in eliminating this proarrhythmic factor. Placebo-controlled trials with the angiotensin-converting enzyme inhibitors have shown a reduction in premature ventricular complexes in patients with severe heart failure (57,85). Although there was no reduction in sudden death in the CONSENSUS trial (85) it still may be that reduction of premature ventricular complexes with the angiotensin-converting enzyme inhibitors could be of benefit in some patients with excess arrhythmias. The mechanism of reduced premature ventricular complexes with the angiotensin-converting enzyme inhibitors is unknown. Factors that might contribute, however, would include an increase in serum potassium, which is frequently seen with the angiotensin-converting enzyme inhibitors; unloading of the ventricle, which may reduce stretch-induced arrhythmias or ischemia; a decrease in myocardial oxygen consumption, which could also decrease episodes of ischemia; and a withdrawal of sympathetic tone. These or other factors may contribute to this beneficial antiarrhythmic effect.

Indications for antiarrhythmic therapy. When all proarrhythmic factors have been ruled out and a patient with

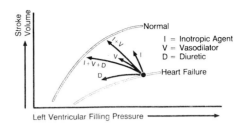

Figure 8.6. Conceptual ventricular function curves showing the effects of single and combined therapy for congestive heart failure. Note that the individual beneficial effects of each of the three classes of drugs are additive when additional drugs are given. This sets the stage for the use of all three classes of drugs to provide maximal beneficial hemodynamic effects in patients with congestive heart failure.

congestive heart failure still has serious arrhythmias the physician must make a decision whether to treat the arrhythmia. One must remember that, in general, antiarrhythmic therapy has a proarrhythmic effect that is seen in approximately 10% of patients, a figure that may, in fact, be closer to 20% in patients with severe heart failure (94). In addition, studies (95) have shown that the efficacy of antiarrhythmic agents appears to be proportionally less as the degree of heart failure increases. At the present time, we do not have any placebo-controlled trials to suggest that antiarrhythmic therapy can prolong life, although such trials are either underway or in the planning stage. The physician is therefore left to his best judgment in regard to antiarrhythmic therapy.

Effect on survival. In a retrospective review (96) of the data in a group of patients whom we treated with potent oral inotropic agents (phosphodiesterase inhibitors) we noted that sudden death appeared to occur less often in patients treated with antiarrhythmic agents as those in patients not so treated. Cleland et al. (97) also suggested that the drug amiodarone may be effective in prolonging life in patients with severe heart failure and arrhythmias. Although such data are uncontrolled, they do suggest the possibility that antiarrhythmic drugs may be of some benefit. Certainly the toxic effects of amiodarone become less important in patients with severe heart failure when life span is generally shortened. Until well controlled studies are available, however, physician judgment must be used in the absence of firm data in determining whether to use antiarrhythmic therapy in selected patients.

Summary

In conclusion, we have learned a tremendous amount about the pathophysiology of congestive heart failure over the past 2 decades. One of the most important principles that has emerged is that compensatory mechanisms that are initially helpful may subsequently become deleterious. Counteracting

Table 8.4. Proarrhythmic Factors in Congestive Heart Failure

1. Arrhythmogenic effects of positive inotropic agents
2. Electrolyte imbalance
3. Ischemia
4. High catecholamines
5. Myocardial damage
6. Myocardial stretch
7. Hypotension
8. Proarrhythmic effects of antiarrhythmic agents

these compensatory mechanisms has formed one of the most important therapeutic approaches to patients with congestive heart failure. Of the three classes of drugs available to treat congestive heart failure, the vasodilator drugs have emerged as the most important, especially because of their demonstrated ability to prolong life. Of the available vasodilator drugs, the angiotensin-converting enzyme inhibitors have emerged as the most important single class of drugs to consider in patients with heart failure. Because of the additive effects of all three classes of drugs, it is reasonable to start with one agent and then sequentially add others as required so that most patients with severe heart failure will be receiving a combination of a diuretic, an inotropic agent and a vasodilator drug. The role of antiarrhythmic agents is not settled as yet, although the prevalence of severe arrhythmias and sudden death suggests the possibility that these agents may be of benefit to some patients with congestive heart failure and serious arrhythmias.

In looking to the future, it is clear that prevention of heart failure should be one of our most important goals as physicians. As with any disease, preventive measures are far more effective in the long run than is treating the end stage of the disease. Because coronary artery disease is the most common cause of congestive heart failure in the United States, preventive measures will be closely linked to the ability to control and alter risk factors in a way that will reduce the incidence of coronary disease and the damaging effects of myocardial infarction. Revascularization procedures both during acute infarction and in chronic coronary disease may also delay the adverse effects of myocardial damage in this syndrome. Unloading agents early in the course of left ventricular dysfunction may also prove to be an effective way to delay the onset of heart failure. It is likely that this emphasis on prevention will, over time, produce greater benefit than the current benefit seen with the use of drugs in patients with established congestive heart failure.

References

1. Cohn JN, ed. Drug Treatment of Heart Failure. Secaucus, NJ: Advanced Therapeutics Communications, 1988.
2. McFate-Smith W. Epidemiology of congestive heart failure. Am J Cardiol 1985;55:3–8A.
3. Savage DD, Garrison RJ, Kannel WB, et al. The spectrum of left ventricular hypertrophy in a general population sample—the Framingham study. Circulation 1983;68(suppl III):III-36.
4. McKee PA, Castelli WP, McNamara PM, et al. The natural history of congestive heart failure: the Framingham study. N Engl J Med 1971;285:1441–6.
5. Francis GS. Development of arrhythmias in the patient with congestive heart failure: pathophysiology, prevalence, and prognosis. Am J Cardiol 1986;57:3–7B.
6. Stamler J. Epidemiology, established major risk factors, and the primary prevention of coronary heart disease. In: Parmley WW, Chatterjee K, eds Cardiology, Vol. 2, Ch 1, Philadelphia: JB Lippincott Company. 1988.
7. Kannel WB, Castelli WP, McNamara PM. Role of blood pressure in the development of congestive heart failure: the Framingham Study. N Engl J Med 1972;287:781–7.
8. Franciosa JA, Wilen M, Ziesche S, et al. Survival in men with severe chronic left ventricular failure due to either coronary heart disease or idiopathic dilated cardiomyopathy. Am J Cardiol 1983;51:831–6.
9. Sonnenblick EH, Yellin E, LeJemtel TH. Congestive heart failure and intact systolic ventricular performance. Heart Failure 1988;4:164–73.
10. Chatterjee K, Raff G, Anderson D, Parmley WW. Hypertrophic cardiomyopathy—therapy with slow channel inhibiting agents. Prog Cardiovasc Dis 1982;25:193–210.
11. Wicker P, Fouad FM, Tarazi RC. Effects of antihypertensive treatment of left ventricular hypertrophy and coronary blood flow. In: Ref. 6: Ch 25
12. Pfeffer MA, Lamas GA, Vaughan DE, Parisi AF, Braunwald E. Effect of captopril on progressive ventricular dilatation after anterior myocardial infarction. N Engl J Med 1988;319:80–6.
13. Spann JF, Covell JW, Eckberg DL, et al. Contractile performance in the hypertrophied and chronically failing cat ventricle. Am J Physiol 1972;2223:1150–7.
14. Entman ML, Michael LH. Molecular and cellular basis for myocardial failure. In: Ref. 6: Ch 4.
15. Barany M. ATPase activity of myosin correlated with speed of muscle shortening. J Gen Physiol 1967;50:197–201.
16. Buccino RA, Harris E, Spann JF Jr, et al. Response of myocardial connective tissue to development of experimental hypertrophy. Am J Physiol 1968;216:425–30.
17. Wikman-Coffelt J, Sievers R, Parmley WW, Jasmin G. Verapamil preserves adenine nucleotide pool in cardiomyopathic Syrian hamster. Am J Physiol 1986;19:1422–8.
18. Whitmer JT, Pankaj K, Solaro RJ. L Calcium transport properties of cardiac sarcoplasmid reticulum from cardiomyopathic Syrian hamsters (BIO 53.58 and 14.6): evidence for a quantitative defect in dilated myopathic hearts not evidenced in hypertrophic hearts. Circ Res 1988;62:81–5.
19. Wikman-Coffelt J, Sievers R, Parmley WW, Jasmin G. Verapamil preserves adenine nucleotide pool in cardiomyopathic Syrian hamster. Am J Physiol 1986;19:H22–8.
20. Factor SM, Sonnenblick EH. Hypothesis: is congestive cardiomyopathy caused by a hyperreactive myocardial microcirculation (microvascular spasm)? Am J Cardiol 1982;50:1149–52.
21. Sole MJ, Lien CC. Catecholamines, calcium and cardiomyopathy. Am J Cardiol 1988;62:20–4G.
22. Levine TB, Francis GS, Goldsmith SR, et al. Activity of the sympathetic nervous system and renin-angiotensin system assessed by plasma hormone levels and their relationship to hemodynamic abnormalities in congestive heart failure. Am J Cardiol 1982;49:1659–66.
23. Spann JF Jr, Chidsey CA, Pool PE, et al. Mechanism of norepinephrine depletion in experimental heart failure produced by aortic constriction in guinea pig. Circ Res 1965;17:312.
24. Pool PE, Covell J, Levitt M, et al. Reduction of tyrosine hydroxylase activity in experimental congestive heart failure. Circ Res 1967;20:349.
25. Bristow MR. Myocardial beta-adrenergic receptor down regulation in heart failure. Int J Cardiol 1984;5:648.
26. Swedberg K, Hjalmarson A, Waagstein F, et al. Beneficial effects of long-term beta blockade in congestive cardiomyopathy. Br Heart J 1980;44:117.
27. Rona G, Chappel CI, Balazs T, Gaudry R. An infarct-like myocardial lesion and other toxic manifestations produced by isoproterenol in the rat. Arch Pathol 1959;67:443–5.
28. Greenberg B, Massie B, Bristow D, Cheitlin M, Siemienczuk D, et al: Long-term vasodilator therapy of chronic aortic insufficiency: a random-

ized double-blinded, placebo-controlled clinical trial. Circulation 1988;78: 92–103.

29. Curtiss C, Cohn NJ, Vrobel T. Role of the renin-angiotensin system in the systemic vasoconstriction of chronic congestive heart failure. Circulation 1978;58:763–70.

30. Goldsmith SR, Francis GS, Cowley AW, et al. Increased plasma arginine vasopressin in patients with congestive heart failure. J Am Coll Cardiol 1983;1:1385–90.

31. Cohn JN, Levine TB, Francis GS, et al. Neurohumoral control mechanisms in congestive heart failure. Am Heart J 1981;509–14.

32. Goldsmith SR, Francis GS, Levine TB, et al. Regional blood flow response to orthostasis in patients with congestive heart failure. J Am Coll Cardiol 1983;1:1391–5.

33. Levine TB, Francis GS, Goldsmith SR, et al. Activity of the sympathetic nervous system and renin-angiotensin system assessed by plasma hormone levels and their relationship to hemodynamic abnormalities in congestive heart failure. Am J Cardiol 1983;49:1659–66.

34. Francis GS, Goldsmith SR, Ziesche SM, et al. Response of plasma norepinephrine and epinephrine to dynamic exercise in patients with congestive heart failure. Am J Cardiol 1982;49:1152–6.

35. Goldsmith SR, Cowley AW, Francis GS, et al. Arginine vasopressin and the renal response to water loading in congestive heart failure. Am J Cardiol 1986;58:295–9.

36. Raine AEG, Erne P, Burgisser E, et al. Atrial natriuretic peptide and atrial pressure in patients with congestive heart failure. N Engl J Med 1986;315:533–7.

37. Cody RJ, Kubo SH, Atlas SA, et al. Direct demonstration of the vasodilator properties of atrial natriuretic factor in normal man and heart failure patients (abstr). Clin Res 1986;34:476A.

38. Packer M, Medina N, Yushak M. Relation between serum sodium concentration and the hemodynamic and clinical responses to converting enzyme inhibition with captopril in severe heart failure. J Am Coll Cardiol 1984;3:1035–43.

39. Packer M, Lee WH, Kessler PD, et al. Role of neurohormonal mechanisms in determining survival in patients with severe chronic heart failure. Circulation 1987;75(suppl IV):IV-80–92.

40. Creager MA, Faxon DP, Cutler SS, Kohlmann O, Ryan TJ, Gavras H. Contribution of vasopressin to vasoconstriction in patients with congestive heart failure: comparison with the renin-angiotensin system and the sympathetic nervous system. J Am Coll Cardiol 1986;7:758–65.

41. Zelis R, Mason DT, Braunwald E. A comparison of the effects of vasodilator stimuli on peripheral resistance vessels in normal subjects and in patients with congestive heart failure. J Clin Invest 1968;47:960–70.

42. Just H, Drexler H, Zelis R. Regional blood flow in congestive heart failure. Am J Cardiol 1988;62:1–114E.

43. McCall D, O'Rourke R. Congestive heart failure. Mod Concepts Cardiovasc Dis 1985;52:55–60.

44. Grossman W, Braunwald E. High cardiac output states. In: Braunwald E, ed. Heart Disease. Philadelphia: WB Saunders, 1988;778–92.

45. Hollenberg NK. The role of the kidney in heart failure. In: Ref. 1:53–72.

46. Dikshit K, Vyden JK, Forrester JS, et al. Renal and extrarenal hemodynamic effects of furosemide in congestive heart failure after acute myocardial infarction. N Engl J Med 1971;288:1087.

47. Puschett JB. Physiologic basis for the use of new and older diuretics in congestive heart failure. Cardiovasc Med 1977;2:119–34.

48. Hull SM, MacIntosh A. Discontinuation of maintenance therapy in general practice. Lancet 1977;2:1054–5.

49. Fonrose HA, Ahlbaum N, Bugatch E, et al. The efficacy of digitalis withdrawal in an institutional aged population. J Am Geriatr Soc 1974;22:208–11.

50. Griffiths BE, Penny WI, Lewis MI, et al. Maintenance of the inotropic effect of digoxin on long-term treatment. Br Med J 1982;284:1819–22.

51. Lee DC, Johnson RA, Bingham JB. Heart failure in out-patients: a randomized trial of digoxin vs. placebo. N Engl J Med 1982;306:699.

52. Dobbs SM, Kenyon WL, Dobbs RJ. Maintenance digoxin after an episode of heart failure: placebo-controlled trial in outpatients. Br Med J 1977;1:749–52.

53. Kimmelstiel C, Benotti JR. How effective is digitalis in the treatment of congestive heart failure. Am Heart J 1988;116:1063–70.

54. Bigger JT Jr, Fleiss JL, Rolitsky LM, Merab JB, Ferrick KJ. Effect of digitalis treatment on survival after acute myocardial infarction. Am J Cardiol 1985;55:623.

55. Moss AJ, Davis HT, Conrad DL, DeCamila JJ, Odoroff CL. Digitalis-associated cardiac mortality after myocardial infarction. Circulation 1981;64:1150.

56. Ryan TJ, Bailey KR, McDabe CH, et al. The effects of digitalis on survival in high-risk patients with coronary artery disease. Circulation 1983;67:735.

57. Captopril-Digoxin Multicenter Research Group. Comparative effects of captopril and digoxin in patients with mild to moderate heart failure. JAMA 1988;259:539–44.

58. Francis GS. Inotropic agents in the management of heart failure. In Ref. 1: Ch 8.

59. Kereiakes D, Chatterjee K, Parmley WW, Atherton B, Curran D, Kereiakes A. Intravenous and oral MDL 17043 (a new inotrope-vasodilator agent) in congestive heart failure: hemodynamic and clinical evaluation in 38 patients. J Am Coll Cardiol 1984;4:844.

60. Weber KT, Andrews V, Janicki JS, et al. Amrinone and exercise performance in patients with chronic heart failure. Am J Cardiol 1981;48:164–9.

61. Packer M, Medina N, Yushak M. Hemodynamic and clinical limitations of long-term inotropic therapy with amrinone in patients with severe chronic heart failure. Circulation 1984;70:1038.

62. Rajfer SL, Anton AH, Rossen JD, et al. Beneficial hemodynamic effects of oral levodopa in heart failure: relation to the generation of dopamine. N Engl J Med 1984;310:1357–62.

63. Rude RE, Turi Z, Brown EJ, et al. Acute effects of oral pirbuterol on congestive heart failure. Circulation 1981;64:139.

64. Wahr DW, Swedberg K, Rabbino M, et al. Intravenous and oral prenalterol in congestive heart failure. Effects on systemic and coronary hemodynamics and myocardial catecholamine balance. Am J Med 1984;76:999–1055.

65. Sharma B, Goodwin JF. Beneficial effect of salbutamol on cardiac function in severe congestive cardiomyopathy. Circulation 1978;58:449.

66. Liang Chang-Seng, Sherman LG, Doherty JU, Wellington K, Lee VW, Hood WB. Sustained improvement of cardiac function in patients with congestive heart failure after short-term infusion of dobutamine. Circulation 1984;69:113.

67. Chatterjee K, Ports TA, Brundage BH, et al. Oral hydralazine in chronic heart failure: sustained beneficial hemodynamic effects. Ann Intern Med 1980;92:600.

68. Franciosa JA, Weber KT, Levine TB, et al. Hydralazine in the long-term treatment of chronic heart failure: lack of difference from placebo. Am Heart J 1982;104:587.

69. Greenberg BH, Massie BM, Brundage BH, Botvinick EH, Parmley WW, Chatterjee K. Beneficial effects of hydralazine in severe mitral regurgitation. Circulation 1978;58:273–9.

70. Greenberg B, DeMot H, Murphy E, et al. Beneficial effects of hydralazine on rest and exercise hemodynamics in patients with severe aortic insufficiency. Circulation 1980;62:49.

71. McKay C, Chatterjee K, Ports TA, et al. Minoxidil in chronic congestive heart failure: a hemodynamic and clinical study. Am Heart J 1982;104:575.

72. Franciosa JA, Jordan RA, Wilen MM, et al. Minoxidil in patients with chronic left heart failure: contrasting hemodynamic and clinical effects in a controlled trial. Circulation 1984;70:63.

73. Franciosa JA, Norstrom LA, Cohn JN. Nitrate therapy for congestive heart failure. J Am Med Assoc 1978;240:443.

74. Franciosa JA, Goldsmith SR, Cohn JN. Contrasting immediate and long-term effects of isosorbide dinitrate on exercise capacity in congestive heart failure. Am J Med 1980;69:559.

75. Leier CV, Huss P, Magorien RP, et al. Improved exercise capacity and differing arterial and venous tolerance during chronic isosorbide dinitrate therapy for congestive heart failure. Circulation 1983;67:817.

76. Massie B, Chatterjee K, Werner J, Greenberg B, Hart R, Parmley WW. Hemodynamic advantage of combined oral hydralazine and nonparenteral nitrates in the vasodilator therapy of chronic heart failure. Am J Cardiol 1977;40:794–801.

77. Cohn JN, Archibald DG, Ziesche S, et al. Effect of vasodilator therapy on mortality in chronic congestive heart failure. N Engl J Med 1986;314:1547.

78. Olivari MT, Cohn JN. Cutaneous administration of nitroglycerin: a review. Pharmacotherapy 1983;3:149–57.

79. Miller RR, Awan NA, Maxwell KS, et al. Sustained reduction of cardiac impedance and preload in congestive heart failure with the antihypertensive vasodilator, prazosin. N Engl J Med 1977;297:303.

80. Arnold SB, Williams RL, Ports TA, et al. Attenuation of prazosin effect on cardiac output in chronic heart failure. Ann Intern Med 1979;91:345–49.

81. Parmley WW. Angiotensin converting-enzyme inhibitors in the treatment of heart failure. In Ref 1: Ch 10, 227–250.

82. Ader R, Chatterjee K, Ports T, et al. Immediate and sustained hemodynamic and clinical improvement in chronic heart failure by an oral angiotensin-converting enzyme inhibitor. Circulation 1980;61:931–7.

83. Chatterjee K, Parmley WW, Cohn JN, et al. A cooperative multicenter study of captopril in congestive heart failure: hemodynamic effects and long-term response. Am Heart J 1985;110 (suppl 2):439–47.

84. White HD, Ribeiro JP, Hartley LH, Colucci WS. Immediate effects of milrinone on metabolic and sympathetic response to exercise in severe congestive heart failure. Am J Cardiol 1985;56:93.

85. CONSENSUS Trial Study Group. Effects of enalapril on mortality in severe congestive heart failure. N Engl J Med 1987;316.

86. Dennick LG, Maskin CS, Meyer JH, et al. Enalapril for congestive heart failure (letter). N Engl J Med 1987;317:1350.

87. Packer M, Lee WH, Yushak M, et al. Comparison of captopril and enalapril in patients with severe chronic heart failure. N Engl J Med 1986;315:847–53.

88. Chalmers JP, West MJ, Cyran et al. Placebo controlled study of lisinopril in congestive heart failure: a multicenter study. J Cardiovasc Pharmacol 1987;9 (suppl 3):589–97.

89. Gheorghiade M, St. Clair J, St. Clair C, Beller GA. Hemodynamic effects of intravenous digoxin in patients with severe heart failure initially treated with diuretics and vasodilators. J Am Coll Cardiol 1987;9:849–57.

90. Massie BM, Packer M, Hanlon JT, et al. Hemodynamic responses to combined therapy with captopril and hydralazine in patients with severe heart failure. J Am Coll Cardiol 1983;2:338–44.

91. Packer M. Vasodilator and inotropic drugs for the treatment of chronic heart failure: distinguishing hype from hope. J Am Coll Cardiol 1988;12:1299–317.

92. Francis GS. Development of arrhythmias in the patient with congestive heart failure: pathophysiology, prevalence, and prognosis. Am J Cardiol 1986;57:3B–7B.

93. The CAPS Investigators. The cardiac arrhythmia pilot study (CAPS). Am J Cardiol 1986;57:91–5.

94. Parmley WW, Chatterjee K. Congestive heart failure and arrhythmias: an overview. Am J Cardiol 1986;57(suppl B):34B–7B.

95. Hohnloser SH, Raeder EA, Podrid PJ, Graboys TB, Lown B. Predictors of antiarrhythmic drug efficacy in patients with malignant ventricular tachyarrhythmias. Am Heart J 1987;114:1–7.

96. Simonton CA, Daly P, Kereiakes D, Sata H, Modin G, Chatterjee K. Survival in severe congestive heart failure treated with the new nonglycosidic nonsympathomimetic oral inotropic agents. Chest 1987;92:118–23.

97. Cleland JGJ, Dargie HJ, Ford I. Mortality in heart failure: clinical variables of prognostic value. Br Heart J 1987;58:572–82.

CHAPTER 9

Changing Strategies in the Management of Heart Failure

ARNOLD M. KATZ, MD

"The heart muscle supplies the force which maintains the circulation. In the normal condition, the mechanism of the circulation is so adjusted that all parts combine to facilitate the work of the heart and to attain the object of the circulation. Any disturbance of that adjustment must at once entail more work upon the heart muscle, inasmuch as a departure from the normal means the embarrassment of the heart in maintaining normal arterial pressure. So long as the heart can overcome the impediment, and maintain the circulation in a normal manner, no symptoms are evoked, but if the heart is no longer able to carry on the circulation efficiently, then certain phenomena at once arise, and these phenomena we call 'symptoms of heart failure.' "

Sir James MacKenzie
Diseases of the Heart
Oxford University Press, 1908

"It is hard to see . . . how a man will be more of a physician by having thought about the ideal of the good, for the physician does not appear to investigate health in this way, but instead studies the health of man; or rather, of a particular man. For he cares for each man as an individual."

Aristotle
The Nicomachean Ethics
Translated by P. B. Katz

Introduction

This is a time of dramatic change in the management of congestive heart failure. Rapid developments in our understanding of normal cardiac function and the pathogenesis of this common condition illustrate the growing impact of the basic sciences on clinical practice, and the way that concepts developed in the research laboratory come to influence strategies for the care of the patient (1). This article reviews current understanding of the regulation of cardiac function, and the way that clinical applications of these basic principles are changing the treatment of patients with congestive heart failure.

What Is Heart Failure?

A simple definition of heart failure is not possible as this condition arises from a variety of pathophysiologic processes; furthermore, the clinical manifestations of heart failure may differ considerably, even among patients in whom the condition arises from a single process like mitral stenosis (2). Most definitions focus on the clinical presentation of the patient with heart failure and especially on the syndromes that appear when the failing heart becomes unable to meet the hemodynamic demands of the body. I believe, however, that this hemodynamic approach to the definition of heart failure perpetuates an outdated tradition that, by emphasizing the circulatory impairment, inadequately recognizes important cellular changes in the hypertrophied and failing heart. For these myocardial cellular abnormalities, rather than the disordered circulation, are largely responsible for the poor prognosis in these patients, about 50% of whom die within 5 years after an initial diagnosis of heart failure (3). Definitions of heart failure that focus on disorders of the circulation, which in fact represent not the cause but the consequences of an impaired ability of the heart to meet the demands of the body, are therefore incomplete. It can even be argued that to define heart failure in terms of abnormal hemodynamics inappropriately diverts attention from important cellular abnormalities that develop in the hypertrophied heart. Such definitions, by not recognizing a *cardiomyopathy of overload* as one of the major causes of clinical deterioration and death, can misdirect therapeutic strategies for this common and deadly condition.

MacKenzie's definition of heart failure, which is reproduced at the beginning of this article, highlights the interplay between the heart and circulation. MacKenzie clearly understood the primary role of the myocardial abnormalities in heart failure when he wrote:

"The more I study the symptoms of heart failure, and the more I reflect on the part played by the heart muscle, the more convinced I am that the explanation of heart failure can be summed up in the general statement that heart failure is due to the exhaustion of the reserve force of the heart muscle . . ." (4).

Although the "reserve force of the heart muscle" could not be understood in terms of the science of 1908, research over the past 81 years has clarified the mechanisms that control the contractile processes in the heart. Today, this knowledge provides the foundation for new therapeutic strategies that, when individualized to treat specific abnormalities present in each patient with heart failure, both relieve symptoms and improve prognosis.

Three Mechanisms That Regulate the Work of the Heart

Current approaches to the therapy of heart failure are based on the new understanding that the work of the heart is regulated by at least three fundamentally different mecha-

Table 9.1. Three Mechanisms That Regulate the Work of the Heart

Regulation by changing end-diastolic fiber length (Starling's law of the heart).
  Beat to beat responses to altered hemodynamics; adjustment of cardiac output to changing preload and afterload, and equalization of the outputs of the two ventricles.
Regulation by biochemical changes within the myocardial cell (excitation-concentration coupling and myocardial contractility).
  Short-term responses of the heart to physiologic and pharmacologic interventions; e.g., neurotransmitters and cardiac drugs.
Regulation by altered gene expression (molecular biology).
  Long-term adaptation of myocardial cells to the functional heterogeneity of the heart, and to chronic changes in cardiac loading, endocrinopathies and aging.

nisms (Table 9.1). Although each plays a unique role in adjusting the performance of the heart to the needs of the body, it is their interplay that defines cardiac and circulatory regulation in health and disease (5).

Forty years ago, only the role of changing *end-diastolic fiber length* (Starling's law of the heart) was understood; this mechanism operates at the organ level to adjust the output of the heart to changing preload and afterload on a beat to beat basis. Changes in *myocardial contractility*, which regulate cardiac performance over a slower time course largely by altering the calcium fluxes involved in excitation-contraction coupling, came to be understood over the past 25 years. This biochemical mechanism allows individual myocardial cells to respond to humoral stimuli, such as the sympathetic neurotransmitters released during exercise. Regulation by *variable gene expression*, the third of these mechanisms, brings about changes in myocardial protein composition that

alter cardiac function over an even slower time course; for example, in the response to chronically altered cardiovascular function as occurs in endocrinopathies, aging and chronic hemodynamic overloading (6–8). Regulation by variable gene expression also makes possible a remarkable cellular and molecular heterogeneity that underlies the essential functional homogeneity of the heart as an organ (5,9).

The evolution of our understanding of the regulatory mechanisms listed in Table 9.1 has contributed to the changing management of congestive heart failure summarized in Table 9.2. Starling's law of the heart and alterations in myocardial contractility, which until recently dominated thinking in cardiology, had initially determined strategy for managing patients with congestive heart failure. However, it is now apparent that optimal therapy for these patients must also be based on knowledge of the altered composition and behavior of the overloaded cells of the failing heart. Thus, to treat the patient with congestive heart failure, the physician must understand the interplay between all three of the regulatory mechanisms that determine the state of the circulation, the heart and the individual cells of the myocardium.

Strategies for the Management of Congestive Heart Failure. Phase I: Digitalis and Diuretics

Forty years ago, treatment of heart failure focused largely on two groups of drugs, the cardiac glycosides and mercurial diuretics. The former had been in use for >150 years, since Withering (10) had identified the foxglove as the active ingredient in a secret family recipe used to treat dropsy. Calomel (mercurous chloride), like digitalis, had been rec-

Table 9.2. Changing Strategies in the Management of Congestive Heart Failure

Phase I (1949 to 1969): Digitalis and Diuretics	
Cardiac glycosides	Increase inotropy; reduce dromotropy in atrial fibrillation
Diuretics	Reduce preload
Phase II (1969 to 1979): Vasodilators	
Alpha-adrenergic blockers	Reduce preload and afterload
Nitrates	Reduce preload
Arteriolar dilators	Reduce afterload
Calcium channel blockers	Reduce afterload
Phase III (1979 to 1989): Inotropic stimulation	
Beta–adrenergic agonists	Increase inotropy and lusitropy
Calcium sensitizing agents	Increase inotropy
Phosphodiesterase inhibitors	Increase inotropy and lusitropy
Phase IV (1989–): Preserve the failing heart	
Converting enzyme inhibitors	Reduce preload and afterload
	Reduce inotropic stimulation
Beta-adrenergic blockers	Reduce inotropy
Phase V (?): Correct the myocardial abnormality	
??	Modify synthesis of abnormal gene products

Data are approximations.

ognized to induce diuresis in patients with dropsy since the latter half of the 18th century; however, the toxicity and unpredictable effects of this inorganic mercurial precluded its routine use. It was not until 1920 that the diuretic effect of the organic mercurials was discovered accidentally in a patient who was receiving one of these compounds for the treatment of syphilitic aortitis (11). Supplemented by the weaker diuretic actions of the xanthines, the organic mercurials had joined digitalis as standard therapy for heart failure when the American College of Cardiology was founded in 1949.

Strategies for the Management of Congestive Heart Failure. Phase II: Vasodilators

Heart Failure as a Hemodynamic Abnormality

It is possible to trace the beginnings of the second phase in the evolution of our strategy for the management of heart failure to the introduction of cardiac catheterization into clinical medicine shortly after World War II. This Nobel prize-winning advance made it possible to evaluate heart failure in terms of basic hemodynamic principles and overall cardiac energetics, topics once viewed as only of theoretical interest. Measurements of cardiac output and pressures in the cardiac catheterization laboratory, and the development of flow-directed catheters in the coronary care unit, made it possible to characterize hemodynamic abnormalities in patients with both chronic and acute heart failure. This approach provided the basis for the second phase in the evolving strategy for managing heart failure (Table 9.2) when measurements of peripheral resistance in patients with heart failure made it possible to understand how vasoconstriction, long known to be compensatory in acute heart failure (12), contributed to the clinical disability in patients with chronic heart failure (13). Recognition of the detrimental effects of vasoconstriction in turn provided a foundation for later demonstrations that afterload reduction could relieve symptoms (14) and prolong life (15) in patients with heart failure. Today, of course, vasodilator therapy has joined digitalis and diuretics as standard therapy for this condition.

Strategies for the Management of Congestive Heart Failure. Phase III: Inotropic Stimulation

Heart Failure as an Abnormality of Myocardial Cell Biochemistry: Depressed Contractility in the Failing Heart

At the same time that improved understanding of the interplay between the heart and circulation refined strategies for the management of heart failure through manipulation of the peripheral vasculature, it was becoming apparent that the cardiac abnormality in patients with heart failure involved more than abnormal cardiac metabolism (16–18) and

the descending limb of the Starling curve (19). Yet as recently as the mid 1960s, the importance, and indeed the existence, of cardiac muscle abnormalities in the patient with heart failure had not been established, and myocardial contractility had not been shown to be depressed in these patients. Thus, in summarizing the deliberations of a distinguished group of cardiologists and cardiovascular physiologists who examined this question in 1964, I was forced to write: ". . . the basic question: 'Is the failure of chronically overloaded hearts the result of abnormalities within the cardiac fiber?' remains unanswered . . ." (20). This question was answered only when myocardial contractility (MacKenzie's "reserve force"), came to be understood in biochemical and biophysical terms (Table 9.1). Characterization of the state of the myocardium in patients with congestive heart failure became possible when the work of the heart was recognized to be regulated by changes in *myocardial cell biochemistry*, which were expressed clinically as abnormalities in *myocardial contractility*.

Our present understanding of the role of depressed myocardial contractility in the pathogenesis of heart failure is based on two lines of research, both of which were stimulated by the observation that factors other than end-diastolic fiber length determined the performance of the heart (5,21). Recognition that changing properties of individual myocardial cells played a major role in controlling the work of the heart (Table 9.2) stimulated efforts to characterize the mechanical behavior of the heart in terms of skeletal muscle mechanics (22,23). At the same time, rapid progress in our understanding of the biochemical and biophysical processes that regulate myocardial contractility made clear the central role of Ca^{2+} in cardiac excitation-contraction coupling (24). Application of this new understanding to evaluate myocardial function in humans led to the demonstration that myocardial contractility was, in fact, depressed in patients with heart failure (25).

The Search for the Ideal Inotropic Agent

A seemingly obvious corollary to the depressed myocardial contractility in patients with heart failure, which until recently dominated strategy for management of this syndrome, was that the condition of these patients would be improved by increasing contractility in the failing heart. The conclusion that more powerful inotropic stimulation would be beneficial to these patients gained support from clinical experience in the coronary care unit, where temporary inotropic support of the failing left ventricle was of clear value in treating the acute heart failure that followed massive myocardial infarction. The view that survival could be similarly improved by increasing myocardial contractility in chronic congestive heart failure stimulated a search for improved means to increase contractility in these patients.

Cardiac glycosides. Forty years ago, the cardiac glycosides were the only useful positive inotropic agent for the treatment of heart failure. I suspect, however, that the benefit of these agents was due, in large part, to their ability to slow ventricular rate in atrial fibrillation. Such a view had been expressed by two of the giants of British cardiology. Sir James MacKenzie wrote in 1918:

"In searching the records in literature for the evidence of the good effects of digitalis, I feel fairly certain that it is in patients with auricular fibrillation, particularly when it is subsequent to rheumatic fever, that the extraordinarily good results have been obtained. If one reads carefully the records given by Withering in the first valuable account of digitalis in 1785, though he used it as a diuretic, yet he noted its good effects in heart cases; and several of his successful cases had undoubtedly auricular fibrillation" (26).

Twenty years later, Sir Thomas Lewis wrote: "It is to their striking effect in cases of auricular fibrillation that drugs of the digitalis group almost conclusively owe their well-founded reputation" (27). Even in the 1940s, rheumatic heart disease was the leading cause of heart failure, affecting about 2% of the population (28), and atrial fibrillation was found in about 40% of patients with mitral stenosis (29).

Regardless of the basis for their wide acceptance, the cardiac glycosides were given as a matter of course to virtually every patient who appeared to be suffering from congestive heart failure. However, the low therapeutic/toxic ratio of the cardiac glycosides had, for years, stimulated unsuccessful efforts to identify a safer drug of this class. This search ended only recently when it was realized that the therapeutic and toxic effects of the cardiac glycosides both arose from the same molecular interaction of these drugs with the cardiac cell, which by inhibiting the sodium pump (30), increases intracellular sodium concentration and so promotes calcium entry by Na/Ca exchange (31).

Early inotropic agents. Although the benefit derived from the positive inotropic actions of the catecholamines in the short-term management of patients with acute myocardial infarction suggested their possible usefulness in chronic congestive heart failure, most inotropic drugs available 40 years ago were poorly suited for long-term administration. The sympathomimetic amines of that time had chronotropic and arrhythmogenic side effects that precluded their routine use in the management of chronic congestive heart failure, whereas phosphodiesterase inhibitors like aminophylline were short-acting and sometimes caused arrhythmia and sudden death.

Paired pulse stimulation. The inotropic effect of postextrasystolic potentiation enjoyed a brief moment in the spotlight of clinical cardiology over 20 years ago (32). This now almost forgotten inotropic therapy attempted to use the marked potentiation of the contraction after a premature systole, a manifestation of the positive (Bowditch) staircase, to treat heart failure. Although paired pulse stimulation was once viewed as having clinical potential in the management

of patients with heart failure, the risk of inducing arrhythmias and interference with ventricular filling by the premature systoles was quickly recognized and this hazardous approach to therapy was abandoned.

New inotropic agents. The search for new inotropic drugs was facilitated by rapid advances in our understanding of the ability of cyclic adenosine monophosphate (AMP), the second messenger that mediates the cellular effects of sympathomimetic amines, to modify the Ca^{2+} fluxes responsible for cardiac excitation-contraction coupling. It now appears that, with the notable exception of the cardiac glycosides, most inotropic agents that have been examined clinically act by increasing the rate of cyclic AMP production or decreasing the rate of breakdown of this second messenger (33). Whereas the bipyridines, introduced a decade ago as "novel" inotropic drugs, are now generally accepted to be phosphodiesterase inhibitors, another class of new agents, the imidazopyridines, increase the Ca^{2+} sensitivity of the contractile proteins (34). Clinical applications of drugs that modify various ion channels in the cardiac sarcolemma are still to be found; examples are agents that prolong sodium channel opening, and so promote calcium entry through exchange of the increased cellular Na^+ with extracellular Ca^{2+} by way of Na/Ca exchange (35). Other inotropic drugs delay the closing of the potassium channels that cause membrane repolarization; the resulting increase in action potential duration prolongs calcium channel opening and so increases cellular Ca^{2+}. Although these mechanisms are of promise in the development of truly novel inotropic drugs, new knowledge of the pathophysiology of heart failure is bringing this phase in the management of congestive heart failure to a close.

Limitations on the Use of Inotropic Agents for the Management of Congestive Heart Failure

Major conceptual advances in our understanding of the cardiac abnormalities in patients with congestive heart failure are now shifting therapeutic strategies away from efforts to increase contractility. This redirection of the goals of therapy is due in part to the recognition of the role of relaxation abnormalities in these patients and to the realization that relaxation is especially sensitive to an imbalance between energy production and energy utilization in the myocardium.

Importance of relaxation (lusitropic) abnormalities. Emphasis on inotropic abnormalities during the "phase of inotropic stimulation" (Table 9.2) reflected the widely held view that heart failure was due entirely, or at least largely, to impaired ability of the heart to contract. This focus on systolic abnormalities was, in no small measure, a reflection of the utilization of intraventricular pressure measurements as the reference standard for evaluating ventricular function. As the indexes most easily derived from pressure curves occur during the isovolumic phase of systole, such estimates of myocardial contractility as positive first derivative of left ventricular pressure (+dP/dt), V_{max}, and V_{CE} once dominated the assessment of cardiac dysfunction in patients with heart failure. Because of difficulties in evaluating relaxation by the use of pressure-derived indexes based on catheterization data, it was not until the introduction of noninvasive methods for the study of ventricular wall motion (echocardiography) and volume changes (nuclear cardiology) that simple and accurate evaluations of diastolic function became feasible in the failing human ventricle (36). Over the past decade, these new clinical methods revealed that relaxation abnormalities played a much greater role in the pathogenesis of heart failure than had previously been suspected (37).

Energy is required for the heart to relax. Recognition of the importance of relaxation abnormalities in the pathogenesis of congestive heart failure highlighted the clinical significance of the fact that relaxation, like contraction, is an energy-requiring process (38). This raised the possibility that the lusitropic abnormalities commonly encountered in these patients might be due to a lack of energy in the overloaded myocardium, and so added to earlier concerns (39) that inotropic stimulation, by increasing energy expenditure in the failing heart, might represent an inappropriate strategy for routine therapy of congestive heart failure (40,41).

Is the failing heart an energy-starved heart? In most patients with heart failure, whether due to hemodynamic overloading, loss of functional myocardial tissue or a valve abnormality, the work of the active myocardial cells, and so their expenditure of energy, are increased on a long-term basis. However, there is abundant evidence, albeit mostly indirect, that the cells of the hypertrophied and failing heart are unable to generate sufficient energy to provide for this increased rate of energy expenditure; as a result, the failing heart is likely to be in an energy-starved state (42).

A number of changes that occur in the failing heart can impair the ability of the hypertrophied myocardial cells to meet their increased energy needs. Intercapillary distance is increased (43) and there is a decreased number of transverse capillary profiles per square millimeter (44); both would increase the distance required for the diffusion of substrates, notably oxygen, to the cells of the hypertrophied heart. A resulting predisposition to a state of energy deficiency would be especially severe in the relatively underperfused subendocardial regions of the hypertrophied ventricle (45).

Changes in the composition of the cells in the chronically overloaded myocardium represent another possible cause for an energy-starved state in the failing heart. Several experimental studies (44,46,47) have shown that the fraction of cell volume occupied by myofibrils in the hypertrophied heart is increased, whereas mitochondrial mass decreases; changes that could exacerbate an energy deficit by increasing the number of adenosine triphosphate (ATP)-consuming myofibrils that must be supported by each ATP-generating mitochondrion.

Myocardial high energy phosphate content has been *found to be decreased* in the pressure-overloaded left (48) and right (49) ventricles in animal models of heart failure. Cardiac biopsies in patients with congestive heart failure have also shown that reduced content of high energy phosphate compounds (50) correlates with the extent of impairment of both contraction and relaxation (51). These data are consistent with the view that a chronic myocardial energy deficit contributes to the deterioration in patients with chronic congestive heart failure.

Strategies for the Management of Congestive Heart Failure. Phase IV: Preserve the Failing Heart

Much like the once prevalent "senescence" theory of atherosclerosis as an inevitable consequence of the aging process (52), the progressive deterioration in patients with congestive heart failure was, until a few years ago, thought to be unavoidable and untreatable. This fatalistic view was heightened by the fact that heart failure often results from clinical conditions, such as some of the cardiomyopathies, that are themselves progressive. As recently as the mid 1980s, therapy of severe congestive heart failure was believed to have little likelihood of improving the poor prognosis in these patients (53).

This hopeless view of congestive heart failure was dramatically reversed by recent demonstrations that medical therapy could, in fact, significantly prolong life (15,54) and slow cardiac deterioration (55) in these patients. This realization has stimulated a new emphasis on efforts to preserve the failing heart and added significance to studies of the molecular biology of the overloaded myocardium.

Spontaneous Deterioration of the Hypertrophied Heart

Almost a century ago, Osler (56) recognized that the clinical state in patients with a hemodynamically overloaded heart follows a predictable course. The first response to a lesion like acute aortic regurgitation is a period of "development," during which the myocardium hypertrophies to meet the increased load. This leads into a stage of "compensation," in which acute heart failure caused by the increased load is alleviated as hypertrophy distributes the increased load among a larger number of cardiac fibers. Osler recognized, however, that the hypertrophied heart tends to undergo spontaneous, progressive deterioration in a final stage of "broken compensation."

The cardiomyopathy of overload. The modern era of understanding the causes of deterioration of the overloaded heart began with the monumental work of Meerson (57), who found that experimental aortic coarctation causes the myocardium to undergo a sequence of structural and biochemical changes that lead to fibrosis and cell death (Table 9.3).

Hypertrophy, which begins during the initial phase in this sequence (analogous to Osler's "development"), represents a beneficial response as the increased mass of heart muscle distributes the overload among a greater number of sarcomeres (analogous to Osler's "compensation"). However, this response carries with it a heavy price; much like Faust's bargain with the devil, a brief period of pleasure is followed by an eternity of pain! This occurs because the cells of the hypertrophied heart are not normal and, in the face of sustained overloading, deteriorate and die (analogous to Osler's "broken compensation"), thereby initiating a vicious cycle by further increasing the load on the surviving cells (Fig. 9.1). The response of the heart in patients with congestive heart failure therefore resembles that of the circulation described by Harris (12), where mechanisms like vasoconstriction and sodium retention are compensatory for the short term, but come to have deleterious long-term effects. It is clear that, as stated over 20 years ago: "the failing heart is not simply an enlarged version of the normal heart" (58). On the contrary, the cells of the hypertrophied heart undergo a progressive deterioration that can be viewed as a "cardiomyopathy of overload," which may become a major determinant of the downhill course in patients with this condition (59).

Possible role for energy starvation. A clue to the mechanisms responsible for the progressive deterioration of the overloaded myocardium is found in the "stone heart syndrome." This form of ischemic contracture was described by Cooley et al. (60) in patients with severe left ventricular hypertrophy who underwent open heart surgery with inadequate cardioplegia. This syndrome, which appears to result from high energy phosphate depletion that occurs when the severely overloaded heart becomes ischemic (61), may represent a model for the slower myocardial cell deterioration seen when patients with chronic congestive heart failure are treated medically.

A word of caution is in order, however. If the past is any guide to the future (1,5,21), the final answer to the important question of what causes the progressive deterioration in the overloaded heart is likely to be far more complex than can be imagined today. For example, it is by no means impossible that accelerated senescence accompanies the hypertrophy that develops in the cells of the overloaded heart.

Morphologic changes in the hypertrophied heart. Complex morphologic abnormalities in hypertrophied and failing hearts have long been recognized. Using light microscopy, Linzbach (62) observed that the myocardial cells are uniformly and moderately enlarged in the mildly hypertrophied heart ("concentric hypertrophy"), whereas he attributed thinning of the wall of the heart in more severe heart failure ("eccentric hypertrophy") to weakening of connective tissue and destruction of myofibers. It is now apparent that changes in the extracellular matrix of the hypertrophied heart reflect very complex processes; for example, fibrosis involves not only changes in the amount of collagen, but also

the appearance of different types of collagen during the different phases of the response to overload (63). Evidence that chronic overloading of the heart leads to changes in cardiac composition (44,46,47) and alterations in the number of beta-adrenergic receptors (64) provides further examples of important changes in the composition of the hypertrophied and failing heart.

Heart Failure as an Abnormality of Gene Expression in the Myocardium

Molecular changes now recognized to occur in the individual proteins of the hypertrophied and failing heart have functional consequences that can be both compensatory and deleterious in the patient with congestive heart failure. Alpert and Gordon (65) first suggested such molecular changes when they reported that cardiac myosin adenosine triphosphate (ATPase) activity is depressed in congestive heart failure. Subsequent demonstrations that cardiac myosin ATPase activity changes not only in response to chronic overload, but also in aging and the endocrinopathies (66), suggested that altered protein structure represents a "tonic" mechanism (6) by which myocardial function becomes adapted to long-term circulatory changes (Table 9.1). These early concepts have recently been incorporated into the fast-moving fields of "molecular biology," which are demonstrating a hitherto unimagined degree of molecular heterogeneity in the proteins of the myocardium (9).

Variability of gene expression in the heart. Growing knowledge of the mechanisms responsible for the remarkable variability of gene expression in the heart has defined a key role for changes in the cardiac proteins in determining the myocardial response in patients with heart failure. Although this field is still in its infancy, characterization of cardiac myosin, the major protein of the thick filament that is readily isolated in pure form and in large amounts from heart muscle, illustrates a number of important functional and biochemical features of these changes in gene expression (67–69). These focus on the myosin "heavy chains," which determine the rate of energy liberation by myosin both in vitro (ATPase activity) and in vivo (muscle shortening velocity).

The myosin heavy chains, which are encoded by several gene families, are expressed differently among different muscles and at different times in a single muscle during ontogeny (68). In the adult heart, chronic hemodynamic overloading and heart failure are among the most important causes of altered cardiac myosin gene expression (67,70–76). This is readily apparent in the rat ventricle, which can express several myosin heavy chain isoforms; the V_1 (alpha) myosin heavy chain determines a high myosin ATPase activity and rapid shortening velocity, whereas the V_3 (beta) myosin heavy chain determines low myosin ATPase activity and slow shortening velocity. In the overloaded, hypertrophied myocardium, the preferential synthesis of the messenger ribonucleic acid that encodes the low ATPase V_3 heavy

Table 9.3. Three Stages in the Response to a Sudden Hemodynamic Overload

Stage 1 (days): Transient breakdown
    Circulatory: Acute heart failure; pulmonary congestion, low output
    Cardiac: Acute left ventricular dilation, early hypertrophy
    Myocardial: Increased content of mitochondria relative to myofibrils

Stage 2 (weeks): Stable hyperfunction
    Circulatory: Decreased pulmonary congestion and improved cardiac output
    Cardiac: Established hypertrophy
    Myocardial: Increased content of myofibrils relative to mitochondria

Stage 3 (months): Exhaustion and progressive cardiosclerosis
    Circulatory: Progressive left ventricular failure
    Cardiac: Further hypertrophy with progressive fibrosis
    Myocardial: Cell death

This table is based on experimental studies of the response of the heart to aortic constriction described by Meerson (57).

chain (75) leads to the replacement of fast myosin with slow myosin, which decreases the rate of cross-bridge cycling and so reduces myocardial contractility. However, at the same time that this alteration in gene expression has a negative inotropic effect, mechanical efficiency is increased (8,39). Thus, one result of the changing expression of different myosin heavy chain genes in hypertrophy is an energy-sparing effect that facilitates the adaptation of the heart to the chronically increased hemodynamic load. Although the human ventricle is now recognized to contain only one myosin heavy chain isoform, a similar change in myosin gene expression has been observed in overloaded human atria, where a decreased proportion of fast (alpha) atrial myosin heavy chain parallels the extent of left atrial enlargement (77).

Expression of different protein isoforms in the hypertrophied heart has also been reported for two proteins of the thin filament; actin (78,79) and tropomyosin (79). This response represents more than a simple "up-regulation" of sarcomere synthesis, as is apparent from evidence that expression of altered myosin and actin isoforms follows different time courses (78,79).

Isoform changes in the hypertrophied heart have also

Figure 9.1. By increasing the number of contractile units, and so reducing the loading on each sarcomere of the overloaded heart (−), hypertrophy is beneficial. However, hypertrophy also initiates myocardial changes that lead ultimately to cell death. As a result, hypertrophy perpetuates a vicious cycle that, by reducing the number of contractile units, increases the load on each of the surviving cells (+).

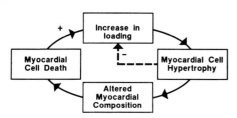

been reported for lactate dehydrogenase (80), creatine kinase (81,82) and the sarcolemmal sodium pump (83). That this list is incomplete is evidenced by major functional changes in the failing heart that have not yet been explained at a molecular level. Among the latter is the severely impaired relaxation seen when heart muscle from patients with dilated or hypertrophic cardiomyopathy is studied in vitro (84). Although this lusitropic abnormality may be due in part to a deficit in chemical energy, the mechanism appears to be more complex and may involve increased sensitivity of the energy-dependent reactions that relax the heart to as yet poorly understood energetic abnormalities in the hypertrophied myocardium (85).

Therapeutic implications of excessive energy demands by the hypertrophied heart. Demonstration that changes in the synthesis of specific myocardial proteins reduce contractility in the hypertrophied heart raises fascinating questions as to whether these changes are compensatory or deleterious. I believe that they are both (39). Insofar as the changes in myosin heavy chain isoforms synthesized by the overloaded heart reduce myocardial contractility, the alterations in gene expression are detrimental to pumping by the failing heart. This view has, in the past, provided a rationale for efforts to increase myocardial contractility in patients with heart failure. At the same time, however, the important energy-sparing effect of depressed contractility could preserve myocardial cell viability in an energy-starved heart and so, like afterload reduction, might prolong survival in patients with congestive heart failure.

A logical corollary to the interpretation that depression of contractility in the overloaded heart has a potentially beneficial energy-sparing effect is that negative inotropic agents could be of value in preserving cell viability in the chronically overloaded heart (39). Such an interpretation is supported by the ability of vasodilators to prolong survival and preserve myocardial function in patients with congestive heart failure (15,54,55), a beneficial effect that may be due, at least in part, to a reduced rate of energy utilization by the overloaded cells of the failing heart (42). The ability of negative inotropic drugs to produce a similar energy-sparing effect may explain the results of several clinical trials (86–91) that indicate that beta-adrenergic blocker therapy can prolong survival and slow deterioration in patients with heart failure. Although these observations in no way deny the hazards of negative inotropic therapy in heart failure, especially when it is acute as in cardiogenic shock, they offer hope that means are at hand to alter further the bleak prognosis in patients with chronic congestive heart failure.

Strategies for the Management of Congestive Heart Failure. Phase V: Correct the Myocardial Abnormality

Should efforts be made to modify the evolution of hypertrophy in the failing heart? We have seen how the remarkable plasticity in cellular composition of the myocardium gives rise to important functional changes in the hypertrophied, failing heart. By providing more sarcomeres to aid the heart in meeting the overload caused by a variety of disease processes, hypertrophy is initially compensatory; however, because hypertrophy also initiates processes that may lead to myocardial cell death, this response can lead to a cardiomyopathy of overload that becomes part of the pathologic process itself (Fig. 9.1). Although attempts to modify detrimental changes in gene expression in the patient with congestive heart failure are not yet feasible, the likely existence of a cardiomyopathy of overload should stimulate efforts to formulate new strategies to modify gene expression in the failing heart.

Conclusions

As it is essential to understand the past before attempting to predict the future, this article has focused largely on the history of strategies for the therapy of congestive heart failure. Three important points can be drawn from this historic survey. *The first, apparent when Table 9.2 is examined in light of Table 9.1, is that new clinical strategies, although often initiated by thoughtful and careful clinical observation, become established when they find support in concepts derived from basic research.* I do not mean to imply that innovations in clinical practice depend on basic research; more often, it is the other way around in that novel observations in patients frequently direct basic research to important clinical problems. In fact, new ideas in medicine find clinical application most rapidly when basic and clinical science advance together.

The second point of this review is that the pace of scientific advance is accelerating (Table 9.2). It is no exaggeration that we have learned more of value about the therapy of heart failure in the past 10 years than had been learned previously since the dawn of time (92).

Finally, the history of science teaches us that important advances come from unexpected directions. This caveat notwithstanding, it seems safe to predict that better understanding of regulation of gene expression, coupled with new knowledge about the biochemistry of the hypertrophied and failing heart, will provide means by which myocardial composition can be altered so as to benefit the patient with congestive heart failure. Such a capability could allow the fifth of the strategies set forth in Table 9.2 to be achieved; but how to restore normal structure and function in the myocardium of the patient with congestive heart failure is, of course, a question for future research.

I thank my colleagues and the fellows, residents and students at the University of Connecticut, with whom this topic has been elucidated through ongoing discussion and debate. I thank especially Frank C. Messineo, MD and W. David Hager, MD for their careful reading of this manuscript and help in clarifying many salient points of this review.

References

1. Katz AM. Role of the basic sciences in the practice of cardiology. J Mol Cell Cardiol 1987;19:3–17.
2. Wood P. An appreciation of mitral stenosis. Br Med J 1954;1:1051–63, 1113–24.
3. Kannel WB. Epidemiology and prevention of congestive heart failure: Framingham Study insights. Eur Heart J 1987;8(suppl F):23–39.
4. MacKenzie J. Diseases of the Heart. Oxford: Oxford University Press, 1908.
5. Katz AM. Molecular biology in cardiology, a paradigmatic shift. J Mol Cell Cardiol 1988;20:355–66.
6. Katz AM. Tonic and phasic mechanisms in the regulation of myocardial contractility. Basic Res Cardiol 1976;71:447–55.
7. Bugaisky L, Zak R. Biological mechanisms of hypertrophy. In: Fozzard H, Haber E, Katz A, Jennings R, Morgan HE, eds. The Heart and Cardiovascular System. New York: Raven, 1986:1491–506.
8. Hamrell BB, Alpert NA. Cellular basis of the mechanical properties of hypertrophied myocardium. In Ref. 7:1507–24.
9. Katz AM, Katz PB. Homogeneity out of heterogeneity. Circulation 1989;79:712–17.
10. Withering W. An Account of the Foxglove and Some of its Medical Uses: With Practical Remarks on Dropsy and other Diseases. London: CGJ Robinson, 1785.
11. Saxl P, Heilig R. Übar die diuretische Wirkung von Novasurol und andern Quecksilberinjecktionen. Wein Klin Wochenschr 1920;33:943.
12. Harris P. Evolution and the cardiac patient. Cardiovasc Res 1983;17: 313–9, 373–8, 437–45.
13. Ross J Jr. Afterload mismatch and preload reserve: a conceptual framework for the analysis of ventricular function. Prog Cardiovasc Dis 1976;18:255–64.
14. Cohn J, Franciosa JA. Vasodilator therapy of cardiac failure. N Engl J Med 1977;297:27–31, 254–57.
15. Cohn JN, Archibald DG, Ziesche S, et al. Effect of vasodilator therapy on mortality in chronic congestive heart failure: results of a Veterans Administration cooperative study (V-HeFT). N Engl J Med 1986;314: 1547–52.
16. Katz LN. Analysis of the several factors regulating the performance of the heart. Physiol Rev 1955;35:91–106.
17. Olson RE. Myocardial metabolism in congestive heart failure. J Chronic Dis 1959;9:442–64.
18. Bing RJ. Cardiac metabolism. Physiol Rev 1965;45:171–213.
19. Katz AM. The descending limb of the Starling curve and the failing heart. Circulation 1965;32:871–5.

20. Katz AM. Fundamental mechanisms in myocardial failure. In: The Heart and Circulation. Second National Conference on Cardiovascular Diseases. Research. Washington, DC: FASEB J 1965;1:533–7.

21. Katz AM. Regulation of myocardial contractility, 1958–1983: an odyssey. J Am Coll Cardiol 1983;1:42–51.

22. Abbott BC, Mommaerts WHFM. A study of inotropic mechanisms in the papillary muscle preparation. J Gen Physiol 1959;42:533–51.

23. Sonnenblick EH. Implications of muscle mechanics in the heart. Fed Proc 1962;21:975–90.

24. Katz AM. Regulation of cardiac muscle contractility. J Gen Physiol 1967;50:185–96.

25. Braunwald E, Ross J Jr, Sonnenblick EH. Mechanisms of Contraction of the Normal and Failing Heart. 2nd ed. Boston: Little, Brown, 1975.

26. MacKenzie J. Diseases of the Heart. 3rd ed. Oxford: Oxford University Press, 1918.

27. Lewis T. Diseases of the Heart. New York: Macmillan, 1933.

28. Wilson MG. Rheumatic Fever. New York: The Commonwealth Fund, 1940.

29. Wood P. Diseases of the Heart and Circulation. 2nd ed. Philadelphia: JB Lippincott, 1956.

30. Katz AM. Effects of digitalis on cell biochemistry: sodium pump inhibition. J Am Coll Cardiol 1985;5:16A–21A.

31. Lee CO, Abete P, Pecker M, Sonn JK, Vasalle M. Strophanthidin inotropy: role of intracellular sodium ion activity and sodium-calcium exchange. J Mol Cell Cardiol 1985;17:1043–53.

32. Cranefield P, ed. Conference on paired pulse stimulation and postextrasystolic potentiation in the heart. Bull NY Acad Med 1965;41:417–748.

33. Scholz H. Inotropic drugs and their mechanisms of action. J Am Coll Cardiol 1984;4:289–97.

34. Solaro JR, Ruegg JC. Stimulation of Ca^{++} binding and ATPase activity of dog cardiac myofibrils by AR-L115BS. Circ Res 1968;51:290–4.

35. Luellman H, Peters J, Ravens U. Pharmacological approaches to influence cardiac inotropism. Pharmacol Ther 1983;21:229–45.

36. Smith VE, Katz AM, Weisfeldt ML. Relaxation and diastolic properties of the heart. In: Ref. 7:803–18.

37. Grossman W, Lorell BH. Diastolic Relaxation of the Heart. Boston: Martinus Nijhoff, 1988.

38. Katz AM. Potential deleterious effects of inotropic agents in the therapy of chronic heart failure. Circulation 1986;73(suppl III):III-184–8.

39. Katz AM. Biochemical "defect" in the hypertrophied and failing heart: deleterious or compensatory? Circulation 1973;47:1076–9.

40. Katz AM. A new inotropic drug: its promise and a caution. N Engl J Med 1978;299:1409–10.

41. LeJemtel TH, Sonnenblick EH. Should the failing heart be stimulated? N Engl J Med 1984;310:1384–5.

42. Katz AM. The myocardium in congestive heart failure. Am J Cardiol 1989;63:12A–6A.

43. Roberts JT, Wearn JT. Quantitative changes in the capillary-muscle relationship in human hearts during normal growth and hypertrophy. Am Heart J 1941;21:617–23.

44. Anversa P, Olivetti G, Melissari M, Loud AV. Stereological measurement of cellular and subcellular hypertrophy and hyperplasia in the papillary muscle of adult rat. J Mol Cell Cardiol 1980;12:781–95.

45. Hoffman JEI. Transmural myocardial perfusion. Prog Cardiovasc Dis 1987;29:429–64.

46. Page E, McCalister LP. Quantitative electron microscopic description of heart muscle cells: application to normal, hypertrophied and thyroxin-stimulated hearts. Am J Cardiol 1973;31:172–81.

47. Rabinowitz M. Protein synthesis and turnover in normal and hypertrophied heart. Am J Cardiol 1973;31:202–10.

48. Furchgott RF, Lee KS. High energy phosphates and the force of contraction of cardiac muscle. Circulation 1961;24:416–28.

49. Pool PE, Spann JF, Buccino RA, Sonnenblick EH, Braunwald E. Myocardial high energy phosphate stores in cardiac hypertrophy and heart failure. Circ Res 1967;1:365–73.

50. Swain JL, Sabina RL, Peyton RB, et al. Derangements in myocardial purine and pyrimidine nucleotide metabolism in patients with coronary artery disease and left ventricular hypertrophy. Proc Natl Acad Sci USA 1982;79:655–9.

51. Bashore TM, Magorien DJ, Letterio J, Shaffer P, Unverferth DV. Histologic and biochemical correlates of left ventricular chamber dynamics in man. J Am Coll Cardiol 1987;9:734–42.

52. Katz LN. Experimental atherosclerosis. Circulation 1952;5:101–14.

53. Braunwald E. Newer positive inotropic agents: concluding comments. Circulation 1986;73(suppl III):III-237.

54. CONSENSUS Trial Study Group. Effects of enalapril on mortality in severe congestive heart failure: results of the Cooperative North Scandinavian Enalapril Survival Study (CONSENSUS). N Engl J Med 1987;316:1429–35.

55. Pfeffer MA, Lamas GA, Vaughan DE, Parisi AF, Braunwald E. Effect of captopril on progressive ventricular dilatation after anterior myocardial infarction. N Engl J Med 1988;319:80–6.

56. Osler W. The Principles and Practice of Medicine. D Appleton, 1892:634.

57. Meerson FZ. On the mechanism of compensatory hyperfunction and insufficiency of the heart. Cor Vasa 1961;3:161–77.

58. Katz LN, Schaffer AB. Hemodynamic aspects of congestive heart failure. In: Blumgart H, ed. Symposium on Congestive Heart Failure. 2nd ed. Monograph No. 1, Dallas, Texas: American Heart Association, 199:12–31.

59. Katz AM. Cardiomyopathy of overload: a major determinant of prognosis in congestive heart failure. N Engl J Med 1990;322:100–10.

60. Cooley DA, Reul GJ, Wukasch DC. Ischemic contracture of the heart: stone heart. Am J Cardiol 1972;29:571–3.

61. Katz AM, Tada M. The "stone heart": a challenge to the biochemist. Am J Cardiol 1972;29:578–80.

62. Linzbach AJ. Über das Langenwachstum der Herzmuskelfasern und ihrer Kerne in Beziehung zur Herzdilatation. Virchows Arch Pathol Anat Physiol Klin Med 1956;328:165–81.

63. Weber KT, Janicki JS, Schroff SG, Pick R, Chen RM, Bashey RI. Collagen remodeling of the pressure-overloaded, hypertrophied nonhuman primate myocardium. Circ Res 1988;62:757–65.

64. Bristow MR, Ginsburg R, Minobe WA, et al. Decreased catecholamine sensitivity and β-adrenergic receptor density in the failing heart. N Engl J Med 1982;307:205–11.

65. Alpert NR, Gordon MS. Myofibrillar adenosine triphosphatate activity in congestive heart failure. Am J Physiol 1962;202:940–6.

66. Katz AM. Contractile proteins of the heart. Physiol Rev 1970;50:58–163.

67. Swynghedauw B. Developmental and functional adaptation of contractile proteins in cardiac and skeletal muscles. Physiol Rev 1986;66:710–71.

68. Emerson CP Jr, Bernstein SI. Molecular genetics of myosin. Annu Rev Biochem 1987;56:695–726.

69. Breitbart RE, Andreadis A, Nadal-Ginard B. Alternative splicing: a ubiquitous mechanism for the generation of multiple protein isoforms from single genes. Annu Rev Biochem 1987;56:467–95.

70. Lompre AM, Schwartz K, D'Albis A, Lacombe G, Van Thiem N, Swynghedauw B. Myosin isoenzyme redistribution in chronic heart overload. Nature 1979;282:105–7.

71. Rupp H. The adaptive changes in the isoenzyme pattern of myosin from hypertrophied rate myocardium as a result of pressure overload and physical training. Basic Res Cardiol 1981;76:79–88.

72. Scheuer J, Malhotra A, Hirsch C, Capasso J, Schaible TF. Physiologic cardiac hypertrophy corrects contractile protein abnormalities associated with pathologic hypertrophy in rats. J Clin Invest 1982;70:1300–5.

73. Litten RZ, Martin BJ, Low RB, Alpert NR. Altered myosin isozyme pattern from pressure-overloaded and thyrotoxic hypertrophied rabbit hearts. Circ Res 1982;50:856–64.

74. Tsuchimochi H, Kuro-o M, Takaku F, et al. Expression of myosin isozymes during the developmental stage and their redistribution induced by pressure overload. Jpn Circ J 1986;50:1044–52.

75. Izumo S, Lompre A-M, Matsuoka R, et al. Myosin heavy chain messenger RNA protein isoform transitions during cardiac hypertrophy. J Clin Invest 1987;79:970–7.

76. Bugaisky L, Zak R. Biological mechanisms of hypertrophy. In: Ref. 7:1491–506.

77. Mercadier JJ, de la Bastie D, Menasche P, et al. Alpha-myosin heavy chain isoform and atrial size in patients with various types of mitral valve dysfunction: a quantitative study. J Am Coll Cardiol 1987;9:1024–30.

78. Schwartz K, de la Bastie D, Bouveret P, et al. *a*-skeletal muscle actin mRNAs accumulate in hypertrophied adult rat hearts. Circ Res 1986;59: 551–5.

79. Izumo S, Nadal-Ginard B, Mahdave V. Protooncogene induction and reprogramming of cardiac gene expression produced by pressure overload. Proc Natl Acad Sci USA 1988;85:339–43.

80. Fox AC. High-energy phosphate compounds and LDH isozymes in the hypertrophied right ventricle. In: Alpert NR, ed. Cardiac Hypertrophy. New York: Academic, 1971:203–12.

81. Meerson FZ, Javick MP. Isozyme pattern and activity of myocardial creatine phosphokinase under heart adaptation to chronic overload. Basic Res Cardiol 1982;77:349–58.

82. Ingwall JS, Kramer MF, Fifer MA, et al. The creatine kinase system in normal and diseased human myocardium. N Engl J Med 1985;313:1050–4.

83. Charlemagne D, Maixen J-M, Preteseille M, Lelievre LG. Ouabain binding sites and (Na$^+$, K$^+$)-ATPase activity in rat cardiac hypertrophy: expression of neonatal forms. J Biol Chem 1986;261:185–9.

84. Gwathmey JK, Copelas L, MacKinnon R, et al. Abnormal intracellular calcium handling in myocardium from patients with end-stage heart failure. Circ Res 1987;61:70–6.

85. Wexler LF, Lorell BH, Monomura S-i, Weinberg EO, Ingwall JS, Apstein CS. Enhanced sensitivity to hypoxia-induced diastolic dysfunction in pressure-overload left ventricular hypertrophy in the rat: role of high-energy phosphate depletion. Circ Res 1988;62:766–75.

86. Svedberg K, Hjalmarson A, Waagstein F, Wallentin I. Prolongation of survival in congestive cardiomyopathy by beta-receptor blockade. Lancet 1979;1:1374–6.

87. Furberg CD, Hawkins CM, Lichstein E. Effect of propranolol in postinfarction patients with mechanical or electrical complications. Circulation 1984;69:761–5.

88. Anderson JL, Lutz JR, Gilbert EM, et al. A randomized trial of low-dose beta-blockade therapy for idiopathic dilated cardiomyopathy. Am J Cardiol 1985;55:471–5.

89. Engelmeier RS, O'Connell JB, Walsh R, Rad N, Scanlon PJ, Gunnar RM. Improvement in symptoms and exercise tolerance by metoprolol in patients with dilated cardiomyopathy: a double-blind, randomized, placebo-controlled trial. Circulation 1985;72:536–46.

90. Gilbert EM, Anderson JL, Deitchman D, et al. Chronic beta blockade with bucindolol improves resting cardiac function in dilated cardiomyopathy (abstr). Circulation 1987;76(suppl IV):IV-358.

91. The German and Austrian Xamoterol Study Group. Double-blind placebo-controlled comparison of digoxin and xamoterol in chronic heart failure. Lancet 1988;1:489–93.

92. Packer M. Vasodilator and inotropic drugs for the treatment of chronic heart failure: distinguishing hype from hope. J Am Coll Cardiol 1988;12: 1299–317.

CHAPTER 10

Treatment of Acute Myocardial Infarction in the Era of Thrombolysis

DONALD W. DIXON, MD, ROLF M. GUNNAR, MD

Treatment of acute myocardial infarction now includes thrombolysis, but much of the data regarding concomitant therapy are data generated in the prethrombolysis era. This review attempts to put these data in perspective.

It is now accepted that an immediate invasive strategy in patients without persistent angina or recurrent ischemia after thrombolysis for acute myocardial infarction has no positive effect on outcome and may be detrimental. However, the mortality rate after hospital discharge is dependant on myocardial function, electrical stability and coronary anatomy. Only coronary anatomy can be altered sufficiently to significantly alter long-term outcome. To accomplish this, better knowledge of the coronary pathology, including knowledge of the lesions in the noninfarct-related arteries, is needed. Coronary angiography appears to be the best strategy to obtain this information. Revascularization by angioplasty or surgery based on criteria developed in patients with chronic angina may be our best current strategy. This approach needs to be tested in a long-term study to facilitate development of cost containment strategies that could include routine angiography in the management of the patient recovering from acute myocardial infarction.

Thrombolysis early in the course of acute myocardial infarction is now accepted therapy (where not contraindicated) and appears to reduce the incidence of death significantly (1). However, after thrombolysis, the patient cannot be easily equated with prior historic patient groups that had completed their infarction. If thrombolysis is successful in opening the infarct-related artery, a very active lesion remains and is subject to reocclusion in up to 20% of patients (2). Some patients will have critical fixed stenosis, whereas others may have minimal occlusion or, in a small percent of patients, no remaining obstruction (3). Because most cardiologists were unwilling to perform angiography on patients with acute infarction before the report of DeWood et al. (4), there are few data available to help understand the dynamics of the occlusive process in the era before thrombolytic therapy. For this reason, we must design our postthrombolysis therapeutic strategy to a major extent utilizing recent studies (5–9) that include angiographic evaluation in the early postinfarction period. Because of the frequency of subsequent reperfusion by angioplasty or bypass surgery in patients so studied, we are without the benefit of knowing the natural history of the disease correlated with the underlying coronary anatomy and ventricular function and not modified by an invasive intervention. This is a new era.

With these reservations in mind, however, we do have to define a perithrombolysis strategy for the individual patient. In this report, we attempt to develop such a strategy on the basis of a review of the design and results of current published studies.

Heparin

Heparin has been a part of the therapy in most trials of thrombolysis, being started immediately or within the first 24 h of thrombolysis (2,3,10–18). With a short half-life thrombolytic agent such as recombinant-type tissue plasminogen activator (rt-PA), heparin is best started in conjunction with or at the termination of the thrombolytic infusion. To delay its use beyond 90 min may leave the patient with a highly active endothelial surface and no protection from reocclusion. There is no evidence, however, that heparin infusion beginning with the rt-PA infusion is any more effective than if delayed to 90 min after the onset of the thrombolytic infusion (19). Conversely, the incidence of cerebral hemorrhage has been significant in some series (16,20). For this reason, it is imperative to avoid over anticoagulation by keeping the partial thromboplastin time between 1.5 and 2 times normal. This infusion should be continued for 48 to 96 h.

It is not known to what extent heparin therapy contributes to the incidence of hemorrhagic stroke in patients with acute myocardial infarction who have been treated with thrombolytic agents. The incidence of stroke in acute myocardial infarction before thrombolytic therapy was reported to be 3% (21,22). The observed 1.5% rate of hemorrhagic stroke in the early Thrombolysis in Myocardial Infarction (TIMI) Trial (20) was judged to be due to the use of a 150 mg dose of rt-PA, and the incidence was reduced to 0.5% in a subsequent series of patients treated with a 100 mg dosage. There are some trade-offs at these levels, however, between a reduction in thrombotic stroke and an increase in hemorrhagic stroke and thrombolytic success (23). As one expands the exclusion criteria to limit rt-PA to younger patients, patients without hypertension on one or more readings in the emergency room and without a history of hypertension and patients without a history of prior stroke, there can be a reduction in the incidence of hemorrhagic stroke, but at the expense of denying increasingly effective therapy to some patients with acute myocardial infarction. When outside a research protocol, each patient becomes a problem of risk versus benefit for the clinician. The patient seen early with a large area of myocardium in jeopardy will benefit greatly from thrombolysis, so perhaps he or she can be older and have a somewhat higher blood pressure than the patient seen late or with less myocardium at risk, or both. There are no studies of thrombolysis that correlate the baseline changes in hypertension with the risk of hemorrhagic stroke, but a look at the retinal vessels may be of help when one is deciding for or against thrombolysis in the older, moderately hypertensive patient.

Aspirin

The Second International Study of Infarct Survival (ISIS-2) (24) showed a clear advantage of low dose aspirin in acute myocardial infarction. There was a 21% reduction in the mortality rate with aspirin alone compared with placebo, very similar to the 23% reduction with streptokinase alone. When both agents were combined, there was a 39% reduction in the mortality rate. This augmentation of the effect of streptokinase when aspirin was added is not surprising because thrombolytic agents have been shown to activate platelets and release thromboxane A_2, as demonstrated by the appearance of thromboxane A_2 metabolites in the serum and urine (25). Such platelet activation can be a significant factor in reocclusion. Since the ISIS-2 report (24), most new trials include low dose aspirin as standard therapy for acute infarction. The small dose used during ISIS-2 (160 mg/day) is most likely sufficient for long-term therapy, although recent long-term studies (26) have used $\geq$330 mg/day and have not compared the various dosage levels (26). A dose of 160 mg/day has the advantage of being associated with very little gastrointestinal irritation and appears to be sufficient to inhibit reocclusion.

Thus, standard therapy for acute myocardial infarction now includes thrombolysis (where not contraindicated), low dose aspirin and heparin after thrombolysis. The controversy over which thrombolytic agent to use continues and is not dealt with here because currently published studies have been inconclusive in establishing clear survival differences between agents. They have, however, established the value of thrombolysis, the need for identification of the patient qualifying for thrombolysis at the earliest time after the onset of the acute infarct syndrome and the necessity of omitting all administrative procedures that can delay infusion of the thrombolytic agent (1).

Beta-Blocker Therapy

Large-scale trials (27,28) of beta-adrenergic blocker therapy in acute myocardial infarction have suggested that their intravenous use early in acute myocardial infarction may improve survival and preserve myocardium. The largest trial (28) of >16,000 patients showed a clear improvement in survival at 7 days, with a reduction in the mortality rate from 4.6% to 3.9% (p < 0.02). The patients in the treatment arm of the study were given atenolol intravenously at a dose of 5 to 10 mg, followed by an oral dose of 100 mg/day. Patients were entered into the study an average of 5 h after the onset of pain. The second largest trial (27) of >5,700 patients failed to show more than a trend, with the mortality rate at 15 days being reduced from 4.9% to 4.3%. This latter trial showed most of its mortality reduction in the "high risk" subgroup. This may represent the difficulty of further reducing an already low acute mortality rate in this disease. Both of these trials and 28 other smaller studies (29) of early intravenous beta-blocker therapy have generally accepted the use of these agents for long-term therapy and thus have given oral beta-blockers to patients in both arms of the study after 7 to 15 days.

It becomes apparent that early intravenous beta-blockade has only a minor effect on the early mortality rate. It may have a greater but still not well-defined effect on protecting myocardium from irreversible ischemic damage. Also, beta-blockers can only be used in a portion of patients who do not have one of the rather long list of contraindications. These contraindications include heart rate <60 beats/min, systolic blood pressure <100 mm Hg, moderate to severe left ventricular failure, signs of peripheral hypoperfusion, atrioventricular (AV) conduction abnormalities (PR internal >0.22 s), AV block and severe chronic obstructive lung disease. There is also a list of relative contraindications, including history of asthma, severe peripheral vascular disease, difficult to control insulin-dependent diabetes and caution for patients already on beta-blockers or calcium channel blockers (1). It has been suggested that when in doubt, one can use a short-acting beta-blocker such as esmolol as a test (30). Concern about adverse effects has been confirmed by a significant increase in the need for inotropic agents and an increased but not statistically significant incidence of complete heart block in patients treated with aterolol (28).

In an analysis (29) of 28 reported randomized trials of early intravenous beta-blocker therapy of acute myocardial infarction, in addition to a 16% reduction in the mortality rate, there was also an 18% reduction in early reinfarction or extension and a 15% reduction in ventricular fibrillation. One would have to conclude that in the prethrombolysis era, there was an advantage to the use of intravenous beta-blockers in acute myocardial infarction if they could be given early and were not contraindicated. This still holds for the patient who is denied thrombolysis because of hypertension or bleeding propensity. Such therapy has an advantage in reducing the incidence of death, recurrent ischemia and ventricular fibrillation.

Current recommendations must be modified in accordance with the acceptance of thrombolysis as the keystone of therapy. From these previous studies, one cannot infer any significant benefit of early beta-blockade for those patients receiving reperfusion with thrombolytic agents. Animal studies (31,32) suggest that such a therapy would preserve myocardium, but it is not clear that this would translate to use in the naturally occurring syndrome in humans.

A subprotocol of the TIMI IIB Study (3) was designed to determine the effect on mortality and ventricular function of immediate versus deferred beta-blockade after thrombolytic therapy in patients with acute myocardial infarction. Patients were excluded from this part of the trial if they were already on oral beta-blockers, verapamil or diltiazem or if they had a ventricular rate <55 beats/min, a systolic pressure <90 mm Hg, advanced AV block, rales above the lower third of the lungs or a history of asthma, and only 48.4% of the patients qualified for therapy. Metoprolol was randomly assigned and administered as three 5 mg intravenous injections at 2 min intervals, followed by 50 mg orally twice a day on the first day and 100 mg twice a day thereafter. Those randomized to deferred therapy were begun on the oral therapy on hospital day 6. Preliminary reports from this trial (3) indicate that metoprolol was well tolerated in 90% of the patients. At follow-up study, there was no difference in survival or ventricular function between the groups given immediate beta-blockade compared with those with deferred therapy. The investigators, however, did demonstrate a significant reduction in reinfarction and recurrent ischemia during the 6 day interval, during which the immediate treatment group was the only one receiving beta-blockade. The incidence of recurrent ischemia decreased from 21.2% to 15.4% (p < 0.005) and nonfatal reinfarction from 4.5% to 2.3% (p < 0.02). Death or reinfarction decreased from 6.9% to 4.7% (p < 0.08) with early intravenous metoprolol therapy. For the patients who received therapy within 2 h of the onset of symptoms, death or reinfarction decreased from 12.1% in the placebo group to 5% in the metoprolol group (p < 0.01). In a low risk subgroup, there were no deaths at 42 days in the intravenous metoprolol-treated patients and a 2.8% mortality rate in those in whom therapy was deferred (p < 0.007), just the reverse of the experience from the metoprolol in acute myocardial infarction (MIAMI) Trial (27), which found most benefit in the high risk group. When the 100 mg dose of rt-PA was utilized, there was no intracranial hemorrhage during the initial 6 days in the patients randomized to receive immediate intravenous metoprolol, whereas five patients in the deferred treatment group had such an event (p = 0.03). These data suggest a potential indication for immediate beta-blockade, but the number of patients is too small to be considered statistically significant (33).

Thus, the recommendation for early intravenous beta-blockade in patients with acute myocardial infarction seen within the first 6 h of pain onset and without contraindications seems based on adequate data, but the advantages of such therapy are small (34). It is probable that one is dealing with three different effects of such therapy. In the patients seen very early (first 2 h), there may be myocardial preservation as seen in animal models of coronary occlusion (31,32). During the first several days, beta-blockers may tend to prevent recurrent ischemia (3), cardiac rupture (34,35) and primary ventricular fibrillation (36), whereas the longer-term positive effects may be preponderantly due to the antiarrhythmic effect of the agent (37,38). Only the first of these effects would require intravenous administration of the beta-blocker. Thus, for those who do not wish to give intravenous beta-blockers to the patient with early acute myocardial infarction >2 h old, it may be prudent to initiate oral therapy earlier to capture the effect on recurrent ischemia and the antiarrhythmic effects of these agents.

Nitroglycerin

Nitroglycerin has also become standard therapy in acute myocardial infarction (1). Recently a randomized trial (39) confirmed previous clinical trials and demonstrated a reduction in the in-hospital mortality rate from 26% to 14% with use of intravenous nitroglycerin. With the endothelial disruption seen after acute infarction and thrombolysis, the infarct-related artery has a propensity for spasm. Therefore, the use of nitroglycerin even in the absence of symptoms is becoming recognized in patients after thrombolytic therapy. Intravenous nitroglycerin has been recommended for the 1 or 2 days after thrombolysis (1). Because of the ease of dosage titration, intravenous use is preferable to transdermal and sublingual administration. In patients who may have right ventricular infarction, however, one must be cautious with the use of nitroglycerin because it may decrease filling pressure in a damaged right ventricle that may be dependent on an elevated filling pressure.

Calcium Channel Entry Blockers

Calcium channel entry blockers may be helpful for coronary spasm not controlled with intravenous nitroglycerin. As routine therapy after thrombolysis, however, we cannot recommend their use on the basis of currently available data. A review of several studies (40) suggests that routine use of nifedipine has an adverse effect on acute myocardial infarction. The Diltiazem Reinfarction Study Group (41) reported efficacy of diltiazem in preventing early reinfarction and recurrent angina in patients with non-Q wave myocardial infarction. This 14 day trial done before the era of thrombolysis showed a reduction in creatine kinase MB isoenzyme (CK-MB) evidence of reinfarction from 9.3% of patients in the placebo group to 5.2% of patients in the treatment group. Diltiazem was started within 24 to 72 h of the onset of infarction (mean 53 h). The dosage was 90 mg every 6 h, with the first and second doses being modified to 30 and 60 mg, respectively. The reduction in the incidence of refractory angina with diltiazem therapy was also significant. This study, however, did not demonstrate a difference in mortality and cannot be used as an argument for prolonged medical therapy in these patients. Almost all of the benefit from diltiazem therapy occurs after day 6. It may well be that early (5 to 6 days) angiography and revascularization, where indicated, would be more beneficial than diltiazem in preventing ischemia and reinfarction in patients with non-Q wave myocardial infarction.

The Multicenter Diltiazem Postinfarction Research Group (42) reported on the use of diltiazem (60 mg given orally four times a day, beginning 3 to 15 days after the onset of myocardial infarction). This was also a prethrombolysis era study. There was a 3:1 ratio between Q wave and non-Q wave infarction. The patients were followed up for at least 1 year, with an average follow-up period of 25 months. The investigators reported what appeared to be an adverse effect of diltiazem in patients with pulmonary congestion and left ventricular dysfunction, which they felt obscured a beneficial effect for the entire group of patients. Patients were blocked at randomization into those randomized at ≤5 days and those >5 days. Because of a litany of exclusions and frequent lack of patient consent, only 2,466 patients from a total of 13,618 eligible patients were actually randomized. There was no difference in mortality between the diltiazem and the placebo groups, even though there was a slight but statistically insignificant benefit in reducing the first cardiac event rate in the diltiazem group. Of greatest interest was the adverse effect diltiazem had on the mortality rate in patients with left ventricular dysfunction severe enough to cause pulmonary congestion.

Of additional note was the low surgery or angioplasty intervention rate reported during the first year (17% and 0.2%, respectively) in a group of patients with a mortality rate of 10% over 25 months. Most of these deaths occurred in the first year. All the patients had survived at least 5 days after infarction, and 70% had an ejection fraction ≥0.40. It would appear from other studies (43) that these patients should have had a much better survival outlook.

The routine use of diltiazem or any other calcium channel blocker in patients with transmural infarction appears to have little proven value and may perhaps be deleterious. A reduction in ischemic events might be better achieved by a more invasive strategy of revascularization. If a calcium channel blocker is to be used for treatment of recurrent ischemia, however, one should be particularly cautious in patients with evidence of left ventricular dysfunction.

Lidocaine

On the basis of data then available, prophylactic infusion of lidocaine was recommended by the Bethesda Conference on Emergency Cardiac Care (44). More recent data (45), however, suggest that the increased incidence of asystole during lidocaine infusion may counter the beneficial effects of reducing unheralded ventricular fibrillation. A meta analysis (46) of 14 randomized trials of prophylactic lidocaine in acute myocardial infarction failed to show a reduction in the overall mortality, even though there was a decreased incidence of ventricular fibrillation. Therefore, although prophy-

lactic lidocaine is an option for preventing unheralded ventricular fibrillation in patients <70 years of age within 6 h of acute infarction and without cardiac failure, it is no longer recommended as a routine infusion (1). It has been a standard therapy in the TIMI (2), Thrombolysis and Angioplasty in Myocardial Infarction (TAMI) (47) and New Zealand (48) Trials and may help suppress reperfusion arrhythmias in patients receiving thrombolysis, even though these arrhythmias are unpredictable and can usually be treated as they arise. It has not been a routine therapy in the Gruppo Italiano per lo Studio Della Streptochinasi Nell'Infarto Myocardico (GISSI) (49), ISIS-2 (24) or APSAC Intervention Mortality Study (AIMS) (14) Trials. Lidocaine remains the first line therapy in patients with frequent and complex ventricular premature beats, and this applies to patients after thrombolysis (1).

The current recommended indicators for lidocaine use in acute myocardial infarction, based on the Delphi process, are frequent premature ventricular beats (>6/min), couplets, multifocal premature ventricular beats and runs of premature beats (44). These clinical indicators are still accepted, even though they have never been subjected to scientific trial in either the pre- or postthrombolytic era. A single bolus injection of 50 to 100 mg, followed by a 2 mg/min infusion, will frequently lead to subtherapeutic levels at 20 min to 1 h in the average adult (50). A second bolus injection during this hiatus may be necessary to suppress arrhythmias. Caution is advised, however, in the elderly, patients with liver disease and those with congestive failure or shock. The diagnosis of "intensive care unit disorientation of the elderly" should not be made in a patient with a running lidocaine infusion. As the infusion continues past 24 h, the half-life increases and the infusion rate should be slowed. In withdrawing lidocaine, there is no need to "wean" the drug because decay in blood levels will occur naturally over many minutes to hours, depending on the volume of distribution of the drug and the patient's ability to metabolize the agent.

Long-Term Anticoagulation

The decision to initiate anticoagulant therapy has been settled when the patient with acute myocardial infarction receives a thrombolytic agent. These patients, as already discussed, should receive heparin for at least 48 to 96 h and then continue on low dose aspirin (1). Those with a large infarct involving the left ventricular apex are in jeopardy of systemic embolization from a mural thrombus (51). Although echocardiography is excellent in detecting such thrombi, the dynamic nature of the process gives no assurance that a thrombus absent early will not develop later (52). The use of thrombolytic therapy may only delay the appearance of a thrombus and, except as it limits infarct size, there is no reason to conclude that data from the prethrombolytic era do not pertain to these patients as well, although the time frame may be postponed. The incidence of systemic embolization after anterior infarction is 4% to 6% (53). The incidence of such embolization has been shown to be reduced by the use of heparin, followed by oral anticoagulation with warfarin (51,53). Waiting for echocardiographic evidence of mural thrombus before initiating therapy may result in inadequate protection. When on warfarin, it is sufficient to keep the prothrombin time between 1.3 and 1.5 times the control value (54). Although oral anticoagulants may be stopped safely after 3 months (55), patients with diffuse left ventricular dysfunction should be continued on such therapy indefinitely (56).

Aspirin has been shown to reduce the mortality rate by 15% and late recurrence of myocardial infarction by 31% (26). In an analysis of nine controlled trials (57,58), warfarin after acute myocardial reinfarction was also demonstrated to reduce reinfarction and death by 30% and 20%, respectively.

These results confirm that patients recovering from myocardial infarction should receive aspirin or warfarin. It may be that they should be on both, but this has not been tested. The fear of gastrointestinal or other bleeding complications has made clinicians cautious of such a regimen. However, if a small dose of aspirin (160 mg/day) and warfarin at a lower dose than has been traditionally used in the United States are utilized, bleeding might be less of an adverse factor. It is now accepted that the effect of warfarin can be adequate when the prothrombin time is between 1.3 and 1.5 times the control value, and at this level adverse bleeding is reduced (54).

Arrhythmias

A discussion of arrhythmias in the postthrombolytic era can be done more intelligently than discussion of antiarrhythmic therapy. When atrial fibrillation/flutter or ventricular arrhythmias appear >48 h after the onset of acute myocardial infarction, there is a good correlation with left ventricular dysfunction (59). Prognosis may be determined primarily by the left ventricular dysfunction, but there is good evidence (60) that ventricular arrhythmias are also an independent predictor of poor outcome. There is no evidence that random treatment or even therapeutic efficacy-directed treatment will positively effect outcome. There are studies (61,62) that show that programmed stimulation can identify patients who have inducible ventricular tachycardia and that these patients have a significantly increased incidence of sudden death in the 12 months after acute myocardial infarction, but therapy has not been shown to change the outcome. The Cardiac Arrhythmia Suppression Trial (CAST) (63) showed that even the use of a type IC antiarrhythmic agent demonstrated to be effective against premature ventricular beats during the prerandomization period resulted in an excess of deaths in the treated group compared with the placebo control group during the randomized portion of the trial. The patients studied were asymptomatic, with premature beats and symptomless nonsustained runs of ventricular tachycardia. It must be remembered that the previous data (64) that supported therapy of nonsustained symptomatic ventricular tachycardia with an agent shown to suppress inducibility of the ventricular tachycardia were developed in patients with chronic ischemic heart disease and may not apply to the patient recovering from myocardial infarction.

Failure of Thrombolytic Therapy

Patients with acute infarction continuing to have pain and ST segment elevation despite thrombolytic therapy should, if possible, have coronary angiography and reperfusion. Although there are and probably will be no randomized trials, clinical experience suggests that these patients are in serious difficulty and have a poor prognosis (65), particularly if the area of infarction is anterior. Rescue angioplasty (66) and emergency surgical revascularization (67) should be considered in such patients. Repeated unsuccessful attempts at angioplasty should not be pursued if coronary bypass surgery is available within 6 h of the onset of pain. To delay surgery beyond 6 h increases the incidence of death and closes the "window of opportunity" for salvage of ischemic myocardium in these unstable patients (67).

Conservative Versus Invasive Strategy After Thrombolysis

The TIMI Phase II Trial (3,68,69) was designed to test an invasive strategy of angiography and percutaneous transluminal coronary angioplasty at 18 to 48 h after thrombolytic therapy compared with a conservative strategy where angiography and angioplasty were done only if there was a recurrence of angina or ischemia during a predischarge exercise test. This study was preceded by several studies, including at least three randomized trials that are discussed here. The European Cooperative Study Group (70) conducted a trial in which 367 patients were randomized after thrombolysis with rt-PA to a conservative strategy or immediate angioplasty. The patients in the conservative treatment group were found to have a lower incidence of recurrent ischemia, bleeding complications, hypotension and ventricular fibrillation. The mortality rate at 14 days was 3% in the conservative treatment group and 7% in the invasive treatment group. These investigators (70) concluded that there was no benefit from early angioplasty. Another randomized trial (71) of elective coronary angioplasty after rt-PA delayed angioplasty until the third hospital day. This study was conducted by the Johns Hopkins investigators (71) and demonstrated a low 5.6% mortality rate in both groups without a significant difference between the groups. Although the number of patients randomized was small, results of this study did suggest that elective coronary angioplasty on day 3 after infarction reduced the incidence of recurrent ischemia and resulted in improved ventricular function as measured at hospital discharge by radionuclide ventriculography during submaximal exercise testing.

The TAMI Study Group (47) randomized 197 patients to either immediate or delayed angioplasty after intravenous rt-PA. They studied 386 patients with acute myocardial infarction seen within 6 h of the onset of chest pain (mean time to rt-PA administration 2.95 ± 1.1 h) and randomized the 197 patients who were shown at catheterization 90 min later to have TIMI grade 2 or 3 patency of the infarct-related artery. Patients were randomized to immediate or elective angioplasty at 7 to 10 days. All patients underwent repeat catheterization at 7 to 10 days. Of the 99 patients assigned to immediate angioplasty, the procedure was successful in 90 patients, there was closure of the infarct-related artery in 9 patients and 7 of these went to emergency coronary bypass surgery. Five patients with successful angioplasty had to have emergency angioplasty after leaving the catheterization laboratory. In the 98 patients assigned to the elective strategy, angioplasty was performed emergently in 16 and electively in 35. Eleven patients were referred for bypass surgery, 20 were discharged on medical therapy and 14 were found to have resolution of their stenosis to <50%. The incidence of reocclusion was similar in the two groups. The investigators (47) conclude that in patients who have had successful thrombolysis, there is no advantage of immediate angioplasty over a strategy of delayed elective angioplasty.

There were additional nonrandomized studies (72–74) suggesting that early coronary angioplasty was safe and reduced the overall mortality rate. A report (72) of 342 patients with acute myocardial infarction, all of whom were treated with thrombolysis followed by emergency coronary angioplasty, demonstrated an in-hospital mortality rate of 11%. However, the 1 year survival rate for hospital survivors was 98% and the infarct-free survival rate at 1 year was 94%. Four percent of the patients required emergency coronary bypass surgery. Thus, the in-hospital mortality rate may appear high, but 13% of these patients were in cardiogenic shock, which carried a 42% in-hospital mortality rate. In addition, several patients in this series had suffered cardiac arrest or ventricular fibrillation before entry, which would have eliminated them from most of the randomized trials.

The TIMI Phase IIA Trial (75) was a three-way randomization comparing immediate with delayed catheterization and angioplasty and a conservative noninvasive strategy. The investigators randomized 586 patients between immediate angioplasty, angioplasty delayed to 48 h and a conservative strategy where angioplasty was done only if there was recurrence of ischemia. All patients had coronary angiography and contrast ventriculography just before discharge. No difference was found between the groups in their baseline characteristics. However, the immediate angioplasty group experienced an increased need for emergent coronary bypass surgery, an increased frequency of bleeding and no

statistically significant advantage in reduced mortality or recurrent ischemia over either the delayed invasive or conservative strategy groups.

On the basis of these findings, the TIMI Phase II Trial (3) randomized 3,262 patients between conservative and invasive treatment (including 389 patients not in the immediate invasive strategy of the TIMI-IIA Substudy). The thrombolytic agent used was rt-PA at a dose of 150 mg in the first 520 patients, 100 mg in the remainder. The details of this significant study are very important to our current understanding of treatment during the acute phase of myocardial infarction. Because of recurrent ischemia, 66 of the 1,636 patients assigned to the invasive strategy had angiography emergently before the assigned 18 to 48 h period. Of the 1,636 patients, 1,461 had angiography and 878 had angioplasty during the specified interval. The reasons for not performing angioplasty in the remaining 692 patients were as follows: no infarct-related artery >60% occluded in 12.6% of patients, total occlusion in the infarct-related artery without continuous ischemia in 12.1%, an infarct-related artery unsuitable for angioplasty in 13.4% and miscellaneous reasons in 2%. The success rate for angioplasty in the 878 patients was 93.3%.

Of the 1,626 patients assigned to the conservative strategy, 25.8% had recurrent ischemia, 32.7% had cardiac catheterization, 13.3% had angioplasty and 10.5% had coronary bypass surgery. Thus, 23.8% of the patients in the conservative strategy group had revascularization, whereas 43.3% in the invasive strategy group did not. If one includes the 50 patients in the invasive strategy group in whom angioplasty was attempted during the 18 h before the prescribed time in the protocol, then 928 (56.7%) of the patients randomized to the invasive strategy had angioplasty. The results of angioplasty in these 928 patients revealed that the procedure was successful in 92.6% of the patients, with complications occurring in 22%. After angioplasty, 7.9% of patients developed total occlusion of the infarct-related artery or one of its branches, 5.4% had reinfarction and 0.5% died. Coronary bypass surgery was required in 4.5% of these patients with total occlusion of the infarct-related artery. Thus, of the entire group assigned to the invasive strategy, only 47.7% appeared to have had a successful outcome from angioplasty.

Of the patients assigned to the conservative strategy, 33% had angiography and 13.3% had angioplasty. The complication rate for angioplasty was similar to that in patients in the invasive strategy group who required emergency angioplasty for recurrent ischemia in the initial 18 h of the infarction. Approximately 20% had total occlusion of the infarct-related artery or reinfarction. The almost doubled complication rate in patients having emergency angioplasty suggests that these lesions are unstable and, although they may need revascularization, success is not as assured as if one can wait to 18 to 48 h. The overall mortality rate was 5.9% in patients assigned to the invasive strategy and 4.7% in those assigned to the conservative strategy. The incidence of nonfatal reinfarction also was not statistically different between the groups. Only when bypass surgery after angioplasty was considered as an adverse end point was a statistical difference observed. Deaths at 24 h were identical between the two groups, amounting to 2.3% of the overall group. This probably represents an irreducible minimal mortality rate during this period.

The final study end point for the main trial occurred at 6 weeks after acute myocardial infarction. In the TIMI Phase II Trial (3), 19.4% of the conservative treatment group had a positive exercise test at the 6 week follow-up study. This occurred despite the fact that 19% had had a revascularization procedure (either angioplasty or bypass surgery). In the invasive strategy group, 16.8% of patients had a positive exercise test at 6 weeks. It should not be surprising that a number of patients in both the invasive and conservative strategy groups would still have exercise-induced ischemia because the study was designed to perform angioplasty only on the infarct-related artery. What is surprising is that the difference between the groups was not greater. However, 50% of the patients with acute myocardial infarction would be expected to have multivessel coronary artery disease, as suggested by Kulick and Rahimtoola (76). Therefore, if only 57% of the patients in the invasive strategy group had angioplasty and 19% of the patients in the conservative strategy group had revascularization, it becomes less surprising that potential differences between the groups were obscured. What the TIMI Phase II Study most effectively demonstrated was that current treatment of acute myocardial infarction should include thrombolysis for all patients who qualify, followed by angioplasty in those who have recurrent ischemia. The 5% overall in-hospital mortality rate attests to the efficacy of this therapy, particularly when one considers that almost 50% of deaths occur within the first 24 h. The TIMI Phase II demonstrated no advantage to an invasive strategy applied early after infarction unless required by recurrent ischemia. It also demonstrated that coronary angiography can be safely performed in the acute phase of myocardial infarction. Because 12.6% of patients in the invasive strategy group had an infarct-related artery <60% occluded at angiography, this study suggested that delaying angiography may allow spontaneous clot dissolution and make it easier to identify those patients who have had myocardial infarction without significant underlying coronary artery stenosis and who thus do not need revascularization. In addition, because a significant number of patients still had a positive exercise test at 6 weeks, such a finding should not be used to conclude that these patients do not need coronary angiography.

Waters et al. (77) observed a 23% mortality rate from hospital discharge to 1 year after acute myocardial infarction in patients with ST segment depression on a limited exercise test done at the time of hospital discharge. This continues to increase to 2 years, but is a poor predictor for death between 2 and 5 years.

There are numerous clinical variables that tend to predict the incidence of death in the first year after acute myocardial infarction, including prior myocardial infarction, ability to reach the target heart rate or work load, ventricular arrhythmias during exercise and a QRS score that is used to define infarct size on the basis of the standard 12 lead electrocardiogram. Angina appearing ≥48 h after admission is also a significant variable, but is weaker than the other variables. The Multicenter Postinfarction Research Group (43) reported on risk stratification in patients surviving myocardial infarction. They enrolled 866 patients <70 years of age who met strict criteria for acute myocardial infarction. The follow-up period was between 1 and 3 years. This study (77) identified four factors that significantly predicted an adverse mortality rate: ejection fraction <0.40, >10 premature ventricular beats/min, pulmonary rales and a history consistent with New York Heart Association functional class II to IV before hospitalization. These predicted a cardiac mortality rate ranging from 3% when no factors were present to 60% when all four factors were present. All these factors really relate to left ventricular dysfunction, including ventricular premature beats, which in addition to being an independent predictor of death (60) also are an index of poor ventricular function (77).

There are indications that coronary angiography can predict survival after myocardial infarction. Schulman et al. (78) evaluated 143 patients <67 years of age with documented acute myocardial infarction; patients were followed up for 5 years. Although there was no attempt to standardize medical therapy, surgical therapy in this group of patients was restricted to those with medically refractory angina or significant left main coronary artery stenosis. On the basis of their data, these authors made three important observations. They demonstrated that as left ventricular function deteriorates, the prognosis for event-free survival also deteriorates. Angiographic evidence of myocardial segments at risk and the coronary anatomy can be shown to predict survival over a 5 year period. When these two variables are combined with ejection fraction as an index of left ventricular function, the ability to predict survival is further enhanced. Myocardial segments at risk are defined as segments of viable myocardium lying behind partially occluded coronary vessels. Patients with an ejection fraction of 0.55, no segments of myocardium at risk and not having combined left anterior descending and right coronary artery disease have a near normal 5 year survival rate. Patients with segments at risk, an ejection fraction of 0.25 and combined left anterior descending and right coronary artery disease have a 5 year survival rate of 5%. These studies suggest the need to define coronary anatomy as well as left ventricular function in determining prognosis.

A third element is electrical instability manifested by ventricular premature beats. Even though in many patients, this may just reflect left ventricular dysfunction, it has been shown to be an independent risk factor and does identify patients at risk for sudden death (79).

Of these three elements—left ventricular dysfunction, electrical instability and coronary artery obstruction—we propose that only coronary artery obstruction is sufficiently amenable to change to improve survival significantly. Patients with severe left ventricular dysfunction can have their prognosis altered somewhat with the use of angiotensin converting enzyme inhibitors (80). It may be important to treat most patients with even modest left ventricular dysfunction with angiotensin converting enzyme inhibitors early after infarction (81,82), even though it has not as yet been conclusively shown that such early treatment will prevent heart failure or death. It has been demonstrated that ventricular arrhythmias can be suppressed pharmacologically, but it has not been shown that this improves outlook (63). The Westmead Group (61) and others (62) have demonstrated that an increased mortality rate can be predicted in patients with inducible ventricular tachycardia in the early postinfarction period, but they failed to show that drug therapy makes any difference.

There is good evidence (83) that coronary artery bypass surgery can affect outcome in patients with coronary disease. Studies done by the Veterans Administration Coronary Artery Bypass Surgery Cooperative Study Group (84), the European Coronary Surgery Study Group (85) and the Coronary Artery Surgery Study (CASS) Group (86) have shown that certain subsets of patients have improved longevity after surgical treatment as compared with medical therapy. That surgery in patients with left main coronary artery disease improves survival has been accepted universally (87). Patients with triple vessel disease and good left ventricular function in the European Coronary Surgery Study (85) had improved survival after coronary bypass surgery. Patients with poor left ventricular function and triple vessel disease in both the Veterans Administration Study (84) and CASS (88) also had improved survival when treated surgically. The European Study (85) showed improved survival in patients treated surgically with double vessel disease in which one of the vessels involved was the proximal left anterior descending coronary artery. These latter patients had good ventricular function, but one would suspect from other studies that with poor left ventricular function, this particular effect would be amplified. Unfortunately, there is evidence that vein grafts deteriorate within 7 to 10 years, and this may significantly effect survival (84). Reported randomized studies of such length, however, have not used internal mammary arteries for bypass grafts (84,85), and there is increasing evidence (89) that such grafts continue to do well for many years and do not deteriorate as rapidly as vein grafts.

Surgery during the early postinfarction period now appears to be reasonably safe. In our experience (90), after acute transmural myocardial infarction, the operative mortality rate in patients with unstable angina is 3%, even if surgery is performed during the second to fourth weeks. At our institution, the overall mortality rate in those after their first bypass surgery was 2.2% during 1988 and 1989. Long-term results after bypass surgery in patients with acute myocardial infarction are quite good, with few deaths occurring during the period from hospital discharge to 52 months (67). This outlook was confirmed by Phillips et al. (91,92) in a smaller series of patients followed up for a shorter period. If one can use the long-term follow-up data from patients operated for stable angina as proxy for the posthospital survival in patients undergoing surgery after acute myocardial infarction, then the survival curve to 5 years would be nearly flat.

Can these results from cardiovascular surgery be applied to angioplasty? This question has not been answered. Some might suggest that if angioplasty is successful, the outlook could be similar to that after successful bypass surgery. However, there are no data as yet to support this. There are those (93) who believe that surgical revascularization will result in a better long-term survival rate than angioplasty. The TIMI Trials (3,68,69) were directed toward angioplasty, and bypass surgery was considered an adverse event. We suggest that bypass surgery might have been a better alternative than angioplasty in some patients. Certainly, it is a better alternative than prolonged and repetitive attempts at angioplasty, which use up time during which surgical reperfusion could still salvage myocardium. Again, we cannot use the positive treadmill test findings at the conclusion of the TIMI Trial as evidence for poor results from angioplasty because angioplasty was limited to the infarct-related artery by the study protocol. If there are other lesions that supply viable segments of myocardium, they need to be opened before the incidence of inducible ischemia after postmyocardial infarction angioplasty can be assessed. It is probable that patients who have had a single infarct-related vessel successfully opened and still have another vessel that needs to be opened could have the second procedure done when they are stable and at least a week or so after the acute event.

If we decide that reasonably complete revascularization is the best strategy to obtain the lowest incidence of death after acute myocardial infarction, all patients with acute myocardial infarction should have angiography at some stage during their initial hospitalization or perhaps immediately thereafter. There is solid evidence (3) to support angiography and consideration of revascularization in patients with poor left ventricular function, angina or exercise-induced ischemia after infarction. If the remainder of the patients do indeed have a mortality rate of approximately 2% during the subsequent year, conservative management without invasive study would be acceptable treatment. There are those (76), however, who propose that even these patients should have their coronary anatomy defined. It has been demonstrated that patients with inferior infarction have

>50% incidence of disease in the left anterior descending or left main coronary artery, and exercise testing may not identify all of these patients (94). Although not universally accepted, it can be defended that all patients with a non-Q wave infarction should have angiography. This issue is subject to a trial currently in progress. If Gibson et al. (95) are correct in concluding that 60% of patients with a non-Q wave infarction have redistribution abnormalities during exercise, there would be little added benefit to screening this subcategory of patients with this expensive test.

There are data (96) suggesting that as many as 47% of patients with a negative exercise test at discharge have multivessel disease. If we cannot rely on noninvasive testing to identify patients with multivessel disease, then what data can we use? It is accepted that all patients with postinfarction angina should have angiography (1,97) and a revascularization procedure, if such a procedure is feasible (78). Conversely, if the patient has an uneventful course and performs an exercise test at the termination of or 3 weeks after hospitalization without evidence of inducible ischemia, current guidelines do not call for angiography (1). There is evidence (76), however, that some of these patients will have coronary anatomy that needs revascularization to achieve the best long-term survival. Thallium perfusion scanning during exercise and exercise radionuclide ventriculography to make certain that these patients do not have ischemia may be far more costly than performing coronary angiography to define the coronary anatomy. Because we know that progression of coronary artery disease is uncommon in totally normal coronary arteries over a 5 year period, one can feel fairly relaxed about a patient with single vessel disease and good left ventricular function (98). If the only evidence for a lack of ischemia is from an indirect test, how often must the test be repeated to be certain that nonobstructive lesions are not progressing?

Before coming to any conclusion regarding the need for angiography, we must decide for what purpose it should be performed. There are no long-term randomized studies specific to the effect of coronary bypass surgery early after infarction. Furthermore, even though we could propose that such data might be extrapolated from data for chronic stable angina and perhaps to angioplasty, there are no long-term randomized comparisons to justify this linkage. However, the physician living in 1990 must make this judgment on the basis of whatever data are currently available. This has to be linked to the individual patient using intuitive clinical logic based on the understanding of the details of the studies, how they are analyzed and, with randomized studies, how many patients were excluded and why.

It is not acceptable to have a 7% mortality rate during the period from hospital discharge to 1 year in patients with acute myocardial infarction treated by thrombolysis, as was reported by GISSI (48). The ISIS-II Trial (24) reported a 5.7% and 6.2% mortality rate between 5 weeks and 1 year in the streptokinase and placebo groups, respectively. Neither of these studies was done with an emphasis on revascularization by angioplasty or surgery in the interim after infarction. The AIMS Trial (14) using APSAC showed a mortality rate of 4.4% and 7.2% between 30 days and 1 year in the treated and placebo groups, respectively. The TIMI-IIA Trial (68) comparing invasive and noninvasive strategies revealed a 2% to 2.6% mortality rate between 21 days and 1 year. This approach included the evaluation of patients at discharge, with those demonstrating ischemia receiving revascularization. By 1 year, 84.4% of the patients in the immediate invasive, 72.3% in the delayed (18 to 48 h) invasive and 38.6% in the conservative strategy groups had had revascularization. The TAMI Investigators (99), who followed an aggressive immediate or deferred angioplasty strategy, reported a 1.9% mortality rate between hospital discharge and 1 year.

From studies to date, it appears that the 1 year mortality rate in patients who survive hospitalization for their first myocardial infarction should be approximately 2% if residual ischemia is properly identified and treated. Thus, treatment that limits infarct size during the acute phase provides a window of opportunity to prevent new ischemia and permits a stable period from discharge to 1 year during which there is an opportunity for secondary prevention by risk factor modification. There is a need for a study of patients after acute myocardial infarction in which *all* patients have coronary angiography, with carefully documented descriptions of the other coronary lesions in addition to the description of the infarct-related artery. We then need to test whether aggressively pursuing total revascularization in the weeks after myocardial infarction improves long-term survival. Some of these data may be able to be generated from the long-term follow-up study of patients in the TIMI Trial (68), but it is not clear whether any of these patients had aggressive pursuit of total revascularization in any systematic fashion. For those who believe that angiography in all patients recovering from infarction would be too costly, we argue that if this clinical strategy is shown to be superior, unit costs for angiography should be reduced. We need to test this approach in a long-term study as we develop cost-containment strategies that include routine angiography in the management of the patient recovering from acute myocardial infarction. Perhaps, we also need to develop experienced clinical centers where large numbers of these patients can have their angiography, costs can be contained, quality can be assured and access to such care can be available to all.

References

1. Gunnar RM, Bourdillon PDV, Dixon DW, et al. Guidelines for the early management of patients with acute myocardial infarction: A report of the American College of Cardiology/American Heart Association Task Force on Assessment of Diagnostic and Therapeutic Cardiovascular Procedures (Subcommittee to Develop Guidelines for the Early Management of

Patients With Acute Myocardial Infarction). J Am Coll Cardiol 1990;16: 249–92.

2. Chesebro JH, Knatterud G, Roberts R, et al. Thrombolysis in Myocardial Infarction (TIMI) trial phase I: a comparison between intravenous tissue plasminogen activator and intravenous streptokinase. Circulation 1987; 76:142–54.

3. The TIMI Study Group. Comparison of invasive and conservative strategies after treatment with intravenous tissue plasminogen activator in acute myocardial infarction. N Engl J Med 1989;320:618–27.

4. DeWood MA, Spores J, Notske R, et al. Prevalence of total coronary occlusion during the early hours of transmural myocardial infarction. N Engl J Med 1980;303:897–902.

5. Mathey DG, Kuck K-H, Tilsner V, Krebber H-J, Bleifeld W. Nonsurgical coronary artery recanalization in acute transmural myocardial infarction. Circulation 1981;63:489–97.

6. Merx W, Dorr R, Rentrop P, et al. Evaluation of the effectiveness of intracoronary streptokinase infusion in acute myocardial infarction: postprocedure management and hospital course in 204 patients. Am Heart J 1981;102:1181–7.

7. Khaja F, Walton J, Brymer J, et al. Intracoronary fibrinolytic therapy in acute myocardial infarction. N Engl J Med 1983;308:1305–11.

8. Leiboff RH, Katz R, Wasserman AG, et al. A randomized, angiographically controlled trial of intracoronary streptokinase in acute myocardial infarction. Am J Cardiol 1984;53:404–7.

9. Kennedy JW, Ritchie JL, Davis KB, Stadius ML, Maynard C, Fritz JK. The Western Washington randomized trial of intracoronary streptokinase in acute myocardial infarction. N Engl J Med 1985;312:1073–8.

10. Topol EJ, Morris DC, Smalling RW, et al. A multicenter, randomized, placebo-controlled trial of a new form of intravenous recombinant tissuetype plasminogen activator (Activase) in acute myocardial infarction. J Am Coll Cardiol 1987;9:1205–13.

11. White HD, Norris RM, Brown MA, et al. Effect of intravenous streptokinase on left ventricular function and early survival after acute myocardial infarction. N Engl J Med 1987;317:850–5.

12. Topol EJ, Bates ER, Walton JA, et al. Community hospital administration of intravenous tissue plasminogen activator in acute myocardial infarction: improved timing, thrombolytic efficacy and ventricular function. J Am Coll Cardiol 1987;10:1173–7.

13. Kennedy JW, Martin GV, Davis KB, et al. The Western Washington intravenous streptokinase in acute myocardial infarction randomized trial. Circulation 1988;77:345–52.

14. AIMS Trial Study Group. Effect of intravenous APSAC on mortality after acute myocardial infarction: preliminary report of a placebo-controlled clinical trial. Lancet 1988;1:545–9.

15. Wilcox RG, Olsson CG, Skene AM, et al. Trial of tissue plasminogen activator for mortality reduction in acute myocardial infarction. Lancet 1988;2:525–30.

16. Van de Werf F, Arnold AER, for the European Cooperative Study Group for Recombinant Tissue Type Plasminogen Activator. Intravenous tissue plasminogen activator and size of infarct, left ventricular function, and survival in acute myocardial infarction. Br Med J 1988;297:1374–9.

17. White HD, Rivers JT, Maslowski MB, et al. Effect of intravenous streptokinase as compared with that of tissue plasminogen activator on left ventricular function after first myocardial infarction. N Engl J Med 1989;320:817–21.

18. Magnani B, for the PAIMS Investigators. Plasminogen Activator Italian Multicenter Study (PAIMS): comparison of intravenous recombinant single-chain human tissue-type plasminogen activator (rt-PA) with intravenous streptokinase in acute myocardial infarction. J Am Coll Cardiol 1989;13:19–26.

19. Topol EJ, George BS, Kereiakes DJ, et al. A randomized controlled trial of intravenous tissue plasminogen activator and early intravenous heparin in acute myocardial infarction. Circulation 1989;79:281–86.

20. Braunwald E, Knatterud GL, Passamani E, et al. Update from the Thrombolysis in Myocardial Infarction Trial (letter). J Am Coll Cardiol 1987;970.

21. Thompson PL, Robinson JS. Stroke after acute myocardial infarction: relation to infarct size. Br Med J 1978;2:457–9.

22. Komrad MS, Coffey CE, Coffey KS, et al. Myocardial infarction and stroke. Neurology 1984;34:1403–9.

23. Tiefenbrunn AJ, Ludbrook PA. Coronary thrombolysis. It's worth the risk. JAMA 1989;261:2107–8.

24. ISIS-2 (Second International Study of Infarct Survival) Collaborative Group. Randomised trial of intravenous streptokinase, oral aspirin, both, or neither among 17,187 cases of suspected acute myocardial infarction: ISIS-2. Lancet 1988;8:350–60.

25. Fitzgerald DJ, Catella F, Roy L, Fitzgerald GA. Marked platelet activation in vivo after intravenous streptokinase in patients with acute myocardial infarction. Circulation 1988;77:142–50.

26. Acheson J, Archibald D, Barnett H, et al. Secondary prevention of vascular disease by prolonged antiplatelet treatment: antiplatelet trialists' collaboration. Br Med J 1988;296:320–31.

27. The MIAMI Trial Research Group. Mortality. Am J Cardiol 1985;56:15G–22G.

28. ISIS-1 (First International Study of Infarct Survival) Collaborative Group. Randomised trial of intravenous atenolol among 16,027 cases of suspected acute myocardial infarction: ISIS-1. Lancet 1986;2:57–66.

29. Yusuf S, Peto R, Lewis J, Collins R, Sleight P. Beta blockade during and after myocardial infarction: an overview of the randomized trials. Prog Cardiovasc Dis 1985;27:335–71.

30. Lange R, Kloner RA, Braunwald E. First ultra-short-acting betaadrenergic blocking agent: its effect on size and segmental wall dynamics of reperfused myocardial infarcts in dogs. Am J Cardiol 1983;51:1759–67.

31. Hammerman H, Kloner RA, Briggs LL, Braunwald E. Enhancement of salvage of reperfused myocardium by early beta-adrenergic blockade (timolol). J Am Coll Cardiol 1984;3:1438–43.

32. Van de Werf F, Vanhaecke J, Jang I-K, Flameng W, Collen D, DeGeest H. Reduction in infarct size and enhanced recovery of systolic function after coronary thrombolysis with tissue-type plasminogen activator combined with β-adrenergic blockade with metoprolol. Circulation 1987;75: 830–6.

33. Roberts R, Rogers WJ, Mueller HS, et al. Immediate versus deferred beta-blockade following thrombolytic therapy in patients with acute myocardial infarction: results of the thrombolysis in myocardial infarction (TIMI) II-B study. Circulation (in press).

34. Roberts R, Croft C, Gold HK, et al. Effect of propranolol on myocardial infarct size in a randomized blinded multicenter trial. N Engl J Med 1984;311:218–25.

35. ISIS-1 (First International Study of Infarct Survival) Collaborative Group. Mechanisms for the early mortality reduction produced by betablockade started early in acute myocardial infarction: ISIS-1. Lancet 1988;1:92–3.

36. Norris RM, Brown MA, Clarke ED, et al. Prevention of ventricular fibrillation during acute myocardial infarction by intravenous propranolol. Lancet 1984;2:883–6.

37. The Norwegian Multicenter Study Group. Timolol-induced reduction in mortality and reinfarction in patients surviving acute myocardial infarction. N Engl J Med 1981;304:802–7.

38. β-Blocker Heart Attack Trial Research Group. A randomized trial of propranolol in patients with acute myocardial infarction. JAMA 1982;247: 1707–14.

39. Jugdutt BI, Warnica JW. Intravenous nitroglycerin therapy to limit myocardial infarct size, expansion, and complications. Circulation 1988; 78:906–19.

40. Moss AJ. Secondary prevention with calcium channel-blocking drugs in patients after myocardial infarction: a critical review. Circulation 1987; (suppl V):V-148–53.

41. Gibson RS, Boden WE, Theroux P, et al. Diltiazem and reinfarction in patients with non-Q-wave myocardial infarction: results of a double-blind, randomized, multicenter trial. N Engl J Med 1986;315:423–9.

42. The Multicenter Diltiazem Postinfarction Trial Research Group. The effect of diltiazem on mortality and reinfarction after myocardial infarction. N Engl J Med 1988;319:385–92.

43. The Multicenter Postinfarction Research Group. Risk stratification and survival after myocardial infarction. N Engl J Med 1983;309:331–6.

44. Gunnar RM, Lambrew CT, Abrams W, et al. Task force IV: pharmacologic interventions. Am J Cardiol 1982;50:393–408.

45. Wyse DG, Kellen J, Rademaker AW. Prophylactic versus selective lidocaine for early ventricular arrhythmias of myocardial infarction. J Am Coll Cardiol 1988;12:507–13.

46. MacMahon S, Collins R, Peto R, Koster RW, Yusuf S. Effects of prophylactic lidocaine in suspected acute myocardial infarction: an overview of results from the randomized controlled trials. JAMA 1988;260: 1910–6.

47. Topol EJ, Califf RM, George BS, et al. A randomized trial of immediate versus delayed elective angioplasty after intravenous tissue plasminogen activator in acute myocardial infarction. N Engl J Med 1987;317:581–8.

48. White HD, Norris RM, Brown MA, et al. Effect of intravenous streptokinase on left ventricular function and early survival after acute myocardial infarction. N Engl J Med 1987;317:850–5.

49. Gruppo Italiano per lo Studio Della Streptochinasi Nell'Infarto Miocardico (GISSI). Long-term effects of intravenous thrombolysis in acute myocardial infarction: final report of the GISSI study. Lancet 1987;2: 871–4.

50. Wyman MG, Lalka D, Hammersmith L, Cannom DS, Goldreyer BN. Multiple bolus technique for lidocaine administration during the first hours of an acute myocardial infarction. Am J Cardiol 1978;41:313–7.

51. Meltzer RS, Visser CA, Fuster V. Intracardiac thrombi and systemic embolization. Ann Intern Med 1986;104:689–98.

52. Fuster V, Halperin JL. Left ventricular thrombi and cerebral embolism. N Engl J Med 1989;320:392–3.

53. Resnekov L, Chediak J, Hirsh J, Lewis J. Antithrombotic agents in coronary artery disease. Chest 1989;95(suppl):52S–72S.

54. Hirsh J, Deykin D, Poller L. "Therapeutic range" for oral anticoagulant therapy. Chest 1989;95(suppl):5S–11S.

55. Lapeyre AC III, Steele PM, Kazmier FJ, Chesebro JH, Vliestra RE, Fuster V. Systemic embolism in chronic left ventricular aneurysm: incidence and the role of anticoagulation. J Am Coll Cardiol 1985;6: 534–8.

56. Stratton JR, Nemanich JW, Johannessen KA, Resnick AD. Fate of left ventricular thrombi in patients with remote myocardial infarction or idiopathic cardiomyopathy. Circulation 1988;78:1388–93.

57. An International Anticoagulant Review Group. Collaborative analysis of long-term anticoagulant administrative after acute myocardial infarction. Lancet 1970;1:203–9.

58. Report of the Sixty Plus Reinfarction Study Research Group. A double-blind trial to assess long-term oral anticoagulant therapy in elderly patients after myocardial infarction. Lancet 1980;2:989–94.

59. James TN. Myocardial infarction and atrial arrhythmias. Circulation 1961;24:761–76.

60. Bigger JT, Fleiss JL, Kleiger R, Miller JP, Rolnitzky LM and The Multicenter Post-Infarction Research Group. The relationships among ventricular arrhythmias, left ventricular dysfunction, and mortality in the 2 years after myocardial infarction. Circulation 1984;69:250–8.

61. Richards DA, Cody DV, Denniss AR, Russell PA, Young AA, Uther JB. Ventricular electrical instability: a predictor of death after myocardial infarction. Am J Cardiol 1983;51:75–80.

62. Cripps T, Bennett ED, Camm AJ, Ward DE. Inducibility of sustained monomorphic ventricular tachycardia as a prognostic indicator in survivors of recent myocardial infarction: a prospective evaluation in relation to other prognostic variables. J Am Coll Cardiol 1989;14:289–96.

63. The Cardiac Arrhythmia Suppression Trial (CAST) Investigators. Preliminary report: effect of encainide and flecainide on mortality in randomized trial of arrhythmia suppression after myocardial infarction. N Engl J Med 1989;321:406–12.

64. Horowitz LN, Josephson ME, Farshidi A, Spielman SR, Michelson EL, Greenspan AM. Recurrent sustained ventricular tachycardia. 3. Role of the electrophysiologic study in selection of antiarrhythmic regimens. Circulation 1978;58:986–97.

65. Schuster EH, Bulkley BH. Early post-infarction angina. N Engl J Med 1981;305:1101–5.

66. Califf RM, Topol EJ, George BS, et al. Characteristics and outcome of patients in whom reperfusion with intravenous tissue-type plasminogen activator fails: results of the Thrombolysis and Angioplasty in Myocardial Infarction (TAMI) I trial. Circulation 1988;77:1090–9.

67. DeWood MA, Spores J, Notske RN, et al. Medical and surgical management of myocardial infarction. Am J Cardiol 1979;44:1356–64.

68. The TIMI Research Group. Immediate vs delayed catheterization and angioplasty following thrombolytic therapy for acute myocardial infarction: TIMI IIA results. JAMA 1988;260:2849–58.

69. Chaitman BR, Thompson BW, Kern MJ, Vandormael MG, et al. Tissue plasminogen activator followed by percutaneous transluminal coronary angioplasty: one-year TIMI phase II pilot results. Am Heart J 1990;119: 213–23.

70. Simoons ML, Betriu A, Col J, et al. Thrombolysis with tissue plasminogen activator in acute myocardial infarction: no additional benefit from immediate percutaneous coronary angioplasty. Lancet 1988;1:197–203.

71. Guerci AD, Gerstenblith G, Brinker JA, et al. A randomized trial of intravenous tissue plasminogen activator for acute myocardial infarction with subsequent randomization to elective coronary angioplasty. N Engl J Med 1987;317:1613–8.

72. Stack RS, Califf RM, Hinohara T, et al. Survival and cardiac event rates in the first year after emergency coronary angioplasty for acute myocardial infarction. J Am Coll Cardiol 1988;11:1141–9.

73. Flaker GC, Webel RR, Meinhardt S, et al. Emergency angioplasty in acute anterior myocardial infarction. Am Heart J 1989;118:1154–60.

74. O'Keefe JH, Rutherford BD, McConahay DR, et al. Early and late results of coronary angioplasty without antecedent thrombolytic therapy for acute myocardial infarction. Am J Cardiol 1989;64:1221–30.

75. Rogers WJ, Baim DS, Gore JM, et al. Comparison of immediate invasive, delayed invasive, and conservative strategies after tissue-type plasminogen activator. Circulation 1990;81:1457–76.

76. Kulick DL, Rahimtoola SH. Is noninvasive risk stratification sufficient, or should all patients undergo cardiac catheterization and angiography after a myocardial infarction? In: Melvin D, Cheitlin MD, eds. Dilemmas in Clinical Cardiology. Philadelphia: FA Davis, 1990, pp 3–25.

77. Waters DD, Bosch X, Bouchard A, et al. Comparison of clinical variables and variables derived from a limited predischarge exercise test as predictors of early and late mortality after myocardial infarction. J Am Coll Cardiol 1985;5:1–8.

78. Schulman SP, Achuff SC, Griffith LSC, et al. Prognostic cardiac catheterization variables in survivors of acute myocardial infarction: a 5 year prospective study. J Am Coll Cardiol 1988;11:1164–72.

79. Mukharji J, Rude RE, Poole WK, et al. Risk factors for sudden death after acute myocardial infarction: two-year follow-up. Am J Cardiol 1984;54: 31–6.

80. The Consensus Trial Study Group. Effects of enalapril on mortality in severe congestive heart failure. N Engl J Med 1987;316:1429–35.

81. Sharpe N, Smith H, Murphy J, Hannon S. Treatment of patients with symptomless left ventricular dysfunction after myocardial infarction. Lancet 1988;2:255–9.

82. Pfeffer MA, Lamas GA, Vaughn DE, Parisi AF, Braunwald E. Effect of captopril on progressive ventricular dilatation after anterior myocardial infarction. N Engl J Med 1988;319:80–6.

83. Gunnar RM, Loeb HS. An alternative interpretation of the results of the coronary artery surgery study (editorial). Circulation 1985;71:193–4.

84. The Veterans Administration Coronary Artery Bypass Surgery Cooperative Study Group. Eleven-year survival in the Veterans Administration randomized trial of coronary bypass surgery for stable angina. N Engl J Med 1984;311:1333–9.

85. Varnauskas E and the European Coronary Surgery Study Group. Twelve-year follow-up of survival in the randomized European Coronary Surgery Study. N Engl J Med 1988;319:332–7.

86. CASS Principal Investigators and Their Associates. Coronary Artery Surgery Study (CASS): a randomized trial of coronary artery bypass surgery. Circulation 1983;68:939–50.

87. Takaro T, Hultgren HN, Lipton MJ, Detre KM and Participants in the Study Group. The VA cooperative randomized study of surgery for coronary arterial occlusive disease. II. Subgroup with significant left main lesions. Circulation 1976;54(suppl III):III-107–17.

88. Passamani E, Davis KB, Gillespie MJ, Killip T and the CASS Principal Investigators and Their Associates. A randomized trial of coronary artery bypass surgery. N Engl J Med 1985;312:1665–71.

89. Loop FD, Irarrazaval MJ, Bredee JJ, Siegel W, Taylor PC, Sheldon WC. Internal mammary artery graft for ischemic heart disease. Am J Cardiol 1977;39:516–22.

90. Jones RN, Pifarre R, Sullivan HJ, et al. Early myocardial revascularization for postinfarction angina. Ann Thorac Surg 1987;44:159–63.

91. Phillips SJ, Kongtahworn C, Zeff RH, et al. Emergency coronary artery revascularization: a possible therapy for acute myocardial infarction. Circulation 1979;60:241–6.

92. Phillips SJ, Zeff RH, Skinner JR, et al. Reperfusion protocol and results in 738 patients with evolving myocardial infarction. Ann Thorac Surg 1986;41:119–25.

93. Hochberg MS, Gielchinsky I, Parsonnet V, et al. Coronary angioplasty versus coronary bypass. J Thorac Cardiovasc Surg 1989;97:496–503.

94. Miller RR, DeMaria AN, Vismara LA, et al. Chronic stable inferior myocardial infarction: unsuspected harbinger of high-risk proximal left coronary arterial obstruction amenable to surgical revascularization. Am J Cardiol 1977;39:954–60.

95. Gibson RS, Beller GA, Gheorghiade M, et al. The prevalence and clinical significance to residual myocardial ischemia 2 weeks after uncomplicated non-Q wave infarction: a prospective natural history study. Circulation 1986;73:1186–98.

96. Griffith LSC, Varnauskas E, Wallin J, Bjuro T, Ejdeback J. Correlation of coronary arteriography after acute myocardial infarction with predischarge limited exercise test response. Am J Cardiol 1988;61:201–7.

97. Ross J, Brandenburg RO, Dinsmore RE, et al. Guidelines for coronary angiography: a report of the American College of Cardiology/American Heart Association Task Force on assessment of diagnostic and therapeutic cardiovascular procedures. J Am Coll Cardiol 1987;10:935–50.

98. Palac RT, Hwang MH, Loeb HS, Gunnar RM. The influence of medical and surgical therapy on the progression of coronary artery disease. In: Rowlands DJ, ed. Recent Advances in Cardiology 9. Edinburgh: Churchill Livingston, 1984:213.

99. Califf RM, Topol EJ, George BS, et al. One-year outcome after therapy with tissue plasminogen activator: report from the Thrombolysis and Angioplasty in Myocardial Infarction Trial. Am Heart J 1990;119:777–85.

CHAPTER 11

Platelet Inhibitor Drugs in Cardiovascular Disease: An Update

BERNARDO STEIN, MD,* VALENTIN FUSTER, MD,* DOUGLAS H. ISRAEL, MD,*
MARC COHEN, MD,* LINA BADIMON, PhD,* JUAN J. BADIMON, PhD,*
JAMES H. CHESEBRO, MD†

Platelets interact with the coagulation and fibrinolytic systems in the maintenance of hemostasis and play a fundamental role in the response of the organism to different forms of vascular injury. However, these physiologic mechanisms may become pathologic by participating in the processes of atherosclerosis and thromboembolism.

Aspirin reduces the mortality and infarction rate in unstable angina and significantly decreases cardiovascular mortality in acute myocardial infarction. Platelet inhibitors reduce mortality and recurrent cardiovascular events in the chronic phase after myocardial infarction. They also decrease the vein-graft occlusion rate after coronary bypass surgery. Although platelet inhibitors are beneficial in preventing acute vessel occlusion during coronary angioplasty, they are ineffective in preventing late restenosis. Emerging evidence suggests that these drugs may reduce the incidence of myocardial infarction in patients with stable coronary disease. Antiplatelet agents combined with warfarin reduce thromboembolic events in patients with a mechanical prosthesis. Platelet inhibitors are effective in the secondary prevention of vascular events in patients with cerebrovascular disease. In addition, recent data suggest that aspirin reduces stroke and systemic embolism in patients with nonvalvulopathic atrial fibrillation. Finally, the value of aspirin in the primary prevention of cardiovascular disease is being recognized and appears useful, particularly for individuals with risk factors for coronary artery disease.

In the late 1960s, aspirin was found to have platelet inhibitory effects and its role in the prevention of coronary platelet thrombosis, then considered the cause of heart attacks, was anticipated. During the 1970s, however, the antithrombotic effects of aspirin were viewed with pessimism, mainly because of two factors. First, the role of coronary thrombosis in the pathogenesis of myocardial infarction was questioned. Second, the effects of platelet inhibitors (including aspirin) in the secondary prevention of coronary disease did not meet with the expectations of the investigators. In the 1980s, an enthusiastic support for platelet inhibitors, especially aspirin, has reemerged. This renewed interest results from a better understanding of the important role of platelets and thrombosis in the pathogenesis of coronary disease. In addition, the results of better designed trials of aspirin in patients with coronary disease have lent further support to the use of antiplatelet therapy in

unstable angina, acute myocardial infarction, coronary angioplasty and saphenous vein bypass surgery. Furthermore, the role of aspirin in the secondary prevention of coronary and cerebrovascular disease has become apparent and its usefulness for stroke prevention in atrial fibrillation and in the primary prevention of cardiovascular pathology is emerging.

Platelets are not the only elements involved in thrombotic and thromboembolic processes, which result from an interaction between platelets and the coagulation and fibrinolytic systems. In this review, we attempt to analyze: 1) the role of platelets in thrombogenesis, 2) the pharmacology of platelet inhibitor agents, and 3) the results of randomized controlled trials of platelet inhibitors in coronary artery disease, saphenous vein-graft disease, prosthetic valve replacement, cerebrovascular disease and other cardiovascular disorders. A complete discussion of anticoagulant and fibrinolytic therapy is beyond the scope of this review and has been undertaken elsewhere (1,2). However, specific aspects of anticoagulation and fibrinolysis will be briefly mentioned when pertinent.

Role of Platelets in Thrombogenesis

Platelets are fragments of membrane-enclosed megakariocytic cytoplasm that travel in the periphery of the circulating mass and do not adhere to intact endothelium. After superficial endothelial injury, only a monolayer of platelets adheres to the exposed subendothelium. When endothelial damage is more severe, exposure of collagen and other elements of the vessel wall to the circulating blood stimulates the activation of platelets and the coagulation system and leads to thrombus formation (3). In this section, we examine the processes of platelet adhesion and spreading, platelet secretion and aggregation, activation of the clotting system and endogenous inhibitors of thrombosis.

Platelet adhesion and spreading. Platelets do not attach to the intact endothelium, but they firmly adhere to a disrupted or damaged endothelial surface (Fig. 11.1). Subendothelial collagen and fibronectin stimulate platelet adhesion. Platelets adhere more avidly to collagen fibrils that lie deep within the vascular wall, such as in ulcerated atherosclerotic plaques, than to those found immediately beneath the endothelium (4). Platelet membrane receptors are essential in the

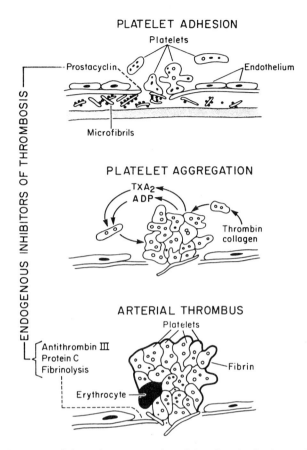

Figure 11.1. Schematic representation of the microscopic phases of arterial thrombus formation: platelet adhesion and spreading, platelet aggregation, activation of the coagulation system and thrombus formation and activation of the endogenous inhibitors of thrombosis. **Dashed line** denotes an inhibitory reaction. ADP = adenosine diphosphate; TXA_2 = thromboxane A_2.

processes of adhesion and aggregation (Fig. 11.2). Glycoprotein Ia binds collagen at low shear rates and may contribute to platelet adherence to the area of damage. Glycoprotein Ib serves as the binding site for von Willebrand factor, especially at high shear rates (5). Glycoprotein IIb-IIIa not only plays an essential role in platelet aggregation by binding fibrinogen and von Willebrand factor, but also participates in the process of adhesion (5).

After adhesion, platelets lose their discoid shape, form pseudopods and spread out over the injured surface. Parallel association of actin filaments leads to pseudopod formation, spread of the platelet surface membrane into a thin film, platelet contraction and stabilization of the hemostatic plug (6).

Platelet secretion and aggregation. Platelets contain different types of secretory granules, including dense and alpha granules, lysosomes and peroxisomes (Table 11.1). The first two are particularly important in aggregation and thrombogenesis. Dense granules contain adenosine diphosphate, serotonin, calcium and phosphate. Of these, adenosine diphosphate is the most important proaggregating compound. Alpha granules contain fibrinogen, fibronectin, von Willebrand factor, platelet factor 4, platelet-derived growth factor, thrombospondin and other compounds. Fibrinogen, von Willebrand factor and fibronectin are not only found in platelet granule secretions, but also in plasma. It is not yet known whether the platelet or the plasmatic components are physiologically more important in aggregation. Fibrinogen and von Willebrand factor bind to their receptor—glycoprotein IIb-IIIa—on adjacent platelets and form stable platelet aggregates (Fig. 11.2) (5,7). Platelet-derived growth factor is a potent mitogen and chemotactic agent for smooth muscle cells; it also attracts neutrophils and is a vasoconstrictor (8,9). Platelet factor 4 (antiheparin factor) attracts

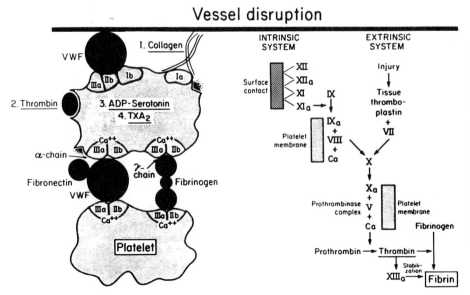

Figure 11.2. Left, Schematic representation of the interactions among platelet membrane receptors (glycoproteins Ia, Ib and IIb-IIIa), adhesive macromolecules and the disrupted vessel wall. Numbers indicate the different pathways of platelet activation, dependent on (1) collagen, (2) thrombin, (3) adenosine diphosphate (ADP) and serotonin and (4) thromboxane A_2 (TXA_2). **Right,** The intrinsic and extrinsic systems of the coagulation cascade. Note the interaction between clotting factors and the platelet membrane. Ca^{++} = calcium; VWF = von Willebrand factor.

Table 11.1. Content of Platelet Granules

Dense granules
  Adenosine diphosphate, serotonin, calcium, phosphate
Alpha granules
  Proteins not present in plasma: platelet-derived growth factor, platelet
  factor 4, beta-thromboglobulin
  Proteins present in plasma: fibrinogen, von Willebrand factor, fibronectin,
  albumin, thrombospondin, platelet factor 5
Lysosomes
  Acid hydrolases, cathepsin D, E
Peroxisomes
  Catalase

neutrophils and monocytes, perhaps serving as a stimulus to leukocyte accumulation in areas of endothelial injury (10).

The first pathway. How does the overall process of platelet aggregation take place? Through the action of several extrinsic activators such as collagen and thrombin (when there is vascular damage) and epinephrine, platelets change their shape from discs to spiney spheres. Calcium is then released from the dense tubular system into the cytoplasm by the action of phospholipase on platelet membrane phosphatidylinositol. This in turn is associated with the activation of the actin-myosin system, which results in platelet contraction and release of adenosine diphosphate, serotonin and thromboxane A_2. It appears that collagen and thrombin not only contribute to platelet aggregation indirectly (through the release of these compounds), but also have a direct effect on platelets, possibly through a platelet-activating factor. For the purpose of this discussion, these reactions, which are dependent on collagen and thrombin, constitute the first pathway of platelet activation, leading to the exposure of platelet membrane receptors.

The second pathway. This pathway is mediated by serotonin and adenosine diphosphate, which are released from the platelet dense granules after contraction. Adenosine diphosphate is a potent inducer of platelet aggregation in the presence of calcium and fibrinogen. It stimulates neighboring platelets to expose their binding sites for fibrinogen and von Willebrand factor (7), thus promoting aggregation. The high shear stress found in stenotic areas and at branching points within the arterial tree facilitates the deposition of platelets and the development and growth of thrombi (11). Furthermore, the turbulence present in these areas promotes red cell lysis, with the subsequent release of adenosine diphosphate, which in turn activates platelets and promotes their aggregation.

The third pathway. This pathway is mediated by arachidonic acid, which is released from the platelet membrane by the action of phospholipase A_2 on phosphatidylcholine. Cyclooxygenase converts arachidonic acid into the proaggregating prostaglandin endoperoxide intermediates (prostaglandins G_2 and H_2); thromboxane A_2 is formed by the action of thromboxane synthetase, particularly on prostaglandin H_2. Thromboxane A_2 is both a potent platelet-

aggregating substance and a vasoconstrictor. It stimulates platelet aggregation by promoting the mobilization of intracellular calcium and causing a conformational change in the glycoprotein IIb-IIIa complex, which results in the exposure of previously occult fibrinogen and von Willebrand factor binding sites (12,13).

Collagen that becomes exposed after vessel injury, thrombin generated by activation of the coagulation system and products of platelet secretion such as adenosine diphosphate and thromboxane A_2 can enhance the thrombotic process by stimulating adjacent platelets and facilitating the exposure of their membrane receptors to fibrinogen and von Willebrand factor. These reactions in turn promote further platelet aggregation and thrombus growth.

Prostacyclin. Vascular tissue synthesizes prostacyclin (prostaglandin I_2) from arachidonic acid (14) or platelet-derived prostaglandin G_2. Prostacyclin is a potent inhibitor of platelet aggregation by stimulating adenyl cyclase, which leads to an increase in cyclic adenosine monophosphate levels and a reduction in calcium mobilization from intracellular storage sites (15). Prostaglandins, cyclic adenosine monophosphate and intracellular calcium control platelet activity by interacting in a number of complex ways. Cyclic adenosine monophosphate inhibits both platelet secretion and aggregation, and its concentration depends on the activity of two enzymes—adenyl cyclase and phosphodiesterase. Whereas prostacyclin inhibits platelet aggregation by stimulating adenyl cyclase, thromboxane A_2 has the opposite biologic effect.

Leukotrienes. The other metabolic pathway of arachidonic acid is mediated by the enzyme lipoxygenase, which results in the production of leukotrienes. These compounds have been associated with a number of pathophysiologic reactions, including immune-mediated reactions, chemotaxis for neutrophils, constrictor actions on various smooth muscle beds (particularly the coronary vessels) and platelet aggregation. Our understanding of the effects of leukotrienes on the cardiovascular system is evolving.

Activation of the coagulation system. In addition to adhering to the injured vascular wall and forming aggregates, activated platelets markedly accelerate the generation of thrombin (16). Perhaps by rearranging their surface lipoproteins during contraction, activated platelets promote interactions among clotting factors (16). It is on the platelet surface where the interactions between factors IX and VIII and factors X and V occur (Fig. 11.2). Furthermore, the binding of thrombin and other activated clotting factors to platelets may protect them from inhibition (17).

The intrinsic coagulation pathway is initiated when blood comes in contact with the deendothelialized vascular surface. In the extrinsic pathway, a lipoprotein called tissue factor or tissue thromboplastin is released into the plasma and initiates the coagulation process. Aside from the intrinsic and extrinsic activation, the negatively charged phospholipids on the platelet surface and calcium are both essential

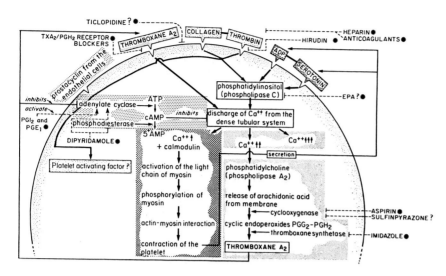

Figure 11.3. Mechanisms of platelet activation and presumed sites of action of various platelet inhibitor drugs. Platelet agonists lead to the mobilization of calcium (Ca^{++}), which functions as a mediator of platelet activation by means of metabolic pathways dependent on adenosine diphosphate (ADP), thromboxane A_2 (TxA_2), thrombin and collagen. Cyclic adenosine monophosphate (cAMP) inhibits calcium mobilization from the dense tubular system. Note that thrombin and collagen may independently activate platelets by means of a platelet-activating factor. **Dashed line** indicates the presumed site of drug action. * = platelet inhibitor; ATP = adenosine triphosphate; EPA = eicosapentaenoic acid; PGE_1 = prostaglandin E_1; PGH_2 = prostaglandin H_2; PGI_2 = prostaglandin I_2.

for maximal activation of factor X. Once factor X is activated, prothrombin is converted to thrombin, which cleaves fibrinogen to fibrin and activates factor XIII. This factor catalyzes the cross-linking reaction of fibrin. Polymerized fibrin in turn stabilizes the platelet mass and allows the arterial thrombus to withstand the high intraarterial pressure and force of blood flow. In addition, it should be emphasized that thrombin itself is a powerful platelet activator. Therefore, it appears that platelets and the coagulation system interact with each other in the development of intravascular thrombosis.

Endogenous inhibitors of thrombus formation. During platelet activation and fibrin formation, endogenous mechanisms tend to limit thrombus formation (Fig. 11.1). The most important of these are prostacyclin (discussed earlier), antithrombin III, protein C and the fibrinolytic system. Prostacyclin inhibits platelet aggregation by increasing platelet cyclic adenosine monophosphate and reducing the mobilization of calcium from its storage sites (15). Antithrombin III is an important endogenous anticoagulant that inhibits thrombin and activated factors IX, X, XI and XIII (18). Its inhibitory action is markedly increased by heparin.

Protein C is activated by the association of thrombin with thrombomodulin. In addition to being a potent anticoagulant, protein C initiates fibrinolysis by activating plasminogen and neutralizing a circulating inhibitor of tissue plasminogen activator (19). Once activated, plasminogen is converted to plasmin, which hydrolyzes fibrin into soluble fragments and degrades fibrinogen, prothrombin and factors VIII and V (20). The proteolytic activity of plasmin remains localized to the fibrin surface; as fibrin degradation proceeds to completion, plasmin is rapidly inactivated by alpha$_2$-plasmin inhibitor. A specific plasminogen activator inhibitor (type I) has been identified in human platelets (21) and the extracellular matrix of cultured endothelial cells (22). Recent findings underscore the importance of the fibrinolytic system in maintaining normal hemostasis and suggest that the bal-

ance between plasminogen activators and inhibitors may be important in both arterial and venous thrombotic disorders.

Pharmacology of Platelet Inhibitor Drugs

There has been continuous interest in the mechanism of action of drugs that interfere with platelet function in atherosclerosis, thrombosis and embolism. Platelet inhibitors may exert their effects through several different mechanisms, including (among others) direct inhibition of the arachidonic acid pathway, an increase in platelet cyclic adenosine monophosphate levels and inhibition of thrombin formation and action (Fig. 11.3).

Inhibitors of the Arachidonic Acid Pathway

Inhibitors of platelet cyclooxygenase: aspirin. Aspirin and other nonsteroidal anti-inflammatory drugs acetylate the platelet enzyme cyclooxygenase and thus inhibit the formation of thromboxane A_2. Aspirin only partially inhibits platelet aggregation induced by adenosine diphosphate, collagen or thrombin (at low concentrations). The adherence of the initial layer of platelets to the subendothelium and the release of granule contents are not inhibited by aspirin (23). Consequently, the effects of platelet-derived growth factor and other mitogens on smooth muscle cell proliferation may still occur in the presence of cyclooxygenase inhibitors (24). In contrast, these drugs have the ability to inhibit platelet aggregate formation on the layer of adherent platelets, presumably by blocking thromboxane A_2 synthesis.

The acetylation of cyclooxygenase in platelets exposed to aspirin is permanent (25) and thus the effects of the drug persist for the life of the platelets. The long-term administration of 1 mg/kg per day of aspirin effectively inhibits platelet cyclooxygenase and thromboxane A_2 formation. In contrast, aspirin inhibition of vascular endothelial cyclooxygenase is not irreversible because these cells are capable of synthesizing new enzyme, though they may require several hours to do so. Although earlier studies suggested that platelet cyclooxygenase was more sensitive to the inhibitory effects of low dose aspirin than vascular wall cyclooxygenase, more recent experimental data (26) have challenged the concept that low dose aspirin can selectively inhibit platelet thromboxane A_2 production but spare vascular prostacyclin synthesis.

The antithrombotic effect of aspirin can be achieved with a dose of 80 to 325 mg/day and therefore the toxic side effects associated with higher doses can be avoided (27–29). Side effects are dose-related and predominantly involve the gastrointestinal tract (30). Although higher doses of aspirin (>1,000 mg/day) are effective in terms of antithrombotic activity, they are associated with substantial gastrointestinal toxicity (30,31). For these reasons, an aspirin dose of 80 to 325 mg/day for the prevention of thromboembolic disease is currently recommended. Aspirin rarely causes significant generalized bleeding unless it is combined with an anticoagulant. When the risk of thrombosis is high (as in unstable angina), thrombolysis for acute myocardial infarction and during coronary revascularization and the use of the combination of low dose aspirin ($\leq$325 mg/day) and an anticoagulant are attractive and are currently undergoing clinical testing. The use of higher doses of aspirin, however, can result in significant gastrointestinal bleeding and is not recommended.

Although nonsteroidal anti-inflammatory drugs reversibly inhibit cyclooxygenase, the antithrombotic activity of these compounds has not been properly tested in large randomized trials and therefore its use cannot be recommended (32). Furthermore, one of the nonsteroidal anti-inflammatory agents, indomethacin, has been found to increase coronary vascular resistance and exacerbate ischemic attacks in patients with coronary disease (33).

Drugs that alter platelet membrane phospholipids: omega-3 fatty acids. Both eicosapentaenoic acid and docosahexaenoic acid are present in high concentration in most saltwater fish and may account for the lower incidence of coronary heart disease in Greenland Eskimos and populations that consume large amounts of fish (34,35). Eicosapentaenoic acid competes with arachidonic acid for platelet cyclooxygenase. This leads to the formation of two endoperoxidases (prostaglandins G_3 and H_3) and thromboxane A_3, which have minimal biologic activity (36). Furthermore, eicosapentaenoic acid does not inhibit endothelial prostacyclin production and stimulates the formation of prostaglandin I_3, which has antiplatelet activity (36). The net result is a shift in the hemostatic balance toward an antiaggregative and vasodilative state. Docosahexaenoic acid also has platelet inhibitory effects and undergoes retroconversion to eicosapentaenoic acid (37). Although fish consumption may decrease the incidence of coronary heart disease, administration of pharmacologic doses of fish oils is associated with some potentially adverse events such as increased bleeding

diathesis and reduced inflammatory and immune responses (37). Before fish oils are recommended for the prevention of atherosclerosis, properly designed and controlled human trials are necessary (36). The role of fish oils in the prevention of restenosis after coronary angioplasty is reviewed later in this chapter.

Inhibitors of thromboxane synthetase. Imidazole-analogue thromboxane synthetase inhibitors have been developed with the expectation of not only suppressing thromboxane A_2 biosynthesis, but sparing or even enhancing the formation of prostacyclin by the vascular endothelium. The rationale behind this hypothesis was that in the presence of a thromboxane synthetase inhibitor, platelet-derived prostaglandin G_2 would be transferred to the endothelial cells and used in the production of prostacyclin. Although thromboxane synthetase inhibitors have shown some benefit in experimental models (38,39), their effects in clinical trials (40,41) in patients with coronary artery disease have been controversial. This may be the result of two factors: first, thromboxane A_2 may not be completely suppressed by the available compounds, and second, the prostaglandin endoperoxide intermediates that result from thromboxane synthetase inhibition have their own significant proaggregating effects.

Blockers of thromboxane and prostaglandin endoperoxide receptors. Because it is difficult to inhibit thromboxane synthetase completely, agents have been developed to block the receptor of both thromboxane A_2 and its cyclic endoperoxide precursors (41,42). An interesting approach consists of combining a thromboxane synthetase inhibitor and a thromboxane A_2 receptor or endoperoxide receptor antagonist to block the aggregating effects of the endoperoxidases and any remaining thromboxane (41–43). Despite their theoretical appeal, it remains to be proved that this combination is more effective than aspirin alone. In addition, antiplatelet agents that operate on the thromboxane A_2 pathway are limited because this pathway is not absolutely necessary for the exposure of glycoprotein IIb-IIIa, which is the critical event in the process of platelet aggregation.

Drugs That Increase Platelet Cyclic Adenosine Monophosphate Levels

Dipyridamole. Dipyridamole may increase platelet cyclic adenosine monophosphate by three mechanisms: 1) it blocks its breakdown by inhibiting phosphodiesterase, 2) it activates adenylate cyclase by a prostacyclin-mediated effect on the platelet membrane (44), and 3) it increases the levels of plasma adenosine by inhibiting its uptake by vascular endothelium and erythrocytes (45,46). Adenosine in turn enhances platelet adenylate cyclase activity. In addition, the vasodilatory effects of dipyridamole appear to be related to the elevation in plasma adenosine levels. Although there are in vitro data to support the mechanisms of action of dipyridamole on platelets, there is no firm clinical evidence that such mechanisms contribute to a significant antithrombotic effect in humans (46).

In contrast to aspirin, the antithrombotic effects of dipyridamole are more evident on prosthetic materials (artificial heart valves [47,48] and arteriovenous cannulae [49]) than on biologic surfaces. Although one study (50) showed that aspirin potentiates the efficacy of dipyridamole in experimental thromboembolism on prosthetic surfaces, other studies (46) have yielded conflicting results with regard to the pharmacologic interaction between these two agents. Furthermore, aspirin alone was shown to be as effective as the combination of aspirin and dipyridamole in recent antithrombotic trials (51–55) in myocardial infarction, saphenous vein-graft disease and stroke. On the basis of these findings, there is little evidence to support the use of dipyridamole as an antithrombotic agent except in combination with warfarin in high risk patients with a mechanical prosthesis (56–60) and possibly before operation in patients with coronary artery bypass surgery (61,62).

The main side effects of dipyridamole are headache, epigastric discomfort and nausea, which occur in >10% of patients but subsequently subside. This agent is not associated with gastritis or gastroduodenal ulcers and does not increase the bleeding tendency, even when combined with an anticoagulant (60).

Prostaglandins E_1 and I_2. These prostaglandins are powerful systemic vasodilators and inhibitors of platelet aggregation by virtue of their ability to increase platelet cyclic adenosine monophosphate. Intravenous infusions of prostaglandin E_1 are commonly used in neonates with congenital heart disease, who are dependent on the persistence of a patent ductus arteriosus until surgical correction is done. It has also been used to improve myocardial function in patients with acute myocardial infarction and to treat peripheral vascular disease (63).

Prostacyclin is a potent naturally occurring platelet inhibitor. Its clinical use has been limited by its instability at neutral pH and its propensity to cause significant systemic hypotension at the doses required for platelet inhibition. Its duration of action is very short, and the pharmacologic effects disappear in 30 min. Infusion of prostacyclin strongly limits platelet interaction with artificial surfaces and preserves platelet number and function during cardiopulmonary bypass (64,65). The effects of prostacyclin in patients with ischemic heart disease and peripheral vascular insufficiency are controversial (63). Some studies (66,67), however, suggest that these prostanoids may improve the results of intracoronary thrombolysis in acute myocardial infarction. Further research in this area is needed.

Iloprost, a newly synthetized prostacyclin analogue, is chemically stable at neutral pH. In an in vitro comparison with equimolar concentrations of prostaglandins I_2 and E_1, iloprost was found to be more potent in increasing the levels of platelet cyclic adenosine monophosphate and inhibiting platelet aggregation by various agonists, particularly throm-

bin (68). In contrast, other animal (69) and human (70) studies of acute myocardial infarction failed to show any benefit from the combination of tissue plasminogen activator and iloprost over the thrombolytic agent alone. Another prostacyclin analogue, ciprostene, was found to reduce the rate of ischemic events in patients after coronary angioplasty and was associated with a trend toward a lower restenosis rate (71). Although chemically stable analogues of prostacyclin may be effective for temporary control of platelet activity in the management of thromboembolic disorders, further investigation is necessary.

Thrombin Inhibitors

By inhibiting thrombin formation with heparin or oral anticoagulant agents, the effects of thrombin on platelets and fibrinogen activation can be partially prevented.

Heparin. Aside from the antithrombotic effects of heparin, mainly by enhancing antithrombin III activity, its effects on platelet reactions are complex and contradictory (72), partly because of the variability among different commercially available preparations. There is evidence that suggests that fractions of high molecular weight (approximately 20,000 daltons) are more reactive with platelets than are fractions of lower molecular weight (approximately 7,000 daltons). Therefore, antithrombotic therapy may be enhanced by selecting heparin fractions of low molecular weight and high antithrombin III activity. In addition to its antithrombotic effects, the inhibitory effects of heparin on smooth muscle cell proliferation have been demonstrated experimentally (73,74). This opens interesting therapeutic opportunities, particularly with respect to restenosis after coronary angioplasty.

Peptide blockers of thrombin. An alternative strategy involves the synthesis of peptides that specifically block thrombin-mediated platelet activation. Several studies have demonstrated the effectiveness of thrombin inhibitors in the prevention of platelet-rich thrombosis in arteries (75) and vascular grafts (76). However, no clinical experience is yet available. Another potent selective thrombin inhibitor, hirudin, initially isolated from the salivary secretions of the medicinal leech, has been recently synthesized by deoxyribonucleic acid recombinant technology. Hirudin prevents the activation of clotting factors V, VIII and XIII; in addition, by being a powerful thrombin inhibitor, hirudin blocks the metabolic pathway of platelet activation that is dependent on thrombin. Hirudin has been recently shown to prevent thrombosis in an animal model of carotid angioplasty and was found to have a more potent antithrombotic effect than heparin (77). Because these agents may effectively inhibit platelet activation by blocking thrombin, their potential for clinical use is enormous. Intensive research in this area is currently underway.

Other Platelet Inhibitors

Ticlopidine. Ticlopidine is chemically unrelated to other antiplatelet drugs; its mechanism of action is not completely understood. It may act on the platelet membrane to alter its reactivity, perhaps by blocking the interaction of von Willebrand factor and fibrinogen with platelets (78). It inhibits platelet aggregation induced by adenosine diphosphate and most other agonists, prolongs bleeding time and normalizes shortened platelet survival (79). Optimal efficacy is reached only 3 days after its administration, and its effects last for several days after the drug has been stopped.

Clinical evaluation of this drug is now underway. Evidence from an Italian multicenter trial (Study of Ticlopidine in Unstable Angina) (80) suggests that it is effective in unstable angina for the prevention of myocardial infarction and cardiovascular death. Another recent study (81) showed a reduction in the incidence of acute occlusion and thrombosis after coronary angioplasty in patients treated with ticlopidine. This agent was also found to be effective in reducing vein-graft closure in patients after aortocoronary bypass surgery (82).

In addition, recently published data suggest that ticlopidine reduces cardiac and cerebrovascular morbidity and mortality in patients with recent ischemic stroke (83) and may be even more effective than aspirin for secondary prevention in patients with transient ischemic attacks or mild stroke (84). In these studies, however, ticlopidine was associated with several toxic effects, including diarrhea, rash and reversible neutropenia.

Sulfinpyrazone. Sulfinpyrazone is structurally related to phenylbutazone, but has minimal anti-inflammatory activity. In contrast to aspirin, sulfinpyrazone is a competitive inhibitor of platelet cyclooxygenase, but the exact mechanism for its antithrombotic activity is not well understood (50). It inhibits the formation of thrombi on subendothelium and protects the endothelium for chemical injury in vitro and possibly in vivo. In addition, sulfinpyrazone produces a dose-dependent inhibition of experimental thromboembolism in artificial cannulas (50), reduces the rate of thrombotic events in patients with arteriovenous cannulas (85) and normalizes platelet survival in patients with artificial heart valves (86). Overall, beneficial effects have been more consistent on prosthetic than on biologic surfaces. Despite a beneficial trend in decreasing vascular events after myocardial infarction (87) and reducing the occlusion rate in saphenous vein coronary artery bypass (55,88), sulfinpyrazone offered no additional benefit to patients with unstable angina (31) or stroke (89). Side effects include increased sensitivity to warfarin, hypoglycemia when combined with sulfonylureas, exacerbation of peptic ulcer and precipitation of uric acid stones.

Dextran. Dextran of a molecular weight of 65,000 to 80,000 daltons prolongs the bleeding time after intravenous infusion of ≥1 liter. Its mechanism of action is unclear. It may involve some alteration of platelet membrane function (90) or interference with factor VIII-von Willebrand factor complex (91). Although some experimental studies (92) have shown an antithrombotic effect of dextran, no effect was found in a randomized trial (93) in patients undergoing coronary angioplasty. Furthermore, dextran has been associated with a low but disturbing incidence (0.6%) of anaphylactoid reactions (94). Data supporting the role of dextran as antithrombotic agent on foreign materials (that is, arterial stents and vascular grafts) are emerging.

Future developments. Currently available drugs do not interfere with all the platelet metabolic pathways that lead to their activation; therefore, these agents are unable to entirely prevent thrombus formation. As previously discussed, the exposure of receptors in the platelet membrane (glycoprotein IIb-IIIa) that bind fibrinogen and von Willebrand factor seems to play a pivotal role in platelet aggregation (Fig. 11.2). Therefore, short-term total inhibition of platelet aggregation may depend on the use of agents such as monoclonal antibodies, which block either the platelet membrane receptor glycoprotein IIb-IIIa (95–97), or the adhesive macromolecules such as von Willebrand factor (98,99). Similarly, agents that inhibit platelet membrane receptors responsible for platelet adhesion may be useful for short-term therapy. However, long-term therapy may be hazardous because of the increased bleeding tendency. Finally, agents that block the biochemical steps responsible for platelet contraction and granular release may plan an important role in inhibiting platelet secretion and aggregation and deserve investigation.

Role of Platelet Inhibitor Drugs in Cardiovascular Disease

With a better understanding of the pathogenetic mechanisms involved in cardiovascular disease, the role of platelets in thrombosis and thromboembolism has been established, and a more extensive role for antithrombotic therapy has emerged. We review the available data on antithrombotic therapy in different cardiovascular syndromes, with particular emphasis on the indications for platelet inhibitors based on the results of clinical trials.

Coronary Atherosclerotic Disease

The natural history of coronary atherosclerotic disease includes a long initial asymptomatic period that lasts three to four decades and may be characterized by benign, raised, nonobstructive fatty streaks in the coronary vessels. In the presence of a genetic predisposition and certain coronary risk factors, these raised plaques grow and may either remain silent or produce clinical symptoms of angina pectoris. The acute coronary syndromes, namely, unstable angina, myocardial infarction and ischemic sudden death, may occur when growing plaques undergo a rapid morphologic

Table 11.2. Proposed Pathophysiologic Mechanisms in Coronary Atherosclerotic Disease

Early lesions (asymptomatic stage)
  Hemodynamic factors: endothelial damage
  Platelet and monocyte deposition
  Smooth muscle cell migration and proliferation
  Connective tissue synthesis
  Lipid transformation and deposition

Growing lesions (asymptomatic or stable angina stage)
  Slow process
    Chronic endothelial injury
    Platelet and monocyte interaction with vessel wall
    Smooth muscle cell proliferation, collagen synthesis, lipid accumulation
  Rapid process
    Intermittent fissuring of coronary plaques
    Nonocclusive thrombus formation*
    Fibrotic organization of thrombus

Plaque rupture (acute coronary syndromes)
  Unstable angina
    Plaque rupture with transient thrombosis*
    Vasospasm
    Increased myocardial oxygen demand
  Myocardial infarction
    Plaque rupture with thrombotic occlusion*
    Vasospasm
    Spontaneous recanalization and rethrombosis*
  Sudden ischemic death
    Plaque rupture with thrombotic occlusion*
    Coronary microembolism of platelet-fibrin aggregates

*Denotes events that may be prevented or diminished by use of antithrombotic therapy.

change after they rupture, with significant occlusive or near occlusive thrombus formation (Table 11.2). Finally, extensive coronary artery disease or myocardial infarction may lead to left ventricular dysfunction. The roles of platelets and platelet inhibitors in the asymptomatic phase of coronary atherosclerosis and in the phases of stable angina and acute ischemic syndromes are reviewed.

Asymptomatic and stable angina phases. Knowledge of the pathogenesis of atherosclerosis, although still incomplete, is rapidly evolving. The process is multifactorial in origin and involves the interaction of genetic factors, platelets, smooth muscle cells, endothelium, cholesterol and lipoproteins.

Concepts in atherogenesis. Platelet deposition in areas of subtle endothelial injury may constitute one of the initiating factors in the development of atheromatous plaques. Areas of increased turbulence, such as branching points, are particularly susceptible to endothelial injury. Through the interaction of von Willebrand factor, collagen, fibronectin and other proteins, platelets become firmly attached to gaps between endothelial cells or to injured vascular wall and may release several mitogens, including platelet-derived growth factor, epidermal growth factor and transforming growth factor beta. These factors stimulate the proliferation and migration of smooth muscle cells and fibroblasts from the media to the intima of the vessel wall. Platelet interaction with injured endothelium may induce a rapid proliferative response, whereas other sources of growth factors, including activated macrophages and endothelial cells, may be responsible for stimulating smooth muscle cells at a slower rate and produce atherosclerosis even in the absence of endothelial disruption (100).

In the experimental hyperlipidemic model of atherosclerosis (100), monocytes attach to the endothelium early after the induction of hypercholesterolemia. These monocytes then localize subendothelially, accumulate lipid and become foam cells, eventually leading to the development of fatty streaks. After several months, the endothelium that covers the fatty streaks retracts and allows the attachment of platelets to areas of endothelial desquamation or to the subendothelium (100). All principal cells involved in the atherosclerotic process—endothelium, platelets, monocytes and smooth muscle cells—are capable of releasing chemotactic and mitogenic factors. In hyperlipidemia, interaction of monocytes with the vessel wall and monocyte-dependent growth factor or factors may be more important than platelet-dependent factors.

If platelet adherence to the vessel wall plays a role in atherogenesis, inhibition of platelet adhesion may be beneficial in preventing atherosclerosis. Unfortunately, no drugs with this property are currently available. If platelet adhesion was to be completely prevented by a pharmacologic agent, as occurs in pigs with an absence or alteration of von Willebrand factor (101), the risk of bleeding would prohibit its long-term use. In contrast, such an agent may prove beneficial when short-term inhibition of platelet adhesion is desired (such as during coronary angioplasty or after coronary thrombolysis).

Primary prevention. Results from a double-blind placebo-controlled trial (102) of >22,000 male physicians in the United States assigned to receive aspirin (325 mg every other day) for 5 years revealed a 44% reduction in the incidence of myocardial infarction from approximately 0.4% to 0.2% per year (p < 0.00001). This effect was limited to individuals >50 years old. The incidence of cardiovascular death was similar in the aspirin and placebo groups; however, aspirin was associated with a slight increase in hemorrhagic stroke.

In a randomized primary prevention trial (103) of >5,000 male physicians in the United Kingdom, two-thirds were randomly assigned to take aspirin (500 mg/day) and one-third were instructed to avoid it (no placebo used). After 6 years, no difference in the rate of myocardial infarction or cardiovascular death was detected. Although the number of enrolled subjects was smaller than in the U.S. trial, cardiovascular event rates were 5 to 10 times higher. When both studies are considered together, there appears to be reduction in coronary events with aspirin, but at the price of increased risk of hemorrhagic stroke.

Table 11.3. Antithrombotic Therapy in Unstable Angina

Trial (ref)	No. of Patients	Follow-up	Drug	(%) Reduction Death + MI	p Value
Telford and Wilson (118)	214	7 days	Heparin	80	<0.05
VACS (27)	1,266	12 weeks	Aspirin	51	<0.001
McMaster (31)	555	18 months	Aspirin	51	<0.01
			Sulfinpyrazone	−6	
Montreal Heart Institute (116)	479	6 days	Aspirin	72	<0.01
			Heparin	89	<0.001
			Aspirin + heparin	88	0.001
STAI (80)	652	6 months	Ticlopidine	53	<0.01
Wallentin (117)	794	3 months	Aspirin	63	<0.01
			Heparin	15	
			Aspirin + heparin	70	<0.001

MI = Myocardial infarction; ref = reference; STAI = Italian Study of Ticlopidine in Unstable Angina; VACS = Veterans Administration Cooperative Study.

Given the available data, aspirin for primary prevention cannot be universally recommended. Based on risk/benefit analysis, aspirin at a dose of 160 to 325 mg/day seems prudent for patients >50 years old with clear risk factors for coronary disease or with evidence of cerebrovascular or peripheral artery disease (104). Because long-term aspirin may be associated with some toxicity (105), it should not be used indiscriminately, particularly for patients without risk factors or evidence of atherosclerosis in other vascular territories. The ongoing Thrombosis Prevention Trial (106) is comparing the value of low dose aspirin warfarin or the combination of both for men at high risk of coronary disease. The results of this trial will further define the role of antithrombotic agents in primary prevention.

Stable coronary disease. Rupture of small atherosclerotic plaques, with subsequent mural thrombosis and fibrotic organization of thrombus, may contribute to the progression of coronary atherosclerosis. Support for this concept comes from the pathologic finding of old organized thrombi within the coronary arteries that are difficult to distinguish from atherosclerotic changes seen in the arterial wall (107). A more recent study (108) demonstrated the presence of fibrinogen and fibrin and their degradation products in areas of advanced atherosclerotic plaque. On the basis of these observations, recurrent episodes of plaque disruption and thrombosis do not necessarily lead to an acute ischemic syndrome, but rather to progressive narrowing of the coronary arteries. Although it is not yet known how prevalent this process is, its clinical significance is potentially enormous because thrombotic episodes may be prevented by platelet inhibitors or anticoagulant agents. In this context, preliminary evidence (109) from a 5 year trial of aspirin plus dipyridamole for prevention of progression of coronary disease in patients with stable angina revealed that platelet inhibitors reduced the incidence of myocardial infarction and new lesion formation, but had no effect on the progression of pre-existing lesions.

Acute coronary syndromes. Angiographic (110,111), angioscopic (112) and pathologic (113,114) studies have demonstrated the presence of complex ulcerated plaques with or without thrombus formation in a large proportion of patients with unstable angina, myocardial infarction or ischemic sudden death. The causes of plaque rupture are unknown, but may be related to the physiocochemical properties of the plaque (fragility of the fibrous cap, infiltration by foam cells, abnormal elastin), hemodynamic factors (wall shear stress, changes in vasotonicity and blood pressure) and continuous arterial bending and twisting with each cardiac cycle. Plaque rupture exposes collagen fibrils and tissue thromboplastin, promoting the development of thrombus. The degree, suddenness and duration of the obstruction and the size of the involved vessel probably determine the nature of the clinical event.

Unstable angina (Table 11.3). Plaque disruption in areas of mild coronary stenosis may lead to an acute change in plaque configuration and a reduction in coronary blood flow, resulting in progressive ischemic symptoms. Transient episodes of thrombotic vessel occlusion at the site of injury may occur, resulting in rest angina (112). Additionally, blood supply may be further compromised by intermittent vasoconstriction related to the release of vasoactive substances from platelets or abnormal endothelial vasodilative properties in areas of atherosclerosis (115). Alternatively, transient increases in myocardial oxygen demand may explain some of the episodes of unstable angina.

Aspirin: There have been four large, randomized, placebo-controlled, double-blind studies of aspirin in unstable angina. In the Veterans Administration Cooperative Study (27), 1,266 men with unstable angina were randomized to receive buffered aspirin (324 mg/day) or placebo for 12 weeks. During the treatment period, the incidence of death and acute myocardial infarction was reduced from 10.1% to 5% in the aspirin-treated group, and the overall benefits of aspirin were maintained during the 1 year follow-up period.

No increase in gastrointestinal side effects was seen in the aspirin-treated group. In the Canadian Multicenter Trial (31), 555 patients (73% male) with unstable angina were randomized to receive aspirin (1,300 mg/day), sulfinpyrazone (800 mg/day), the combination of both or placebo. After 2 years, the incidence of death and myocardial infarction was reduced in the aspirin-treated groups from 17% to 8.6%, a risk reduction of 51%. Sulfinpyrazone conferred no benefit and did not interact with aspirin. Gastrointestinal toxicity was more frequently seen in the aspirin-treated groups, probably related to the high dose used.

In the Montreal Heart Institute Study (116), 479 patients with unstable angina were randomized to receive aspirin (325 mg twice daily), intravenous heparin, the combination of both or placebo. The study was ended after a mean of 6 days, when a final therapeutic decision for the individual patient was made on the basis of the results of cardiac catheterization. Aspirin significantly reduced the rate of myocardial infarction by 72% compared with placebo. In a more recent trial published in preliminary fashion, Wallentin (117) randomized 794 men with unstable angina or non-Q wave infarction to receive aspirin (75 mg/day) for 3 months, intravenous heparin for 5 days, both or neither. At 3 month follow-up study, the risk of myocardial infarction or death was significantly reduced by aspirin (risk ratio 0.41) and by the combination of aspirin and heparin (risk ratio 0.23), but not by heparin alone (Fig. 11.4). Aspirin use was associated with decreased recurrence of ischemia and need for revascularization (117).

Further support for the use of antiplatelet agents in unstable angina comes from the recently published Italian Study of Ticlopidine in Unstable Angina (80). Ticlopidine at a dose of 250 mg twice daily for 6 months reduced the incidence of death and myocardial infarction by 46%.

Anticoagulant therapy: Evidence of a beneficial effect of heparin in unstable angina was suggested by Telford and Wilson (118), who demonstrated an 80% reduction in the incidence of myocardial infarction in patients with unstable angina treated with heparin for 7 days. Deficiencies in patient recruitment, however, left the conclusions of this study less convincing. The strongest support for immediate anticoagulation in unstable angina comes from the Montreal Heart Institute Study (116). Heparin decreased the rate of infarction by 89% and the incidence of refractory angina by 50%. Although no statistically significant differences among patients treated with aspirin, heparin or their combination were found, there was a trend favoring heparin over aspirin. The combination was not better than heparin alone and was associated with a slight increase in bleeding complications. In contrast, in the preliminary report from Wallentin (117), heparin alone was not as effective as aspirin, whereas the combination was more effective than either agent alone. Differences in baseline characteristics of the patients studied could perhaps explain the different results obtained in these studies. At present, there is enough evidence to support the

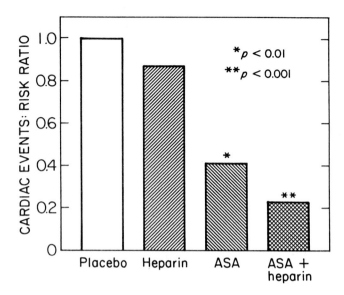

Figure 11.4. Efficacy of low dose aspirin (ASA) (75 mg/day) alone and aspirin plus intravenous heparin (but not of heparin alone) in reducing the risk of myocardial infarction or death, or both, in patients with unstable angina or non-Q wave myocardial infarction over a follow-up period of 3 months. Data obtained from a preliminary report by Wallentin (117).

use of aggressive antithrombotic treatment in patients with unstable angina. A multicenter randomized trial of anticoagulant agents plus low dose aspirin in unstable angina is currently underway.

Non-Q wave infarction. The angiographic configuration of the responsible lesion in non-Q wave infarction is similar to that seen in unstable angina (119), which suggests that plaque disruption is common in both syndromes. The presence of ST segment elevation on the electrocardiogram (120), early peak in plasma creatine kinase (120,121) and high angiographic patency rates of the infarct-related artery (120–122) suggest that complete coronary occlusion followed by early reperfusion is important in the pathogenesis of non-Q wave infarction. Reperfusion may occur as a result of spontaneous thrombolysis or resolution of vasospasm, or both. Furthermore, contraction band necrosis, which is the hallmark of reperfusion, is more often found in patients dying of non-Q wave versus Q wave infarction (123). When complete coronary occlusion persists, however, the presence of adequate collateral flow may limit the extent of myocardial necrosis and prevent the development of Q wave infarction (122). Given the relatively high incidence of reinfarction and vascular death in these patients, not unlike those with unstable angina, aggressive antithrombotic therapy with a combination of aspirin and intravenous heparin has been proposed and appears beneficial, as suggested by a preliminary report from a recent randomized trial (117).

Q wave infarction (no thrombolytic therapy). In Q wave infarction, atherosclerotic plaque rupture leads to fixed and persistent occlusive thrombus formation (113). Quantitative angiographic studies (124) have shown that the coronary lesion responsible for the infarction may be only mild to moderately stenotic. This suggests that plaque rupture with thrombus formation rather than the severity of the underlying stenosis may be the primary determinant in the development of acute coronary syndromes (124–127). Myocardial infarction may also be favored by alterations in hemostasis, such as increased activation of the coagulation system, increased platelet aggregability, elevated fibrinogen, increased factor VII activity or deficient fibrinolytic mechanisms (128,129).

Platelet inhibitor therapy: The strongest evidence supporting the use of platelet inhibitors in the acute stage of myocardial infarction comes from the Second International Study of Infarct Survival (ISIS-2) (29). In this study, >17,000 patients with suspected acute myocardial infarction were randomized to receive aspirin (160 mg/day), intravenous streptokinase, both or placebo. At 5 weeks, the vascular mortality rate was significantly reduced by aspirin alone (by 23%) and nonfatal reinfarction and nonfatal stroke by almost 50%. Because a certain number of patients with acute infarction undergo spontaneous vessel recanalization, aspirin probably owes its beneficial effects to a reduction in early reinfarction. It should be noted that because admission into this trial did not require electrocardiographic confirmation of acute infarction, some patients probably had unstable angina, a situation for which aspirin has clearly proved to be beneficial (27,31,116,117). On the basis of this trial, in the absence of contraindications, aspirin (160 to 325 mg/day) should be considered for all patients with acute infarction.

Anticoagulant therapy: Although the purpose of this review is to analyze the value of platelet inhibitor therapy in cardiovascular disease, it is important to mention briefly the results obtained with the use of anticoagulant therapy. The role of anticoagulant agents in the prevention of coronary rethrombosis, infarct extension and death in patients with acute infarction has not been settled. Of the large number of studies conducted, only three randomized trials (130–132) have been sufficiently large to be able to detect a significant effect of therapy. Although all three studies showed a beneficial trend toward reduced mortality and reinfarction, only the Bronx Municipal Hospital trial (131) found a significant 30% reduction in the case fatality rate. In contrast, all these trials clearly showed that anticoagulant agents reduce pulmonary and systemic embolism after infarction (130–132), as well as left ventricular mural thrombosis in cases of acute anterior infarction (133,134). Therefore, clinical studies (29,135) have demonstrated benefit from both aspirin and anticoagulant agents in patients with acute myocardial infarction.

Q wave infarction (thrombolytic therapy). The benefits of adjuvant treatment with aspirin in patients receiving a thrombolytic agent were confirmed by ISIS-2 (29). The cardiovascular mortality rate was reduced by 25% with streptokinase and by 42% with the combination of aspirin and streptokinase. The excess of nonfatal reinfarction observed with streptokinase was eliminated by the use of aspirin, probably through prevention of thrombotic vessel reocclusion. The effects of aspirin and streptokinase on mortality reduction were additive, and the benefit was maintained at the 15-month follow-up evaluation.

With regard to anticoagulant therapy, the recent Italian Studio sulla Calciparina nell'Angina e nella Thrombosi Ventricolare nell'Infarto (SCATI) (134) randomized 711 patients within 24 h of the onset of myocardial infarction to receive heparin intravenously (2,000 U bolus) and subcutaneously (12,500 U twice daily) or no anticoagulant therapy. In addition, 433 of these patients admitted within 6 h of infarction received intravenous streptokinase. Heparin reduced in the hospital mortality from 9.9% to 5.8% (p = 0.03); however, no significant reduction in the incidence of reinfarction was observed. Even though the need for anticoagulant therapy after thrombolysis is not completely settled, the presence of a highly thrombogenic surface (the ruptured plaque and the partially lyzed thrombus) and the substantial risk of recurrent ischemia and reinfarction in these patients justify the use of intravenous heparin after administration of the thrombolytic agent. Two additional studies (136,137) clearly suggest that adjuvant treatment with heparin improves the early coronary artery patency rate in patients with acute infarction treated with tissue plasminogen activator.

Secondary prevention after myocardial infarction. In the first years after acute myocardial infarction, cardiac morbidity and mortality are related to a number of factors, including left ventricular dysfunction, ventricular arrhythmias and reinfarction. Therefore, proving that antithrombotic drugs are beneficial in this group of patients has been difficult, generating enormous controversy over the last few decades.

Antiplatelet therapy. With respect to the use of antiplatelet agents for the secondary prevention of vascular events, several large, randomized, placebo-controlled, double-blind trials (51,87,138–144) in patients recovering from myocardial infarction have been conducted (Table 11.4). In seven of these trials, aspirin (at a dose of 300 to 1,500 mg/day) was used alone or in combination with dipyridamole. In the remaining two trials, sulfinpyrazone was used. Despite the large total number of patients studied (>17,000), no clear evidence of benefit from therapy was shown in any single study. The reduction in the cardiac mortality rate varied from 5% to 42% and in the nonfatal reinfarction rate from 12% to 57% (Table 11.4). The largest single trial, the Aspirin Myocardial Infarction Study (142), showed no benefit from therapy, but unbalanced randomization introduced an inadvertent bias against aspirin. Three of the trials (87,141,144) disclosed a beneficial trend from therapy in terms of a lower mortality rate, and, in some cases, a significant reduction in the coronary event rate.

A pooled analysis of antiplatelet therapy in secondary prevention after myocardial infarction was recently pub-

Table 11.4. Randomized Trials of Platelet Inhibitors for Secondary Prevention of Myocardial Infarction

| Trial (ref) | No of Patients | Drug (mg/day) | Reduction in Event Rate With Therapy (%) | | |
			Total Mortality	Cardiac Mortality	Coronary Events
MRC-I (138)	1,239	ASA (300)	24	NA	NA
CDP (139)	1,529	ASA (972)	30	28	22
GARS (140)	626	ASA (1,500)	18	42	37
MRC-II (141)	1,682	ASA (900)	17	22	28†
AMIS (142)	4,524	ASA (1,000)	(−10)	(−8)	5
PARIS-I (51)	2,206	ASA (972)	18	21	24
		ASA (972) + Dip (225)	16	24	25
PARIS-II (144)	3,128	ASA (990) + Dip (225)	3	6	24†
ART (143)	1,558	Sulf (800)	28*	24*	NA
ARIS (87)	727	Sulf (800)	5	5	56‡

*Lower total and cardiac mortality rates are due to a marked reduction in early sudden death. †p < 0.05; ‡p < 0.01. AMIS = Aspirin Myocardial Infarction Study; ARIS = Anturane Reinfarction Italian Study; ART = Anturane Reinfarction Trial; ASA = aspirin; CDP = Coronary Drug Project; Dip = dipyridamole; GARS = German-Austrian Reinfarction Study; MRC-I = Medical Research Council Study; MRC-II = Medical Research Council Study (1979); NA = not available; PARIS-I = Persantine-Aspirin Reinfarction Study (1980); PARIS-II = Persantine-Aspirin Reinfarction Study (1986); Sulf = sulfinpyrazone.

lished (145). It suggested that in survivors of myocardial infarction, platelet inhibitors significantly reduced the vascular mortality rate by 13%, nonfatal reinfarction rate by 31%, nonfatal stroke rate by 42% and all important cardiovascular events by 25%. Although no statistically significant differences among the antiplatelet agents used were found, current evidence does not justify the additional expense and increased frequency of administration of dipyridamole or sulfinpyrazone (46,145). At present, the best studied, most convenient and least expensive antiplatelet drug appears to be aspirin at a dose of ≤325 mg/day.

Anticoagulant therapy. Numerous studies have assessed the usefulness of long-term anticoagulant therapy in the secondary prevention of cardiovascular disease after myocardial infarction, but only five randomized controlled trials (140,146–149) were large enough to be able to detect a significant effect from therapy. Among the earlier trials (140,146,147), only the Medical Research Council Study (146) was able to show a reduction in the reinfarction rate by as much as 60%. Utilizing a different design, the Sixty Plus Reinfarction Study (148) entered patients >60 years of age who had been maintained on anticoagulant agents for a median of 6 years after infarction. Patients were randomized to continuation of anticoagulant therapy or to placebo substitute for 2 additional years. By intention to treat analysis, patients receiving anticoagulant therapy had a 26% lower death rate (p = 0.07) and an impressive 55% reduction in reinfarction (p = 0.0005). Efficacy analysis showed a more substantial reduction in death and reinfarction rates of 43% and 66%, respectively. A trend toward reduced frequency of cerebrovascular events was observed in the group receiving anticoagulant therapy; however, bleeding was more common, perhaps as a result of higher intensity anticoagulant therapy used.

The firmest evidence supporting the use of anticoagulant agents after infarction derives from the large Warfarin Re-

Infarction Study (WARIS), published recently (149). This study randomly allocated 1,214 patients to receive warfarin or placebo, with a follow-up period of about 3 years. Warfarin was shown to reduce the mortality rate by 24% (p = 0.026), reinfarction by 34% (p = 0.0007) and stroke by 55% (p = 0.0015). Major bleeding episodes occurred in only 2% of treated patients. Thus, this is the first large and well-conducted study to show unequivocally that long-term anticoagulant treatment reduces cardiovascular mortality and morbidity after myocardial infarction.

The French Enquete de Prevention Secondaire de l'Infarctus du Myocarde (EPSIM) (150) trial attempted to compare anticoagulant therapy with aspirin in patients recovering from myocardial infarction; however, no control group was included. At 29 months of follow-up evaluation, no significant difference between both treatment arms emerged with regard to total and cardiac mortality and reinfarction rate. When the trials of aspirin and anticoagulant therapy for the secondary prevention of cardiac disease are analyzed together, both treatments appear to convey protection against death and reinfarction. The advantage of aspirin over anticoagulant agents resides not on higher effectiveness, but on lower cost, ease of administration, less need for monitoring and lower incidence of hemorrhagic side effects. For patients intolerant to aspirin, those at risk of embolism from the left ventricle (those with mural thrombi or severe myocardial dysfunction) or left atrium (those with atrial fibrillation) and those with prior embolism, oral anticoagulant treatment is preferred.

Current recommendations. 1) The preferred platelet inhibitor drug in patients with unstable angina is aspirin at a dose of 325 mg/day and its beneficial effect is still present during a 2 year follow-up period. In addition, recent trials suggest that high dose anticoagulant therapy with heparin (116) or a combination of low dose aspirin and heparin (117) significantly reduce the incidence of infarction and refractory angina in these patients. The short-term combination of aspirin (80 mg/day) and low dose warfarin is currently being evaluated.

2) Recent evidence (29) suggests that aspirin (160 mg/day) is beneficial in patients with acute myocardial infarction by reducing reinfarction, stroke and early cardiovascular death. In addition, short-term anticoagulant therapy may also be beneficial in decreasing the mortality rate (134). Aggressive antithrombotic management with aspirin (160 to 325 mg/day) and intravenous heparin is recommended in patients treated with a thrombolytic agent for acute myocardial infarction. Anticoagulant agents are particularly effective in reducing left ventricular mural thrombosis and perhaps systemic embolism in patients with anterior myocardial infarction.

3) For secondary prevention in survivors of myocardial infarction, aspirin therapy reduces vascular death, reinfarction and stroke (145). Although doses ranging from 300 to 1,500 mg/day have been used, the lower dosage is as effective as the larger one, but produces fewer side effects. Available data do not support the use of sulfinpyrazone or dipyridamole. Long-term anticoagulant therapy has also shown significant benefit in reducing death, reinfarction and stroke (149), but is associated with a higher cost, need for frequent monitoring and hemorrhagic side effects.

4) Platelet inhibitors appear to reduce the rate of infarction and atherosclerotic lesion formation in patients with stable coronary disease or stable angina (109). Aspirin at a dose of 80 to 325 mg/day may be beneficial in these patients.

5) Aspirin for primary prevention is still controversial. At present, it may be recommended only in individuals at high risk of developing significant coronary disease, in whom the potential benefits of aspirin outweigh the risk of hemorrhagic stroke.

Saphenous Vein Bypass Graft Disease

Coronary vein-graft disease is the most important contributor to cardiac morbidity and mortality after coronary artery surgery. Occlusion rates of 8% to 18% per distal anastomosis at 1 month postoperatively and 16% to 26% at 12 months have been reported (151). At the end of 10 years, up to 50% of vein grafts will be occluded. Vein-graft disease can be divided into three phases: an early postoperative phase of thrombotic occlusion; an intermediate phase characterized by intimal hyperplasia, resulting in a form of accelerated atherosclerosis; and a late phase composed of graft atherosclerosis similar to that affecting the native coronary arteries (152). The last two phases of vein-graft disease probably represent a continuum of the hyperplastic response to injury with superimposed thrombotic tendency, which may develop at any point during the disease process.

Early phase. *Pathogenesis.* The initial endothelial damage to saphenous vein grafts occurs when the vein is removed from the leg during surgery and is suddenly ex-

posed to the high pressure arterial system. Saphenous vein endothelium is injured during harvesting from the leg, surgical handling, suturing and immediately after anastomosis when the vein is abruptly exposed to arterial shear forces (152,153). As blood starts to flow through the graft, platelets activated after passing through the extracorporeal oxygenator adhere to areas of damaged endothelium and release their thrombogenic factors. With the understanding that early vein-graft occlusion is mainly thrombotic in origin and that platelet deposition begins intraoperatively (154), platelet inhibitor drugs are indicated for the prevention of early graft occlusion; this therapy should be started before or immediately after surgery.

Prevention. Several studies (54,55,61,62,155–157) have convincingly demonstrated the importance of initiating platelet inhibitor therapy in the perioperative period, preferably before but no later than 48 h after surgery. Indeed, when therapy was started >48 h after surgery, no reduction in the vein-graft occlusion rate was observed (158–161). Experimentally, preoperative treatment with dipyridamole appears to decrease platelet activation by the extracorporeal pump, maintains the platelet count during cardiopulmonary bypass and does not increase bleeding during surgery (154,162). Accordingly, in a randomized, double-blind placebo-controlled trial (61), patients received dipyridamole (100 mg four times daily) for 2 days before operation, followed by aspirin (325 mg) and dipyridamole (75 mg) three times daily, started 7 h after operation and continued for 1 year. There was no increased incidence of bleeding complications in the treatment group. At vein-graft angiography 1 month after operation, there was a significant reduction in graft occlusion in the treated group from 10% to 2% per distal graft anastomosis and from 22% to 6% per patient. This was true even in patients at high risk for early graft occlusion.

In another study (82), ticlopidine (250 mg twice daily) started on the second postoperative day significantly reduced the incidence of vein-graft occlusion by approximately 40%, as assessed angiographically at 10, 180 and 360 days after surgery. In the recently published Veterans Administration Cooperative Study (55), 555 patients were randomized into five groups: aspirin (325 mg/day), aspirin (325 mg three times daily), aspirin (325 mg) plus dipyridamole (75 mg) three times daily, sulfinpyrazone (267 mg three times daily) and placebo. Except for aspirin, which was started 12 h preoperatively, therapy was initiated 48 h before surgery. Graft patency was assessed angiographically between 6 and 60 days after surgery (median 9) (Fig. 11.5). Early graft patency was significantly higher in the aspirin-treated groups (92% to 93.5%) compared with placebo (85%). There was a nonstatistically significant trend toward an improved patency rate with sulfinpyrazone, but this therapy was associated with transient renal insufficiency in 5% of patients. It is important to note that one daily dose of aspirin was as effective as aspirin given three times daily and

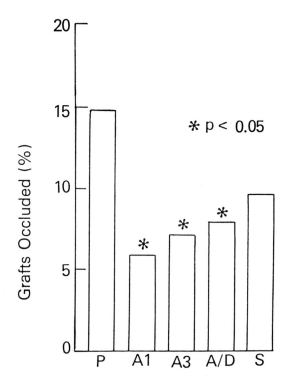

Figure 11.5. Percent of occluded vein grafts within 60 days after bypass surgery in different treatment groups. Only the aspirin-containing regimens improved graft patency (by cluster analysis). A1 = aspirin (325 mg/day); A3 = aspirin (325 mg three times daily); A/D = aspirin plus dipyridamole (325 and 75 mg three times daily, respectively); p = placebo; s = sulfinpyrazone (267 mg three times daily). Reproduced from Goldman et al. (55), with permission from the American Heart Association, Inc.

that dipyridamole conferred no additional benefit over aspirin alone. Because aspirin was given preoperatively, bleeding during and after surgery, transfusion requirements and reoperation rate were significantly greater in the aspirin-treated patients (163).

Intermediate and late phases. *Pathogenesis.* These phases probably represent a continuum of the pathologic process that affects vein grafts when exposed to the arterial circulation. The pathogenesis is most likely multifactorial. As already stated, platelet deposition in areas of endothelial damage occurs as soon as the graft is exposed to arterial shear forces (162,164). Smooth muscle cell proliferation leading to intimal hyperplasia may follow (153,165), probably as a result of chronic endothelial injury and release of mitogenic factors from platelets or other cells. Occlusive or nonocclusive thrombus formation may occur at any point during the disease process, as documented in surgical specimens (166), autopsy studies (152,153,165) and experimental models (154). Finally, lipid accumulation in intra- and extracellular sites, connective tissue synthesis by smooth muscle cells and fibroblasts and foci of calcification become evident at the end of the first year after surgery (152,165). These fibrous plaques are indistinguishable from the athero-

sclerotic plaques that occur in the native coronary arteries. In a recent study (166), two-thirds of vein grafts removed during a second coronary artery bypass operation showed evidence of mural or occlusive thrombosis. This was particularly prevalent in atherosclerotic grafts and those with aneurysmal dilation, which suggests that late thrombosis is not an uncommon event in chronically injured grafts.

Prevention. Available platelet inhibitors do not prevent platelet adherence to the injured endothelium or the release of their mitogenic factors. Thus, smooth muscle cell proliferation and intimal hyperplasia are not affected by these drugs (151). In contrast, antiplatelet agents have been beneficial in reducing the rates of early and late vein-graft occlusion (62). This benefit is most likely a result of the effect of these drugs in limiting superimposed thrombus formation, rather than through a direct effect on the primary occlusive proliferative process. Trials (62,82,167) that have followed up patients beyond the early postoperative phase have demonstrated that the early benefit of platelet inhibitors on graft patency is maintained at 1 year. Furthermore, a recent randomized trial (168) of low dose aspirin plus dipyridamole or an anticoagulant in patients after bypass surgery showed that graft patency rates were significantly higher in patients continued on either of the two antithrombotic regimens for 12 months compared with those withdrawn from therapy at 3 months.

No currently available agent prevents graft atherosclerosis, although control of risk factors such as hyperlipidemia and cigarette smoking may be beneficial (166). Furthermore, aggressive treatment of hyperlipidemia resulted in reduction of progression and even regression of atherosclerosis in a selected group of patients after bypass surgery (169). In a new trial sponsored by the National Institutes of Health for prevention of vein-graft atherosclerosis, the use of aspirin and lipid-lowering therapy, either alone or in combination, will be tested.

Current recommendations. 1) For prevention of early thrombotic occlusion of saphenous vein bypass grafts, platelet inhibitor therapy appears mandatory. Because preoperative aspirin is associated with increased intraoperative bleeding (163), dipyridamole, which prevents activation of platelets by the extracorporeal pump and does not increase bleeding, appears to be a safer agent. However, whether this agent offers additional benefit over postoperative aspirin alone is unknown. Most importantly, aspirin (at a dose of 325 mg/day) should be started immediately after surgery and continued for ≥1 year. Postoperative dipyridamole confers no additional benefit over that of aspirin (54,55).

2) It is not yet clear whether aspirin should be continued indefinitely. However, on the basis of the previously reviewed available data on native coronary artery disease and the positive results from a randomized trial (168), long-term antithrombotic treatment for prevention of chronic coronary artery or graft thrombotic disease is probably justified.

3) The control of coronary risk factors is essential. After

Table 11.5. Trials of Antiplatelet Agents for Prevention of Acute Complications During Coronary Angioplasty

Trial (ref)	Design	No. of Patients	Treatment	Rate of Acute Complications (%)	Results
White et al. (81)	Prospective randomized	333	ASA + Dip	5.0	Reduction in abrupt vessel closure,
			Ticlopidine	2.0	thrombosis or dissection (p < 0.005)
			Placebo	14.0	
Schwartz et al. (174)	Prospective randomized	376	ASA	1.6	Reduction in acute myocardial infarction
			Placebo	6.9	(secondary end point, p = 0.01)*
Chesebro et al. (175)	Prospective randomized	207	ASA + Dip	11.0	Trend toward lower acute complication rate
			Placebo	20.0	(p = 0.07)†
Barnathan et al. (176)	Retrospective	220	ASA	1.8	Reduction in clinically significant thrombi
			ASA + Dip	0	producing total occlusion or requiring
			None	10.7	surgery (p = 0.005)
Kent et al. (177)	Retrospective	500	ASA	1.3	Reduction in acute myocardial infarction and
			None	6.5	emergency bypass surgery (p < 0.001)

*Primary end point = effect of therapy on late restenosis; †complications included coronary occlusion, infarction, repeat angioplasty and urgent surgery. ASA = Aspirin; Dip = Dipyridamole.

the first postoperative year, vein-graft atherosclerotic disease is conditioned by similar risk factors that predispose to native coronary artery disease.

Postangioplasty Occlusion and Restenosis

Percutaneous transluminal coronary angioplasty is an important alternative to surgical revascularization in suitable patients with coronary artery disease, and its use has been greatly expanded in the last few years. Fracture or splitting of the stenotic lesion, medial disruption and stretching or expansion of the external diameter of the artery are probably necessary for successful angioplasty (170,171). Endothelial denudation, platelet deposition and mural thrombus formation occur immediately after angioplasty and may lead to acute occlusion and restenosis (172).

Acute occlusion. *Pathogenesis.* The pathogenesis of acute occlusion probably involves one or several mechanisms, including formation of large, folded intimal flaps due to intimal-medial dissection; arterial damage associated with residual stenosis, which facilitates platelet and clotting activation and thrombosis; vasospasm or relaxation of overstretched vessel wall segments; or subintimal plaque hemorrhage, especially after thrombolytic therapy (173). Experimental angioplasty (172) has shown that when arterial injury is mild, it is associated with endothelial denudation and subintimal deposition of platelets. In contrast, extensive arterial wall damage or dissection leads to exposure of media and collagen, which are profoundly thrombogenic despite systemic heparinization.

Prevention. Three prospective (81,174,175) and two retrospective (176,177) angiographic studies have clearly

shown that pretreatment with aspirin alone, aspirin plus dipyridamole or ticlopidine alone significantly reduces the incidence of acute thrombotic occlusion and periprocedural Q wave infarction in patients undergoing coronary angioplasty (Table 11.5). A recent prospective study (178) indicated that aspirin alone was as effective as the combination of aspirin and dipyridamole.

The role of heparin in the prevention of acute vessel occlusion during angioplasty has not been properly tested clinically, but there is experimental evidence (179) that suggests an inverse relation between the dose of heparin and the degree of platelet deposition and vascular thrombosis. In addition, several studies (180–183) have suggested that prolonged intravenous heparin before the procedure in patients with unstable angina and intracoronary thrombi improves the angioplasty success rate and reduces the risk of thrombotic coronary occlusion. Given the substantial risk of acute thrombotic complications associated with plaque disruption during angioplasty, pretreatment with aspirin combined with adequate heparinization throughout the procedure is strongly recommended. The value of intracoronary administration of a thrombolytic agent before angioplasty in patients with unstable angina or recent infarction is currently being investigated.

Late restenosis. Restenosis is the major complication after successful angioplasty, with an incidence rate of 25% to 40%. Although its definition varies among investigations, a number of clinical, anatomic and procedural variables that predispose to restenosis have been identified (184,185). Factors associated with higher restenosis rates include recent onset of crescendo or unstable angina, diabetes mellitus, presence of severe preangioplasty stenosis, proximal as opposed to distal dilations, lesions in the left anterior descending artery or saphenous vein grafts, dilation of multiple lesions in the same vessel, high postangioplasty residual stenosis and severe vessel injury with large and complicated intimal dissection (186–189).

Pathogenesis. The pathogenesis of restenosis is not entirely understood and may involve several different mechanisms. Increased residual luminal stenosis after dilation produces a high local shear rate and favors platelet deposition and thrombosis (184). Deep arterial injury with subsequent exposure of fibrillar collagen and release of tissue thromboplastin favors platelet aggregation, activation of the coagulation system and thrombus formation (172,190). Furthermore, vessel wall injury may lead to the release of growth factors from platelets, endothelium, smooth muscle cells or macrophages (100). These growth factors are potent mitogens for smooth muscle cells and fibroblasts. As a result of balloon injury, smooth muscle cells migrate from the media to the intima and proliferate. In addition, excessive amounts of connective tissue matrix can be synthesized, resulting in recurrent arterial stenosis. Finally, the release of vasoactive substances by aggregating platelets (191), loss of endothelium-derived relaxing factor as a consequence of endothelial damage and alteration in prostaglandin metabolism (192) may result in vasoconstriction and potentially contribute to restenosis.

Antithrombotic agents. Adequate antithrombotic therapy started before the procedure is necessary to reduce the hemostatic response to arterial wall injury and prevent acute thrombotic occlusion. Unfortunately, results of clinical trials using different antiplatelet drugs and anticoagulant agents aimed at reducing the restenosis rate have been disappointing. Recent clinical studies using aspirin plus dipyridamole (174,175,193) or ticlopidine (193) failed to reduce the rate of restenosis.

Because heparin was shown to suppress smooth muscle cell proliferation in an animal model of vascular injury (73) and in vitro cell culture (74), interest in this agent for the prevention of restenosis after angioplasty has emerged. A recent study (194) compared short-term heparin (given for 18 to 24 h) versus placebo after angioplasty and found no difference in restenosis rate at 6 months. Long-term subcutaneous heparin after angioplasty has not been properly tested in humans. Similarly, anticoagulant therapy with warfarin for 6 months was unable to prevent restenosis (195,196).

Omega-3 fatty acids. The use of omega-3 fatty acids in patients who have had angioplasty has generated a great deal of interest, but available studies (197–201) have yielded conflicting results. The most carefully conducted of these studies (197) found a significant reduction in the restenosis rate as assessed angiographically. In this trial, fish oils were initiated 7 days before angioplasty, and the effects of therapy on platelet fatty acid concentration were evaluated. Two other trials (198,199) using mostly nonangiographic defini-

tions of restenosis also observed a benefit from fish oil therapy. In contrast, the other two studies (200,201) that employed angiographic follow-up study found no benefit from therapy. Although no definite recommendations can be made given available conflicting data, there is some evidence that suggests that pretreatment with large doses of omega-3 fatty acids may be beneficial in selected patients.

Other unsuccessful attempts aimed at reducing restenosis rates have included administration of high dose steroids (202,203), prostacyclin (204) and calcium channel blocking agents (205,206).

New intravascular technologies. Intensive research has focused on the development of mechanical devices, with the expectation of reducing the process of restenosis. These include intracoronary stents, devices that deliver laser, ultrasonic or radiofrequency energy, atherectomy catheters and infusion devices for local delivery of antithrombotic or antiproliferative agents. The widespread use of these devices awaits the results of large-scale clinical trials.

Current recommendations. 1) Until the results of ongoing and future clinical trials are available, the best antiplatelet agent for prevention of acute occlusion is aspirin, which should be started 1 day before angioplasty, followed by a dose of 325 mg 1 h before the procedure and daily thereafter. Ticlopidine also appears effective.

2) All patients should receive a bolus injection of heparin (100 U/kg) at the beginning of the procedure, followed by an intravenous infusion (at approximately 15 U/kg per h), which should be continued for several hours; the length of heparin therapy will depend on whether a thrombus or large vessel wall dissection is detected at the end of the procedure.

3) Antiplatelet therapy reduces the incidence of acute occlusion, but its effect on late restenosis is doubtful. A technically good result from the angioplasty procedure itself, with minimal or no postdilatation residual stenosis, probably reduces the restenosis rate.

4) Future approaches that may be valuable in decreasing the incidence of restenosis include omega-3 fatty acid therapy, blockers of receptors in smooth muscle cells, inhibitors of growth factors that stimulate smooth muscle cell proliferation, thrombin inhibitors and monoclonal antibodies against platelet membrane receptors and adhesive macromolecules such as von Willebrand factor.

Prosthetic Heart Valves

Thromboembolism. There is a long-term risk of arterial thromboembolism in patients with prosthetic heart valves; progressively fewer patients remain free of embolic events over time. In a long-term study (207) of patients with a mitral or aortic Starr-Edwards prosthesis, only 66% were free of thromboembolic events at 10 years and 58% at 15 years of follow-up study. Of the embolic events, 85% were cerebral, resulting in a 10% mortality rate. Of patients who received inadequate anticoagulant therapy, 40% had thromboembo-

Table 11.6. Randomized Trials of Platelet Inhibitors Added to Anticoagulant Therapy in Mechanical Prosthetic Valves

Trial (ref)	Treatment	No. of Patients	Embolic Events (%)	Results of Therapy
Sullivan et al. (56)	A/C + placebo	84	14	
	A/C + Dip	79	1	Reduction in embolism (p < 0.01)
Kasahara (57)	A/C	39	21	
	A/C + Dip	40	5	Favorable trend
PACTE (58)	A/C	154	5	
	A/C + Dip	136	3	Favorable trend
Rajah et al. (59)	A/C	87	13	
	A/C + Dip	78	4	Favorable trend
Chesebro et al. (60)	A/C	183	4	
	A/C + Dip	181	1	Reduction in embolism (p < 0.05)
	A/C + ASA	170	4	No added benefit*
Altman et al. (212)	A/C	65	20	
	A/C + ASA	57	5	Reduction in embolism (p < 0.05)
Dale et al. (213)	A/C + placebo	73	12	
	A/C + ASA	75	2	Reduction in embolism (p < 0.01)

*Significant increase in gastrointestinal hemorrhage observed. A/C = anticoagulants; PACTE = Prevention des Accidents Thromboemboliques Systemiques Recherche Groupe; other abbreviations as in Table 11.4.

lism. Patients with a Björk-Shiley prosthesis have a lower incidence of thromboembolism, but when thrombotic occlusion of the valve occurs, it may rapidly lead to cardiogenic shock and death. Among the mechanical valves, the St. Jude Medical valve has the lowest risk of thromboembolism.

Although bioprosthetic valves are less thrombogenic, this complication sometimes occurs, particularly in patients not taking anticoagulant agents with atrial fibrillation, a mitral prosthesis or poor left ventricular function (208). Overall, there has been a reduction in the incidence of thromboembolism after valve replacement in recent years, probably because patients are being operated on at an earlier stage in their disease process and new mechanical prosthetic valves have better hemodynamic characteristics.

Mechanical prostheses. Studies (208–210) in patients with mechanical valves have consistently shown that appropriate anticoagulation significantly reduces the incidence of valvular thrombosis and embolism. Without long-term anticoagulation, the incidence of thromboembolism increases by two- to six-fold (208). Platelet inhibitors alone have not been found to confer protection against embolism in patients with a mechanical prosthesis. Several studies (209–211) of aspirin plus dipyridamole in these patients have shown an incidence of thromboembolism as high as 10% per year.

Prevention. Because of the persistent risk of thromboembolism in patients with a mechanical prosthesis and anticoagulant therapy, the addition of a platelet inhibitor has been prospectively studied (56–60,212,213) (Table 11.6).

The addition of dipyridamole to an oral anticoagulant has been shown to decrease the incidence of thromboembolism in five trials (56–60). In addition, the combination of aspirin and an oral anticoagulant was found to be beneficial in two other trials (212,213) but not in a third one (60), which found an increased incidence of gastrointestinal bleeding with aspirin (500 mg/day) plus warfarin. In patients who cannot tolerate dipyridamole and aspirin, sulfinpyrazone (200 mg four times daily) may be empirically added to warfarin, although no randomized prospective trials of this combination have been conducted. Uncontrolled studies (86), however, do suggest that this agent is effective.

Bioprostheses. *Mitral bioprosthesis.* Although bioprostheses are less thrombogenic than mechanical devices, thromboembolism still occurs, especially in the first 3 months after surgery, more often in patients with a mitral prosthesis and those with atrial fibrillation or prior embolism (208). These patients should receive oral anticoagulant therapy postoperatively for 1 to 3 months unless atrial fibrillation persists, in which case long-term warfarin therapy is required. Long-term aspirin therapy 3 months after surgery has been suggested in patients with a mitral bioprosthesis who do not have any of the risk factors of embolism already mentioned (214), but its value remains to be proved. Valve repair instead of replacement in selected patients is rapidly becoming an acceptable alternative and is probably associated with a lower incidence of thromboembolism.

Aortic bioprosthesis. The appropriate therapy for aortic bioprostheses is still controversial. Although some investigators have recommended warfarin for 3 months, others advocate the use of antiplatelet drugs or no therapy at all because the embolic risk of these patients is low as long as normal sinus rhythm is maintained (208). Earlier surgical intervention and better protection of the bioprosthetic material to prevent valvular degeneration have lead to increased use of homograft and heterograft bioprostheses.

Current recommendations. 1) All patients with a mechanical prosthetic heart valve require long-term anticoagulant therapy, which should be commenced in the early postoperative period. The dose of warfarin should be tightly controlled to avoid thromboembolic or bleeding complications. Therapy is aimed at prolonging the prothrombin time (PT) to 1.5 to 2.0 × control (equivalent to an International Normalized Ratio of prothrombin suppression [INR] of 3.0 to 4.5).

2) Because of the persistent embolic risk, the addition of dipyridamole may be beneficial in patients at high risk of thromboembolism, including those with a mechanical prosthesis implanted before the mid-1970s and certainly those with prior embolism. In patients who cannot tolerate dipyridamole, low dose aspirin (80 to 160 mg/day) added to warfarin may be a good alternative; however, higher doses of aspirin (>500 mg/day) are contraindicated because of the significant risk of gastrointestinal bleeding.

3) Patients with a mitral bioprosthesis should probably receive anticoagulant therapy for 1 to 3 months after surgery. Anticoagulation is recommended indefinitely to patients with prior embolic events or atrial fibrillation. No antithrombotic treatment appears necessary for patients with an aortic bioprosthesis in sinus rhythm.

4) Patients with recurrent thromboembolism despite adequate antithrombotic therapy should be considered for repeat valve replacement.

Cerebrovascular Disease

Approximately 85% of acute strokes are ischemic in origin, whereas 15% are due to intracranial hemorrhage. Eighty percent of ischemic strokes result from atherosclerotic disease in the carotid or large cerebral arteries by means of embolism of plaque material or platelet-fibrin thromboemboli or the presence of flow-restricting stenosis that may lead to thrombosis and occlusion. Of all ischemic strokes, only 15% are caused by cardiogenic emboli. These emboli usually arise from thrombi in the left atrium, left ventricle and native or prosthetic mitral or aortic valves (215).

Stroke. *Antiplatelet therapy.* The effectiveness of platelet inhibitor drugs in the secondary prevention of stroke recurrence has been controversial. One study (52) showed that aspirin had a significant beneficial effect, whereas another large study (216) using 1,500 mg/day of aspirin failed to demonstrate any benefit in the reduction of stroke recur-

rence or death. In a recent, randomized, double-blind, placebo-controlled trial (217), 2,500 patients with a recent ischemic neurologic event (60% with stroke, 33% with transient ischemic attack and 6% with reversible ischemic neurologic deficit) were randomized to receive aspirin (325 mg) plus dipyridamole (75 mg) three times daily. After 2 years, the treated group had a striking 33% reduction in the combined rate of stroke and death (p < 0.001).

In another large, randomized, placebo-controlled trial (83) of 1,072 patients with a recent ischemic stroke, the novel antiplatelet agent ticlopidine was found to decrease the combined rate of recurrent stroke, myocardial infarction and vascular death by 23% at the end of 3 years (p = 0.02). However, treatment with ticlopidine was associated with an 8% incidence of significant side effects that include neutropenia, rash and diarrhea (83).

A pooled analysis (145) of 13 randomized trials of antiplatelet therapy in cerebrovascular disease (including patients with stroke and transient ischemic attacks) clearly showed that treatment reduced the incidence of nonfatal stroke by 22%, nonfatal myocardial infarction by 35% and vascular death by 15%. Therefore, long-term antiplatelet treatment for secondary prevention is recommended in survivors of stroke.

Anticoagulant therapy. With respect to anticoagulant therapy in stroke, several trials have shown that this approach is potentially hazardous because of the increased risk of bleeding or that it is without benefit, and thus is not recommended (215). In contrast, the use of long-term anticoagulant therapy in patients with cardiogenic embolism is mandatory and will not be discussed further in this review.

Transient ischemic attacks. Numerous studies (28,52,84, 89,217–221) have compared aspirin with placebo or other antithrombotic therapy in patients with transient ischemic attacks (Table 11.7). Although the smaller trials (218–221) showed no advantage of aspirin over placebo, the small number of patients limits the significance of these results. More importantly, all four larger trials (28,52,89,217) demonstrated that aspirin significantly reduced the rate of stroke and death by 18% to 40%.

Preliminary results from the large, randomized, controlled United Kingdom Transient Ischemic Attack (UK-TIA) Aspirin Trial (28) revealed a significant 18% reduction in the combined rate of nonfatal stroke, nonfatal myocardial infarction and death in patients treated with aspirin. However, there was a nonsignificant reduction in the odds of disabling stroke and vascular death. In this study, 300 and 1,200 mg/day of aspirin were equally effective, but the lower dose caused substantially less gastric toxicity (28). This evidence coupled with the results of the pooled analysis (145) of platelet inhibitor trials in the secondary prevention of vascular disease clearly suggests that aspirin reduces the incidence of stroke and vascular death in patients with transient ischemic attacks.

In a recently published trial (84), >3,000 patients with recent transient or mild persistent focal cerebral ischemia were

Table 11.7. Randomized Trials of Platelet Inhibitors in Patients With Transient Ischemic Attacks

Trial (ref)	Treatment	No. of Patients	Follow-up (mo)	Stroke/Death No. (%)	Results of Therapy
AITIA-I (218)	ASA	88	24	13 (15)	Beneficial trend (small trial)
	Placebo	90		19 (21)	
AITIA-II (219)	ASA	65	24	8 (12)	No benefit (small trial)
	Placebo	60		8 (13)	
German (220)	ASA	29	24	0 (0)	No benefit (very small trial)
	Placebo	29		4 (14)	
CCSG (89)	ASA	290	26	46 (16)	Only ASA was beneficial (p < 0.05)
	Sulf/placebo	295		68 (23)	
Danish (221)	ASA	101	25	21 (21)	No benefit (small trial)
	Placebo	102		17 (17)	
AICLA (52)	ASA	400	36	35 (9)	Reduction in event rate (p < 0.02)
	Placebo	204		31 (15)	
ESPS (217)	ASA + Dip	1,250	24	190 (15)	Marked reduction in event rate (p < 0.001)
	Placebo	1,250		283 (23)	
UK-TIA (28)	ASA	1,621	48	171 (11)	Reduction in combined vascular event rate (p < 0.05)
	Placebo	814		109 (13)	
TASS (84)	Ticlopidine	1,529	36	306 (17)	Lower event rate with ticlopidine (p < 0.05), but increased side effects
	ASA	1,540		349 (19)	

AICLA = Accidents Ischemiques Cerebraux lies L'atherosclerose (half of the aspirin-treated patients received dipyridamole); AITIA-I = Aspirin in Transient Ischemic Attacks (Medical); AITIA-II = Aspirin in Transient Ischemic Attacks (Surgical); ASA = aspirin; CCSG = Canadian Cooperative Study Group; Danish = Danish Cooperative Study; Dip = dipyridamole; ESPS = European Stroke Prevention Study (included patients with stroke and ischemic attacks); German = German Transient Ischemic Attack Trial; TASS = Ticlopidine Aspirin Stroke Study; UK-TIA = United Kingdom Transient Ischemic Attack Trial (aspirin doses used: 300 and 1,200 mg/day).

randomly allocated to receive ticlopidine (500 mg/day) or aspirin (1,300 mg/day). At the end of 3 years, death or nonfatal stroke occurred in 17% of patients in the ticlopidine-treated group and 19% in the aspirin-treated group (p < 0.05). Fatal and nonfatal stroke were 21% lower in the ticlopidine-treated patients (0 = 0.024). However, adverse reactions were more common in the ticlopidine-treated group, including diarrhea (20%), rash (12%) and severe neutropenia (1%).

The use of anticoagulant therapy in transient ischemic attacks is still controversial since both beneficial and harmful trends have been observed (215). Because available evidence supporting the use of aspirin is stronger than that supporting anticoagulant agents and the risks of treatment are lower, aspirin is preferred.

Current recommendations. 1) In patients with transient ischemic attacks, aspirin is recommended for prevention of stroke, myocardial infarction and cardiovascular death. A recent study (28) showed that a dose of 300 mg/day is as effective as 1,200 mg/day, but is less toxic. In a recent large trial (84), ticlopidine was found somewhat more effective than aspirin in preventing stroke, but was associated with a higher incidence of side effects.

2) In patients with completed stroke, antiplatelet treatment with aspirin plus dipyridamole (217) or with ticlopidine (83) was found to be effective in reducing the incidence of recurrent stroke or cardiovascular death. Available data (145) suggest that aspirin alone is as effective as the combination of aspirin and dipyridamole and thus is recommended at a dose of 325 mg/day. Whereas ticlopidine is also effective, the higher incidence of severe side effects may limit its usefulness.

3) Anticoagulant therapy is not recommended in patients with a transient ischemic attack or completed stroke. However, patients with cerebral embolism from a cardiac source should receive long-term anticoagulant therapy.

Other Cardiovascular Conditions

Nonvalvular atrial fibrillation. The incidence of stroke is higher in patients with atrial fibrillation, even in the absence of valvular heart disease. In patients at the highest risk (namely, those with embolism in the previous 2 years), the incidence of stroke is >10% per year (215). For these patients, moderate intensity anticoagulation (prothrombin time [PT] range 1.5 to 2.0 × control, International Normalized Ratio of prothrombin suppression [INR] 3.0 to 4.5) is recommended (1). Patients with atrial fibrillation and mitral stenosis are also at high risk and should be managed with long-term anticoagulant therapy aimed at a PT of 1.3 to 1.5 × control (INR 2.0 to 3.0). Patients at low risk for embolism (namely, those <60 years old and no associated heart disease [lone fibrillators]) usually do not require anticoagulation (222).

Between these two clinical settings poles exists a large group of patients with an intermediate but incompletely defined risk of embolism (namely, those with nonvalvular atrial fibrillation associated with various forms of cardiovascular disease). Three prospective randomized studies (223,224,224a) of antithrombotic treatment have been published. The Copenhagen Atrial Fibrillation, Aspirin, Anticoagulation Study (223) randomly allocated 1,007 patients to receive warfarin, aspirin (75 mg/day) or placebo. At the end of 2 years, the incidence of stroke, transient ischemic attack and systemic embolism was significantly lower in the warfarin group (1.5%) compared with the aspirin and placebo groups (6% each) (p < 0.05). However, bleeding side effects and withdrawal from treatment were more common in patients receiving anticoagulant therapy.

Preliminary results from the Stroke Prevention in Atrial Fibrillation (SPAF) Study (224) recently became available. This study randomized 588 patients to receive warfarin, aspirin (325 mg/day) or placebo. In addition, 656 patients not eligible for warfarin received aspirin or placebo in a double-blind fashion. At the end of 1 year, the placebo arm of the study was terminated because active treatment (either warfarin or aspirin) reduced the risk of stroke and systemic embolism by an impressive 81% (p < 0.00005). In addition, the study revealed that aspirin reduced stroke and embolism by 50% (p = 0.014), but was not effective in patients >75 years of age. Finally, the Boston Area Anticoagulation Trial for Atrial Fibrillation (BAATAF) (224a) demonstrated that low-dose warfarin therapy (target prothrombin time ration, 1.2–1.5) significantly reduced the incidence of strokes and death by 86% and 62%, respectively, compared with placebo. In summary, these 3 trials have clearly shown that warfarin reduces the stroke rate in patients with nonvalvular atrial fibrillation. In addition, the SPAF Study (224) revealed the beneficial effects of aspririn. These investigators are currently comparing the benefits of aspirin and warfarin.

Peripheral vascular disease. The combination of aspirin and dipyridamole reduced the progression of peripheral atherosclerosis in a 2 year study (225) of patients with peripheral vascular disease. Other studies (226) suggest a beneficial effect of ticlopidine in patients with chronic arterial insufficiency. Despite encouraging results from some studies (227), there are no convincing data from properly designed, large trials showing that antithrombotic therapy delays the progression of peripheral vascular disease.

Arteriovenous cannulas. Thrombosis of arteriovenous cannulas results in significant morbidity in patients with chronic renal failure on hemodialysis. Anticoagulant agents may decrease the incidence of thrombosis, but are hazardous in uremic patients. Two studies using aspirin (160 mg/day) (228) or sulfinpyrazone (85) demonstrated a reduction in the incidence of thrombosis of arteriovenous shunts in these patients.

Mitral valve prolapse. Patients with mitral valve prolapse, particularly those with myxomatous valves, are at somewhat higher risk of stroke than the general population (229,230). Because the risk is low, prophylaxis is not indicated in the absence of additional risk factors for embolism. If an embolic event occurs or there is evidence of recurrent embolism, oral anticoagulation may be empirically instituted, although there is no clear evidence that this is beneficial.

We are indebted to Stephanie Lipson Stein for her invaluable help in the preparation of the manuscript.

References

1. Dalen JE, Hirsh J. Second ACCP National Conference on Antithrombotic Therapy. Chest 1989;95(suppl):1S–169S.
2. Topol EJ, Califf RM. Symposium on myocardial reperfusion 1988: practical considerations. J Am Coll Cardiol 1988;12(suppl A):1A–92A.
3. Fuster V, Badimon L, Cohen M, Ambrose JA, Badimon JJ, Chesebro JH. Insights into the pathogenesis of acute ischemic syndromes. Circulation 1988;77:1213–20.
4. Crowley JG, Pierce RA. The affinity of platelets for subendothelium. Am J Surg 1981;47:529–32.
5. Hawiger J. Formation and regulation of platelet and fibrin hemostatic plug. Hum Pathol 1987;18:111–22.
6. Escolar G, Krumwiede M, White JG. Organization of the actin cytoskeleton of resting and activated platelets in suspension. Am J Pathol 1986;123:86–94.
7. Peerschke EIB. The platelet fibrinogen receptor. Semin Hematol 1985; 22:241–59.
8. Antoniades HN, Hunkapiller MW. Human platelet-derived growth factor (PDGF): aminoterminal aminoacid sequence. Science 1983;220: 963–5.
9. Berk BC, Alexander RW, Brock TA, et al. Vasoconstriction: a new activity for platelet-derived growth factor. Science 1986;232:87–90.
10. Deuel TF, Senior RM, Chang D, et al. Platelet factor 4 is chemotactic for neutrophiles and monocytes. Proc Natl Acad Sci USA 1981;78:4584–7.
11. Badimon L, Badimon JJ. Mechanism of arterial thrombosis in nonparallel streamlines: platelet thrombi grow on the apex of the stenotic severely injured vessel wall. Experimental study in the pig model. J Clin Invest 1989;84:1134–44.
12. Shattil SJ, Brass LP. Induction of the fibrinogen receptor on human platelets by intracellular mediators. J Biol Chem 1987;262:992–1000.
13. Coller BS. Activation affects access to the platelet receptor for adhesive glycoproteins. J Cell Biol 1986;103:451–6.
14. Moncada S, Vane JR. Arachidonic acid metabolites and the interactions between platelets and blood-vessel walls. N Engl J Med 1979;300: 1142–7.
15. Haslam RJ, Davidson MML, Fox JEB, Lynham JA. Cyclic nucleotides in platelet function. Thromb Haemost 1978;40:232–40.
16. Walsh PN, Schmaier AH. Platelet-coagulation protein interactions. In: Colman RW, Hirsh J, Marder VJ, Salzman EW, eds. Hemostasis and Thrombosis. Philadelphia: JB Lippincott, 1987;689–709.

17. Ofosu FA, Cerskus AL, Hirsh JA, et al. The inhibition of the anticoagulant activity of heparin by platelets, brain phospholipids and tissue factor. Br J Haematol 1984;57:229–38.

18. McNeely TB, Griffith MJ. The anticoagulant mechanism of action of heparin in contact-activated plasma: inhibition of factor X activation. Blood 1985;65:1226–31.

19. Van Hinsbergh VWM, Bertina RM, van Wijngaarden A, et al. Activated protein C decreases plasminogen activator-inhibitor activity in endothelial cell-conditioned medium. Blood 1985;65:444–51.

20. Collen D. On the regulation and control of fibrinolysis. Thromb Haemost 1980;43:77–89.

21. Erickson LA, Ginsberg MH, Loskutoff DJ. Detection and partial characterization of an inhibitor of plasminogen activator in human platelets. J Clin Invest 1984;74:1465–72.

22. Mimuro J, Schleef RR, Loskutoff DJ. Extracellular matrix of cultured bovine aortic endothelial cells contains functionally active type I plasminogen activator inhibitor. Blood 1987;70:721–8.

23. Tschopp TB. Aspirin inhibits platelet aggregation on, but not adhesion to, collagen fibrils: an assessment of platelet adhesion and deposited platelet mass by morphometry and ^{51}Cr-labelling. Thromb Res 1977;11: 619–32.

24. Clowes AW, Karnovsky MJ. Failure of certain antiplatelet drugs to affect myointimal thickening following arterial endothelial injury in the rat. Lab Invest 1977;36:452–64.

25. Roth GL, Majerus PW. The mechanism of the effect of aspirin on human platelets. I. Acetylation of a particulate fraction protein. J Clin Invest 1975;56:624–32.

26. Kyrle PA, Eichler HG, Jager U, Lechner K. Inhibition of prostacyclin and thromboxane A_2 generation by low-dose aspirin at the site of plug formation in man in vivo. Circulation 1987;75:1025–9.

27. Lewis HD, David JW, Archibald DG, et al. Protective effects of aspirin against acute myocardial infarction and death in men with unstable angina: results of a Veterans Administration cooperative study. N Engl J Med 1983;309:396–403.

28. UK-TIA Study Group. United Kingdom Transient Ischaemic Attack (UK-TIA) Aspirin Trial: Interim results. Br Med J 1988;296:316–20.

29. ISIS-2 (Second International Study of Infarct Survival) Collaborative Group. Randomized trial of intravenous streptokinase, oral aspirin, both, or neither among 17187 cases of suspected acute myocardial infarction: ISIS-2. Lancet 1988;2:349–60.

30. Graham DY, Smith LJ. Aspirin and the stomach. Ann Intern Med 1986;104:390–8.

31. Cairns JA, Gent M, Singer J, et al. Aspirin, sulfinpyrazone, or both in unstable angina. N Engl J Med 1985;313:1369–75.

32. Neri Serneri GG, Castellani S. Platelet and vascular prostaglandins: pharmacological and clinical implications. In: Born GVR, Neri Serneri GG, eds. Antiplatelet Therapy: Twenty Years' Experience. Proceedings of a European Conference. Amsterdam: Elsevier (Excerpta Medica), 1987;37–51.

33. Friedman PL, Brown EJ, Gunther S, et al. Coronary vasoconstrictor effect of indomethacin in patients with coronary artery disease. N Engl J Med 1981;305:1171–5.

34. Kromhout D, Bosschieter EB, Coulander CDL. The inverse relation between fish consumption and 20-year mortality from coronary heart disease. N Engl J Med 1985;312:1205–9.

35. Shekelle RB, Missel L, Paul O, Shryock AM, Stamler J. Fish consumption and mortality from coronary heart disease (letter). N Engl J Med 1985;313:820.

36. Von Schacky C. Prophylaxis of atherosclerosis with marine omega-3 fatty acids: a comprehensive strategy. Ann Intern Med 1987;107:890–9.

37. Leaf A, Weber PC. Cardiovascular effects of n-3 fatty acids. N Engl J Med 1988;318:549–57.

38. Mullane KM, Fornabaio D. Thromboxane synthetase inhibitors reduce infarct size by a platelet-dependent, aspirin-sensitive mechanism. Circ Res 1988;62:668–78.

39. Willerson JT, Golino P, Eidt J, Campbell WB, Buja LM. Specific platelet mediators and unstable coronary artery lesions: experimental evidence and potential clinical implications. Circulation 1989;80:198–205.

40. Thaulow E, Dale J, Myhre E. Effects of a selective thromboxane synthetase inhibitor, dazoxiben, and of acetylsalicylic acid on myocar-

41. Fiddler GI, Lumley P. Preliminary clinical studies with thromboxane synthase inhibitors and thromboxane receptor blockers: a review. Circulation 1990;81(suppl I):I-69–78.

42. Oates JA, FitzGerald GA, Branch RA, Jackson EK, Knapp HR, Roberts LJ. Clinical implications of prostaglandin and thromboxane A_2 formation. N Engl J Med 1988;319:689–98, 761–7.

43. Gresele P, Arnout J, Deckmyn H, Huybrechts E, Pieters G, Vermylen J. Role of proaggregatory and antiaggregatory prostaglandins in hemostasis: studies with combined thromboxane synthase inhibition and thromboxane receptor antagonism. J Clin Invest 1987;80:1435–45.

44. Moncada S, Korbut R. Dipyridamole and other phosphodiesterase inhibitors act as antithrombotic agents by potentiating endogenous prostacyclin. Lancet 1978;1:1286–9.

45. Crutchley DJ, Ryan US, Ryan JW. Effects of aspirin and dipyridamole on the degradation of adenosine diphosphate by cultured cells derived from bovine pulmonary artery. J Clin Invest 1980;66:29–35.

46. FitzGerald GA. Dipyridamole. N Engl J Med 1987;316:1247–57.

47. Harker LA, Slichter SJ. Studies of platelet and fibrinogen kinetics in patients with prosthetic heart valves. N Engl J Med 1970;283:1302–5.

48. Weily HS, Steele PP, Davies H, Pappas G, Genton E. Platelet survival in patients with substitute heart valves. N Engl J Med 1974;290:534–7.

49. Harker LA. Platelet survival time: its measurement and use. Prog Hemost Thromb 1978;4:321–47.

50. Hanson SR, Harker LA, Bjornsson TD. Effect of platelet-modifying drugs on arterial thromboembolism in baboons: aspirin potentiates the antithrombotic actions of dipyridamole and sulfinpyrazone by mechanism(s) independent of platelet cyclooxygenase inhibition. J Clin Invest 1985;75:1591–9.

51. The Persantine-Aspirin Reinfarction Study Group. Persantine and aspirin in coronary heart disease. Circulation 1980;62:449–61.

52. Bousser MG, Eschwege E, Haugenau M, et al. "AICLA" controlled trial of aspirin and dipyridamole in the secondary prevention of atherothrombotic cerebral ischemia. Stroke 1983;14:5–14.

53. American-Canadian Cooperative Study Group. Persantine-aspirin trial in cerebral ischemia. Part II: endpoint results. Stroke 1985;16:406–15.

54. Brown BG, Cukingnan RA, DeRouen T, et al. Improved graft patency in patients treated with platelet-inhibiting therapy after coronary bypass surgery. Circulation 1985;72:138–46.

55. Goldman S, Copeland J, Moritz T, et al. Improvement in early saphenous vein graft patency after coronary artery bypass surgery with antiplatelet therapy: results of a Veterans Administration cooperative study. Circulation 1988;77:1324–32.

56. Sullivan JM, Harken DE, Gorlin R. Pharmacologic control of thromboembolic complications of cardiac-valve replacement. N Engl J Med 1971;284:1391–4.

57. Kasahara T. Clinical effect of dipyridamole ingestion after prosthetic heart valve replacement—especially on the blood coagulation system. Nippon Kyobu Geka Gakkai Zarshi 1977;25:1007–21.

58. Groupe de Recherche PACTE. Prevention des accidents thromboemboliques systemiques chez les porteurs de prosthesis valvulaires artificielles: essai cooperatif controle du dipyridamole. Arch Mal Coeur 1978;9:915–69.

59. Rajah SM, Sreeharan N, Joseph A, et al. A prospective trial of dipyridamole and warfarin in heart valve patients (abstr). Acta Therapeutica 1980;6(suppl 93):54.

60. Chesebro JH, Fuster V, Elveback LR, et al. Trial of combined warfarin plus dipyridamole or aspirin therapy in prosthetic heart valve replacement: danger of aspirin compared with dipyridamole. Am J Cardiol 1983;51:1537–41.

61. Chesebro JH, Clements IP, Fuster V, et al. A platelet inhibitor-drug trial in coronary-artery bypass operations: benefit of perioperative dipyridamole and aspirin therapy on early postoperative vein-graft patency. N Engl J Med 1982;307:73–8.

62. Chesebro JH, Fuster V, Elveback LR, et al. Effect of dipyridamole and aspirin on late vein-graft patency after coronary bypass operations. N Engl J Med 1984;310:209–14.

63. Weksler BB. Prostaglandins and vascular function. Circulation 1984; 70(suppl III):III-63–71.

64. Coppe D, Sobel M, Seavans L, Levine F, Salzman E. Preservation of platelet function and number by prostacyclin during cardiopulmonary bypass. J Thorac Cardiovasc Surg 1981;81:274–8.

65. Smith MC, Danviriyasup K, Crow JW, et al. Prostacyclin substitution for heparin in long-term hemodialysis. Am J Med 1982;73:669–78.

66. Uchida Y, Hanai T, Hasewaga K, Kawamura K, Oshima T. Recanalization of obstructed coronary artery by intracoronary administration of prostacyclin in patients with acute myocardial infarction. Adv Prostaglandin Thromboxane Leukotriene Res 1983;11:377–83.

67. Sharma B, Wyeth RP, Heinemann FM, Bissett JK. Addition of intracoronary prostaglandin E_1 to streptokinase improves thrombolysis and left ventricular function in acute myocardial infarction (abstr). J Am Coll Cardiol 1988;11(suppl A):104A.

68. Fisher CA, Kappa JR, Sinha AK, Cottrell ED, Reiser HJ, Addonizio VP. Comparison of equimolar concentrations of iloprost, prostacyclin, and prostaglandin E_1 on human platelet function. J Lab Clin Med 1987;109:184–90.

69. Nicolini FA, Mehta JL, Nichols WW, Saldeen TGP, Grant M. Prostacyclin analogue iloprost decreases thrombolytic potential of tissue-type plasminogen activator in canine coronary thrombosis. Circulation 1990; 81:1115–22.

70. Topol EJ, Ellis SG, Califf RM, et al. Combined tissue-type plasminogen activator and prostacyclin therapy for acute myocardial infarction. J Am Coll Cardiol 1989;14:877–84.

71. Raizner A, Hollman J, Demke D, Wakefield L. Beneficial effects of ciprostene in PTCA: a multicenter, randomized, controlled trial (abstr). Circulation 1988;78(suppl II):II-290.

72. Salzman EW, Rosenberg RD, Smith MH, Lindon JN, Favreau L. Effect of heparin fractions on platelet aggregation. J Clin Invest 1980;65:64–73.

73. Clowes AW, Karnowsky MJ. Suppression by heparin of smooth muscle cell proliferation in injured arteries. Nature 1977;265:625–6.

74. Reilly CF, Fritze LMS, Rosenberg RD. Heparin inhibition of smooth muscle cell proliferation: a cellular site of action. J Cell Physiol 1986; 129:11–9.

75. Jang I-K, Gold HK, Ziskind AA, Leinbach RC, Fallon JT, Collen D. Prevention of platelet-rich arterial thrombosis by selective thrombin inhibition. Circulation 1990;81:219–25.

76. Hanson SR, Harker LA. Interruption of acute platelet-dependent thrombosis by the synthetic antithrombin D-phenylalanyl-L-prolyl-L-arginyl chloromethyl ketone. Proc Natl Acad Sci USA 1988;85:3184–8.

77. Heras M, Chesebro JH, Penny WJ, Bailey KR, Badimon L, Fuster V. Effects of thrombin inhibition on the development of acute platelet-thrombus deposition during angioplasty in pigs. Circulation 1989;79:657–65.

78. Lee H, Paton RC, Ruan C. The in vitro effect of ticlopidine on fibrinogen and factor VIII binding to human platelets (abstr). Thromb Haemost 1981;46:67.

79. O'Brien JR. Ticlopidine, a promise for the prevention and treatment of thrombosis and its complications. Haemostasis 1983;13:1–54.

80. Balsano F, Rizzon P, Violi F, et al. Antiplatelet treatment with Ticlopidine in unstable angina. A Controlled Multicenter Clinical Trial. Circulation 1990;82:17–26.

81. White CW, Chaitman B, Lassar TA, et al. Antiplatelet agents are effective in reducing the immediate complications of PTCA: results from the ticlopidine multicenter trial (abstr). Circulation 1987;76(suppl IV): IV-400.

82. Limet R, David JL, Magotteaux P, Larock MP, Rigo P. Prevention of aorta-coronary bypass graft occlusion. J Thorac Cardiovasc Surg 1987; 94:773–83.

83. Gent M, Blakely JA, Easton JD, et al. The Canadian American Ticlopidine Study (CATS) in thromboembolic stroke. Lancet 1989;1:1215–20.

84. Hass WK, Easton JD, Adams HP, et al. A randomized trial comparing ticlopidine hydrochloride with aspirin for the prevention of stroke in high-risk patients. N Engl J Med 1989;321:501–7.

85. Kaegi A, Pineo GF, Shimizu A, Trivedi H, Hirsh J, Gent M. Arteriovenous-shunt thrombosis: prevention by sulfinpyrazone. N Engl J Med 1974;290:304–6.

86. Steele PP, Rainwater J, Vogel R. Platelet suppressant therapy in patients with prosthetic cardiac valves: relationship of clinical effectiveness to alteration of platelet survival time. Circulation 1979;60:910–3.

87. Report from the Anturane Reinfarction Italian Study. Sulfinpyrazone in post-myocardial infarction. Lancet 1982;1:237–42.

88. Baur HR, Van Tassel RA, Pierach CA, Gobel RL. Effects of sulfinpyrazone on early graft closure after myocardial infarction. Am J Cardiol 1982;49:420–4.

89. Canadian Cooperative Study Group. A randomized trial of aspirin and sulfinpyrazone in threatened stroke. N Engl J Med 1978;229:53–9.

90. Harker LA, Fuster V. Pharmacology of platelet inhibitors. J Am Coll Cardiol 1986;8(suppl B):21B–32B.

91. Oberg M, Hedner U, Bergentz SE. Effect of dextran 70 on factor VIII and platelet function in von Willebrand's disease. Thromb Res 1978;12: 629–34.

92. Weiss HJ. The effect of clinical dextran on platelet aggregation, adhesion and ADP release in man: in vivo and in vitro studies. J Lab Clin Med 1967;69:37–46.

93. Swanson KT, Vlietstra RE, Holmes DR, et al. Efficacy of adjunctive dextran during percutaneous transluminal coronary angioplasty. Am J Cardiol 1984;54:447–8.

94. Brown RIG, Aldridge HE, Schwartz L, Henderson M, Brooks E, Coutanche M. The use of dextran-40 during percutaneous transluminal coronary angioplasty: a report of three cases of anaphylactoid reactions—one near fatal. Cathet Cardiovasc Diagn 1985;11:591–5.

95. Coller BS. A new murine monoclonal antibody reports an activation-dependent change in the conformation and/or microenvironment of the platelet glycoprotein IIb/IIIa complex. J Clin Invest 1985;76:101–8.

96. Hanson SR, Pareti FI, Ruggeri ZM, et al. Effects of monoclonal antibodies against the platelet glycoprotein IIb/IIIa complex on thrombosis and hemostasis in the baboon. J Clin Invest 1988;81:149–58.

97. Gold HK, Coller BS, Yasua T, et al. Rapid and sustained coronary artery recanalization with combined bolus injection of recombinant tissue-type plasminogen activator and monoclonal antiplatelet GPIIb/IIIa antibody in a canine preparation. Circulation 1988;77:670–7.

98. Badimon L, Badimon JJ, Chesebro JH, Fuster V. Inhibition of thrombus formation: blockage of adhesive glycoprotein mechanisms versus blockage of the cyclooxygenase pathway (abstr). J Am Coll Cardiol 1988; 11(suppl A):30A.

99. Bellinger DA, Nichols TC, Read MS, et al. Prevention of occlusive coronary artery thrombus by a mural monoclonal antibody to porcine von Willebrand factor. Proc Natl Acad Sci USA 1987;84:8100–4.

100. Ross R. The pathogenesis of atherosclerosis—an update. N Engl J Med 1986;314:488–500.

101. Fuster V, Griggs TR. Porcine von Willebrand disease: implications for the pathophysiology of atherosclerosis and thrombosis. Prog Hemost Thromb 1986;8:159–83.

102. The Steering Committee of the Physicians' Health Study Research Group. Final report on the aspirin component of the ongoing Physician's Health Study. N Engl J Med 1989;321:129–35.

103. Peto R, Gray R, Collins R, et al. A randomized trial of the effects of prophylactic daily aspirin among male British doctors. Br Med J 1988; 296:313–6.

104. Fuster V, Cohen M, Halperin JL. Aspirin in the prevention of coronary disease. N Engl J Med 1989;321:129–35.

105. Paganini-Hill A, Chao A, Ross RK, Henderson BE. Aspirin use and chronic diseases: a cohort study of the elderly. Br Med J 1989;299:1247–50.

106. Meade TW. Low-dose warfarin and low-dose aspirin in the primary prevention of ischemic heart disease. Am J Cardiol 1990;65(suppl C):7C–11C.

107. Roberts WC, Buja LM. The frequency and significance of coronary arterial thrombi and other observations in fatal acute myocardial infarction: a study of 107 necropsy patients. Am J Med 1972;52:425–43.

108. Bini A, Fenoglio JJ, Mesa-Tejada R, Kudryk B, Kaplan KL. Identification and distribution of fibrinogen, fibrin, and fibrin(ogen) degradation products in atherosclerosis: use of monoclonal antibodies. Arteriosclerosis 1989;9:109–21.

109. Chesebro JH, Webster MWI, Smith HC, et al. Antiplatelet therapy in coronary disease progression: reduced infarction and new lesion formation (abstr). Circulation 1989;80(suppl II):II-266.

110. Levin DC, Fallon JT. Significance of the angiographic morphology of localized coronary stenoses: histopathological correlates. Circulation 1982;66:316–20.

111. Ambrose JA, Winters SL, Stern A, et al. Angiographic morphology and the pathogenesis of unstable angina pectoris. J Am Coll Cardiol 1985;5: 609–16.

112. Sherman CT, Litvak F, Grundfest W, et al. Coronary angioscopy in patients with unstable angina. N Engl J Med 1986;315:913–9.

113. Davies MJ, Thomas AC. Plaque fissuring—the cause of acute myocardial infarction, sudden ischaemic death, and crescendo angina. Br Heart J 1985;53:363–73.

114. Falk E. Unstable angina with fatal outcome, dynamic coronary thrombosis leading to infarction and/or sudden death: autopsy evidence of recurrent mural thrombosis with peripheral embolization culminating in total vascular occlusion. Circulation 1985;71:699–708.

115. Ludmer PL, Selwyn AP, Shook TL, et al. Paradoxical vasoconstriction induced by acetylcholine in atherosclerotic coronary arteries. N Engl J Med 1986;315:1046–51.

116. Theroux P, Ouimet H, McCans J, et al. Aspirin, heparin, or both to treat acute unstable angina. N Engl J Med 1988;319:1105–11.

117. Wallentin L. ASA 75 mg and/or heparin after an episode of unstable coronary artery disease—risk for myocardial infarction and death in a randomized placebo-controlled study (abstr). Circulation 1989;80(suppl II):II-419.

118. Telford AM, Wilson C. Trial of heparin versus atenolol in prevention of myocardial infarction in intermediate coronary syndrome. Lancet 1981; 1:1225–8.

119. Ambrose JA, Hjemdahl-Monsen CE, Borrico S, Gorlin R, Fuster V. Angiographic demonstration of a common link between unstable angina pectoris and non-Q wave myocardial infarction. Am J Cardiol 1988;61: 244–7.

120. Gibson RS, Beller GA, Gheorghiade M, et al. The prevalence and clinical significance of residual myocardial ischemia 2 weeks after uncomplicated non-Q wave infarction: a prospective natural history study. Circulation 1986;73:1186–98.

121. Timmis AD, Griffin B, Crick JCP, Nelson DJ, Sowton E. The effects of early coronary patency on the evolution of myocardial infarction: a prospective arteriographic study. Br Heart J 1987;58:345–51.

122. DeWood M, Stifter WF, Simpson CS, et al. Coronary arteriographic findings soon after non-Q-wave myocardial infarction. N Engl J Med 1986;315:417–23.

123. Freifeld AG, Shuster EH, Bulkley BH. Nontransmural versus transmural myocardial infarction: a morphologic study. Am J Med 1983;75:423–32.

124. Brown BG, Gallery CA, Badger RS, et al. Incomplete lysis of thrombus in the moderate underlying atherosclerotic lesion during intracoronary infusion of streptokinase for acute myocardial infarction: quantitative angiographic observations. Circulation 1986;73:653–61.

125. Ambrose JA, Tannenbaum MA, Alexopoulos D, et al. Angiographic progression of coronary artery disease and the development of myocardial infarction. J Am Coll Cardiol 1988;12:56–62.

126. Little WC, Constantinescu M, Applegate RJ, et al. Can coronary arteriography predict the site of a subsequent myocardial infarction in patients with mild-to-moderate coronary artery disease? Circulation 1988;78:1157–66.

127. Webster MWI, Chesebro JH, Smith HC, et al. Myocardial infarction and coronary artery occlusion: a prospective 5-year angiographic study (abstr). J Am Coll Cardiol 1990;15(suppl A):218A.

128. Meade TW, Brozovic M, Chakrabarti RR, et al. Haemostatic function and ischemic heart disease: principal results of the Northwick Park Heart Study. Lancet 1986;2:533–7.

129. Francis RB, Kawanishi D, Baruch T, Mahrer P, Rahimtoola S, Feinstein DI. Impaired fibrinolysis in coronary artery disease. Am Heart J 1988;115:776–80.

130. Report of the Working Party on Anticoagulation Therapy in Coronary Thrombosis to the Medical Research Council. Assessment of short-term anticoagulation administration after cardiac infarction. Br Med J 1969; 1:335–42.

131. Drapkin A, Merskey C. Anticoagulation therapy after acute myocardial infarction: relation of therapeutic benefit to patient's age, sex and severity of infarction. JAMA 1972;222:541–8.

132. Veterans Administration Hospital Investigators. Anticoagulants in acute myocardial infarction: results of a cooperative clinical trial. JAMA 1973;225:724–9.

133. Turpie AGG, Robinson JG, Doyle DJ, et al. Comparison of high-dose with low-dose subcutaneous heparin to prevent left ventricular mural thrombosis in patients with acute transmural anterior myocardial infarction. N Engl J Med 1989;320:352–7.

134. The SCATI (Studio sulla Calciparina nell'Angina e nella Trombosi Ventricolare nell'Infarto) Group. Randomised controlled trial of subcutaneous calcium-heparin in acute myocardial infarction. Lancet 1989;2: 182–6.

135. Chalmers TC, Matta RJ, Smith H, Kunzler A-M. Evidence favoring the use of anticoagulants in the hospital phase of acute myocardial infarction. N Engl J Med 1977;297:1091–6.

136. Bleich SD, Nichols T, Schumacher R, et al. The role of heparin following coronary thrombolysis with tissue plasminogen activator (abstr). Circulation 1989;80(suppl II):II-113.

137. Hsia J, Hamilton WP, Kleiman N, Roberts R, Chaitman BR, Ross AM. A comparison between heparin and low-dose aspirin as adjunctive therapy with tissue plasminogen activator for acute myocardial infarction. N Engl J Med 1990;323:1433–1437.

138. Elwood PC, Cochrane AL, Burr ML, et al. A randomized controlled trial of acetylsalicylic acid in the secondary prevention of mortality from myocardial infarction. Br Med J 1974;1:436–40.

139. Coronary Drug Project Group. Aspirin in coronary heart disease. J Chronic Dis 1976;29:625–42.

140. Breddin K, Loew D, Lechner K, Oberla K, Walter E. The German-Austrian Aspirin Trial: a comparison of acetylsalicylic acid, placebo and phenprocoumon in secondary prevention of myocardial infarction. Circulation 1980;62(suppl V)V-63–72.

141. Elwood PC, Sweetnam PM. Aspirin and secondary mortality after myocardial infarction. Lancet 1979;2:1313–5.

142. Aspirin Myocardial Infarction Study Research Group. A randomized, controlled trial of aspirin in persons recovered from myocardial infarction. JAMA 1980;243:661–9.

143. The Anturane Reinfarction Trial Research Group. Sulfinpyrazone in the prevention of sudden death after myocardial infarction. N Engl J Med 1980;302:250–6.

144. Klimt CR, Knatterud GL, Stamler J, Meier P and the Persantine-Aspirin Reinfarction Study Research Group. Part II: secondary coronary prevention with persantine and aspirin. J Am Coll Cardiol 1986;7:251–69.

145. Antiplatelet Trialists' Collaboration. Secondary prevention of vascular disease by prolonged antiplatelet treatment. Br Med J 1988;296:320–31.

146. Second Report of the Working Party on Anticoagulant Therapy in Coronary Thrombosis to the Medical Research Council. An assessment of long-term anticoagulant administration after cardiac infarction. Br Med J 1964;2:837–43.

147. Ebert RV, Borden CW, Hipp HR, et al. Long-term anticoagulant therapy after myocardial infarction: final report of the Veterans Administration Cooperative Study. JAMA 1969;207:2263–7.

148. Report of the Sixty Plus Reinfarction Study Research Group. A double-blind trial to assess long-term oral anticoagulant therapy in elderly patients after myocardial infarction. Lancet 1980;2:989–93.

149. Smith P, Arnesen H, Holme I. The effect of warfarin on mortality and reinfarction after myocardial infarction. N Engl J Med 1990;323:147–152.

150. The E.P.S.I.M. Research Group. A controlled comparison of aspirin and oral anticoagulants in prevention of death after myocardial infarction. N Engl J Med 1982;307:701–8.

151. Fuster V, Chesebro JH. Role of platelets and platelet inhibitors in aortocoronary artery vein-graft disease. Circulation 1986;2:227–32.

152. Bulkley BH, Hutchins GM. Accelerated "atherosclerosis": a morphologic study of 97 saphenous vein coronary artery bypass grafts. Circulation 1977;55:163–9.

153. Unni KK, Kottke BA, Titus JL, Frye RL, Wallace RB, Brown AL. Pathologic changes in aortocoronary saphenous vein grafts. Am J Cardiol 1974;34:526–32.

154. Josa M, Lie JT, Bianco RL, Kaye MP. Reduction of thrombosis in canine coronary bypass vein grafts with dipyridamole and aspirin. Am J Cardiol 1981;47:1248–54.

155. Lorenz RL, Weber M, Kotzur J, et al. Improved aortocoronary bypass patency by low-dose aspirin (100 mg/daily): effects on platelet aggregation and thromboxane formation. Lancet 1984;1:1262–4.

156. Rajah SM, Salter MCP, Donaldson DR, et al. Acetylsalicylic acid and dipyridamole improve the early patency of aorta-coronary bypass grafts: a double-blind, placebo-controlled, randomized trial. J Thorac Cardiovasc Surg 1985;89:373–7.

157. Mayer JE, Lindsay WG, Castaneda W, Nicoloff DM. Influence of aspirin and dipyridamole on patency of coronary artery bypass grafts. Ann Thorac Surg 1981;31:204–10.

158. Brooks N, Wright J, Sturridge M, et al. Randomised placebo controlled trial of aspirin and dipyridamole in the prevention of coronary vein graft occlusion. Br Heart J 1985;53:201–7.

159. McEnany MT, Salzman EW, Mundth ED, et al. The effect of antithrombotic therapy on patency rates of saphenous vein coronary artery bypass graft. J Thorac Cardiovasc Surg 1982;83:81–9.

160. Pantely GA, Goodnight SH, Rahimtoola SH, et al. Failure of antiplatelet and anticoagulant therapy to improve patency of grafts after coronary-artery bypass: a controlled randomized study. N Engl J Med 1979;301:962–6.

161. Sharma GVRK, Khuri SF, Josa M, Folland ED, Parisi AF. The effect of antiplatelet therapy on saphenous vein coronary artery bypass graft patency. Circulation 1983;68(suppl II):II-218–21.

162. Fuster V, Dewanjee MK, Kaye MP, Josa M, Metke MD, Chesebro JH. Noninvasive radioisotopic technique for detection of platelet deposition in coronary artery bypass grafts in dogs and its reduction with platelet inhibitors. Circulation 1979;60:1508–12.

163. Sethi GK, Copeland JG, Goldman S, Mortiz T, Zadina K, Henderson WG. Implications of preoperative administration of aspirin in patients undergoing coronary artery bypass grafting. J Am Coll Cardiol 1990;15:15–20.

164. Dewanjee MK, Tago M, Josa M, Fuster V, Kaye MP. Quantification of platelet retention in aortocoronary femoral vein bypass graft in dogs treated with dipyridamole and aspirin. Circulation 1984;69:350–6.

165. Lie JT, Lawrie GM, Morris GC. Aortocoronary bypass saphenous vein graft atherosclerosis. Am J Cardiol 1977;40:906–14.

166. Solymoss BC, Nadeau P, Millette D, Campeau L. Late thrombosis of saphenous vein coronary bypass grafts related to risk factors. Circulation 1988;78(suppl I):I-140–3.

167. Goldman S, Copeland JG, Moritz T, et al. Saphenous vein graft patency 1 year after coronary artery bypass surgery and effects of antiplatelet therapy: results of a Veterans Administration cooperative study. Circulation 1989;80:1190–7.

168. Pfisterer M, Burkart F, Jockers G, et al. Trial of low-dose aspirin plus anticoagulants for prevention of aortocoronary vein graft occlusion. Lancet 1989;2:1–7.

169. Blankenhorn DH, Nessim SA, Johnson RL, Sanmarco ME, Azen SP, Casinh-Hemphill L. Beneficial effect of combined colestipol-niacin therapy on coronary atherosclerosis and coronary venous bypass grafts. JAMA 1987;257:3233–40.

170. Faxon DP, Weber VJ, Haudenschild C, Gottsman SB, McGovern WA, Ryan TJ. Acute effects of transluminal angioplasty in three experimental models of atherosclerosis. Arteriosclerosis 1982;2:125–33.

171. Block PC, Myler RK, Stertzer S, Fallon JT. Morphology after transluminal angioplasty in human beings. N Engl J Med 1981;305:382–5.

172. Steele PM, Chesebro JH, Stanson AW, et al. Balloon angioplasty: natural history of the pathophysiological response to injury in a pig model. Circ Res 1985;57:105–12.

173. Waller BF. "Crackers, breakers, stretchers, drillers, scrapers, shavers, burners, welders and melters"—the future treatment of atherosclerotic coronary artery disease? A clinical-morphologic assessment. J Am Coll Cardiol 1989;13:969–87.

174. Schwartz L, Bourassa MG, Lesperance J, et al. Aspirin and dipyridamole in the prevention of restenosis after percutaneous transluminal coronary angioplasty. N Engl J Med 1988;318:1714–9.

175. Chesebro JH, Webster MWI, Reeder GS, et al. Coronary angioplasty:

176. antiplatelet therapy reduces acute complications but not restenosis (abstr). Circulation 1989;80(suppl II):II-64.

176. Barnathan ES, Schwartz JS, Taylor L, et al. Aspirin and dipyridamole in the prevention of acute coronary thrombosis complicating coronary angioplasty. Circulation 1987;76:125–34.

177. Kent KM, Ewels CJ, Kehoe MK, Lavelle JP, Krucoff MV. Effect of aspirin on complications during transluminal coronary angioplasty (abstr). J Am Coll Cardiol 1988;11(suppl A):132A.

178. Lembo JN, Black AJ, Roubin GS, et al. Effect of pretreatment with aspirin versus aspirin plus dipyridamole on frequency and type of acute complications of percutaneous transluminal coronary angioplasty. Am J Cardiol 1990;65:422–6.

179. Heras M, Chesebro JH, Penny WJ, et al. Importance of adequate heparin dosage in arterial angioplasty in a porcine model. Circulation 1988;78:654–60.

180. Lukas Laskey MA, Deutsch E, Hirshfeld JW, Kussmaul WG, Barnathan E, Laskey WK. Influence of heparin therapy on percutaneous transluminal coronary angioplasty outcome in patients with coronary artery thrombus. Am J Cardiol 1990;65:179–82.

181. Pow TK, Varricchione TR, Jacobs AK, et al. Does pretreatment with heparin prevent abrupt closure following PTCA? (abstr). J Am Coll Cardiol 1988;11(suppl A):238A.

182. Douglas JS, Lutz JF, Clements SD, et al. Therapy of large intracoronary thrombi in candidates for percutaneous transluminal coronary angioplasty (abstr). J Am Coll Cardiol 1988;11(suppl A):238A.

183. Hettleman BD, Aplin RL, Sullivan PR, Lemal H, O'Connor GT. Three days of heparin pretreatment reduces major complications of coronary angioplasty in patients with unstable angina (abstr). J Am Coll Cardiol 1990;15(suppl A):154A.

184. Kent KM. Restenosis after percutaneous transluminal coronary angioplasty. Am J Cardiol 1988;61(suppl G): 67G–70G.

185. McBride W, Lange RA, Hillis LD. Restenosis after successful coronary angioplasty: pathophysiology and prevention. N Engl J Med 1988;318:1734–7.

186. Block PC. Percutaneous transluminal coronary angioplasty: role in the treatment of coronary artery disease. Circulation 1985;72(suppl V):V-161–5.

187. Leimgruber PP, Roubin GS, Hollman J, et al. Restenosis after successful coronary angioplasty in patients with single-vessel disease. Circulation 1986;73:710–7.

188. Roubin GS, King SB, Douglas JS. Restenosis after percutaneous transluminal coronary angioplasty: the Emory University Hospital experience. Am J Cardiol 1987;60(suppl B):39B–43B.

189. Guiteras Val P, Bourassa MG, David PR, et al. Restenosis after successful percutaneous transluminal coronary angioplasty: the Montreal Heart Institute experience. Am J Cardiol 1987;60(suppl B):50B–5B.

190. Lam JTY, Chesebro JH, Steele PM, et al. Deep arterial injury during experimental angioplasty: relations to a positive indium-III-labelled platelet scintigram, quantitative platelet deposition and mural thrombosis. J Am Coll Cardiol 1986;8:1380–6.

191. Lam JYT, Chesebro JH, Steele PM, Badimon L, Fuster V. Is vasospasm related to platelet deposition? Relationship in a porcine preparation of arterial injury in vivo. Circulation 1987;75:242–8.

192. Cragg A, Einzig S, Castaneda-Zuniga W, et al. Vessel wall arachidonate metabolism after angioplasty: possible mediators of postangioplasty vasospasm. Am J Cardiol 1983;51:1441–5.

193. White CW, Knudson M, Schmidt D, et al. Neither ticlopidine nor aspirin-dipyridamole prevents restenosis post PTCA: results from a randomized placebo-controlled multicenter trial (abstr). Circulation 1987;76(suppl IV):IV-213.

194. Ellis SG, Roubin GS, Wilentz J, Douglas JS, King SB. Effect of 18- to 24-hour heparin administration for prevention of restenosis after uncomplicated coronary angioplasty. Am Heart J 1989;117:777–82.

195. Thornton MA, Gruentzig AR, Hollman J, King SB, Douglas JS. Coumadin and aspirin in the prevention of recurrence after transluminal coronary angioplasty: a randomized study. Circulation 1984;69:721–7.

196. Urban P, Buller N, Fox K, Shapiro L, Bayliss J, Rickards. Lack of effect of warfarin on the restenosis rate or on clinical outcome after balloon coronary angioplasty. Br Heart J 1988;60:485–8.

197. Dehmer GJ, Popma JJ, van den Berg EK, et al. Reduction in the rate of early restenosis after coronary angioplasty by a diet supplemented with n-3 fatty acids. N Engl J Med 1988;319:733–40.

198. Milner MR, Gallino RA, Leffingwell A, et al. Usefulness of fish oil supplements in preventing clinical evidence of restenosis after percutaneous transluminal coronary angioplasty. Am J Cardiol 1989;64:294–9.

199. Slack JD, Pinkerton CA, Vantaseel J, et al. Can oral fish oil supplement minimize re-stenosis after percutaneous transluminal coronary angioplasty? (abstr). J Am Coll Cardiol 1987;9(suppl A):64A.

200. Grigg LE, Kay TWH, Valentine PA, et al. Determinants of restenosis and lack of effect of dietary supplementation with eicosapentaenoic acid on the incidence of coronary restenosis after angioplasty. J Am Coll Cardiol 1989;13:665–72.

201. Reis GJ, Boucher TM, Sipperly ME, et al. Randomised trial of fish oil for prevention of restenosis after coronary angioplasty. Lancet 1989;2:177–81.

202. Rose TE, Beauchamp BG. Short term, high dose steroid treatment to prevent restenosis in PTCA (abstr). Circulation 1987;76(suppl IV):IV-371.

203. Pepine CJ, Hirshfeld JW, Macdonald RG, et al. A controlled trial of corticosteroids to prevent restenosis after coronary angioplasty. Circulation 1990;81:1753–1761.

204. Knudtson ML, Flintoft VF, Roth DL, Hansen JL, Duff HJ. Effect of short-term prostacyclin administration on restenosis after percutaneous transluminal coronary angioplasty. J Am Coll Cardiol 1990;15:691–7.

205. Faxon DP, Sanborn TA, Haudenschild CC, et al. Effect of nifedipine on restenosis following experimental angioplasty (abstr). Circulation 1984;70(suppl II):II-175.

206. Corcos T, David PR, Val PG, et al. Failure of diltiazem to prevent restenosis after PTCA. Am Heart J 1985;109:926–31.

207. Fuster V, Pumphrey CW, McGoon MD, Chesebro JH, Pluth JR, McGoon DC. Systemic thromboembolism in mitral and aortic Starr-Edwards prostheses: a 10-19 year follow-up. Circulation 1982;66(suppl I):I-157–61.

208. Edmunds LH. Thrombotic and bleeding complications of prosthetic heart valves. Ann Thorac Surg 1987;44:430–45.

209. Chaux A, Czer LSC, Matloff JM, et al. The St. Jude bileaflet valve prosthesis: a 5 year experience. J Thorac Cardiovasc Surg 1984;88:706–17.

210. Myers ML, Lawrie GM, Crawford ES, et al. The St. Jude valve prosthesis: analysis of the clinical results in 815 implants and the need for systemic anticoagulation. J Am Coll Cardiol 1989;13:57–62.

211. Mok CK, Boey J, Wang R, et al. Warfarin versus dipyridamole-aspirin and pentoxifylline-aspirin for the prevention of prosthetic heart valve thromboembolism: a prospective randomized clinical trial. Circulation 1985;72:1059–63.

212. Altman R, Boullon F, Rouvier J, et al. Aspirin and prophylaxis of thromboembolic complications in patients with substitute heart valves. J Thorac Cardiovasc Surg 1976;72:127–9.

213. Dale J, Myhre E, Storstein O, et al. Prevention of arterial thromboembolism with acetylsalicyclic acid: a controlled clinical study in patients with aortic ball valves. Am Heart J 1977;94:101–11.

214. Nunez L, Gil Aguado M, Larrea JL, et al. Prevention of thromboembolism using aspirin after mitral valve replacement with porcine bioprosthesis. Ann Thorac Surg 1984;37:84–7.

215. Sherman DG, Dyken ML, Fisher M, Harrison MJG, Hart RG. Antithrombotic therapy in cerebrovascular disorders. Chest 1989;95(suppl): 140S–55S.

216. A Swedish Cooperative Study. High dose acetylsalicylic acid after cerebral infarction. Stroke 1987;18:325–34.

217. The ESPS Group. The European Stroke Prevention Study: principal end-points. Lancet 1987;2:1351–4.

218. Fields WS, Lemak NA, Frankowski RF, Hardy RJ. Controlled trial of aspirin in cerebral ischemia. Stroke 1977;8:301–16.

219. Fields WS, Lemark NA, Frankowski RF, Hardy RJ. Controlled trial of aspirin in cerebral ischemia: part II. Surgical group. Stroke 1978;9:309–18.

220. Ruether R, Dorndorf W. Aspirin in patients with cerebral ischemia and normal angiograms or non-surgical lesions: the results of a double-blind trial. In: Breddin K, Dorndorf W, Loew D, Marx R, eds. Acetylsalicylic Acid in Cerebral Ischemia and Coronary Heart Disease. Stuttgart: Schattauer Verlag, 1978;97–106.

221. Sorensen PS, Pedersen H, Marquardsen J, et al. Acetylsalicylic acid in the prevention of stroke in patients with reversible cerebral ischemic attacks: a Danish cooperative study. Stroke 1983;14:15–22.

222. Kopecky SL, Gersh BJ, McGoon MD, et al. The natural history of lone atrial fibrillation: a population-based study over three decades. N Engl J Med 1987;317:669–74.

223. Petersen P, Godtfredsen J, Boysen G, Andersen ED, Andersen B. Placebo-controlled, randomised trial of warfarin and aspirin for prevention of thromboembolic complications in chronic atrial fibrillation: the Copenhagen AFASAK Study. Lancet 1989;1:175–9.

224. Preliminary report of the Stroke Prevention in Atrial Fibrillation Study. N Engl J Med 1990;322:863–8.

224a. The Boston Area Anticoagulation Trial for Atrial Fibrillation Investigators. The effect of low-dose warfarin on the risk of stroke in patients with nonrheumatic atrial fibrillation. N Engl J Med 1990;323:1505–1511.

225. Hess H, Mietaschk A, Deichsel G. Drug-induced inhibition of platelet function delays progression of peripheral occlusive arterial disease: a prospective double-blind arteriographically controlled trial. Lancet 1985;1:415–21.

226. Katsumura T, Mishima Y, Kamiya K, Sakaguchi S, Tanabe T, Sakuma A. Therapeutic effect of ticlopidine, a new inhibitor of platelet aggregation on chronic arterial occlusive diseases: a double-blind study versus placebo. Angiology 1982;33:357–67.

227. Clagett GP, Genton E, Salzman EW. Antithrombotic therapy in peripheral vascular disease. Chest 1989;95(suppl):128S–39S.

228. Harter HR, Burch JW, Marjerus PW, et al. Prevention of thrombosis in patients on hemodialysis by low-dose aspirin. N Engl J Med 1979;301:577–9.

229. Barnett HJM, Jones MW, Boughner DR, Kostuk WJ. Cerebral ischemic events associated with prolapsing mitral valve. Arch Neurol 1976;33:777–82.

230. Nishimura RA, McGoon MD, Shub C, Miller FA, Ilstrup DM, Tajik AJ. Echocardiographically documented mitral valve prolapse: long-term follow-up of 237 patients. N Engl J Med 1985;313:1305–9.

CHAPTER 12

After Coronary Thrombolysis and Reperfusion, What Next?

NILS U. BANG, MD, OLAF G. WILHELM, MD, MICHAEL D. CLAYMAN, MD

Present Status of Thrombolytic Therapy

After 30 years of clinical trials of thrombolysis for acute myocardial infarction (1,2), much accelerated over the last decade (3), the beneficial effects of such therapy are now firmly established. The majority of patients given recombinant tissue-type plasminogen activator (rt-PA) will exhibit reperfusion of the infarct-related artery. Streptokinase also produces reperfusion, particularly when given very early after the acute occlusion. Streptokinase and rt-PA have both been shown to reduce infarct size, improve myocardial performance and reduce at least the immediate and probably the late mortality rates in myocardial infarction. However, serious problems with thrombolytic therapy in acute myocardial infarction remain. First, the incidence of reperfusion, which was 100% in early dog experiments (4), varies between 60% and 80% in patients. Second, the interval between the start of treatment and coronary reperfusion can be shortened. Third, the incidence of reocclusion after successful reperfusion is too high. Finally, the incidence of bleeding complications with rt-PA is far higher than originally anticipated and, in fact, is no different from that with the older agents, streptokinase and urokinase.

Because of these shortcomings, improved therapies are being vigorously investigated. Two areas are being intensively explored: the development of better thrombolytic agents of higher efficiency and less bleeding liability than rt-PA, and the development of adjunctive therapy with agents superior to those currently available. In theory, adjunctive pharmacotherapy could encompass anticoagulants, antiplatelet agents, beta-adrenergic blockers, calcium channel blockers, vasodilators, antiarrhythmic drugs, free radical scavengers and other agents capable of suppressing possible reperfusion injury.

In this review, we have elected to focus on compounds that have an impact on the fibrinolytic enzyme system and the clotting cascade or platelet function, or both, to provide a framework for discussing therapy aimed at enhancing thrombolysis and maintaining patency once reperfusion has occurred. This does not imply that other pharmacologic approaches are of less interest but that, in the stricter sense, drugs used as an adjunct to thrombolysis should complement that process and preclude clot recurrence. In the following discussion, we will summarize clinical data on currently available thrombolytic agents, anticoagulants and antiplatelet agents and their advantages and limitations. We will cover the theoretical reasons why current regimens are suboptimal, and summarize data on experimental agents that are appealing from a conceptual standpoint. Although several agents and regimens look promising, it should be emphasized that the available data are largely from preclinical pharmacology and in only a few instances have these new approaches been tested in preliminary clinical experiments.

What Is the Current Data Base?

Time to Reperfusion

Reperfusion rates. The Thrombolysis in Myocardial Infarction (TIMI) group (5) demonstrated that when predominantly single-chain tissue plasminogen activator was given at its currently approved dose of 100 mg over 3 h (60, 20 and 20 mg/h, with an initial bolus of 6 mg), reperfusion rates of 24% at 30 min, 57% at 60 min and 71% at 90 min were obtained. When the dose was increased to 150 mg, earlier reperfusion was obtained in more patients (42% at 30 min, 68% at 60 min and 76% at 90 min). Interestingly, the 90 min value was only slightly improved over that obtained with the 100 mg dose. Unfortunately, the incidence of intracranial hemorrhage at this high dose was subsequently observed in TIMI-2 (6) to be 1.6%, more than twice that at the 100 mg dose. This resulted in the higher dose being abandoned. The TIMI-1 trial (7) also demonstrated that streptokinase given in the currently approved dose of 1.5 million U over 1 h resulted in substantially lower reperfusion rates compared with rt-PA at 30 min (8%), 60 min (23%) and 90 min (31%). However, in TIMI-1, the interval between the onset of symptoms and the start of treatment averaged 4.7 h. Whereas such delays in therapy do not affect reperfusion rates with rt-PA, they profoundly reduce the efficacy of streptokinase. Thus, in TIMI-1, the 90 min reperfusion rate for patients treated with streptokinase within 4 h of the onset of symptoms was twice that for patients treated at >4 h after symptom onset (7,8).

It is clear that faster reperfusion of the infarct-related artery is beneficial. Both the empiric observation that thrombolytic therapy administered within the 1st h of symptom onset has marked survival advantages over later therapy (9) and the theoretical concerns that 15% of myocardium at risk dies for every 30 min of persistent occlusion (10) strongly support the notion that faster reperfusion improves outcome.

Role of antithrombotic and antiplatelet therapy. The possibility that adjunctive anticoagulant or antiplatelet therapy may effect faster infarct-related artery thrombolysis is consistent with the hypothesis that coronary thrombolysis is accompanied by procoagulant events (that is, that accretion of new platelets and fibrin onto the coronary thrombus takes place as thrombolysis proceeds). Similarly, the observation that coronary thrombolysis is attended by intermittent patency in some patients (11) suggests a possible human equivalent to cyclic flow variations in animal models (12), which is a platelet-dependent phenomenon.

Unfortunately, current data that address the impact of anticoagulation or antiplatelet therapy on time to reperfusion are limited and not illuminating. To obtain such data, sequential angiographic data before and during thrombolytic and thrombolytic adjunctive therapy are needed and, in many quarters, it is now considered unacceptable to impose a delay of 60 min to prepare the patient for angiography before definitive therapy for acute myocardial infarction is provided.

Noninvasive diagnosis of reperfusion. The most obvious solution to this investigative dilemma is to develop noninvasive means of diagnosing reperfusion. Although the commonly used bedside markers of reperfusion have recently been shown (13) to be relatively specific, they are not sensitive or useful for making pronouncements regarding the reperfusion status of individual patients or groups of patients (14). The development of noninvasive markers for reperfusion is particularly important because early cardiac catheterization and angioplasty appear to offer no significant advantages over conservative management in patients in whom reperfusion has been achieved (15–18). However, without the 90 min angiogram, it may be difficult to identify patients who are left with an occluded vessel at that time and who might be candidates for salvage angioplasty (18–20) or bypass surgery.

Reperfusion/Patency Rate

Patency rates. Patency is typically defined as TIMI grade 2 or 3 patency of the infarct-related artery on a 90 min angiogram. Unless one knows that the vessel was occluded before the administration of the thrombolytic agent, the patency rate (not the reperfusion rate) is the variable examined. With rt-PA, patency rates have ranged from 61% to 79% (15,17,21–25); with intravenous streptokinase, a 90 min patency rate of 55% has been documented (24). Regardless of the intravenous thrombolytic regimen used, the infarct-related coronary artery remains occluded in at ≥20% of patients on the 90 min angiogram (although reperfusion rates of 85% to 90% have been reported [26,27] with the use of intracoronary thrombolytic regimens). The exact reasons for this residual of lesions resistant to therapy are not known. Postulated mechanisms include bleeding into the atheromatous plaque with rapid enlargement of the lesion, spasm at the site of the plaque with little contribution to occlusion by clot and the occurrence of very platelet-rich thrombi, which have recently been shown (28) experimentally to be highly resistant to lysis by rt-PA.

Influence of heparin and aspirin. Only very limited data focus on the influence of available anticoagulant and antiplatelet agents, heparin and aspirin on time to reperfusion and patency rates. Available data (23,25) indicate that heparin plays no role in either the time to reperfusion or the initial patency rate associated with rt-PA therapy. The recently published Thrombolysis and Angioplasty in Myocardial Infarction (TAMI-3) study (23) examined the influence of heparin on the 90 min patency rate in a randomized prospective trial of patients given rt-PA for acute myocardial infarction. Patients allocated to heparin treatment received a 10,000 unit bolus of heparin concurrent with rt-PA administration, and those assigned to the no heparin arm did not receive heparin until after a 90 min angiogram was performed. There was no significant difference in patency rates (73% in the no heparin and 79% in the heparin group).

Similar data are not available for adjunctive aspirin therapy. The majority of rt-PA studies include aspirin as a matter of routine in treated as well as control patients and, thus, it is not possible to ascertain whether aspirin influences the time to or rate of reperfusion. The only data suggesting that aspirin may favorably affect outcome come from the Second International Study of Infarct Survival (ISIS-2), in which death was the end point, as discussed later.

Reocclusion

Clinical documentation. Reocclusion of the infarct-related artery after successful thrombolysis can be documented either angiographically or clinically. In angiographic studies, repeat cardiac catheterization is typically performed 24 h to several days after thrombolytic administration. Because of the "time slice" nature of these observations and because spontaneous reperfusion is common (>75% of placebo-treated patients in the recent European Cooperative Study Group trial (29) had a patent index vessel at follow-up angiography 10 to 22 days after admission), it is impossible to know if a vessel may have at least transiently reoccluded and then recanalized. Thus, it is likely that angiographic reocclusion rates may underestimate the real incidence of this phenomenon.

Clinically, reocclusion may be manifested by recurrent angina and, in particular, by reinfarction in the same myocardial location as that observed at the initial presentation. Clinical reocclusion rates are less than angiographically documented reocclusion rates because cases of reocclusion are asymptomatic.

Angiographic reocclusion rates for rt-PA therapy in recent publications (7,15,23,25) have been in the 5% to 24% range. In TIMI-1 (30), reocclusion after streptokinase therapy occurred in 4 (14%) of 29 patients with reperfusion. Pooled data from 10 studies (as discussed in [25]) suggest a reocclusion rate after intracoronary streptokinase of 17%.

Reinfarction rates after thrombolytic therapy have been documented in numerous recent studies. For patients receiving rt-PA, this rate has ranged from 2.4% to 13% (7,16–18,21–25,29,31–33) and for those receiving streptokinase 2.8% to 12% (7,9,24,34–38).

Role of heparin and aspirin. The role of in-hospital heparinization in the prevention of reocclusion and reinfarction is not clear. In the TAMI-3 trial (23), the use of heparin concomitantly with rt-PA as opposed to rt-PA alone as the initial therapy resulted in no improvement in reocclusion rate, reinfarction rate, emergency coronary bypass surgery and recurrent ischemic events during hospitalization. Another study (39) indicated that delaying heparinization for 12 h after beginning thrombolytic therapy had no adverse effect on reinfarction or reocclusion rates. With a 12 h heparin delay, however, bleeding complications were significantly less common and less severe. Data from the Gruppo Italiano per lo Studio della Streptochinasi Nell'Infarto (GISSI) trial (9), which examined the effects of streptokinase versus placebo on mortality rates, are also of some interest. Concomitant medication in that trial was left to the discretion of the investigators, and approximately 80% of patients did not receive therapeutic anticoagulation with heparin. Reinfarction rates in the GISSI trial were no different between patient groups that did and did not receive heparin therapy. Not until the completion of two trials that randomize patients to heparin or no heparin for the duration of hospitalization (GISSI-2 and ISIS-3) will the role of heparin in adjunctive therapy to thrombolysis be determined.

With respect to the role of aspirin in preventing reocclusion, only the large ISIS-2 trial (34) provides data of interest. In this study, patients receiving streptokinase plus aspirin had a substantially lower chance of experiencing reinfarction (1.8%) than that of patients who received streptokinase but no aspirin (2.9%).

Bleeding Complications

Incidence. The incidence of bleeding complications in selected studies (7) comparing rt-PA and streptokinase in addition to three prospective trials focusing on rt-PA with or without other treatment modalities (angioplasty, urokinase or heparin in TAMI-1 [15], TAMI-2 [21] and TAMI-3 [23], respectively) are enumerated in Table 12.1. As mentioned, the incidence of bleeding complications with the "fibrin-specific" rt-PA was surprisingly high. In fact, in all studies cited, rt-PA caused bleeding complications at a rate that was not statistically different from that caused by streptokinase. The incidence of major bleeding for rt-PA ranged from 6.3% to 21% in the six studies listed in Table 12.1 and the incidence of all bleeding complications, major and minor, ranged from 30% to 45%. All the studies cited involved invasive procedures and a large proportion of the bleeding complications encountered with either rt-PA or streptokinase occurred at arterial and venous puncture sites. Bleeding from puncture sites is extremely common for any throm-

bolytic agent for reasons to be discussed elsewhere in this review.

Role of heparin or aspirin. It is not clear from the reports cited (7,15,21–23,29) whether the concomitant administration of heparin or aspirin, or both, significantly contributed to bleeding complications. The exception is TAMI-3, in which no difference in the incidence of major bleeding complications was seen between the groups receiving early heparin in combination with rt-PA and the group receiving rt-PA alone.

Mortality

Although thrombolytic therapy clearly improves survival after acute myocardial infarction (9,31,34,40), the contribution of heparin to this process is unknown. Similarly limited data are available for aspirin. In ISIS-2, >17,000 patients with acute myocardial infarction were randomized to placebo, streptokinase, aspirin and aspirin plus placebo therapies. The 5 week vascular mortality rate was reduced by 21% in those taking aspirin compared with those taking placebo. Streptokinase alone reduced the mortality rate by 23% relative to placebo, and when aspirin was given with streptokinase, the mortality rate was reduced by 42% compared with placebo.

In conclusion, available data limit an objective assessment of anticoagulant and antiplatelet therapy as adjuncts to thrombolysis. TAMI-3 demonstrated that heparin probably does not favorably influence the acute patency rate, and ISIS-2 documented that aspirin has a significant beneficial effect on reinfarction and mortality rates when used alone or in conjunction with streptokinase.

Suggested Approaches Toward Improving Results of Therapy in Coronary Thrombolysis

Newer thrombolytic and anticoagulant agents. The following approaches toward reducing the time to reperfusion, reducing the reocclusion rate and reducing bleeding complications are being worked on in many laboratories. First, it has been suggested that simply changing the dose schedule (that is, giving a high dose of rt-PA over 90 min followed by a lower dose over an additional 4 to 6 h) may result in a reduction in reocclusion rates. Second, combination therapy (for example, rt-PA and urokinase or rt-PA and another novel thrombolytic agent, single-chain urokinase [scu-PA]) have been considered. Alternative plasminogen activators have also been suggested. One such novel activator is a chemically modified streptokinase-plasminogen complex, referred to as anisoylated streptokinase-plasminogen activator complex (APSAC). This preparation has already undergone extensive clinical testing. Many additional plasminogen activators have been produced through recombinant DNA (deoxyribonucleic acid) technology and are in various stages

Table 12.1. Incidence of Bleeding Complications in Reported Studies

Study (reference)	Treatment	No. of Patients	Incidence of Bleeding		
			Major (%)	Minor (%)	Stroke (%)
TIMI-1 (7)	SK + H	147	15.6	15.6	?
	rt-PA + H	143	15.4	17.5	0
ECSG-1 (22)	SK + H + A	65	7.7	2.3	1.5
	rt-PA + H	64	6.3	26.5	0
ECSG-2 (29)	Placebo + H + A	366	2.2	5.2	0
	rt-PA + H + A	355	10.2	29.3	1.7
TAMI-1 (15)	rt-PA* + H (±PCTA)	386	21	24	0.5
TAMI-2 (21)	rt-PA + H + A (±uk)	147	14	20	0.7
TAMI-3 (23)	rt-PA (±H)	175	14	22	1.2

*High dose = 150 mg. A = aspirin; ECSG = European Cooperative Study Group; H = heparin; PTCA = percutaneous transluminal coronary angioplasty; SK = streptokinase; TAMI = Thrombosis and Angioplasty in Myocardial Infarction trial; TIMI = Thrombosis in Myocardial Infarction trial; rt-PA = recombinant tissue type plasminogen activator; UK = urokinase.

of preclinical testing. Finally and importantly, many laboratories are focusing their attention on alternative approaches toward adjunctive therapy, improved novel types of antiplatelet agents as well as novel anticoagulant agents that will be more active than heparin in preventing the growth of arterial thrombi. In the following discussion, each of these approaches will be reviewed.

Prolonged rt-PA administration for the prevention of reocclusion. A relatively small recent clinical trial (41) tested the concept that a maintenance infusion of rt-PA plus heparin would reduce the rate of reocclusion. Sixty-eight patients with acute myocardial infarction all received rt-PA at a dose of 1 mg/kg body weight for 90 min. Coronary angiography at 90 min revealed a patent infarct-related coronary artery in 52 patients (76%). These patients were randomized either to treatment by continuous infusion of heparin alone (27 patients) or to treatment by heparin and a maintenance infusion of rt-PA at a dosage of 0.8 mg/kg over 4 h (25 patients). The approach appeared to work, at least immediately. Heparin plus maintenance rt-PA resulted in a zero incidence of reocclusion; in contrast, five patients (19%) receiving continuous heparin infusion alone exhibited reocclusion immediately. This difference is significant at the $p = 0.05$ level; however, the late reocclusion rates were identical in two patients in each group. Also, the incidence of significant bleeding complications was substantially higher in the heparin plus rt-PA maintenance group as opposed to that in the heparin alone group (49% versus 25%, respectively).

These results were different from those obtained in a similar study by the European Cooperative Study Group (25). In the latter study, 40 mg of rt-PA was given over 1 h, followed by the randomized administration of either heparin alone or a maintenance infusion of 5 mg/h of rt-PA with heparin over 6 h. The overall patency rate at 90 min of infusion was 66%. The maintenance rt-PA level in plasma was 0.08 μg/ml, which is about 1/10 of the level obtained by

0.8 mg/kg of rt-PA over 4 h. The early reocclusion rate (6 to 24 h) was only 7% and was not different between the groups. Thus, the approach of prolonged rt-PA infusion for the prevention of reocclusion needs to be refined, and the dose of rt-PA administered immediately, as well as a continuing infusion dose need to be better established to consistently reduce reocclusion rates while avoiding excessive bleeding complications.

New Agents: Some Theoretical Considerations

A basic understanding of the fibrinolytic enzyme system, the consequences of its activation and certain features of the coagulation system is necessary to understand the rationale for the development of new fibrinolytic agents, new anticoagulant drugs and antiplatelet agents. Certain basic concepts pertaining to the mechanism of action of older agents as opposed to agents under development also need to be introduced.

The fibrinolytic enzyme system. In a recently published review (3), we extensively discussed the biochemistry of the fibrinolytic enzyme system. From this review, the following points need to be reemphasized as pertinent to the present discussion.

1) Plasminogen activators. The physiologic activators are rt-PA, single chain urokinase-type plasminogen activator (scu-PA) and two chain urokinase (tcu-PA) usually referred to as urokinase, a term used in this review. In addition to these physiologic plasminogen activators, the bacterial activator streptokinase is widely used clinically. Recombinant tissue-type plasminogen activator (rt-PA) and scu-PA preferentially activate the fibrinolytic proenzyme plasminogen adsorbed to fibrin; consequently, rt-PA and scu-PA given at moderate doses do not activate plasma plasminogen significantly. The older thrombolytic agents streptokinase and urokinase, in contrast, activate plasminogen adsorbed onto fibrin and circulating plasma plasminogen with equal efficiency. The activation of plasma plasminogen results in temporary hyperplasminemia and a profound multifactorial coagulation defect. Although claimed to be fibrin specific, in some patients, rt-PA and scu-PA produce a serious coagulation defect, although less frequently than that observed with streptokinase and urokinase treatment.

With respect to the fibrin specificity of rt-PA, it should be emphasized that this activator is *fibrin* specific, but not *thrombus* specific. Recombinant tissue-type plasminogen activator does not distinguish between the target thrombus and hemostatic plugs consisting of platelets and fibrin occurring any place in the circulation including arterial and venous puncture sites. Therefore, at best, most fibrin-specific agents we can produce still possess a serious liability of causing bleeding from arterial and venous puncture sites and other potential bleeding sites such as stress ulcers and small blood vessels in the cerebral circulation.

2) Plasminogen activator inhibitors, particularly plasminogen activator inhibitor 1 (PAI-1) (summarized in [3]). Plasminogen activator inhibitor 1 is synthesized in and secreted by endothelial cells and megakaryocytes. It is found in plasma at varying concentrations, exists in platelets at high concentrations and is released during platelet activation. Very large quantities of PAI-1 have recently been demonstrated to be present bound to subendothelial connective tissue. Plasminogen activator inhibitors are found at increased concentrations in patients with venous thromboembolism, in patients after acute myocardial infarction (42) and in patients with conditions predisposing to thromboembolic disease. Plasminogen activator inhibitors rapidly and efficiently inhibit rt-PA, urokinase and PAI-1 in plasma, in platelet-rich fibrin thrombi and in subendothelial connective tissue, and may unfavorably change the therapeutic outcome of thrombolytic therapy in some patients.

Activation of clotting and platelets through activation of the fibrinolytic enzyme system. The administration of massive quantities of plasminogen activators results in the activation of coagulation. The major enzyme systems in plasma (Fig. 12.1), the clotting system, the fibrinolytic enzyme system, the kallikrein-kinin system and the complement system are interdependent systems sharing activators as well as inhibitors (43). The earliest steps of the intrinsic coagulation pathway involve factor XII (Hageman factor) plus two proteins from the kallikrein-kinin system, prekallikrein and high molecular weight kininogen. Hageman factor on negatively charged surfaces is activated by plasmin or kallikrein (43). Once Hageman factor is activated, the clotting cascade is set in motion by means of the intrinsic pathway, with activation of factor XI to factor XIa; it causes massive activation of prekallikrein to kallikrein, which works on kininogens to release kinins. Activated factor XIIa also activates clotting factor VII and sets in motion the chain reaction resulting in clotting by means of the extrinsic pathway. Kallikrein also activates scu-PA to urokinase,

which in turn results in additional activation of the fibrinolytic enzyme system. Thus, activation of the fibrinolytic enzyme system causes activation of clotting and of the kallikrein-kinin system, with the potential for hypotensive reactions that do, indeed, occur when too much streptokinase is given too fast.

Fibrinopeptide A, heparin and thrombin generation. That activation of coagulation occurs during rt-PA and streptokinase therapy in acute myocardial infarction was recently shown unequivocally by Owen et al. (44). They demonstrated a five- to sevenfold increase over baseline values of fibrinopeptide A, a reliable marker for activation of the coagulation system. Eisenberg et al. (45) also measured fibrinopeptide A levels in a similar group of patients receiving streptokinase. In their study, they found that increasing levels of fibrinopeptide A during streptokinase therapy correlated with the occurrence of rethrombosis. It is of great interest that in the study by Owen et al. (44), elevations in fibrinopeptide A after either rt-PA or streptokinase administration occurred despite concurrent heparin therapy (5,000 U as a bolus, followed by 1,000 U/h). The observation that thrombin generation occurs despite heparinization raises the possibility that thrombin generation occurs by means of pathways not generally recognized in the classic scheme of blood coagulation. Although never extensively described, on the basis of animal experiments and clinical observations, it has been suspected by many that heparin, even though an extremely effective anticoagulant on the venous side of the circulation, is far less effective on the arterial side. According to a hypothesis, which is being widely examined and for which we have persuasive preliminary evidence (46), alpha-thrombin, the final enzyme in the coagulation cascade, probably exists as different molecular entities in venous, relatively cell-poor thrombi and in arterial, cell-rich thrombi. In venous thrombi, alpha-thrombin predominates. It is in free solution in plasma and is readily inhibited by heparin in consort with the heparin cofactor antithrombin III. In arterial thrombi, the predominant form of thrombin appears to be meizothrombin. Meizothrombin remains attached to cells and has thrombin activity that is not inhibited by antithrombin III or heparin.

Another possibility is that the thrombus itself is the source of preformed thrombin. Fibrin is known to bind (47) and reversibly inactivate thrombin, and this thrombin can be liberated by plasmin digestion of the fibrin clot (48).

Activation of platelets associated with fibrinolytic therapy. It has been known for many years from in vitro experiments (49) that activation of the fibrinolytic enzyme system results in activation of platelets. Activation of platelets was recently confirmed (50) in vivo in patients receiving streptokinase for the treatment of acute myocardial infarction. A 10- to 20-fold increase in the urinary excretion of 2-3-dinor-thromboxane B2 and plasma 11-dehydro-thromboxane B2 was noted early during therapy. These prostaglandins are metabolites of thromboxane A2, and the appearance of thromboxane A2 in

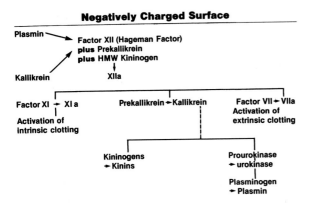

Figure 12.1. Interactions between the contact activation system of coagulation, the fibrinolytic enzyme system and the kallikrein-kinin system of human plasma. For details, see text.

plasma reflects in vivo platelet activation. The implications of these findings are that new accretion of fibrin and platelets onto the thrombus can occur once thrombolysis is underway and that these events may contribute to reocclusion as well as delayed time to reperfusion.

New Agents and Strategies: Preliminary, Preclinical and Clinical Results

Anisoylated plasminogen-streptokinase activator complex (APSAC). Streptokinase itself has neither protease nor esterase activity, but when it interacts with human plasminogen, a one to one stoichiometric complex is formed and the proteolytically active serine of plasmin is exposed; this complex activates plasminogen. A special form of streptokinase-plasminogen activator is prepared from such equimolar complexes of streptokinase and human plasminogen, in which the catalytic center of the plasminogen molecule is bound to an acyl group (51), resulting in an inactive complex. In aqueous solution, the acyl group is hydrolyzed and catalytic activity regained. With the p-anisoyl derivative (anisoylated plasminogen-streptokinase activator complex [APSAC]), the in vivo deacylation half-life is about 90 to 110 min. Thus, APSAC can be considered a sustained release streptokinase activator preparation.

Anisoylated plasminogen-streptokinase activator complex has theoretical advantages. The temporary masking of the catalytic center of the activator complex does not interfere with the capacity of the molecule to bind to fibrin because the fibrin binding sites of plasminogen, "the kringle domains," are located in the plasminogen molecule well separated from the catalytic site. Thus, relative fibrin specificity could be conferred, and has been confirmed in in vitro (52) and animal (53) experiments in which APSAC proved to be more efficient in lysing experimental thrombi and caused less fibrinogen depletion than did streptokinase-plasmin. However, at doses sufficient to cause coronary reperfusion (30 mg as a bolus injection) in humans, APSAC causes

considerable fibrinogen depletion and a rate of bleeding complications not apparently different from that of streptokinase (54). Furthermore, hypotensive reactions have occasionally been reported (55) in patients. Although APSAC has been shown to bind less streptokinase-neutralizing antibody than streptokinase (56), the incidence of clinical allergic anaphylactic reactions is similar to that observed with streptokinase (57). The prolonged half-life for APSAC (90 to 110 min) permits bolus administration. The "sustained release" characteristics of APSAC also ensure relatively constant levels of streptokinase throughout the treatment period. Thus, excessive streptokinase levels capable of completely depleting plasma plasminogen are not reached, and this may explain why reperfusion rates are generally somewhat higher with APSAC than with streptokinase (3).

When instituted early after the onset of symptoms, APSAC therapy has led to a reperfusion rate of approximately 65% and a patency rate of approximately 75% in several clinical studies (summarized in [57]). In the large placebo-controlled APSAC Intervention Mortality Study (AIMS) (58), APSAC administration in acute myocardial infarction resulted in an impressive 47% reduction in mortality rate.

scu-PA thrombolytic combinations. Clot-specific thrombolysis by natural or recombinant scu-PA has been demonstrated in animal models of venous and coronary artery thrombosis (59). In patients with acute myocardial infarction, intravenous infusion of 40 to 70 mg over 1 h resulted in coronary artery reperfusion in 75% of patients, but pronounced fibrinogen depletion in 25% (60).

Synergistic combinations of rt-PA with scu-PA or with urokinase have worked well in animal experiments (61). Combinations of rt-PA and scu-PA have also been efficacious in small uncontrolled studies (62,63) in patients with acute myocardial infarction. In a larger trial (21) evaluating the efficacy of rt-PA–urokinase combined therapy, only high doses of the two agents (1 mg/kg of rt-PA and 2 million U of urokinase) achieved patency rates at 90 min comparable to those achieved with rt-PA alone (73% versus 75%, respectively); additionally, the reocclusion rate was not statistically different among patients receiving the combination therapy than in those receiving rt-PA alone. Thus, the combination of two plasminogen activators to date does not appear to offer clear advantages over rt-PA alone.

Mutant plasminogen activators. Soon after the first successful attempt to clone and express human rt-PA (64), work in many laboratories was initiated to create rt-PA mutants through site-directed mutagenesis in an attempt to create molecules of improved functional properties (65). Recombinant tissue plasminogen activator seems to have evolved through "exon shuffling," and in the rt-PA, protein-specific structures or "domains" encoded by specific exons bear strong structural homology to similar domains in other proteins. Evidence accumulated to date (65) suggests that discrete rt-PA domains possess discrete and specific functional properties.

The domains in rt-PA from the N-terminus to the C-terminus are named: finger, epidermal growth factor, kringle 1, kringle 2 and serine protease. The finger and kringle 2 domains have been shown by several laboratories to be involved in rt-PA binding to fibrin (summarized in [65]). The epidermal growth factor domain may play a role in rt-PA binding to cells. The kringle 1 domain has not been assigned a function with certainty, except that it contains on residue Asn_{117}, a complex, high mannose, branched carbohydrate side chain that is probably responsible for the effective binding, internalization and catabolism of rt-PA by normal hepatocytes (66). The serine protease domain catalyzes the conversion of plasminogen to plasmin.

Attempts to produce rt-PA mutants aim at improving the following less than desirable properties of the enzyme. 1) Recombinant tissue plasminogen activator is a less catalytically efficient plasminogen activator than is urokinase, even when adsorbed to a fibrin clot (67,68). 2) The fibrin specificity, although considerable, is limited as evidenced by the significant incidence of fibrinogen depletion in patients receiving high doses of rt-PA (69). 3) The activity of rt-PA is attenuated by several plasma inhibitors, mainly PAI-1 (42). 4) Like all plasminogen activators, rt-PA activates clotting as well as platelets. 5) Finally, the biologic half-life of rt-PA is very short (<5 min in humans) (70). Therefore, improved plasminogen activators should have a higher catalytic efficiency than has rt-PA, thereby theoretically reducing the time to reperfusion, should be more fibrin-specific than rt-PA and, therefore, theoretically cause less bleeding, and should have a lower affinity for inhibitors to make the molecule more effective than rt-PA. They should not activate clotting or platelets and should possess a longer half-life than rt-PA.

The different strategies involved in creating such molecules include: 1) deletion of one or several domains (71–77); 2) removal of one or more carbohydrate chains by point mutation or by changing appropriate asparagine residues to which N-linked carbohydrate is attached (78); 3) substitution of residue Arg_{275} (79), thereby blocking the conversion of single chain to two chain rt-PA, which normally occurs during purification and in vivo; and 4) creation of hybrid or chimeric proteins in which part or all of the N-terminal portion of rt-PA, which imparts fibrin-specificity to the molecule, is hooked up to the urokinase carboxy terminal serine protease domain (80–83). In an alternative and principally different approach, the serine protease domains of rt-PA or urokinase are conjugated to fibrin-specific monoclonal antibodies either through chemical linkage or protein engineering (84,85). To date, most of these attempts have met with only limited success. Hybrids of rt-PA-urokinase or scu-plasminogen activators have been constructed. These molecules usually possess better catalytic efficiency than rt-PA, but possess significantly lower fibrin specificity.

Mutants of higher fibrin specificity than rt-PA have not been successfully produced so far. However, rt-PA or urokinase-type plasminogen activator fibrin-specific monoclonal antibody chimeras have been shown in vitro and in limited animal experiments (86) to produce rapid thrombolysis without significant fibrinogen depletion. Although certain mutants with decreased affinity for the PAI-1 can be constructed, the manipulations involved also result in loss of fibrin specificity and instability of the protein (87–89). Mutant plasminogen activators that do not cause activation of clotting and platelets in vivo, as predicted, cannot be constructed because these side effects probably result from activation of plasmin, not from the high concentrations of plasminogen activators in the circulation. Thus, these adverse events must be counteracted by appropriate adjunctive therapy. In only one area, the creation of mutants with a prolonged half-life, have attempts in several laboratories (73,90,91) been successful. Mutants that lack Asn_{117} and its attached carbohydrate side chain or mutants that lack epidermal growth factor show varying degrees of prolongation of the half-life up to 10-fold of natural rt-PA in experimental animals (92). Preclinical pharmacologic data from rt-PA mutants with a prolonged half-life strongly suggest that these proteins can shorten the time to reperfusion and can substantially delay or eliminate reocclusion.

Whether such mutants will result in therapeutic gains in acute myocardial infarction in patients cannot be predicted at this time. Only prospective clinical trials can resolve whether these interesting proteins significantly increase the benefit to risk ratio of thrombolytic therapy in acute myocardial infarction (that is, whether an increase in efficacy may occur without increased bleeding complications). A separate issue is whether a plasminogen activator with a prolonged half-life in some instances can be detrimental to the patient if and when, for example, urgent coronary bypass surgery is contemplated.

Adjunctive Therapy

Antiplatelet agents: theoretical considerations. Platelets are activated in vivo and start adhering to subendothelial connective tissue and aggregating to each other through a series of complex and only partly interconnected events. Many agonists can cause platelet activation and aggregation. Among these are thromboxane A_2, a prostaglandin synthesized in the platelet, collagen, thrombin, adenosine diphosphate (ADP), serotonin and epinephrine (reviewed in [93]). Each of these has its own receptors on the platelet and each causes receptor-linked signal transduction to activate several different pathways, resulting in platelet adhesion and aggregation. One can easily block one of the major pathways with a pharmacologic agent, but even if one pathway is blocked, other pathways may prevail such that it is extremely difficult through conventional pharmacologic monotherapy to completely block platelet activation.

Platelet adhesions and aggregations. A change in thinking has come about in recent years, when it became apparent that a common final pathway exists. It is now firmly established that platelets adhere to each other and to the vessel wall by making use of "sticky proteins" contained in plasma, irrespective of the mechanism of platelet activation. The structures in the platelet membranes that allow sticky proteins to attach themselves are receptorlike glycoprotein molecules of the so-called integrin family (94) found on numerous cells. The integrins are of major general importance in bringing about cell-cell adhesion and promoting cell-cell interactions. On the platelet, a glycoprotein called Ib attaches the von Willebrand factor protein to the platelet, and von Willebrand factor also sticks to subendothelial connective tissues, thereby allowing the platelet to adhere at the site of endothelial damage. Another integrin on the platelet is called glycoprotein IIb/IIIa (GPIIb/IIIa). It will bind fibrinogen as well as von Willebrand factor, thereby assuring the sticking together of two or more platelets, resulting in platelet aggregation.

That platelets are important in the pathogenesis of coronary thrombi has long been suspected on the basis of two simple observations. 1) Like all arterial thrombi, coronary thrombi are platelet rich (95) and contain at least 10 to 20 times more platelets per unit mass than do venous thrombi. 2) Many coronary thrombi appear to originate at sites of ruptured atheromatous plaques, where subendothelial connective tissue is exposed, allowing for platelet adhesion and aggregation (96).

Different classes of antiplatelet agents considered as adjunct therapy. As mentioned, the ISIS-2 study (34) established that aspirin, particularly in combination with streptokinase, reduced reinfarction and mortality rates. Aspirin is a cyclooxygenase inhibitor that works during the initial stages in the chain reaction, resulting in thromboxane A_2 synthesis (93). Attempts at synthesizing cyclooxygenase inhibitors more efficient than aspirin have proceeded in many laboratories for many years, but without noticeable success. Thromboxane synthetase inhibitors specifically inhibit the generation of thromboxane A_2, one of the major agonists in platelet activation, but to date, agents of this class have not proved to be effective inhibitors of platelet activation in vivo. Many thromboxane A_2 receptor antagonists have also been synthesized, and are currently being tested and look useful particularly in combination with serotonin 5-HT2 receptor antagonists. Another class of agents includes phosphodiesterase inhibitors, such as dipyridamole, and adenylase cyclase enhancers, such as stable prostacyclin analogs. This class of drugs works through increasing intraplatelet levels of cyclic adenosine monophosphate (AMP), which serves to greatly decrease platelet activation.

Finally, agents that block platelet GPIIb/IIIa and thereby prevent aggregation independent of the pathway of activation of the platelets are being intensively tested. Monoclonal antibodies with GPIIb/IIIa specificity are being tested in experimental animals and in early clinical trials. In addition, fibrinogenomimetic peptides that also prevent the attachment of fibrinogen to the GPIIb/IIIa receptor are being developed and look very promising. The construction of these agents is based on the knowledge of the exact amino acid sequences in fibrinogen that are involved in binding fibrinogen to the GPIIb/IIIa receptors, thereby promoting platelet aggregation. Among these agents, the anti-GPIIb/IIIa monoclonal antibodies, the fibrinogenomimetic peptides and thromboxane A_2 receptor antagonists in combination with 5-HT$_2$ antagonists look the most promising and will be discussed in the next section.

Anti-GPIIb/IIIa monoclonal antibodies. In a series of dog experiments (97), rt-PA was given by repeated bolus injection (0.45 mg/kg every 15 min) and the GPIIb/IIIa monoclonal antibody was given as a single bolus injection in doses ranging from 0.1 to 0.8 mg/kg. The time to reperfusion in the rt-PA-treated control dogs was 33 min, the incidence of reocclusion 100% and the time to reocclusion 11 min. When rt-PA was given in combination with the monoclonal antibody in doses of 0.8, 0.6 and 0.4 mg/kg, striking improvements in treatment results were observed. The time to reperfusion was shortened from 33 min to 6, 8 and 9 min, respectively. Reocclusion occurred in none of six dogs receiving 0.8 mg, one of five receiving 0.6 mg and three of three receiving the 0.4 mg dose of the monoclonal antibody. Doses of the monoclonal antibody <0.4 mg/kg resulted in no differences from the rt-PA control study. It should be noted, however, that the bleeding time in dogs receiving the high doses of the monoclonal antibody was excessively prolonged, indicating platelet dysfunction and increased bleeding risk.

Fibrinogenomimetic peptides. These analogs of the Arg-Gly-Asp-Ser or the gamma-chain carboxy-terminal peptide sequences of fibrinogen have been shown (98) to be highly effective in the prevention of mesenteric artery thrombosis. They are being tested in experimental coronary artery thrombosis with or without rt-PA, but results are not yet known. The peptides do cause prolongation of the bleeding time in animals, but not as marked as that caused by GPIIb/IIIa monoclonal antibodies.

Thromboxane A_2 receptor antagonists (in combination with 5-HT2 antagonists). Reports from several laboratories have suggested that thromboxane A_2 receptor antagonists administered as monotherapy as well as serotonin 5-HT$_2$ antagonists also administered as single agents are effective in preventing or delaying arterial thrombosis. Combination therapy using these two classes of agents was recently reported (99) to be highly effective as adjunctive therapy in dogs after reperfusion with rt-PA. In this study, the incidence of cyclic flow variations and the time to reocclusion were recorded. In control dogs that received heparin after successful reperfusion with rt-PA, the time to reocclusion was 25 min and all dogs showed cyclic flow variations. In dogs receiving a thromboxane A_2 receptor antagonist (SQ29548), the time to reocclusion was prolonged to 86 min, but three of five dogs showed cyclic flow patterns. Dogs receiving only ketanserin, a 5-HT$_2$ antagonist, demonstrated a time to reocclusion of 21 min and all demonstrated cyclic flow variations. A group of dogs receiving an experimental 5-HT$_2$ antagonist (LY53857) demonstrated a significantly prolonged time to reocclusion, but three of four dogs showed cyclic flow variations. However, when serotonin and a thromboxane antagonist were given together, reocclusion was prevented, the time to reocclusion being longer than the duration of the experiment (180 min), and in none of 11 dogs was the cyclic flow variation pattern observed. Whether bleeding occurred with these regimens was not reported.

Novel anticoagulants. Two types of agents must be considered.

Pure thrombin inhibitors. The first type are pure thrombin inhibitors, in contrast to heparin, which in consort with antithrombin III inhibits not only thrombin, but practically every other serine protease in the coagulation cascade. The most potent specific thrombin inhibitor is hirudin, originally purified from the medicinal leech *Hirudo medicinalis* (100) and subsequently cloned and expressed in large quantities through recombinant DNA technology (101). There are also several completely synthetic pure antithrombins; however, limited information about these agents is available. Claims have been made, mostly in abstract form (102,103), that they are effective in preventing arterial thrombosis, but there is also an indication that some of these agents are associated with bleeding problems in experimental animals.

Activated protein C. The second type of agent to be considered is activated protein C, an agent that we have had experience with since protein C was cloned and expressed in the Lilly Research Laboratories (104). Some of its preclinical pharmacology was also studied here (105). Activated protein C is a natural anticoagulant of major physiologic importance. Its mechanism of action is quite elegant in that it displays anticoagulant activity only if, when and where thrombin is being generated (106); it appears to be quite thrombus specific. It has been shown to be effective in the prevention of extension of preformed venous thrombi and also is extremely effective in the treatment of septic shock with disseminated intravascular coagulation. Activated protein C has also been found to be effective in the prevention of arterial thrombi, where it very surprisingly inhibits platelet accumulation as well as fibrin accretion. The major drawback of activated protein C is its relatively short biologic half-life of 12 to 20 min, which could make it expensive in clinical use.

Gruber et al. (107) recently reported results obtained with activated protein C in a baboon arterial thrombosis model. The deposition of platelets in an arterial shunt was quantified by computer-assisted gamma camera imaging in six control animals and in animals receiving two different doses of activated protein C. Platelet deposition was substantially reduced in a dose-dependent fashion in thrombi of animals receiving activated protein C infusion, and continued effects were noted for ≥60 min after the end of the infusion. Occlusion of the arterial shunt occurred in all six control animals between 25 to 50 min, whereas the arteries remained patent in all animals receiving activated protein C for the 2 h duration of the experiment. Bleeding times remained normal in all animals treated with activated protein C and no clinical bleeding was observed. In fact, in all experimental animal studies concluded to date, infusions of activated protein C have been associated with little, if any, bleeding liability. The reasons why activated protein C, which in theory should be a pure anticoagulant, inhibits both platelet function and thrombus formation without increasing bleeding risk are unknown, but they are being intensively investigated at this time.

Conclusions

The results obtained with thrombolytic therapy in acute myocardial infarction to date have been impressive. Nevertheless, many people have been working to further improve results through different strategies, construction of more efficient fibrinolytic enzyme preparations and the development of new and improved adjunctive therapies. The material included in this review strongly suggests that it is possible to design strategies that could shorten the time to reperfusion and perhaps increase the incidence of reperfusion and decrease the incidence of reocclusion, but it is uncertain whether the incidence of bleeding complications can be reduced. Indeed, it is possible that some of these strategies will result in increased bleeding liability. A possible exception is activated protein C, which appears to be therapeutically effective at a dose that does not cause bleeding. What is certain is that many of these strategies and new agents will be tested clinically within the next few years. Our review at this time serves notice that the final chapter in the saga of thrombolytic therapy in acute myocardial infarction is yet to be written.

References

1. Fletcher AP, Sherry S, Alkaersig N, Smyrniotis FE, Jick S. The maintenance of a sustained thrombolytic state in man. II. Clinical observation on patients with myocardial infarction and other thromboembolic disorders. J Clin Invest 1959;38:111–9.
2. Duckert F. Thrombolytic therapy in myocardial infarction. Prog Cardiovasc Dis 1979;21:342–50.
3. Bang NU, Wilhelm OG, Clayman MD. Thrombolytic therapy in myocardial infarction. Annu Rev Pharmacol Toxicol 1989;29:323–41.
4. van de Werf F, Bergman SR, Fox KAA, et al. Coronary thrombolysis with intravenously administered human tissue-type plasminogen activator produced by recombinant DNA technology. Circulation 1984;69:605–10.
5. Mueller HS, Rao AK, Forman SA and the TIMI Investigators. Thrombolysis in Myocardial Infarction (TIMI): comparative studies of coronary reperfusion and systemic fibrinogenolysis with two forms of recombinant tissue-type plasminogen activator. J Am Coll Cardiol 1987;10:479–90.

6. Braunwald E, Knatterud GL, Passamani E. Announcement of protocol change in Thrombolysis in Myocardial Infarction Trial (letter). J Am Coll Cardiol 1987;9:467.

7. Chesebro JH, Knatterud D, Roberts R, et al. Thrombolysis in Myocardial Infarction (TIMI) Trial, phase I: a comparison between intravenous tissue plasminogen activator and intravenous streptokinase. Circulation 1987;76:142–54.

8. Sherry S. Appraisal of various thrombolytic agents in the treatment of acute myocardial infarction. Am J Med 1987;83(suppl 2A):31–46.

9. Gruppo Italiano per lo Studio della Streptochinasi Nell'Infarto Miocardico (GISSI). Effectiveness of intravenous thrombolytic treatment in acute myocardial infarction. Lancet 1986;1:397–401.

10. Hugenholtz PG. Acute coronary artery obstruction in myocardial infarction: overview of thrombolytic therapy. J Am Coll Cardiol 1987;9:1375–84.

11. Grines CL, Topol EJ, Bates ER, et al. Infarct vessel status after intravenous tissue plasminogen activator and acute coronary angioplasty: prediction of clinical outcome. Am Heart J 1988;115:1–7.

12. Golino P, Ashton JH, Glas-Greenwalt P, et al. Medication of reocclusion by thromboxane A$_2$ and serotonin after thrombolysis with tissue-type plasminogen activator in canine preparation of coronary thrombosis. Circulation 1988;77:678–84.

13. Kircher BJ, Topol EJ, O'Neill WW, Pitt B. Prediction of infarct coronary recanalization after intravenous thrombolytic therapy. Am J Cardiol 1987;59:513–5.

14. Califf RM, O'Neill W, Stack RS, et al. Failure of simple clinical measurements to predict perfusion status after intravenous thrombolysis. Ann Intern Med 1988;108:658–62.

15. Topol EJ, Califf RM, George BS, et al. A randomized trial of immediate versus delayed elective angioplasty after intravenous tissue plasminogen activator in acute myocardial infarction. N Engl J Med 1987;317:581–8.

16. Simoons ML, von Essen R, Lubsen J, et al. Thrombolysis with tissue plasminogen activator in acute myocardial infarction: no additional benefit from immediate percutaneous coronary angioplasty. Lancet 1988;1:197–203.

17. The TIMI Study Group. Immediate vs delayed catheterization and angioplasty following thrombolytic therapy for acute myocardial infarction. JAMA 1988;260:2849–58.

18. The TIMI Study Group. Comparison of invasive and conservative strategies after treatment with intravenous tissue plasminogen activator in acute myocardial infarction. N Engl J Med 1989;320:618–26.

19. Califf RM, Topol EJ, George BS, et al. Characteristics and outcome of patients in whom reperfusion with intravenous tissue-type plasminogen activator fails: results of the Thrombolysis and Angioplasty in Myocardial Infarction (TAMI) I Trial. Circulation 1988;77:1090–9.

20. Grines CL, O'Neill WW, Anselmo EG, June JE, Topol EJ. Comparison of left ventricular function and contractile reserve after successful recanalization by thrombolysis versus rescue percutaneous transluminal coronary angioplasty for acute myocardial infarction. Am J Cardiol 1988;62:352–7.

21. Topol EJ, Califf RM, George BS, et al. Coronary arterial thrombolysis with combined infusion of recombinant tissue-type plasminogen activator and urokinase in patients with acute myocardial infarction. Circulation 1988;77:1100–7.

22. Verstraete M, Brower RW, Collen D, et al. Double-blind randomized trial of intravenous tissue-type plasminogen activator versus placebo in acute myocardial infarction. Lancet 1985;2:965–9.

23. Topol EJ, George BS, Kereiakes DJ, et al. A randomized controlled trial of intravenous tissue plasminogen activator and early intravenous heparin in acute myocardial infarction. Circulation 1989;79:281–6.

24. Verstraete M, Bory M, Collen D, et al. Comparative randomized study of the effectiveness of intravenous tissue-type plasminogen activator and intravenous streptokinase in patients with acute myocardial infarction. Klin Wochenschr 1988;66(suppl 12):77–85.

25. Verstraete M, Arnold AE, Brower RW, et al. Acute coronary thrombolysis with recombinant human tissue-type plasminogen activator: initial patency and influence of maintained infusion on reocclusion rate. Am J Cardiol 1987;60:231–7.

26. Ganz W, Buchbinder N, Marcus H, et al. Intracoronary thrombolysis in evolving myocardial infarction. Am Heart J 1981;101:4–13.

27. Markis JE, Malagold M, Parker JA, et al. Myocardial salvage after intracoronary thrombolysis with streptokinase in myocardial infarction. N Engl J Med 1981;305:777–82.

28. Yasuda T, Gold HK, Leinbach RC, et al. Tissue plasminogen activator (t-PA) resistant platelet rich white thrombus (WT) and combination treatment of t-PA and anti-platelet antibody to GPIIb/IIIa receptor (7E3). Circulation 1988;78(suppl II):II-15.

29. van de Werf F, Arnold AE. Intravenous tissue plasminogen activator and size of infarct, left ventricular function, and survival in acute myocardial infarction. Br Med J 1988;297:1374–9.

30. TIMI Study Group. The Thrombolysis in Myocardial Infarction (TIMI) Trial. N Engl J Med 1985;312:932.

31. Wilcox RG, von der Lippe G, Olsson CB, Jensen G, Skene AM, Hampton JR. Trial of tissue plasminogen activator for mortality reduction in acute myocardial infarction: Anglo-Scandinavian Study of Early Thrombolysis (ASSET). Lancet 1988;2:525–30.

32. O'Rourke M, Baron D, Keough A, et al. Limitations of myocardial infarction by early infusion of recombinant tissue-type plasminogen activator. Circulation 1988;77:1311–5.

33. National Heart Foundation of Australia Coronary Thrombolysis Group. Coronary thrombolysis and myocardial salvage by tissue plasminogen activator given up to 4 hours after onset of myocardial infarction. Lancet 1988;1:203–8.

34. ISIS-2 Collaborative Group. Randomized trial of intravenous streptokinase, oral aspirin, both, or neither among 17,187 cases of suspected acute myocardial infarction: ISIS-2. Lancet 1988;2:349–60.

35. Kennedy JW, Martin GV, David KB, et al. The Western Washington Intravenous Streptokinase in Acute Myocardial Infarction Randomized Trial. Circulation 1988;77:345–52.

36. The ISAM Study Group. A prospective trial of intravenous streptokinase in acute myocardial infarction (I.S.A.M.). N Engl J Med 1986;314:1465–71.

37. Schroder R, Neuhaus KL, Leizorovicz A, et al. A prospective placebo-controlled double-blind multicenter trial of intravenous streptokinase in acute myocardial infarction (ISAM): long-term mortality and morbidity. J Am Coll Cardiol 1987;9:197–203.

38. White HD, Norris RM, Brown MA, et al. Effect of intravenous streptokinase on left ventricular function and early survival after acute myocardial infarction. N Engl J Med 1987;317:850–5.

39. Timmis GC, Mammen EF, Ramos RG, et al. Hemorrhage vs rethrombosis after thrombolysis for acute myocardial infarction. Arch Intern Med 1986;146:667–72.

40. The AIMS Trial Study Group. Effect of intravenous APSAC on mortality after acute myocardial infarction. Lancet 1988;1:545–9.

41. Johns JA, Gold HK, Leinbach RC, et al. Prevention of coronary artery reocclusion and reduction in late coronary artery stenosis after thrombolytic therapy in patients with acute myocardial infarction. Circulation 1988;78:546–56.

42. Lucore CL, Sobel BE. Interactions of tissue-type plasminogen activator with plasma inhibitors and their pharmacologic implications. Circulation 1988;77:660–9.

43. Griffin JH, Cochran CHG. Recent advances in the understanding of contact activation reactions. Semin Thromb Hemost 1979;5:254–73.

44. Owen J, Friedman KD, Grossman BA, Wilkins C, Berke AD, Powers ER. Thrombolytic therapy with tissue plasminogen activator or streptokinase induces transient thrombin activity. Blood 1988;72:616–20.

45. Eisenberg PR, Sherman L, Rich N, et al. Importance of continued activation of thrombin reflected by fibrinopeptide A to the efficacy of thrombolysis. J Am Coll Cardiol 1986;7:1255–62.

46. Krishnaswamy S, Mann KG, Nesheim NE. The prothrombinase-catalyzed activation of prothrombin proceeds through the intermediate meizothrombin in an ordered, sequential reaction. J Biol Chem 1986;261:8977.

47. Lin CY, Nossel HL, Kaplan KL. The bindings of thrombin by fibrin. J Biol Chem 1979;254:10421.

48. Francis CW, Markham RE Jr, Barlow GH, Florack TM, Dobrzynski DM, Marder VJ. Thrombin activity of fibrin thrombi and soluble plasmic derivatives. J Lab Clin Med 1983:102–220.

49. Niewiarowski S, Senyi AF, Gillies P. Plasmin-induced platelet aggregation and platelet release reaction. J Clin Invest 1973;52:1647–59.

50. Fitzgerald DJ, Catella F, Roy L, Fitzgerald DG. Marked platelet activation in vivo after intravenous streptokinase in patients with acute myocardial infarction. Circulation 1988;77:142–50.

51. Smith RAG, Dupe RJ, English PD, Green J. Fibrinolysis with acylenzymes: a new approach to thrombolytic therapy. Nature 1981;290:505–8.

52. Fears R, Ferres H, Standring R. Evidence for the progressive up-take of anisoylated plasminogen streptokinase activator complex by clots in human plasma in vitro. Drugs 1987;33:51–6.

53. Matsuo O, Collen D, Verstraete M. On the fibrinolytic and thrombolytic properties of active-side p-anisoylated streptokinase plasminogen complex (BRL26921). Thromb Res 1981;24:347–58.

54. Green J, Harris GS, Smith RAG, Dupe RJ. Acyl-enzymes: a novel class of thrombolytic agents. In: Collen D, Linjen HR, Verstraete M, eds. Thrombolysis: Biological and Therapeutic Properties of New Thrombolytic Agents. Edinburgh: Churchill Livingstone, 1985:124–67.

55. Bossaert LL. Safety and tolerance data from the Belgian multicentre study of anisoylated plasminogen streptokinase activator complex versus heparin in acute myocardial infarction. Drugs 1987;33:287–92.

56. Verstraete M, Vermylen J, Holleman W, Barlow GH. Biological effects of the administration of an equimolar streptokinase-plasminogen complex in man. Thromb Res 1977;11:227–36.

57. Anderson JL. Development and evaluation of anisoylated plasminogen streptokinase activator complex (APSAC) as a second generation thrombolytic agent. J Am Coll Cardiol 1987;10:22–7.

58. The AIMS Trial Study Group. Effects of intravenous APSAC on mortality after acute myocardial infarction: preliminary report of a placebo-controlled clinical trial. Lancet 1988;1:545–9.

59. Lijnen HR, Stump DC, Collen D. Single-chain urokinase-type plasminogen activator: mechanism of action and thrombolytic properties. Semin Thromb Hemost 1987;13:152–9.

60. Collen D. Molecular mechanism of action of newer thrombolytic agents. J Am Coll Cardiol 1987;10:11–5.

61. Collen D, Strassen SM, Stump DC, Verstraete N. In vivo synergism of thrombolytic agents. Circulation 1986;74:838.

62. Collen D, Stump DC, van de Werf F. Coronary thrombolysis in patients with acute myocardial infarction by intravenous infusion of synergistic thrombolytic agents. Am Heart J 1986;112:1083–4.

63. Collen D, van de Werf F. Coronary arterial thrombolysis with low-dose synergistic combinations of recombinant tissue-type plasminogen activator (rt-PA) and recombinant single-chain urokinase-type plasminogen activator (rscu-PA) for myocardial infarction. Am J Cardiol 1987;60: 431–4.

64. Pennica D, Holmes WE, Kohn WD, et al. Cloning and expression of human tissue-type plasminogen activator cDNA in E. coli. Nature 1983;301:214–21.

65. Pannekoek H, de Vries C, van Zonneveld AJ. Mutants of human tissue-type plasminogen activator (t-PA): structural aspects and functional properties. Fibrinolysis 1988;2:123–32.

66. Owensby DA, Sobel BE, Schwartz AL. Receptor-mediated endocytosis of tissue-type plasminogen activator by the human hepatoma cell line Hep G2. J Biol Chem 1988;263:10587–94.

67. Christensen U. Kinetic studies of the urokinase-catalysed conversion of the NH_2-terminal glutamic acid plasminogen to plasmin. Biochim Biophys Acta 1977;481:638–47.

68. Hoylaerts M, Rijken DC, Lijnen HR, Collen D. Kinetics of the activation of plasminogen by human tissue plasminogen activator: role of fibrin. J Biol Chem 1982;257:2912–9.

69. Rao AK, Pratt C, Berke A, et al. Thrombolysis in Myocardial Infarction (TIMI) Trial-phase I: hemorrhagic manifestations and changes in plasma fibrinogen and the fibrinolytic system in patients treated with recombinant tissue plasminogen activator and streptokinase. J Am Coll Cardiol 1988;11:1–11.

70. Seifried E, Tanswell P, Rijken DC, Barrett-Bergshoeff NN, Smith PF, Kluft C. Pharmacokinetics of antigen and activity of recombinant tissue-type plasminogen activator after infusion in healthy volunteers. Arzneim Forsch Drug Res 1988;38:418–22.

71. van Zonneveld AJ, Veerman H, Pannekoek H. Autonomous functions of structural domains on human tissue-type plasminogen activator. Proc Natl Acad Sci USA 1986;83:4670–4.

72. Verheijen JH, Caspers MPM, Chang GTG, de Munk GAW, Pouwels PH, Enger-Valk BE. Involvement of finger domain and Kringle 2 domain of tissue-type plasminogen activator in fibrin binding and stimulation of activity by fibrin. Embo J 1986;5:3525–30.

73. Browne NJ, Carey JE, Chapman CG, et al. A tissue-type plasminogen activator mutant with prolonged clearance in vivo: effect of removal of the growth factor domain. J Biol Chem 1988;263:1599–602.

74. Gething MJ, Adler B, Boose JA, et al. Variants of human tissue-type plasminogen activator that lack specific structural domains of the heavy chain. Embo J 1988:2731–40.

75. Larsen GR, Henson K, Blue Y. Variants of human tissue-type plasminogen activator. J Biol Chem 1988;263:1023–9.

76. Kagitani H, Targawa N, Hatanaka N, et al. Expression in E. coli of finger-domain lacking tissue-type plasminogen activator with high fibrin affinity. FEBS Lett 1985;189:145–9.

77. Kalyan NK, Lee SB, Wilhelm J, et al. Structure-function analysis with tissue-type plasminogen activator. J Biol Chem 1988;263:3971–8.

78. Collen D, Stassen JN, Larsen Y. Pharmacokinetics and thrombolytic properties of deletion mutants of human tissue-type plasminogen activator in rabbits. Blood 1988;71:216–9.

79. Tate KM, Higgins DL, Holmes WE, Winkler ME, Heyneker HL, Vehar GR. Functional role of proteolytic cleavage at arginine-275 of human tissue plasminogen activator as assessed by site-directed mutagenesis. Biochemistry 1987;26:338–43.

80. Gheysen D, Lijnen HR, Pierard L, et al. Characterization of a recombinant fusion protein of the finger domain of tissue-type plasminogen activator with a truncated single-chain urokinase type plasminogen activator. J Biol Chem 1987;262:11779.

81. de Vries C, Veerman H, Blasi F, Pannekoek H. Artificial exon shuffling between tissue-type plasminogen activator (t-PA) and urokinase (u-PA): a comparative study on the fibrinolytic properties of t-PA/u-PA hybrid proteins. Biochemistry 1988;27:2565–72.

82. Lijnen HR, Nelles L, van Hoef B, Demarsin E, Collen D. Characterization of a chimeric plasminogen activator consisting of amino acids 1 to 274 of tissue-type plasminogen activator and amino acids 138 to 411 of single-chain urokinase-type plasminogen activator. J Biol Chem 1988; 263:19083–91.

83. Lee SG, Kalyan N, Wilhelm J, et al. Construction and expression of hybrid plasminogen activators prepared from tissue-type plasminogen activator and urokinase-type plasminogen activator genes. J Biol Chem 1988;263:2917–24.

84. Runge MS, Bode C, Matsueda GR, Haber E. Conjugation to an antifibrin monoclonal antibody enhances the fibrinolytic potency of tissue plasminogen activator in vitro. Biochemistry 1987;27:1153–7.

85. Schnee JM, Runge MS, Matsueda GR, et al. Construction and expression of a recombinant antibody-targeted plasminogen activator. Proc Natl Acad Sci USA 1987;84:G904–8.

86. Runge MS, Bode CH, Matsueda GR, Haber E. Antibody-enhanced thrombolysis: targeting of tissue-plasminogen activator in vivo. Proc Natl Acad Sci USA 1987;84:7659–62.

87. Bang NU, Little SP, Burck PJ, et al. Functional properties of tissue-plasminogen activator. Blood 1985;66:330a.

88. Ehrlich HJ, Bang NU, Little SP, et al. Biological properties of a kringleless tissue-plasminogen activator (t-PA) mutant. Fibrinolysis 1987;1:75–81.

89. Wilhelm OG, Bang NU. Fibrin structural requirements for tissue-plasminogen activator mediated plasminogen activation as studied by t-PA deletion mutants. In: NW Mosesson, et al., eds. Fibrinogen 3, Biochemistry, Biological Functions, Gene Regulation and Expression. Amsterdam: Elsevier Science Publishers BR (Biomedical Division), 1988:185–8.

90. Jackson V, Craft T, Sundboom J, Frank J, Grinnell B, Bobbitt L, Quag J, Smith G. Comparison of a novel plasminogen activator (PA) LY210825, and native t-PA in a canine model of coronary artery thrombosis (abstr). Fed Proc 1988;2:6483.

91. Collen D, Stassen JM, Larsen GR. Pharmacokinetics and thrombolytic properties of deletion mutants of human tissue-type plasminogen activator in rabbits. Blood 1988;71:216–9.

92. Cambier P, van de Werf F, Larsen GR, Collen D. Pharmacokinetics and thrombolytic properties of a non-glycosylated mutant of human tissue-type plasminogen activator, lacking the finger growth factor domains, in

dogs with copper coil-induced coronary artery thrombosis. J Cardiovasc Pharmacol 1988;11:468–72.

93. Bush LR, Patrick D. The role of the endothelium in arterial thrombosis and the influence of antithrombotic therapy. Drug Dev Res 1986;7:319–40.

94. Hawiger J. Adhesive interactions of blood cells and vessel wall. In: Colman R, Hirsch J, Marder V, Salzman E, eds. Hemostasis and Thrombosis. Basic Principles and Clinical Practices. 2nd ed. Philadelphia: JB Lippincott, 182, 1987.

95. Olson PS. Platelets and fibrin in the early development of arterial and venous thrombi. Thesis, Malmo, 1974.

96. Ridolfi RL, Hutchins GM. The relationship between coronary artery lesions and myocardial infarcts: ulceration of atherosclerotic plaques precipitating coronary thrombosis. Am Heart J 1977;93:468–86.

97. Gold HK, Coller BS, Yasuda T, et al. Rapid and sustained coronary artery recanalization with combined bolus injection of recombinant tissue-type plasminogen activator and monoclonal antiplatelet GPIIb/IIIa antibody in a canine preparation. Circulation 1988;77:670–7.

98. Kloczewiak M, Timmons S, Bednarek M, Sakon M, Hawiger J. Platelet receptor recognition domain on the γ-chain of human fibrinogen and its synthetic peptide analogues. Biochemistry 1989;28:2915–19.

99. Golino P, Ashton JH, Glas-Greenwalt P, et al. Mediation of reocclusion by thromboxane A$_2$ and serotonin after thrombolysis with tissue-type plasminogen activator in a canine preparation of coronary thrombosis. Circulation 1988;77:678–84.

100. Markwardt F. Hirudin as an inhibitor of thrombin. Methods Enzymol 1970;19:924–32.

101. Harvey RP, Degryse E, Stefani L, et al. Cloning and expression of a cDNA coding for the anticoagulant hirudo medicinalis. Proc Natl Acad Sci USA 1986;83:1084–8.

102. Jang IK, Tiskind AA, Gold HK, Leinbach RC, Fallon JT, Collen D. Prevention of arterial platelet occlusion by selection thrombin inhibition. Circulation 1988;78(suppl II):1240.

103. Kelly AB, Hanson SR, Marlec U, Harker LA. Recombinant hirudin (r-H) interruption of platelet-dependent thrombus formation. Circulation 1988;78(suppl II):1242.

104. Beckmann RJ, Schmidt RJ, Santerre RF, Plutsky J, Crabtree GR, Long GL. Structure and evolution of a 461 aa human protein C precursor and its messenger RNA based upon the DNA sequence of cloned human liver cDNAs. Nucleic Acids Res 1985;13:5233.

105. Emerick SC, Murayama H, Yan SB, et al. Preclinical pharmacology of activated protein C. In: Holcenberg JS and Winkelhake JS, eds. The Pharmacology and Toxicology of Proteins. New York: Alan R. Liss, 1987:351–67.

106. Esmon CT. The regulation of natural anticoagulant pathways. Science 1987;235:1348–52.

107. Gruber A, Griffin JH, Harker L, Hanson SR. Inhibition of platelet-dependent thrombus formation by human activated protein C in a primate model. Blood 1989;73:639–42.

◆ CHAPTER 13 ◆

Treatment of Coronary Artery Disease

ROBERT L. FRYE, MD, RAYMOND J. GIBBONS, MD, HARTZELL V. SCHAFF, MD,
RONALD E. VLIETSTRA, MD, BERNARD J. GERSH, MD, MICHAEL B. MOCK, MD

It is fascinating to note the progress that has occurred over the past 40 years in our understanding of the pathophysiology of coronary artery disease as well as its treatment. Appreciation of the extraordinary change in the emphasis and approach to coronary artery disease from 1949 to 1989 is provided by review of the Quarterly Cumulative Index Medicus of 1949. A total of 31 papers are referenced under the topic "angina pectoris and its therapy." Of these, six deal with the use of methylthiouracil or thyroidectomy in treatment of angina (1–6), seven report on surgical resection or local injection therapy of the stellate ganglia or aortic nerve plexus (7–14) and two report on experience with vitamin E (15,16). One additional reference cites what must be one of the earliest placebo-controlled trials in evaluating chest pain (17).

The contrast with today's Index Medicus in terms of volume of studies and approach to coronary disease is readily apparent. The advances have been remarkable and associated with a major decline in coronary heart disease mortality (18). Although the basis for this decline is undoubtedly multifactorial, with fascinating geographic variations (19), there seems little doubt that treatment has played a role (20). The object of this article is to provide a review of current approaches to treatment of specific clinical subsets of patients with coronary artery disease.

Approach to Treatment of Individual Patients

Treatment objectives. As is ideal in all physician-patient interactions that result in diagnostic or therapeutic strategy decisions, a clear objective for each intervention needs to be enunciated. Treatment objectives include 1) symptom relief with a minimum of side effects; 2) enhancement of event-free survival; and 3) risk factor control with the objective of reducing progression in the basic disease process.

Risk stratification. The clinician planning therapy for an individual patient must first establish an accurate clinical profile of the patient in terms of symptoms, functional disability, quality of life and risk for subsequent cardiac events. The most important means to establish such a fundamental clinical profile are the history and physical examination. After these are accomplished, it may be appropriate to proceed with selective noninvasive testing to assess prognosis in mildly symptomatic patients or to proceed directly to coronary arteriography in patients with severe or unstable symptoms. Some patients will not require further testing. The approach selected should be based on a clearly stated objective and a pretest review of how the test result will influence decision making. Fundamental to risk stratification is the recognition that left ventricular function is the most powerful predictor of survival (21,22). Simply acquired clinical and rest electrocardiographic (ECG) variables contain important prognostic information, in part because they reflect left ventricular function (23–25). The incremental value of any additional testing should be carefully considered before further testing is performed (26).

Stable Angina Pectoris

Once the clinician has established the presence of angina pectoris by history and identified other complicating medical conditions, an assessment of functional impairment and risk for subsequent cardiac events is necessary. It is impossible to include all possible scenarios that might influence decision making. For an elderly patient with no strenuous demands in work or recreation, a trial of medical therapy may be appropriate without other testing. For patients with severe disabling symptoms, particularly those already on medical therapy, coronary arteriography without other testing is necessary to define suitability for coronary revascularization with either coronary angioplasty or coronary artery bypass grafting. Controlled clinical studies have documented 1) the relief of angina pectoris with bypass surgery (27–29), and 2) improvement in objective indexes of functional capacity and myocardial ischemia (30,31). In the large randomized trials, coronary bypass surgery was demonstrated to be more effective than standard medical therapy alone in relief of angina. However, that advantage diminishes after several years as a result of graft occlusion and progression of native coronary artery disease.

Coronary angioplasty. The transluminal approach to treating coronary artery disease was introduced with coronary angioplasty (32). This technique results in sustained improvement in the majority of appropriately selected patients (33), with low morbidity and little time away from work (34). In patients with multivessel disease, event-free outcomes are more frequent in those with "complete" revascularization (35). An American College of Cardiology/ American Heart Association Task Force recently emphasized that "the approach to every angioplasty procedure requires a knowledgeable judgment that weighs the likelihood of a successful outcome against the likelihood of failure and the risk of complications'' (36). It is important to note the lack of published controlled studies of coronary angioplasty versus other therapies in relief of angina pectoris. Although there are abundant published observational data to support the effectiveness of coronary angioplasty in relief of myocardial ischemia, presumption of applicability of the results of bypass surgery to treatment with angioplasty is unwarranted.

Role of stress testing in assessing prognosis. Stress testing for the purpose of assessing prognosis is appropriate in physically active persons with mild angina and normal ventricular function. Several studies have documented the prognostic value of exercise ECG testing (37,38), radionuclide ventriculography at rest and with exercise (39–41) and stress thallium studies (42,43). Whereas ambulatory monitoring for silent ischemia has been shown to contain important prognostic information in highly selected patients (44–46), its use as a general screening technique in patients at low risk for coronary artery disease in clinical practice has not been established (47). Profound early ischemia with standard stress tests identifies patients at relatively high risk of a subsequent cardiac event and coronary arteriography is indicated. This inference is based on evidence from randomized trials and observational data base studies documenting improved survival of specific angiographic subgroups of patients with stable angina treated with coronary bypass surgery rather than an initial strategy of medical therapy. These studies have emphasized a consistent trend: the higher the risk for subsequent events based on anatomy, left ventricular function and severity of myocardial ischemia, the greater the degree of benefit from coronary artery bypass surgery as compared with medical therapy. Therefore, definition of coronary anatomy and left ventricular global function is necessary in patients with mild symptoms and profound ischemia on stress testing if the patient is a candidate for bypass surgery from a general medical point of view.

Indication for surgery or angioplasty. Patients with angina pectoris associated with >50% luminal diameter narrowing of the left main coronary artery (48) or triple vessel disease and abnormal left ventricular function are generally believed to have better survival with surgery as compared with medical therapy (28,49–53). In the Coronary Artery Surgery Study (CASS) randomized trial, no difference in survival of patients with mild angina and three vessel disease with normal left ventricular function (or single or double vessel disease) was observed in those randomized to an initial strategy of medical therapy compared with those randomized to coronary bypass surgery (54). This observation emphasizes the importance of studies that have documented the value of risk stratification in patients with triple vessel coronary artery disease to define those with a major benefit in survival with bypass surgery (55,56). There are data to support surgical treatment of patients with two vessel disease who have severe angina in association with depressed left ventricular function (57).

Invasive therapy (surgery or angioplasty) is reserved for patients with single vessel disease and disabling symptoms or those with a large area of myocardium at jeopardy with documentation of early profound ischemia on stress testing. Revascularization may be necessary in some patients with single and double vessel disease for control of angina pectoris or protection of large areas of myocardium from subsequent myocardial infarction. However, with the increasing confidence in coronary angioplasty, more patients with single and double vessel disease are coming to angioplasty with less convincing indications. The restenosis rates associated with angioplasty (58,59) should temper enthusiasm for an aggressive approach with angioplasty based solely on anatomic findings in patients at low risk for subsequent events. Most approaches to prevent restenosis have failed (60) and a recent report (61) on the use of fish oil in reducing restenosis needs further study. If the risk for subsequent cardiac events is low in an individual patient, successful accomplishment of angioplasty, while technically satisfying in the short term, may not be in the best interests of the patient. Although criticism from cardiologists regarding surgical treatment of single vessel disease was frequent before angioplasty was available, less is said now that the therapy can be accomplished with coronary angioplasty.

Aggressive invasive treatment of any kind seems doomed to failure if the symptoms are not clearly related to myocardial ischemia (62). Use of angioplasty in patients without definite angina and myocardial ischemia often results in patients with recurrent chest pain, and the multiple subsequent angiographic studies performed to clarify coronary anatomy result in continuing disability and large medical and emotional costs. The same can of course be said of inappropriately applied coronary bypass surgery.

Cost of surgery. Because of the large volume and expense of coronary bypass operations, the procedure remains under close scrutiny in the era of cost containment. It is estimated that in 1986 well over 200,000 coronary bypass procedures were performed (63). An increasing proportion of operations are performed in elderly patients (Fig. 13.1) and those requiring reoperation. The appropriateness of bypass surgery has thus been the subject of considerable debate and study. In one study, Winslow et al. (64) studied the appropriateness of surgery in three randomly selected hospitals in the western United States. In this small sample of patients (n = 386), only 56% of patients were considered ''appropriate'' for coronary bypass surgery by an expert panel. Although this consideration is unfortunate, it demonstrates the need for professional education and guidelines for therapy. When appropriately applied, bypass surgery has been demonstrated to be a highly cost effective therapy (65).

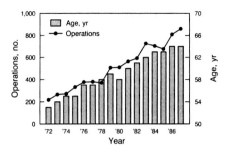

Figure 13.1. Isolated coronary bypass operations at the Mayo Clinic and average age of patients by year (1972 through 1986 inclusive).

Internal mammary versus vein grafts. Although antiplatelet therapy before and after operation improves aortocoronary vein graft patency (66), there remains a major problem with long-term results of vein graft conduits for relief of myocardial ischemia (67). Loop et al. (68) and others have demonstrated that improved late patency of the internal mammary artery increases patient survival over that in patients who receive only saphenous vein grafts. The clinically documented advantages of internal mammary artery versus vein grafting have a physiologic basis as proposed by Luescher et al. (69). The importance of internal mammary artery grafting is further emphasized by the late follow-up data on surgically treated patients in the early large randomized trials with vein grafts as conduits (70,71), which revealed a decline in survival advantages of surgical therapy after 5 to 8 years. These data emphasize the need for careful yearly surveillance of patients after bypass surgery. Equally important is the yearly follow-up of patients treated medically.

Medical treatment. If medical treatment is deemed appropriate for treatment of angina pectoris, the clinician has three classes of drugs available for control of angina pectoris. These are beta-adrenergic blockers, calcium channel entry blockers and nitrates. The choice of these drugs or their use in combination is based on the individual characteristics of the patient (72). Long-acting nitrates may be effective in patients with mild angina, particularly in those who are relatively inactive. There may be a great cost advantage for nitrates if symptom relief is the only objective. Physicians using nitrates must be aware not only of the pharmacology of the multiple products available but also the cost implications of the various modes of administration. Considering the tolerance issue with long-term administration of nitrates, an oral preparation used two to three times daily may have advantages for most patients. However, in more active patients with coexistent hypertension, drugs that control blood pressure and heart rate may optimize the relation between myocardial oxygen demand and supply. A major advance in our understanding of the pathophysiology of angina pectoris occurred with the observations of Chierchia et al. (73) documenting the importance of vasoactivity of the coronary circulation in patients with coronary artery

disease, thus challenging the dogma that myocardial oxygen demand is the most important determinant of myocardial ischemia. This concept provided new approaches for medical therapy (74). The theoretical and objective documentation of beta-blocker efficacy has been indisputably established. Calcium channel blockers have rapidly established their place in the therapeutic armamentarium of angina pectoris. In patients with variant angina, calcium channel blockers and nitrates are the drugs of choice. Enthusiasm for the calcium channel blockers as monotherapy has diminished. However, their synergistic action with beta-blocker drugs may be very helpful, but the increased instance of side effects needs to be borne in mind. The effectiveness of current drugs individually and in combination to provide relief of angina pectoris has been documented in multiple placebo *controlled* trials (75,76).

Revascularization procedures. For patients in whom revascularization is considered appropriate, we still do not have data from *controlled* studies to help choose between coronary angioplasty or bypass surgery as the initial therapy in patients suitable for either procedure. Fortunately a Veterans Administration trial will provide much needed data for patients with single and double vessel disease. There are other studies comparing angioplasty and surgery in multivessel coronary artery disease, including the Emory Angioplasty Surgery Trial (EAST), Bypass Angioplasty Revascularization Investigation (BARI) and several European studies.

Unstable Angina

It has been known for many years that patients with unstable angina are at high risk for subsequent cardiac events (77–79). Whereas some investigators (80) have considered recent onset angina as an exception to this concept, others (81) have provided evidence to support a high risk of subsequent events in such patients. Other patterns of rest pain with ECG changes seem to identify high risk patients (82,83).

Initial management. The patient who presents with increasingly severe angina including episodes of pain at rest is best treated in the hospital with ECG monitoring. Most would agree with an initial effort to provide pain relief with medical therapy before proceeding to coronary arteriography. Use of all three classes of antianginal drugs may be necessary. Intravenous nitroglycerin combined with a beta-blocker represents the first approach unless there is good evidence for coronary vasospasm as a primary mechanism. In addition to beneficial effects on heart rate and blood pressure, beta-blockers have other advantages (84,85). Calcium channel blockers have also been shown to be effective (86,87) but if nifedipine is used, its combination with beta-blocking treatment is wise (88).

Antithrombotic and antiplatelet therapy. Instability of atherosclerotic plaques with thrombus formation (89–93) has been established as the pathogenesis for this syndrome. Thus, it is not surprising that clinical studies are confirming an important role for the use of heparin and antiplatelet treatment. Fitzgerald et al. (94) demonstrated platelet activation in patients with unstable coronary artery disease, and we now have two well designed trials (95,96) establishing the benefit of aspirin therapy in reducing cardiac mortality and other events in patients with unstable angina. Activation of the intrinsic coagulation cascade occurs in patients with unstable angina and is manifested by elevated fibrinopeptide (97). Theroux et al. (98) have also reported a double-blind, randomized, placebo-controlled trial showing independent beneficial effects of heparin and aspirin in reducing cardiac events in the short term (mean of 6 days) in patients with unstable angina. Given the role of thrombus in pathogenesis of unstable angina, the use of fibrinolytic drugs is receiving attention (99) but will require further study in properly designed trials.

Coronary interventions and revascularization. Whereas the aspirin trials in patients with unstable angina have documented one of the few survival benefits of drug therapy in patients with coronary artery disease, most cardiologists favor proceeding with coronary angiography early, though with a patient in stable condition if possible. Inability to stabilize an unstable condition with drugs may require mechanical support with intraaortic balloon pumping. Once coronary anatomy is defined, a decision on invasive revascularization therapy is necessary. Suitability of lesions for either coronary angioplasty or bypass surgery must be decided (36) and then a decision must be made as to advisability of proceeding with either on the basis of an integration of the likelihood of success, risks and the individual patient profile. Most would base the decision to intervene with bypass surgery on accepted anatomic subsets of patients as previously described while preferring angioplasty for single vessel or less extensive multivessel disease in patients with ongoing symptoms of ischemia who are unresponsive to medical treatment. These judgments are influenced importantly by the Veterans Administration study of bypass surgery in unstable angina (100), which demonstrated a benefit in survival only in patients with a moderate decrease in left ventricular function and triple vessel disease. In our own practice, revascularization is recommended in essentially all clinically and anatomically suitable subsets of patients with unstable angina before hospital discharge. Although many observational studies (101) have documented success rates and problems for coronary angioplasty in unstable angina, the assumption that results from surgical trials apply to angioplasty is not proved. This problem further emphasizes the importance of ongoing clinical trials to compare, directly the benefits and adverse effects of an initial angioplasty versus surgical strategy in patients with unstable angina.

Myocardial Infarction

Extraordinary advances have occurred in treating patients with myocardial infarction; these have been based on redefining the primary pathophysiologic events leading to myocardial infarction. Whereas Herrick (102) suggested that thrombus has a primary role in causing myocardial infarction, others (103) considered most thrombi in the infarct-related artery to be secondary events. However, the work of Davies and Thomas (92) and Falk (93) reemphasizing the role of plaque fissuring leading to acute thrombosis at such sites, and the clinical studies of DeWood et al. (104) documenting acute coronary thrombosis in the earliest phase of acute myocardial infarction provided a new stimulus for investigation of thrombolytic therapy.

Thrombolytic and antiplatelet therapy. Excellent data from clinical trials have now been published documenting improved survival after intravenous thrombolytic drug therapy (105–110). In Figure 13.2 early mortality is compared in the placebo versus treatment groups in the large trials of intravenous thrombolytic therapy. There is a consistent trend of enhanced survival in patients receiving thrombolytic therapy as compared with those receiving placebo.

In spite of the survival benefit noted in these trials, a small but definite increase in reinfarction rates followed successful thrombolytic therapy in most trials with use of antiplatelet treatment. Figure 13.3 summarizes a comparison between placebo and treatment groups for several of the trials of intravenous thrombolytic therapy. Note the reduced reinfarction rates in the Second International Study of Infarct Survival (ISIS-2) subgroups treated with aspirin alone or with combined streptokinase and aspirin. These decreases may be the clinical expression of the important observations of Fitzgerald et al. (111) documenting platelet activation as thrombolysis proceeds after streptokinase. Platelet activation with release not only of thromboxane but also of serotonin has been reported after thrombolysis with tissue plasminogen activator (rt-PA) (112). Activation of coagulation with thrombolysis has also been reported (113). It therefore appears that antiplatelet therapy in conjunction with thrombolytic therapy at the onset of acute myocardial infarction prevents or reduces platelet activation in this setting with a reduction in reinfarction rates. The complex nature of the interaction among platelets, ongoing thrombolysis, the actual clot and underlying arterial disease presents other possible approaches to therapy (114).

Combined thrombolysis and angioplasty. With the observed reinfarction rates (115) and the observed high grade residual obstruction evident after successful thrombolysis, a rationale for combining coronary angioplasty with intravenous thrombolysis was proposed. However, data from several trials (116–118) have consistently shown no advantage in routine early angioplasty in the setting of active thrombolytic therapy. The place of coronary angioplasty as a primary modality to open an infarct-related artery is not

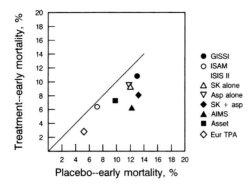

Figure 13.2. Survival data from randomized trials of intravenous thrombolytic therapy in acute myocardial infarction. The early mortality rate is compared for the treatment group on the vertical axis with the placebo group on the horizontal axis. AIMS = APSAC Intervention Mortality Study; Asp = aspirin; Eur TPA = European TPA; GISSI = Gruppo Italiano per lo Studio della Streptochinasi nell'Infarto Miocardico; ISAM = Intravenous Streptokinase in Acute Myocardial Infarction trial; ISIS II = Second International Study of Infarct Survival; SK = streptokinase.

settled primarily because, except for a study by O'Neill et al. (119), we have no controlled studies of angioplasty alone versus thrombolytic therapy alone. Angioplasty as primary therapy to open infarct-related arteries needs further study because 20% to 30% of patients presenting with myocardial infarction may have contraindication to thrombolytic therapy (105). Such patients presenting within 4 h of infarction may benefit from mechanical opening of the infarct-related artery. Feasibility of this approach has been demonstrated in observational studies (120,121), as well as by O'Neill et al. (119), with an approximately 85% success rate in opening the infarct-related artery. Additional advantages may include earlier opening of the infarct-related artery with benefit to patients in cardiogenic shock and less risk of bleeding complications.

Decision protocol. The physician considering thrombolytic therapy for a patient with an acute myocardial infarc-

Figure 13.3. Early reinfarction rates after intravenous thrombolytic therapy in acute myocardial infarction. The treatment group is on the vertical axis and the placebo group on the horizontal axis. Abbreviations as in Figure 13.2.

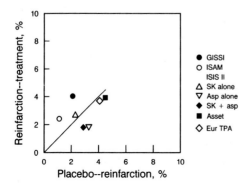

tion must make major decisions decisively and early. First, an accurate diagnosis of myocardial ischemic infarction is mandatory. Age of the patient remains a difficult issue. No trial has sufficient numbers of patients over the age of 80 years to conclude that the benefit of thrombolytic therapy justifies the risk; high complication rates have been reported in at least one major study (122). However, mortality rates in elderly patients with myocardial infarction are high and in some patients the potential benefit of thrombolytic treatment may justify the risk. Although most investigators have concluded that the ideal time for intervention and thrombolytic treatment is ≤4 h after onset of symptoms, in ISIS-2 benefit was noted through 24 h after symptom onset, thus suggesting an increased time frame for intervention. In ISIS-2, however, a significant proportion of the patients did not meet criteria for acute myocardial infarction at time of randomization and represented patients with unstable myocardial ischemia or a slowly evolving infarction. The choice of a thrombolytic drug is controversial. Increased effectiveness in clot lysis has been documented with rt-PA, but clinical effectiveness in reducing mortality of acute infarction has been proved with both streptokinase and rt-PA. Several large randomized trials have been designed to compare streptokinase versus rt-PA with respect to survival and complications to assess whether the early effects of rt-PA on patency will be associated with better survival.

Other advances in management of acute infarction. Although thrombolysis and angioplasty have attracted a great deal of attention, other extremely important advances in managing patients with acute myocardial infarction have occurred. Hemodynamic monitoring has played an important role in managing a subset of patients with hemodynamic instability (123,124). Intravenous nitroglycerin reduces infarct size (125) and mortality (126), but recognition of the problem of nitrate tolerance in prolonged use of the drug is essential (127). Approaches with vasoactive drugs to help stabilize hemodynamically unstable patients are well established and the recognition of hypovolemia as a cause of hypotension in acute infarction has been a major contribution of hemodynamic monitoring. The role of left ventricular assist devices, as a substitute for intraaortic balloon pumping, is receiving increased attention, and these may serve as a bridge to cardiac transplantation in properly selected patients. Another major advance has occurred in recognition and management of patients with right ventricular infarction (128–130).

Role of beta-adrenergic blockers. Documentation of improved survival and reduced reinfarction rates for patients with myocardial infarction treated with a beta-blocker is one of the most effectively documented effects of drug therapy in cardiology (131–133). Although benefit has been observed even when therapy is started several days after the acute event, recent data (134) support administration of a beta-blocker in the acute phase of infarction unless there are contraindications to its use. The major benefit appears to occur in patients with more complicated myocardial infarction (135). Calcium channel blockers have also been tested in the setting of Q wave infarction with either no benefit or adverse effects (136,137), particularly in patients with a left ventricular ejection fraction <40% (138). In spite of the large volume of published data demonstrating the effectiveness of beta-blockers in reducing subsequent cardiac events, especially sudden death and recurrent infarction, many patients who have no contraindication to these agents are still not receiving them after an acute infarction. Failure to provide this treatment is justified only if the patient is demonstrated to be in a low risk category and its occurrence illustrates a continuing problem of inadequate monitoring of the results of continuing education on the actual practice of physicians.

Non-Q wave infarction. The differentiation of non-Q wave from Q wave infarction is now established as important clinically although the ability of the former to predict absolute transmural distribution of myocardial necrosis is recognized as flawed. The clinical features and subsequent outcome of patients with preservation of QRS integrity but with major repolarization abnormalities and elevated creatine kinase (CK) MB isoenzyme levels have been well described. Most investigators (139) agree that the basic coronary anatomic feature is usually an incomplete occlusion of the infarct-related coronary artery. With a persisting high grade stenosis, it is not surprising there is a high rate of subsequent myocardial infarction (140). Diltiazem has been documented to reduce reinfarction rates (141). However, the continued hemodynamic instability of such patients is reflected in a significant rate of reinfarction even with diltiazem and a high proportion of patients who require early coronary angiography and appropriate revascularization. Few studies have examined the role of stress testing for risk stratification after non-Q wave myocardial infarction and further data are needed. The lack of a direct comparison of outcomes between bypass surgery and angioplasty in controlled studies hampers our conclusions on advisability of an initial strategy of angioplasty or surgery. No direct comparisons of invasive treatment versus medical therapy alone in patients with non-Q wave infarction have been published.

Evaluation and therapy of survivors of myocardial infarction. A major issue in management of patients with myocardial infarction is the risk stratification of those who have survived the initial hospital admission and are being prepared for discharge. The three major determinants of late prognosis after an acute myocardial infarction include 1) the extent of left ventricular dysfunction; 2) the presence and severity of residual myocardial ischemia; and 3) ventricular arrhythmias. Post-infarction residual ischemia carries a poor prognosis but is readily amenable to treatment, usually by coronary revascularization. Experimental data in regard to the ability of afterload-reducing agents to modify left ventricular dysfunction are encouraging and clinical studies (142) have documented this in post-myocardial infarction patients. Additional large clinical trials are evaluating this

problem. The adverse impact on prognosis of ventricular arrhythmias is well recognized (143), but the ability of antiarrhythmic therapy to improve survival of symptomatic patients is uncertain and also the subject of current large scale trials.

With this uncertainty in mind, the evaluation of survivors of myocardial infarction should include a measurement of left ventricular function and, in hemodynamically stable patients without angina, noninvasive stress testing before hospital discharge. It is generally accepted that radionuclide studies enhance the sensitivity and specificity of stress testing, but only when they are performed in centers proficient and experienced in using these complex, quantitative imaging modalities. In patients with postinfarction angina, particularly if it occurs with minimal exertion, prompt angiography with a view toward revascularization is indicated and most physicians would perform this study before stress testing. Signal-averaged ECG studies may be useful in the future to identify those patients at risk for malignant ventricular arrhythmias. Additional tests should be obtained only if the information derived is of incremental value beyond data obtained on review of the bedside clinical profile (144).

The question of coronary angiography before hospital discharge, particularly in patients who have had successful thrombolysis, remains controversial (145). Many investigators would compare these patients to patients previously categorized as having non-Q wave infarction, particularly if myocardial salvage has occurred and there is a residual high grade stenosis remaining with demonstrable ischemia in the distribution of this infarct-related artery. Additional studies will be necessary to establish the role of invasive therapy in these asymptomatic patients with a residual high grade lesion after successful thrombolytic therapy.

Sudden Cardiac Death

Of the almost 1 million deaths that occur each year in the United States, half can be attributed to ischemic heart disease, and almost half of these deaths occur suddenly. Our ability to detect patients at risk of experiencing sudden cardiac death and to effectively treat the underlying ischemic heart disease has increased tremendously since 1949 as described in the preceding sections of this review. The development of cardiac defibrillators and cardiopulmonary resuscitation has permitted us to retrieve from certain death many such patients both in and out of the hospital. The availability of electrophysiologic testing and signal-averaged ECGs help us to better understand and treat survivors of sudden cardiac death (146–148). In 1949 we had only quinidine to medically treat patients with ischemic heart disease who presented with life-threatening ventricular arrhythmias. Today we have an extensive array of effective drugs ranging (in potency and toxicity) from lidocaine to amiodarone. When medical treatment of ventricular arrhythmia proves unsuccessful, surgical options are available that include ablation of ventricular scars or resection of ventricular aneurysm with or without coronary bypass surgery (149,150). Implantation of automatic defibrillators is also occurring and the future of the ultimate defibrillator holds real promise. In short, we have altered an attitude of pessimism and futility in our approach to sudden cardiac death as a manifestation of coronary artery disease in 1949 to a very dynamic process with effective treatment options for many patients in 1989.

Congestive Heart Failure

Patients with coronary artery disease may manifest congestive heart failure because of 1) extensive myocardial necrosis leading to pump failure; 2) mechanical complications of myocardial infarction; and 3) reversible myocardial ischemia. The challenge of the clinician managing the patient with coronary artery disease and congestive heart failure is to determine the relative contribution of these factors to the individual patient's problem. Whereas some cases are obvious clinically, others can be frustrating particularly when components of ischemia are present (angina, reversible perfusion defects) in addition to heart failure. The correct classification is important because revascularization may enhance survival and relieve symptoms of heart failure if there is a concomitant component of reversible ischemia (151).

Early recognition of the mechanical complications of myocardial infarction is critically important in the setting of acute infarction because surgical therapy may dramatically improve the outlook. This possibility is particularly likely for papillary muscle rupture (152), postinfarction ventricular septal defect (153) and, rarely, cardiac perforation (154).

Risk Factor Control

A third category of treatment decisions crucial in the long-term management of patients with coronary artery disease, regardless of the treatment for symptom control or enhanced event-free survival, is control of risk factors and establishing a rational life style. It is important for the patient and family to recognize that such efforts are a life-long process and that coronary surgery and angioplasty are only palliative forms of therapy. Abundant evidence is available to support an aggressive approach to risk factor control, although the strength of evidence for benefit with control of each risk factor varies.

Smoking. Avoidance of tobacco is fundamental to the long-term success of any therapeutic program in patients with coronary artery disease. Enhanced survival after cessation of smoking has been demonstrated in large samples of postmyocardial infarction patients (155), those with angiographically documented coronary artery disease (156) and others in large population-based studies (157). Behavior modification remains a major challenge in dealing with patients addicted to tobacco use.

Hypertension. Control of hypertension has failed to affect coronary heart disease mortality directly in large trials (158). However, reduced stroke and overall mortality rates emphasize the importance of hypertension control (158,159). In addition to the benefits of systemic arterial pressure treatment, which should initially be non-pharmacologic, some of the drugs utilized (calcium channel and beta-blockers) provide more direct approaches to relief of associated myocardial ischemia.

Hypercholesterolemia. There are data to support aggressive efforts for lipid-lowering programs, particularly in patients with clearly elevated serum levels (>250 mg) and those with documented coronary heart disease. The data presented thus far suggest some reduction in cardiac mortality (160,161) and reduced rates of progression of coronary artery lesions in patients with high pretreatment serum lipid levels after successful lipid reduction is accomplished (162). Details of a systematic approach to lipid lowering have been published by an expert panel of the National Heart, Lung, and Blood Institute (163). The addition of HMG-CoA reductase inhibitors (Lovastatin) for reduction of cholesterol levels is a major advance (164), particularly in those patients not responsive to more simple dietary measures or other drugs. Reduction in cholesterol appears to benefit patients after coronary bypass surgery in terms of enhancing graft patency and reducing progression of disease (165).

Exercise training. Exercise remains an important part of the overall program for all patients with coronary disease, however treated, as well as in general prevention efforts (166). There is documentation (167) of improvement in myocardial performance and reduction in myocardial ischemia associated with achieving certain training levels. Several surveys (168,169) analyzing objectively the benefits of cardiac rehabilitation are available.

Thoughtful critiques of some of the described trials and an overemphasis of application of population-wide risk factor control should be noted (170,171). Those who are engaged in active patient care are aware of the hazards of unrealistic expectations of some patients with risk factor control, and this applies also to society in general.

Conclusions. Extraordinary advances in the management of patients with coronary artery disease have occurred and we can look forward to continued progress. A disturbing note, however, in the accomplishments of the past 40 years is the recognition that the rate of decline in cardiovascular mortality is being maintained only in white men (172). This fact raises important questions for the medical profession as well as for society in general, and consideration of this must be included in our strategy not only for future developments, but for having an equitable distribution of the benefits of medical science to the entire population.

With ever more choices available, the clinician is challenged to identify the safest and most effective treatment for each individual patient. Steps in this process learned today will be valuable in coming years as many more intravascular devices and biologically sophisticated drugs are introduced.

References

1. Frisk AR, Lindgren I. Methylthiouracil (thiourea derivative) in treatment of congestive heart failure and angina pectoris: results of prolonged treatment. Acta Med Scand 1948;132:69–90.

2. Fisher RL, Zukerman M. Propylthiouracil (thiourea derivative): preliminary report. Am Pract 1949;3:318–20.

3. Sniehotta H. Therapy of angina pectoris associated with coronary sclerosis with methylthiouracil (thiourea derivative). Deutsch Med Wochnschr 1949;74:340–2.

4. Raab W. Propylthiouracil (thiourea derivative). Acta Med Scand 1949; 135:364–73.

5. Pereira A, Tullio de Assis Fiqueiredo M. Thiouracil (thiourea derivative) with special reference to thyroadrenosympathogenic mechanism. Argent Clin 1949;8:79–100.

6. Bolivar J, Rabina P. Thyroidectomy. Rev Cubana Cardiol 1949;10:145–86.

7. Guillaume J, Mazars G. Posterior radicotomies. Presse Med 1948;56:690–1.

8. Danielopolu D. Present status of surgical therapy: necessary anatomicophysiologic concepts. Cardiologia 1949;14:1–25.

9. Danielopolu D. Present status of surgical therapy: physiologic basis and results of method of suppression of pressor reflex: disadvantages of stellectomy. Cardiologia 1949;14:45–80.

10. Stubinger HG, Busse W. Procaine hydrochloride blocking of stellate ganglion with special regard to electrocardiographic findings. Deutsch Med Wochnschr 1949;74:546–9.

11. Welti H, Oury P, Venet A. Late results of posterior, dorsal radicotomies in therapy: 4 cases. Mem Acad Chir 1949;75:364–70.

12. Lian C. New trends in medical and surgical therapy: procaine hydrochloride infiltrations and resection of preaortic nerve plexus. Sem Med 1949;2:82–4.

13. Lian C, Siguier F, Crosnier L, Crosnier J. Procaine hydrochloride infiltration and resection of preaortic nerve plexus. Arch Mal Coeur 1949;42:215–7. Paris Med 1949;39:305–7.

14. Lian C, Siguier F, Crosnier L, Crosnier J. Resection of preaortic nerve plexus in therapy of angina of coronary origin with frequent and painful crises: 19 cases. Bull Mem Soc Med Hop Paris 1948;65:867–77.

15. Ravin IA, Katz KH. Vitamin E. N Engl J Med 1949;240:331–3.

16. Rush HP. Experience with vitamin E in coronary disease. Calif Med 1949;71:391–3.

17. Travell J, Rinzler SH, Bakst H, Benjamin ZH, Bobb AL. Therapy, comparison of effects of alpha-tocopherol and matching placebo on chest pain in patients with heart disease. Ann NY Acad Sci 1949;52:345–53.

18. Havlick RJ, Feinleit M, eds. Proceedings of the Conference on the Decline in Coronary Heart Disease Mortality. Washington, DC: National Institutes of Health, 1979.

19. Raglund K, Selvin S, Merrill DW. The onset of decline in ischemic heart disease mortality in the United States. Am J Epidemiol 1988;127:516–31.

20. Goldman L, Cook EF. The decline in ischemic heart disease mortality rates in the United States: an analysis of the comparative effects of medical interventions and changes in life style. Ann Intern Med 1984; 101:825–36.

21. Vlietstra RE, Assad-Morell JL, Frye RL, et al. Survival predictors in coronary artery disease. Mayo Clin Proc 1977;52:85–90.

22. Nelson GR, Cohn PF, Gorlin R. Prognosis in medically-treated coronary artery disease: influence of ejection fraction compared to other parameters. Circulation 1975;52:408–12.

23. Peduzzi P. Relation of severity of symptoms to prognosis in stable angina pectoris. Am J Cardiol 1984;54:988–93.

24. Califf RM, Mark DB, Harrell FE Jr, et al. Importance of clinical measures of ischemia in the prognosis of patients with documented coronary artery disease. J Am Coll Cardiol 1988;11:20–6.

25. Block WJ Jr, Crumpacker EL, Dry TJ, et al. Prognosis of angina pectoris: observations in 6882 cases. JAMA 1952;150:259–64.

26. Ladenheim ML, Kotler TS, Pollock BH, et al. Incremental prognostic power of clinical history, exercise electrocardiography and myocardial perfusion scintigraphy in suspected coronary artery disease. Am J Cardiol 1987;59:270–7.

27. Peduzzi P, Hultgren HN. Effect of medical vs surgical treatment on symptoms in stable angina pectoris: the Veterans Administration Cooperative Study of surgery for coronary arterial occlusive disease. Circulation 1979;60:888–99.

28. European Coronary Surgery Study Group. Long term results of prospective randomized study of coronary artery bypass surgery in stable angina pectoris. Lancet 1982;2:1173–80.

29. CASS Principal Investigators and their Associates. Coronary Artery Surgery Study (CASS): a randomized trial of coronary artery bypass surgery; quality of life in patients randomly assigned to treatment groups. Circulation 1983;68:951–60.

30. Kloster FE, Kremkau EL, Ritzmann LW, Rahimtoola SH, Rosch J, Hanarek PH. Coronary bypass for stable angina: a prospective randomized study. N Engl J Med 1979;300:149–57.

31. Hultgren HN, Peduzzi P, Detre K, Takaro T and the Study Participants. The five-year effect of bypass surgery on relief of angina and exercise performance. Circulation 1985;72(suppl V):V-79–V-83.

32. Gruntzig HR, Senning A, Seigenthaler WE. Non-operative dilatation of coronary artery stenosis: percutaneous transluminal coronary angioplasty. N Engl J Med 1979;301:61–8.

33. Kent KM, Bentirogio LG, Block PC, et al. Long-term efficacy of percutaneous transluminal coronary angioplasty (PTCA): report from the National Heart, Lung, and Blood Institute PTCA Registry. Am J Cardiol 1984;53:27C–31C.

34. Holmes DR, Van Raden MJ, Reeder GS, et al. Return to work after coronary angioplasty: a report from the National Heart, Lung, and Blood Institute Percutaneous Transluminal Coronary Angioplasty Registry. Am J Cardiol 1984;53:48C–51C.

35. Mabin TA, Holmes DR, Smith HC, et al. Follow-up clinical results in patients undergoing percutaneous transluminal coronary angioplasty. Circulation 1985;71:754–60.

36. ACC/AHA Task Force Report. Guidelines for percutaneous transluminal coronary angioplasty. J Am Coll Cardiol 1988;12:529–45.

37. Mark DB, Hlatky MA, Harrell FE Jr, Lee KL, Califf RM, Pryor DB. Exercise treadmill score for predicting prognosis in coronary artery disease. Ann Intern Med 1987;106:793–800.

38. Rautaharju PM, Prineas RJ, Eifler WJ, et al. Prognostic value of exercise electrocardiogram in men at high risk of future coronary heart disease: multiple risk factor intervention trial experience. J Am Coll Cardiol 1986;8:1–10.

39. Bonow RO, Kent KM, Rosing DR, et al. Exercise-induced ischemia in mildly symptomatic patients with coronary artery disease and preserved left ventricular function: identification of subgroups at risk of death during medical therapy. N Engl J Med 1984;311:1339–45.

40. Pryor DB, Harrell FE Jr., Lee KL, et al. Prognostic indicators from radionuclide angiography in medically treated patients with coronary artery disease. Am J Cardiol 1984;53:18–22.

41. Taliercio CP, Clements IP, Zinsmeister AR, Gibbons RJ. Prognostic value and limitations of exercise radionuclide angiography in medically treated coronary artery disease. Mayo Clin Proc 1988;63:573–82.

42. Kaul S, Lilly DR, Gascho JA, et al. Prognostic utility of the exercise thallium-201 test in ambulatory patients with chest pain: comparison with cardiac catheterization. Circulation 1988;77:745–58.

43. Ladenheim ML, Pollock MPH, Rozanski A, et al. Extent and severity of myocardial hypoperfusion as predictors of prognosis in patients with suspected coronary artery disease. J Am Coll Cardiol 1986;7:464–71.

44. Gottlieb SO, Weisfeldt ML, Ouyang P, Mellits ED, Gerstenblith G. Silent ischemia as a marker for early unfavorable outcomes in patients with unstable angina. N Engl J Med 1986;314:1214–9.

45. Rocco MB, Nabel EG, Campbell S, et al. Prognostic importance of myocardial ischemia detected by ambulatory monitoring in patients with stable coronary artery disease. Circulation 1988;78:877–84.

46. Vaghaiwalla M, Koonlawee N, Intrachot V, et al. Severity of silent myocardial ischemia on ambulatory electrocardiographic monitoring in patients with stable angina pectoris: relation to prognostic determinants during exercise stress testing and coronary angiography. J Am Coll Cardiol 1988;12:1169–76.

47. Berman DS, Roganski A, Knoebel SB. The detection of silent ischemia: cautions and precautions. Circulation 1987;75:101–5.

48. Takaro T, Hultgren HN, Lipton MJ, Detre KM and Participants in the Study Group. The VA cooperative randomized study of surgery for coronary arterial occlusive disease. II. Subgroup with significant left main lesions. Circulation 1976;54(suppl III):III-107–III-16.

49. Takaro T, Hultgren HN, Detre KM, et al. The VA cooperative study on stable angina: current status. Circulation 1982;65(suppl II):II-60–II-67.

50. Kaiser GC, Davis KB, Fisher LD, et al. Survival following coronary artery bypass grafting in patients with severe angina pectoris (CASS): an observational study. J Thorac Cardiovasc Surg 1985;89:513–22.

51. Hlatky MA, Califf RM, Harrell FE, et al. Comparison of predictions based on observational data with the results of randomized controlled clinical trials of coronary artery bypass surgery. J Am Coll Cardiol 1988;11:237–45.

52. DeRouen TA, Hammermeister KE, Dodge HT. Comparisons of the effects on survival after coronary artery surgery in subgroups of patients from the Seattle Heart Watch. Circulation 1981;63:537–45.

53. Passamani E, Davis KB, Gillespie MJ, Killip T and the CASS Principal Investigators and their Associates. A randomized trial of coronary artery bypass surgery: survival of patients with a low ejection fraction. N Engl J Med 1985;312:1665–71.

54. CASS Principal Investigators and Their Associates. Coronary artery surgery study: a randomized trial of coronary artery bypass surgery; survival data. Circulation 1983;68:939–50.

55. Detre K, Peduzzi P, Murphy M, et al. and the Veterans Administration Cooperative Study for Surgery for Coronary Arterial Occlusive Disease. Effect of bypass surgery on survival in patients in low- and high-risk subgroups delineated by the use of simple clinical variables. Circulation 1981;63:1329–37.

56. Weiner DA, Ryan TJ, McCabe CH, et al. Value of exercise testing in determining the risk classification and the response to coronary artery bypass grafting in three-vessel coronary artery disease: a report from the Coronary Artery Surgery Study (CASS) Registry. Am J Cardiol 1987;60:262–6.

57. Mock MB, Fisher LD, Holmes DR Jr, et al. and Participants in the Coronary Artery Surgery Study: comparison of effects of medical and surgical therapy on survival in severe angina pectoris and two-vessel coronary artery disease with and without left ventricular dysfunction: a Coronary Artery Surgery Study Registry study. Am J Cardiol 1988;61:1198–203.

58. Holmes DR Jr, Vlietstra RE, Smith HC, et al. Restenosis after percutaneous transluminal coronary angioplasty (PTCA): a report from the PTCA registry of the National Heart, Lung, and Blood Institute. Am J Cardiol 1984;53(suppl C):C-77–81.

59. Lermgruber PP, Roubin ES, Hollman J, et al. Restenosis after successful coronary angioplasty in patients with single vessel disease. Circulation 1986;73:710–7.

60. Schwartz L, Bourassa MG, Lesperance J, et al. Aspirin and dipyridamole in the prevention of restenosis after percutaneous transluminal coronary angioplasty. N Engl J Med 1988;318:1714–9.

61. Dehmer GJ, Popma JJ, Egerton K, et al. Reduction in the rate of early restenosis after coronary angioplasty by a diet supplemented with n-3 fatty acids. N Engl J Med 1988;319:733–40.

62. Jones RH, Floyd RD, Austin EH, Sabiston DC Jr. The role of radionuclide angiocardiography in the preoperative prediction of pain relief and prolonged survival following coronary artery bypass grafting. Ann Surg 1983;197:743–54.

63. Detailed Diagnosis and Procedures for Patients Discharged from Short Stay Hospitals, U.S. 1986. U.S. Dept. of Health and Human Services publication. National Center for Health Statistics.

64. Winslow CM, Kosecoff JB, Chassin M, Kanouse D, Brook RH. The appropriateness of performing coronary artery bypass surgery. JAMA 1988;260:505–9.

65. Weinstein MC, Stason WB. Cost effectiveness of coronary bypass surgery. Circulation 1982;66(suppl III):III-56–III-66.

66. Chesebro JH, Clements IP, Fuster V, et al. A platelet-inhibitor-drug trial in coronary artery bypass operations: benefit of perioperative dipyridamole and aspirin therapy on early postoperative vein-graft patency. N Engl J Med 1982;307:73–8.

67. Grondin CM, Campeu L, Lesperance J, Enjalbert M, Bourassa MG. Comparison of late changes in internal mammary artery and saphenous vein grafts in two consecutive series of patients 10 years after operation. Circulation 1984;70(suppl I):I-208–I-12.

68. Loop FD, Lytle BW, Cosgrove DM, et al. Influence of the internal-mammary-artery graft on 10-year survival and other cardiac events. N Engl J Med 1986;314:1–6.

69. Luscher TF, Diederich D, Siebermann R, et al. Difference between endothelium-dependent relaxation in arterial and in venous coronary bypass grafts. N Engl J Med 1988;319:462–7.

70. The Veterans Administration Coronary Artery Bypass Surgery Cooperative Study Group. Eleven-year survival in the Veterans Administration randomized trial of coronary bypass surgery for stable angina. N Engl J Med 1984;311:1333–9.

71. Varnauskas E and the European Coronary Surgery Study Group. Twelve-year follow-up of survival in the randomized European Coronary Surgery Study. N Engl J Med 1988;319:332–7.

72. Shub C, Vlietstra RE, McGoon MD. Selection of optimal drug therapy for the patient with angina pectoris. Mayo Clin Proc 1985;60:539–48.

73. Chierchia S, Brunelli C, Simonetti I, et al. Sequence of events in angina at rest: primary reduction in coronary flow. Circulation 1980;61:759–68.

74. Nonogi H, Hess OM, Ritter M, et al. Prevention of coronary vasoconstriction by diltiazem during dynamic exercise in patients with coronary artery disease. J Am Coll Cardiol 1988;12:892–9.

75. de Ponti C, Mauri F, Ciliberto GR, Caru B. Comparative effects of nifedipine, verapamil, isosorbide dinitrate and propranolol on exercise-induced angina pectoris. Eur J Cardiol 1979;10:47–58.

76. Battock DJ, Alvarez H, Chidsey CA. Effects of propranolol and isosorbide dinitrate on exercise performance and adrenergic activity in patients with angina pectoris. Circulation 1969;39:157–69.

77. Russell RO Jr, Moraski RE, Kouchoukos N, et al. Unstable angina pectoris: National Cooperative Study Group to compare surgical and medical therapy. II. In-hospital experience and initial follow-up results in patients with one, two, and three vessel disease. Am J Cardiol 1978;42:839–48.

78. Mulcahy R, Daly L, Graham I, et al. Unstable angina: natural history and determinants of prognosis. Am J Cardiol 1981;48:525–8.

79. Krauss KR, Hutter AM Jr, DeSanctis RW. Acute coronary insufficiency and followup. Arch Intern Med 1972;129:808–13.

80. Duncan B, Fulton M, Morrison SL, et al. Prognosis of new and worsening angina pectoris. Br Med J 1976;1:981–5.

81. Roberts KB, Califf RM, Harrell FE Jr, et al. The prognosis for patients with new-onset angina who have undergone cardiac catheterization. Circulation 1983;68:970–8.

82. Boden WE, Bough EW, Benham I, Shulman RS. Unstable angina with episodic ST segment elevation and minimal creatine kinase release culminating in extensive, recurrent infarction. J Am Coll Cardiol 1983;2:11–20.

83. Blaustein AS, Heller GV, Kolman BS. Adjunctive nifedipine therapy in high-risk, medically refractory, unstable angina pectoris. Am J Cardiol 1983;52:950–4.

84. Campbell WB, Johnson AR, Callahan KS, Graham RM. Anti-platelet activity of beta-adrenergic antagonists: inhibition of thromboxane synthesis and platelet aggregation in patients receiving long-term propranolol treatment. Lancet 1981;2:1382–4.

85. Welman E, Fox KM, Selwyn AP, et al. The effect of established beta-adrenoreceptor blocking therapy on the release of cytoscoloic and lysosomal enzymes after acute myocardial infarction in man. Clin Sci Mol Med 1978;55:549–53.

86. Theroux P, Taeymans Y, Morissette D, Bosch X, Pelletier GB, Waters DD. A randomized study comparing propranolol and diltiazem in the treatment of unstable angina. J Am Coll Cardiol 1985;5:717–22.

87. The Holland Interuniversity Nifedipine/Metroprolol Trial (HINT) Research Group. Early treatment of unstable angina in the coronary care unit: a randomized, double-blind, placebo-controlled comparison of recurrent ischemia in patients treated with nifedipine or metoprolol or both. Br Heart J 1986;56:400–13.

88. Gottlieb SO, Weisfeldt ML, Ouyang P, et al. Effect of the addition of propranolol to therapy with nifedipine for unstable angina pectoris: a randomized, double-blind, placebo-controlled trial. Circulation 1986;73:331–7.

89. Holmes DR Jr, Hartzler GO, Smith HC, Fuster V. Coronary artery thrombosis in patients with unstable angina. Br Heart J 1981;45:411–6.

90. Ambrose JA, Winters SL, Stern A, et al. Angiographic morphology and the pathogenesis of unstable angina pectoris. J Am Coll Cardiol 1985;5: 609–16.

91. Sherman CT, Litvack F, Grundfest W, et al. Coronary angioscopy in patients with unstable angina pectoris. N Engl J Med 1986;315:913–9.

92. Falk E. Unstable angina with fatal outcome: dynamic coronary thrombosis leading to infarction and/or sudden death: autopsy evidence of recurrent mural thrombosis with peripheral embolization culminating in total vascular occlusion. Circulation 1985;71:699–708.

93. Davies MJ, Thomas AC. Plaque fissuring—the cause of acute myocardial infarction, sudden ischaemic death, and crescendo angina. Br Heart J 1985;53:363–73.

94. Fitzgerald DJ, Roy L, Catella F, FitzGerald GA. Platelet activation in unstable coronary disease. N Engl J Med 1986;315:983–9.

95. Lewis HD Jr, Davis JW, Archibald DG, et al. Protective effects of aspirin against acute myocardial infarction and death in men with unstable angina: results of a Veterans Administration Cooperative Study. N Engl J Med 1983;309:396–403.

96. Cairns JA, Gent M, Singer J, et al. Aspirin, sulfinpyrazone, or both in unstable angina: results of a Canadian multicenter trial. N Engl J Med 1985;313:1369–75.

97. Theroux P, Latour JG, Leger-Gauthier C, De Lara J. Fibrinopeptide A and platelet factor levels in unstable angina pectoris. Circulation 1987; 75:156–62.

98. Theroux P, Ouimet H, McCans J, et al. Aspirin, heparin, or both to treat unstable angina. N Engl J Med 1988;319:1105–11.

99. de Zwaan C, Bar FW, Janssen JHA, et al. Effects of thrombolytic therapy in unstable angina: clinical and angiographic results. J Am Coll Cardiol 1988;12:301–9.

100. Luchi RJ, Scott SM, Deupree RH, Principal Investigators and Their Associates of Veterans Administration Cooperative Study No. 28. Comparison of medical and surgical treatment for unstable angina pectoris: results of a Veterans Administration Cooperative Study. N Engl J Med 1987;316:977–84.

101. de Feyter PJ, Suryapranata H, Serruys PW, et al. Coronary angioplasty for unstable angina: immediate and late results in 200 consecutive patients with identification of risk factors for unfavorable early and late outcome. J Am Coll Cardiol 1988;12:324–33.

102. Herrick JB. Clinical features of sudden obstruction of the coronary arteries. JAMA 1912;59:2015.

103. Roberts WC. Coronary arteries in fatal acute myocardial infarction. Circulation 1972;45:215–30.

104. DeWood MA, Spores J, Notske R, et al. Prevalence of total coronary occlusion during the early hours of transmural myocardial infarction. N Engl J Med 1980;303:897–902.

105. Gruppo Italiano per lo Studio della Streptochinasi nell'Infarto Miocardico (GISSI). Effectiveness of intravenous thrombolytic treatment in acute myocardial infarction. Lancet 1986;1:397–402.

106. Wilcox RG, von der Lippe G, Olsson CG, et al. Trial of tissue plasminogen activator for mortality reduction in acute myocardial infarction. Anglo-Scandinavian Study of Early Thrombolysis (ASSET). Lancet 1988;2:525–30.

107. AIMS Trial Study Group. Effect of intravenous APSAC on mortality after acute myocardial infarction: preliminary report of a placebo-controlled clinical trial. Lancet 1988;1:546–9.

108. Van de Werf F, Arnold AER, and the European Cooperative Study Group for Recombinant Tissue-Type Plasminogen Activator (rt-PA). Intravenous tissue plasminogen activator and size of infarct, left ventricular function, and survival in acute myocardial infarction. Br Med J 1988;297:2374–9.

109. ISIS-2 Collaborative Group. Randomized trial of intravenous streptokinase, oral aspirin, both, or neither among 17,187 cases of suspected myocardial infarction. Lancet 1988;2:349–60.

110. Simoons ML, van der Brand M, de Zwabb C, et al. Improved survival after early thrombolysis in acute myocardial infarction. Lancet 1985;2: 578–81.

111. Fitzgerald DJ, Catella F, Roy L, Fitzgerald GD. Marked platelet activation in vivo after intravenous streptokinase in patients with acute myocardial infarction. Circulation 1988;77:142–50.

112. Golino P, Ashton JH, Glas-Greenwalt P, et al. Mediation of reocclusion by thromboxane A2 and serotonin after thrombolysis with tissue-type plasminogen activator in a canine preparation of coronary thrombosis. Circulation 1988;77:678–84.

113. Owen J, Friedman KD, Grossman BA, et al. Thrombolytic therapy with tissue plasminogen activator or streptokinase induces transient thrombin activity. Blood 1988;72:616–20.

114. Gold HK, Coller BS, Yasuda T, et al. Rapid and sustained coronary artery recanalization with combined bolus injection of recombinant tissue-type plasminogen activator and monoclonal antiplatelet GPIIb/IIIa antibody in a canine preparation. Circulation 1988;77:670–7.

115. Schroder R, Neuhaus KL, Leizorovicz A, et al. A prospective placebo-controlled double-blind multicenter trial of Intravenous Streptokinase in Acute Myocardial Infarction (ISAM): long-term mortality and morbidity. J Am Coll Cardiol 1987;9:197–203.

116. Simoons ML, Betriu A, Col J, et al. Thrombolysis with tissue plasminogen activator in acute myocardial infarction: no additional benefit from immediate coronary angioplasty. Lancet 1988;1:197–203.

117. Topol EJ, Califf RM, George BS, et al. A randomized trial of immediate versus delayed elective angioplasty after intravenous tissue plasminogen activator in acute myocardial infarction. N Engl J Med 1987;317:581–8.

118. TIMI Research Group. Immediate vs. delayed catheterization and angioplasty following thrombolytic therapy for acute myocardial infarction. JAMA 1988;260:2849–58.

119. O'Neill W, Timmis GC, Bourdillon PD, et al. A prospective randomized clinical trial of intracoronary streptokinase versus coronary angioplasty for acute myocardial infarction. N Engl J Med 1986;314:812–8.

120. Hartzler GO, Rutherford BD, McConahay MD. Percutaneous transluminal coronary angioplasty: application for acute myocardial infarction. Am J Cardiol 1984;53:117C–21C.

121. Rothbaum DA, Linnemeier TJ, Landin RJ, et al. Emergency percutaneous transluminal coronary angioplasty in acute myocardial infarction: a 3 year experience. J Am Coll Cardiol 1987;10:264–72.

122. Lew AS, Hod H, Cerrek B, Ghah P, Ganz W. Mortality and morbidity rates of patients older than 75 years with acute myocardial infarction treated with intravenous streptokinase. Am J Cardiol 1987;59:1–5.

123. Forrester JS, Diamond G, Chatterjee K, Swan HJC. Medical therapy of acute myocardial infarction by application of hemodynamic subsets. N Engl J Med 1976;295:1356–62.

124. Forrester JS, Diamond G, Chatterjee K, Swan HJC. Medical therapy of acute myocardial infarction by application of hemodynamic subsets. N Engl J Med 1976;295:1404–13.

125. Jugdutt BI, Warnica JW. Intravenous nitroglycerin therapy to limit myocardial infarct size, expansion, and complications: effect of timing, dosage, and infarct location. Circulation 1988;78:906–19.

126. Yusuf S, MacMahon S, Collins R, Peto R. Effect of intravenous nitrates on mortality in acute myocardial infarction: an overview of the randomized trials. Lancet 1988;1:1088–92.

127. May DC, Popma JJ, Black WH, et al. In vivo induction and reversal of nitroglycerin tolerance in human coronary arteries. N Engl J Med 1987;317:805–9.

128. Cohn JN, Guiha NH, Broder MI, et al. Right ventricular infarction. Am J Cardiol 1974;33:209–14.

129. Lorell B, Leinbach RC, Pohost GM, et al. Right ventricular infarction: clinical diagnosis and differentiation from cardiac tamponade and pericardial constriction. Am J Cardiol 1979;43:465–71.

130. Dell'Italia LJ, Starling MR, O'Rourke RA. Physical examination for exclusion of hemodynamically important right ventricular infarction. Ann Intern Med 1983;99:608–11.

131. The Norwegian Multicenter Study Group. Timolol after myocardial infarction. N Engl J Med 1981;304:801–7.

132. Beta-Blocker Heart Attack Trial Research Group. A randomized trial of propranolol in patients with acute myocardial infarction. I. Mortality results. JAMA 1982;247:1707–14.

133. The MIAMI Trial Research Group. Metoprolol in Acute Myocardial Infarction (MIAMI): a randomized placebo-controlled international trial. Eur Heart J 1986;6:199–226.

134. The International Collaboration Study Group. Reduction of infarct size with the early use of timolol in acute myocardial infarction. N Engl J Med 1984;310:9.

135. Furberg CD, Hawkins CM, Lichstein E. Effect of propranolol in postinfarction patients with mechanical or electrical complications. Circulation 1984;69:761–5.

136. Muller JE, Morrison J, Stone PH, et al. Nifedipine therapy for patients with threatened and acute myocardial infarction: a randomized, double-blind, placebo-controlled comparison. Circulation 1984;69:740–7.

137. Sirnes PA, Overskeid K, Pedersen TR, et al. Evolution of infarct size during the early use of nifedipine in patients with acute myocardial infarction: the Norwegian Nifedipine Multicenter Trial. Circulation 1984;70:859–65.

138. The Multicenter Diltiazem Postinfarction Trial Research Group. The effect of diltiazem on mortality and reinfarction after myocardial infarction. N Engl J Med 1988;319:385–92.

139. Madigan NP, Rutherford BD, Frye RL. The clinical course, early prognosis and coronary anatomy of subendocardial infarction. Am J Med 1976;60:634–41.

140. Hutter AM, DeSanctis RW, Flynn T, Yeatman LA. Nontransmural infarction: a comparison of hospital and late clinical course of patients with that of matched patients with transmural anterior and transmural inferior myocardial infarction. Am J Cardiol 1981;48:595–602.

141. The Diltiazem Reinfarction Study Group. Diltiazem and reinfarction in patients with non-Q-wave myocardial infarction. N Engl J Med 1986; 315:423–9.

142. Sharpe N, Murphy J, Smith H, Hannan S. Treatment of patients with symptomless left ventricular dysfunction after myocardial infarction. Lancet 1988;1:255–9.

143. Bigger JT Jr, Fleiss JL, Kleiger R, Miller JP, Rolnitzky LM. The Multicenter Post-infarction Research Group. The relationships among ventricular arrhythmias, left ventricular dysfunction, and mortality in the 2 years after myocardial infarction. Circulation 1984;69:250–8.

144. Tibbits PH, Evaul JE, Goldstein RE, and the Multicenter Post-infarction Research Group. Serial acquisition of data to predict one-year mortality rate after acute myocardial infarction. Am J Cardiol 1987;60:451–5.

145. Dittus RS, Roberts SD, Adolph RJ. Cost-effectiveness analysis of patient management alternatives after uncomplicated myocardial infarction: a model. J Am Coll Cardiol 1987;10:869–78.

146. Roy D, Waxman HL, Kienzle MG, Buxton AE, Marchlinski FE, Josephson ME. Clinical characteristics and long-term follow-up in 199 survivors of out-of-hospital cardiac arrest: relation to inducibility at electrophysiologic testing. Am J Cardiol 1983;52:969–74.

147. Wilber DJ, Garan H, Finkelstein D, Kelly E, et al. Out-of-hospital cardiac arrest: use of electrophysiologic testing in the prediction of long-term outcome. N Engl J Med 1988;318:19–24.

148. Vatterott PJ, Hammill SC, Bailey KR, Berbari EJ, Matheson SJ. Signal-averaged electrocardiography: a new noninvasive test to identify patients at risk of ventricular arrhythmias. Mayo Clin Proc 1988;63:931–42.

149. Swerdlow CD, Mason JW, Stinson EB, Oyer PE, Winkle RA, Derby GC. Results of operations for ventricular tachycardia in 105 patients. J Thorac Cardiovasc Surg 1986;92:105–13.

150. Ostermeyer J, Borggrefe M, Breithardt G, et al. Direct operations for the management of life-threatening ischemic ventricular tachycardia. J Thorac Cardiovasc Surg 1987;94:848–65.

151. Alderman ED, Fisher LD, Litwin P. Results of coronary artery surgery in patients with poor left ventricular function (CASS). Circulation 1983;68:785–95.

152. Nishimura RA, Schaff HV, Shub C, Gersh BJ, Edwards WD, Tajik AJ. Papillary muscle rupture complicating acute myocardial infarction: analysis of 17 patients. Am J Cardiol 1983;51:373–7.

153. Held AC, Cole PL, Lipton B, Gore JM, et al. Rupture of the interventricular septum complicating acute myocardial infarction: a multicenter analysis of clinical findings and outcome. Am Heart J 1988;116:1330–6.

154. Cobbs BW Jr, Hatcher CR Jr, Robinson PS. Cardiac rupture: 3 operations with 2 long-term survivals. JAMA 1973;223:532.

155. Rosenberg L, Kaufman DW, Helmrich SP, Shapiro S. The risk of myocardial infarction after quitting smoking in men under 55 years of age. N Engl J Med 1985;313:1511–4.

156. Vlietstra RE, Kronmal RA, Oberman A, Frye RL, Killip T. Effect of cigarette smoking on survival of patients with angiographically documented coronary artery disease. JAMA 1986;255:1023–7.

157. Gordon T, Kannel WB, McGee D. Death and coronary attacks in men after giving up cigarette smoking: a report from the Framingham Study. Lancet 1974;2:1345–8.

158. Management Committee. The Australian trial in mild hypertension. Lancet 1980;1:1261–7.

159. Hypertension Detection and Follow-up Program Cooperative Group. The effect of treatment on mortality in 'mild' hypertension. N Engl J Med 1982;307:976–80.

160. Lipid Research Clinics Program, National Heart, Lung, and Blood Institute. The Lipid Research Clinics coronary primary prevention trial results: reduction in incidence of coronary heart disease. JAMA 1984; 251:351–64.

161. Manninen V, Elo MO, Frick MH, et al. Lipid alterations and decline in the incidence of coronary heart disease in the Helsinki Heart Study. JAMA 1988;260:641–51.

162. Brensike JF, Levy RI, Kelsey SF, et al. Effects of therapy with cholestyramine on progression of coronary arteriosclerosis: results of the NHLBI Type II Coronary Intervention Study. Circulation 1984;69:313–24.

163. Report of the National Cholesterol Education Program Expert Panel on detection, evaluation, and treatment of high blood cholesterol in adults. Arch Intern Med 1988;148:36–48.

164. The Lovastatin Study Group III. A multicenter comparison of lovastatin and cholestyramine therapy for severe primary hypercholesterolemia. JAMA 1988;260:359–66.

165. Blankenhorn DH, Nessim SA, Johnson RL, et al. Beneficial effects of combined colestipol-niacin therapy on coronary atherosclerosis and coronary venous bypass grafts. JAMA 1987;257:3233–40.

166. Hatziandreu EI, Koplan JP, Weinstein MC, Caspersen CJ, Warner KE. A cost-effectiveness analysis of exercise as a health promotion activity. Am J Public Health 1988;78:1417–21.

167. Ehsani AA, Biello DR, Schultz J, et al. Improvement of left ventricular contractile function by exercise training in patients with coronary artery disease. Circulation 1986;74:350–8.

168. Oldridge NB, Guyatt GH, Fischer ME, Rimm AA. Cardiac rehabilitation after myocardial infarction. JAMA 1988;260:945–50.

169. Dennis C, Houston-Miller N, Schwartz RG, et al. Early return to work after uncomplicated myocardial infarction: results of a randomized trial. JAMA 1988;260:214–20.

170. Oliver MF. Reducing cholesterol does not reduce mortality. J Am Coll Cardiol 1988;12:814–7.

171. Kronmal R. Commentary on the published results of the Lipid Research Clinics Coronary Primary Prevention Trial. JAMA 1985;253:2091–3.

172. Sempos C, Cooper R, Kovar MG, McMillen M. Divergence of the recent trends in coronary mortality for the four major race-sex groups in the United States. Am J Public Health 1988;78:1422–7.

CHAPTER 14

"Crackers, Breakers, Stretchers, Drillers, Scrapers, Shavers, Burners, Welders and Melters"—The Future Treatment of Atherosclerotic Coronary Artery Disease? A Clinical-Morphologic Assessment

BRUCE F. WALLER, MD

During the last few decades, we have seen the development and continued evolution of various pharmacologic and mechanical forms of therapy used in the treatment of atherosclerotic coronary artery disease. Despite significant declines in the last 25 years, atherosclerotic coronary artery disease remains the leading cause of death in the United States. Significant advances have been made in the area of prevention with large scale public education efforts showing the relation between various "risk factors" and the development of coronary atherosclerosis. Recent human studies (1–3) have demonstrated angiographic regression of coronary atherosclerosis after various lipid-lowering therapies. Despite promising efforts in these areas, altering daily habits and risk factors and the use of pharmacologic therapy take several years to decades to accomplish results. Although the future treatment of atherosclerotic coronary disease lies in prevention, the immediate future of therapy will focus on the use of various intervention techniques and devices. This review will examine clinical-morphologic aspects of several of the currently used and developing interventional techniques and devices employed in the treatment of atherosclerotic coronary artery disease, and will describe two new concepts in coronary morphology that will have future impact on treatment modalities.

Many techniques and devices (dilating balloons, perfusion balloons, thermal probes and balloons, lasers, atherectomy devices, stents) have been used or are under study for future use. These techniques and devices can be separated into two main categories based on their effects on coronary luminal shape or obstruction: *remodeling* ("cracking," "breaking," "stretching," "welding") and *removal* ("scraping," "shaving," "burning," "melting").

Remodeling Techniques

Various techniques and devices have been developed that in effect alter the degree of coronary lumen shape or amount of obstruction by "*displacing*" plaque or thrombus, or both, "*cracking*" or "*breaking*" plaque, "*stretching*" a portion or all of the vessel wall to enlarge the lumen or "*welding*" portions of the obstructing material against adjacent walls. All of these methods attempt to increase luminal cross-sectional area and improve blood flow.

Balloon Angioplasty

Since its introduction in 1977 (4), coronary balloon angioplasty has gained wide acceptance as a nonsurgical form of therapy for acutely and chronically obstructed vessels. Increased experience and advances in technology have resulted in an increased primary success rate (90% to 95%) and lowered complication rate (4% to 5%) (5). Despite the therapeutic success of coronary balloon angioplasty, the exact mechanism or mechanisms by which balloon angioplasty improves vessel patency remains unsettled. Morphologic and histologic observations in coronary arteries of patients undergoing percutaneous transluminal balloon angioplasty are limited (6–19), but provide us with clues regarding the mechanism of action. These observations may be divided into two categories: 1) changes observed *early* (acute) (≤30 days) after balloon angioplasty, and 2) changes observed *late* (chronic) (>30 days) after balloon angioplasty.

Early (Acute) Changes

Morphologic changes. Morphologic changes in coronary arteries ≤30 days after dilation have been reported by several investigators (6,8–10,11–15,17,18). Block et al. (6) initially described "splitting" of atherosclerotic plaque in two patients undergoing balloon angioplasty. In one patient, an extension of the plaque "splitting" into the coronary media resulted in a dissecting hematoma. We (9,18) subsequently reported morphologic and histologic observations in several patients undergoing angioplasty procedures 4 h to 30 days before tissue examination. In each patient, an intimal "crack," "tear," "fracture" or "break" was recognized, and each had variable degrees of medial penetration. In some patients, the medial involvement was *localized* (barely penetrating the internal elastic membrane) (Fig. 14.1), and in others, it was *extensive* (dissection anterograde, retrograde or both); adventitial disruption was not observed. We (17) reported nine additional necropsy patients who had undergone a balloon angioplasty procedure alone or in conjunction with a thrombolytic agent in the treatment of evolving acute myocardial infarction. Each of these nine patients had intimal-medial tears, but four patients with combined thrombolytic reperfusion and balloon angioplasty had associated coronary wall and lumen hemorrhage (Fig. 14.2). Mizuno et al. (12) serially sectioned the balloon angioplasty site in one necropsy patient, and observed intimal and medial splitting that led to coronary artery dissection. Soward et al. (14) reported plaque splitting, medial dissection and "lifting" of the atherosclerotic plaque from the medial layer at the site of previous balloon angioplasty. La Delia et al. (19) recently reported histologic findings in the left anterior descending coronary artery of a patient receiving angioplasty and streptokinase for an evolving acute myocardial infarction. Atherosclerotic plaque "cleavage," subintimal leukocytic infiltrations and medial and adventitial fractures with hemorrhage were observed.

Late (Chronic) Changes

Although minimal early morphologic information is available from the coronary arteries of patients undergoing balloon angioplasty, even less morphologic information is available *late* (>30 days) after the procedure (1,18,20–23). To date, late changes observed in human coronary arteries after angioplasty may be divided into two categories: 1) *no morphologic evidence of previous angioplasty injury* (Fig. 14.3), and 2) *intimal fibrous proliferation* (Fig. 14.4).

No morphologic evidence of previous balloon angioplasty injury. We (8,10,13) reported morphologic-histologic changes at the site of angioplasty in three men who died suddenly 80, 90 and 150 days, respectively, after clinically successful coronary angioplasty. In all three the left anterior descending coronary artery had increased angiographic luminal diameter and decreased transstenotic pressure gradient, and each patient had relief of angina pectoris and improved exercise tolerance. Of the two clinically asymptomatic patients, one died suddenly at home (sudden coronary death) and the other was killed in an automobile accident while intoxicated with alcohol (noncardiac cause of death). The symptomatic patient died suddenly at work (sudden coronary death). At necropsy, the site of balloon angioplasty in the left anterior descending coronary artery in each patient was narrowed 76% to 95% in cross-sectional area by fibrous atherosclerotic plaques (Fig. 14.3). Each balloon angioplasty site was free of intraluminal thrombus and mural hemorrhage. Histologic assessment of atherosclerotic plaque in the areas of previous angioplasty compared with other areas of atherosclerotic plaque in the same artery or other arteries in the same patient disclosed no distinctive morphologic differences. No distinctive acute morphologic lesions or healed modifications of these lesions were recognized late in these three patients.

Intimal fibrous proliferation. Essed et al. (7) were the first to report finding, 5 months before death, intimal fibrous hyperplasia at the site of coronary angioplasty. Cross sections of the left anterior descending coronary artery showed evidence of previous disruption of the media, with extensive proximal and distal coronary dissection. A large intimal "crack" with a partial "flap" formation created a "false

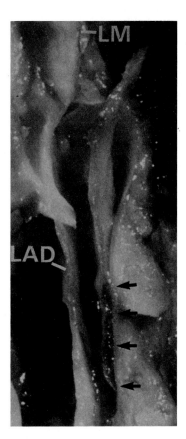

Figure 14.1. Localized coronary artery dissection (**arrows**) is present at the site of transluminal balloon angioplasty in the left anterior descending (LAD) coronary artery. LM = left main. From Waller (8), with permission of the publisher.

channel." After 5 months, the fibrocellular proliferation "coated" surrounding portions of atherosclerotic plaque in addition to the area of previous plaque fracture, producing a severely narrowed coronary artery. Austin et al. (15) observed a late angioplasty site that appeared to have distinct intimal layers: an outer layer composed of hypocellular connective tissue with cholesterol clefts (atherosclerotic plaque), and an inner layer composed of smooth muscle cells, fibroblasts and a basophilic interstitial matrix (intimal fibrous proliferation). The outer atherosclerotic plaque layer contained "gaps" that were presumed to be evidence of the previous balloon angioplasty; these "gaps" were filled with the cellular proliferation of the inner layer. We (16) recently reported histologic evidence of restenosis in the proximal left anterior descending coronary artery 4 months after a clinically successful angioplasty (Fig. 14.4). The site of previous balloon angioplasty had evidence of atherosclerotic plaque "cracks" or "splits" and localized medial dissection (disruption) similar to lesions observed in patients who died acutely after balloon angioplasty. The initial underlying atherosclerotic plaque was still clearly identified, and the luminal channels created by the angioplasty procedure 123 days earlier were filled with fibrocellular tissue that coated

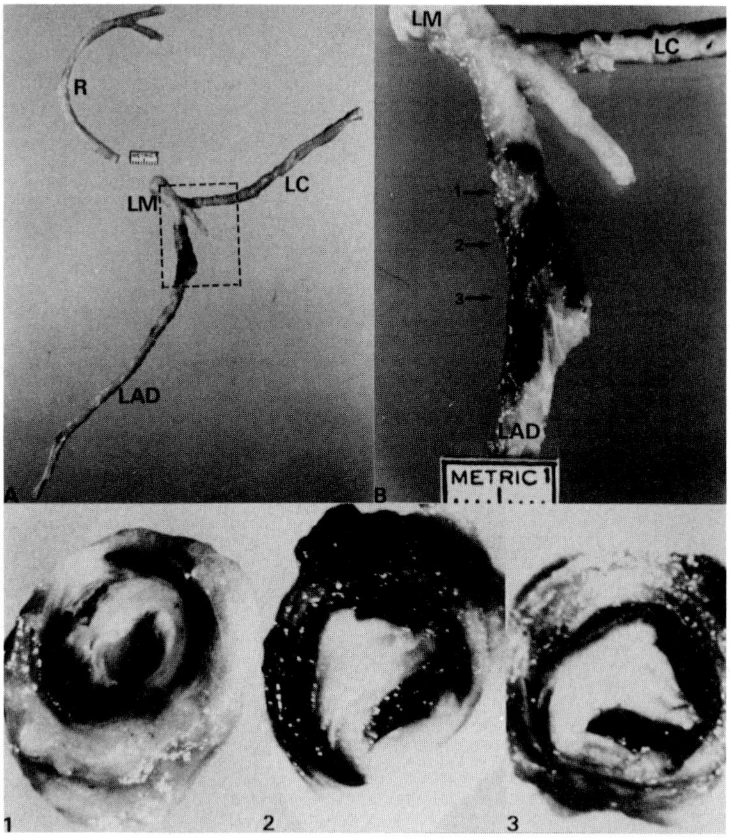

Figure 14.2. Thrombolytic therapy with streptokinase combined with balloon angioplasty. Coronary artery site of angioplasty (**A**) showing marked adventitial hemorrhage (**B**). Numbers in **B** indicate sites of cross sections (**1 to 3**) shown below. **1,** Prominent atherosclerotic plaque "crack" with surrounding hemorrhage. **2 and 3,** Marked bleeding into the area of angioplasty severely narrows the coronary lumen. LAD = left anterior descending artery; LC = left circumflex artery; LM = left main artery; R = right coronary artery. From Waller et al. (17).

the denuded media and narrowed the coronary lumen 96% to 100% in cross-sectional area. Fibrocellular tissue proliferation involved 28 mm of the proximal left anterior descending artery and then abruptly disappeared, covering a distance corresponding to the lengths of the previously used angioplasty balloons.

Thus, in the angioplasty sites seen late after angiographically successful balloon angioplasty, no distinctive lesion or lesions may be seen or, more commonly, a concentric fibrocellular proliferation is observed, which is distinctly different from underlying atherosclerotic plaque. The absence of morphologic signs of previous angioplasty in the former should not be interpreted as indicating "acceleration of underlying atherosclerotic plaque" in a mere 80, 90 or 150 days (8,10).

Mechanism(s) of Balloon Angioplasty

Plaque compression. Dotter and Judkins (24) in their original description of the angioplasty procedure (as well as Gruentzig [25] 12 years later) initially attributed the mechanism of balloon angioplasty to redistribution and compression of intimal atherosclerotic plaque (Fig. 14.5). Inflation of the angioplasty balloon within an arterial stenosis was thought to "compress" atherosclerotic plaque components against the arterial wall, thereby resulting in a larger vessel

lumen. However, the vast majority of atherosclerotic plaque in human coronary arteries is composed of dense fibrocollagenous tissue with varying amounts of calcific deposits and much smaller amounts of intracellular and extracellular lipid (that is, "hard plaques"). Thus, it appears unlikely that plaque compression plays a major role in human coronary artery balloon angioplasty dilation. In experimental animal models, vessel-induced injury plus a high cholesterol diet are used to create atherosclerotic lesions. The atherosclerotic lesions induced in these models are composed almost entirely of lipid-laden foam cells without dense collagen and calcific deposits (that is, "soft plaques") and may be susceptible to compression.

Plaque fracture. Data from angioplasty results in experimental models (26–28), human necropsy coronary arteries (29–31) and human vessels examined after successful or complicated angioplasty procedures (6,12,14) suggest that the major mechanism of human coronary angioplasty is "breaking," "cracking," "splitting" or "fracturing" of atherosclerotic plaque (Fig. 14.5). Plaque fractures, breaks (also called dissection clefts) and cracks extending from the lumen for variable lengths into the plaque provide a means of improving vessel patency by creating additional channels or avenues for coronary blood flow. Healing and repair changes at the angioplasty site eventually may remodel the acute pathologic lesions or lesions to alter or eliminate their distinc-

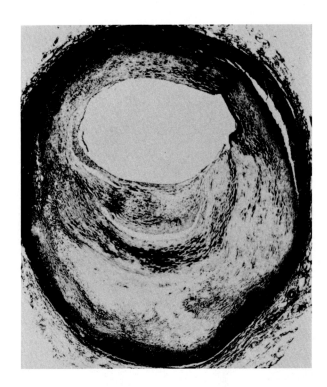

Figure 14.3. Histologic cross section of the left anterior descending coronary artery at the site of transluminal balloon angioplasty 150 days before sudden death, showing severe luminal narrowing by atherosclerotic plaque. From Waller (10), with permission of the publisher.

tive features described previously. The healing process at the angioplasty site itself also may increase (as has been noted angiographically [32]) or decrease luminal size (restenosis).

Plaque fracture, intimal flaps and localized medial dissection. Waller et al. (9) reported plaque fracture, "intimal atherosclerotic flaps" and "localized medial dissection" as the major mechanism of balloon angioplasty in human coronary arteries from patients undergoing angioplasty during life (Fig. 14.5). Initial and persistent luminal cross-sectional area expansion appears to require deep intimal fractures (occasionally creating intimal "flaps") with localized tears or dissection of the underlying media. Failure to obtain localized and limited medial involvement in addition to the intimal cracks may be a cause of early "restenosis" after an initially successful dilation.

Stretching of plaque-free wall segment. An additional mechanism of coronary artery dilation appears to be "stretching" of plaque-free wall segments of eccentric atherosclerotic lesions (Fig. 14.5) (33–35). Inflation of an angioplasty balloon across eccentric plaque lesions may distend or stretch the normal wall segment and produce little or no damage to the plaque on the remaining portions of the arterial wall. Stretching of the plaque-free wall segment may result initially in an increase in coronary lumen diameter and cross-sectional area, but several weeks later gradual relaxation of this overstretched segment ("restitution of tone") decreases the coronary lumen toward the predilation state. This decrease may provide another explanation for early restenosis after an initially angiographically successful dilation (34,35). The high frequency of an eccentric type of coronary lumen in severely diseased vessels (35–37) suggests that stretching of the plaque-free wall segment may be a more frequent mechanism of clinically successful coronary angioplasty than previously thought.

Stretching and compression. A fifth mechanism for balloon angioplasty of coronary arteries is the combination of

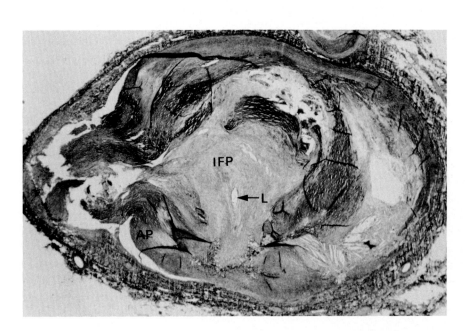

Figure 14.4. Intimal fibrous proliferation (IFP) of the left anterior descending artery "coating" underlying atherosclerotic plaque (AP) 4.5 months after balloon angioplasty. L = lumen. From Waller (16).

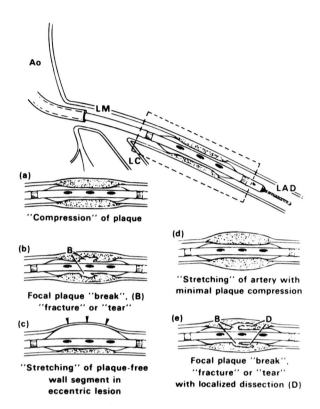

Ao

LM

LC

LAD

(a)

"Compression" of plaque

(b)   B

Focal plaque "break", (B)
"fracture" or "tear"

(c)

"Stretching" of plaque-free
wall segment in
eccentric lesion

(d)

"Stretching" of artery with
minimal plaque compression

(e)   B   D

Focal plaque "break",
"fracture" or "tear"
with localized dissection (D)

Figure 14.5. Diagram of five possible mechanisms of coronary artery balloon angioplasty. Ao = aorta; LAD = left anterior descending artery; LC = left circumflex artery; LM = left main coronary artery. From Waller (34).

vessel stretching with minimal or mild plaque compression (Fig. 14.5). In this situation, an oversized angioplasty balloon may stretch the entire coronary segment that is concentrically narrowed by fibrocollagenous plaque.

Although the technique of balloon angioplasty has been highly successful, the procedure has been plagued with two major problems at the site of angioplasty: 1) early (abrupt) closure (Fig. 14.6), and 2) late closure ("restenosis") (Fig. 14.7). Various new interventional devices and techniques have been used to attempt to solve these problems.

Acute (Abrupt) Closure of the Angioplasty Site

Mechanisms for abrupt closure (Fig. 14.6). Despite improvement in equipment and technique, abrupt closure at the angioplasty site occurs in 2% to 6% of patients treated with balloon angioplasty (38–42). Clinical explanations for the abrupt closure include coronary artery spasm (2%), localized thrombus (8%) and coronary dissection (34%) (42). Morphologic explanations for abrupt closure of the angioplasty site are depicted in Figure 14.6. Acute vessel occlusion from a folded, curled-up, large *intimal flap* accounts for the vast majority of these cases (Fig. 14.6a). This morphologic finding may correspond to the clinical category of "dissection" in that a large intimal flap is created by an extensive

intimal-medial dissection plane. Acute closure may be produced by abrupt *relaxation of an overstretched disease-free wall* of an eccentric plaque (Fig. 14.6b). The coronary artery media of the disease-free wall contains smooth muscle, and is capable of "reacting" to various humoral, neurogenic or traumatic (balloon dilation) stimuli. This morphologic mechanism may correspond to the clinical category of spasm. The potential for dynamic alteration of the coronary lumen (wall spasm) is more likely to occur with *eccentric* than with *concentric* atherosclerotic lesions (35).

Nonocclusive fibrin-platelet thrombus frequently layers the angioplasty site, but *occlusive thrombus* at the site of balloon angioplasty is an uncommon finding in patients who die within hours of coronary dilation (Fig. 14.6c) (8,10,13). Although thrombus may be associated with large, curled-up intimal flaps, the primary mechanism for abrupt closure is the intimal-medial flap. *Subintimal hemorrhage* from traumatic balloon injury of atherosclerotic plaque is a possible cause for abrupt closure. Subintimal plaque bleeding may acutely expand the plaque and severely narrow or occlude the angioplasty site (Fig. 14.6d and 14.8). Intraplaque and intraluminal bleeding can acutely occlude an angioplasty site (Fig. 14.2 and 14.6e), but has been reported (17) only in the setting of combined balloon angioplasty and thrombolytic therapy.

Treatment of abrupt closure (Fig. 14.9 and 14.10). Treatment of sites of abrupt closure has included *repeated balloon angioplasty* and prolonged (30 to 60 min) balloon inflation with the use of *perfusion catheters* ("bailout catheters," hemoperfusion catheters, autoperfusion catheters, shunt catheters [43–48]). Perfusion catheters are placed across the occluded angioplasty site so that arterial blood enters the catheter proximally and exists distally (Fig. 14.9).

Newer devices also may have an important role in the treatment of abrupt closure sites (Fig. 14.10). Large intimal flaps may be "sealed" or "welded" against the adjacent vessel wall with the use of *thermal angioplasty balloons* (Fig. 14.10b). "Pyroplasty" techniques ("thermal welding") may employ laser or radiofrequency energy sources (20,21,49–53). An advantage of pyroplasty techniques over perfusion catheters is the immediate repair of the intimal-medial flap without the need for coronary artery bypass grafting.

Balloon-expandable intravascular stents (an intravascular mechanical support device) have also been used for abrupt closure of an angioplasty site (Fig. 14.10d) (23,54–60). Several types of these metal meshwork devices are being tested, and at least one has been used in the coronary arteries for the treatment of abrupt closure of the angioplasty site (23). The balloon-expandable stent also offers a rapid percutaneous technique to permanently hold the intimal-medial flap against the vessel wall without the use of surgery, and avoids the extra catheterization laboratory equipment necessary for thermal angioplasty.

Thermal angioplasty including stents may also be used at

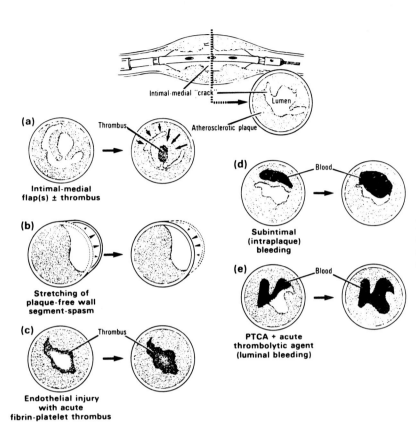

Figure 14.6. Diagram showing causes of *acute* or *early* luminal narrowing or closure ("restenosis") of the percutaneous transluminal coronary balloon angioplasty (PTCA) site.

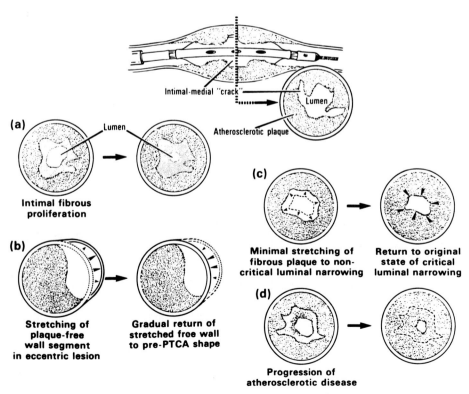

Figure 14.7. Diagram showing causes of *late* luminal narrowing or closure ("restenosis") of the percutaneous transluminal coronary balloon angioplasty (PTCA) site.

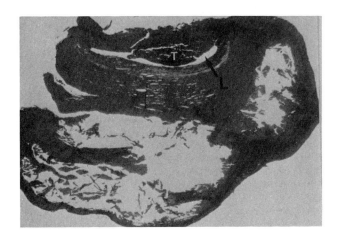

Figure 14.8. Cross section of endarterectomy specimen from a coronary artery undergoing balloon angioplasty, showing extensive plaque hemorrhage and luminal (L) thrombus (T). From Waller (8), with permission of the publisher.

the site of abrupt closure in which "spasm" is the culprit. Thermal injury to the segment of disease-free wall involved in spasm may permit long-term luminal distension. *Hot-tipped lasers* can be used to reopen an angioplasty site occluded by thrombus with or without intimal flaps (Fig. 14.10c) (61–65). *Atherectomy devices* also can be used to remove large intimal-medial flaps, thrombus or both (Fig. 14.10e).

Late (Chronic) Closure ("Restenosis")

Factors responsible for late restenosis. Despite the widespread acceptance and use of balloon angioplasty to treat severely narrowed coronary arteries in patients with symptomatic coronary heart disease, *"recurrence of stenosis"* (*"restenosis"*) at the angioplasty site within several months of the angioplasty procedure has been the major problem. The frequency of clinical restenosis ranges from 17% to 47%, depending on variations in definitions of restenosis (angiographic, clinical, anatomic, physiologic, statistical) (32,66–75). Multiple *clinical-angiographic factors* (number of vessels, site of angioplasty, pre- and postangioplasty diameter stenoses, transstenotic pressure gradients, lesion characteristics [diffuse, long, eccentric, calcified]), *technical factors* (number of inflations, duration of inflation, pressure of inflation, balloon-vessel size ratio, intimal flap or dissection, incomplete revascularization) and *pharmacologic factors* (anticoagulants, vasodilators) have been analyzed to deter-

mine factors responsible for restenosis (72). Despite the large number of variables evaluated, studies diverge on the significance of many and concur on the significance of a few factors (72).

Fibrocellular intimal proliferation (Fig. 14.4 and 14.7a). The most widely accepted theory for the development of the fibrocellular intimal proliferation lesion involves responses from damaged vessel endothelium and media. A major participant in the development of this fibrocellular response appears to be the *smooth muscle cells of the media* and diseased intima (plaque) (7,15,16,76). *The most common mechanism of balloon angioplasty (intimal-medial disruption) is a likely initiating mechanism for restenosis.* Mechanisms for the intimal fibrous proliferation may be precipitated by the release of thromboxane A_2, which leads to platelet deposition, release of platelet-derived growth factors (PDGF) and fibroblast and endothelial growth factors (76). This process results in migration, proliferation and alteration of the smooth muscle cells from the media, resulting in fibrocellular tissue accumulation. The fibrocellular "coating" narrows the vessel lumen.

Other mechanisms of late luminal narrowing at the angioplasty site ("restenosis") involve gradual *elastic recoil* of an overstretched disease-free wall of an eccentric lesion (Fig. 14.7b), return to predilation state of a *stretched concentric lesion* (Fig. 14.7c) and *"progression of atherosclerotic plaque"* (Fig. 14.7d). The latter mechanism appears unlikely in a short interval of 2 to 4 months after angioplasty.

Treatment of chronic closure ("restenosis"). Treatment of restenosed lesions has primarily involved repeated balloon angioplasty procedures two, three and four times after the initial dilation (47,77). Various pharmacologic approaches to prevent restenosis using antiplatelet agents (aspirin, dipyridamole) and calcium channel blockers have been used, but have been unsuccessful in reducing the frequency of restenosis (72). Newer clinical trials with other antiplatelet agents (prostacyclin analogues, omega-3 fatty acids), steroids and platelet-derived growth factor blockers (78) are underway. Newer mechanical devices also may be used to delay or prevent intimal fibrous proliferation at the angioplasty site (Fig. 14.9 and 14.10).

Balloon-expandable intravascular stents (Fig. 14.10d) have been proposed as an alternative approach to prevent restenosis (23,54). The mechanism of restenosis prevention with stents has not been established, but damage of smooth muscle cells of the vessel media or a purely mechanical effect of the stent, or both, is a possible explanation. *Thermal angioplasty* (Fig. 14.10b) may alter the vessel media

Figure 14.9. Diagram showing the use of a distal reperfusion balloon in the treatment of acute vessel closure after balloon angioplasty.

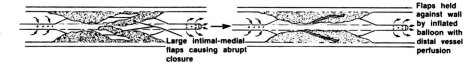

Large intimal-medial flaps causing abrupt closure

Flaps held against wall by inflated balloon with distal vessel perfusion

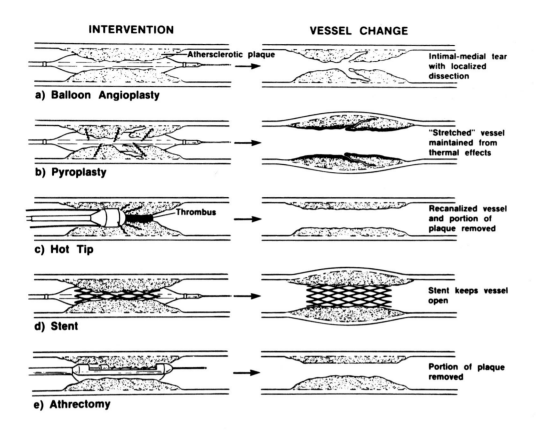

INTERVENTION   **VESSEL CHANGE**

a) Balloon Angioplasty

b) Pyroplasty

c) Hot Tip

d) Stent

e) Athrectomy

Figure 14.10. Diagram showing the effects of various interventional devices used in the treatment of acutely or chronically obstructed coronary arteries.

to prevent or at least delay the smooth muscle response in the development of intimal fibrous hyperplasia. *Prolonged inflation time* (30 to 60 min) with perfusion catheters is also being evaluated as a means of preventing restenosis (Fig. 14.9). Mechanical removal of the intimal fibrous hyperplasia material by atherectomy devices is also a method currently being evaluated (Fig. 14.10e). Simpson et al. (79,80) indicated that if all angiographically visible atheromas are removed, the rate of restenosis is as low as 14%.

Effects of balloon angioplasty on adjacent nondilated vessels. Recent angiographic reports (81,82) have noted accelerated development of coronary artery stenoses *proximal to the site of previous dilation*. In these reports, four patients underwent proximal left anterior descending coronary angioplasty and returned 6 to 14 months later with a severe left main coronary artery lesion. Morphologic evaluation of these lesions was not available. Recently, we (16) reported histologic observations in an accelerated stenosis occurring proximal to a previously dilated lesion. The patient had balloon angioplasty of the proximal left anterior descending

artery 4 months before returning with severe *left main* stenosis. At necropsy, two 5 mm long segments of the left main coronary artery disclosed initial (*old*) atherosclerotic plaque narrowing the lumen 51% to 75% in cross-sectional area, with superimposed (*new*) fibrocellular material further narrowing the cross-sectional luminal area to 77% to 100%. The left main fibrocellular tissue *was histologically identical to that observed in the proximal left anterior descending artery at the site of previous* balloon angioplasty (Fig. 14.11).

Acceleration of left main coronary artery narrowing by fibrocellular tissue proliferation may have resulted from several possible mechanisms involving intimal injury (guiding catheter injury, guide wire injury, dilating balloon injury, combinations of these injuries) or retrograde extension of the fibrocellular tissue from an adjacent site without left main arterial wall injury. The incidence of progressive left main coronary artery narrowing after angioplasty of the left anterior descending or left circumflex artery, or both, is unknown, but is probably low. Of more than 344 patients restudied angiographically within 1 year of previous coronary dilation in whom *specific attention* was given to the left main coronary artery, only 4 patients (1%) were recognized with accelerated left main coronary artery narrowing (81,82).

FUTURE TREATMENT OF CORONARY ARTERY DISEASE 185

Figure 14.11. Composite of consecutive histologic cross sections of the left main (LM 1,2 [**top left** and **top middle**]) and left anterior descending (LAD 1,2,3,4,5 [**top right** and **bottom**]) coronary arteries 123 days after successful balloon angioplasty of the proximal left anterior descending artery. The site of previous angioplasty (LAD 1,2,3) shows initial underlying atherosclerotic plaque (AP) with plaque "fracture" or "cracks" (C) (**arrowheads**) and localized medial dissection. Plaque channels created by the previous angioplasty are filled with fibrocellular (FC) tissue that also extends over the denuded media and narrows the coronary lumen (L) 96% to 100% in cross-sectional area (LAD 1,2,3). The fibrocellular proliferation is histologically distinct from the underlying plaque. Two segments of the left main artery (LM 1,2) show initial (old) atherosclerotic plaque narrowing the lumen 51% to 75% in cross-sectional area, with superimposed (new) fibrocellular tissue (FC) (**arrows**) increasing the luminal cross-sectional area to 76% to 100%. The composition of the fibrocellular tissue in the left main artery is identical to that in the proximal left anterior descending artery. (Elastic stains; original magnification ×4, reduced by 30%). From Waller et al. (17).

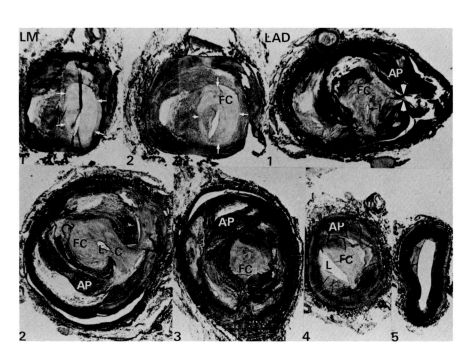

Balloon Pyroplasty (Thermal Balloon Angioplasty, "Biologic Stenting")

Thermal balloon angioplasty (Fig. 14.10b), initially developed as laser balloon angioplasty (83,84), is another method of "remolding" or remodeling a stenotic atherosclerotic vessel to increase luminal area. Thermal balloon angioplasty can use various energy sources (laser, radiofrequency, chemical, ultrasound) to produce a thermal injury on adjacent plaque. Laser balloon angioplasty features traditional balloon angioplasty followed by laser irradiation of the atherosclerotic plaque-lined artery during a final balloon dilation (20,83). In one model, Nd:YAG laser energy fires through an ultrathin central fiber and is transmitted through the balloon and enters the adjacent plaque as heat. Animal (84,85) and cadaver (86,87) studies have indicated that thermal balloon angioplasty decreases vessel elasticity at the dilation site and heat "molds" the arterial segment to the size and shape of the inflated angioplasty balloon (Fig. 14.12). This process essentially creates a "biologic stent." In addition to the acute effects of remolding, thermal effects on the underlying media may destroy smooth muscle cells involved in the late restenosis process.

Lee et al. (87) recently evaluated radiofrequency as an alternate energy source for balloon pyroplasty. Delivery of radiofrequency in combination with angioplasty balloon inflation pressure effectively molded atherosclerotic plaque and vessels. Experimental studies on layers of human cadaver aorta showed tissue fusion ("welding") of previously separated layers, thus indicating its usefulness in the therapy of intraluminal intimal flaps (Fig. 14.13). Balloon pyroplasty has not been associated with subsequent vessel aneurysm or rupture in the experimental model. Thermal angioplasty with lower power, homogeneous heating and simultaneous tissue compression may be better than thermal probes ("hot-tipped probes") that use an instantaneous high heat application to the luminal surface (Fig. 14.10c).

Thermal probes ("G-lazing"). Coronary balloon angioplasty may be followed by a laser thermal probe in an attempt to seal off superficial intimal disruptions (Fig. 14.10c). The low-powered probe skims through the treated vessel, "glazing" the new lumen. No removal of tissue results, but a "finishing touch" type of remodeling occurs (88).

Stents. Placement of balloon-expandable intravascular stents has shown some promise in preventing abrupt closure and restenosis of atherosclerotic vessels (Fig. 14.10d, 14.12 and 14.14). The woven wire stent expands at the target site and becomes permanently embedded within the arterial wall.

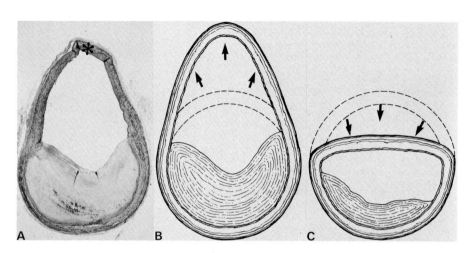

Figure 14.12. Specimen and diagrams showing the beneficial effects of thermal angioplasty (pyroplasty) on eccentric atherosclerotic plaques. **A,** Eccentric atherosclerotic vessel with a segment of disease-free wall (*) "molded" to the size and shape of an inflated balloon, followed by radiofrequency pyroplasty. **B,** Same vessel showing an increase in luminal area (**arrows**) above expected nondilated lumen (**dashed lines**). **C,** Eccentric plaque dilated without pyroplasty. Both vessels were dilated in the fresh state, then fixed in formalin. The vessel treated by thermal angioplasty remains in the stretched state (**A, B**), whereas the vessel dilated by angioplasty alone shrinks with formalin fixation (**C**). From Lee et al. (87), with permission.

After stent implantation, Serruys et al. (54) found an additional increase in cross-sectional area of the previously dilated vessel. Thus, the self-expanding metal meshwork appears to have a "stenting" and an additional "dilating" function. Histologic studies (23,54–60) of implanted stents in animals indicate that a neointimal layer covers the luminal aspect of the stent (Fig. 14.15). Stents appear to reduce luminal obstruction by displacing plaque, stretching vessel walls and maintaining intimal-medial flaps against adjacent vessel wall. Long-term effects of stents on the frequency of balloon angioplasty restenosis are under study. An initial report (80) suggests a marked reduction in the rate of angioplasty restenosis when a stenting device is used.

Removal Techniques

Various techniques and devices have been developed to alter the degree of luminal obstruction by *removal of obstructing tissue* ("scraping or shaving," "drilling," "burning" and "melting").

Laser Therapy

The capacity to conduct tremendous amounts of energy and focus this energy onto a relatively small area of tissue has made laser devices combined with fiberoptic catheters an intriguing way to ablate atherosclerotic plaque. Laser light can be delivered as a continuous beam or as a pulse. Histologic studies of vascular tissue after continuous wave laser therapy show a cone-shaped crater surrounded by concentric zones of protein denaturation and tissue vacuolization (65). The resulting charred, ragged endothelial surface is not desirable because it leads to thrombosis, and thermal diffusion leads to vessel perforation (65). Laser research has now concentrated on ablating tissue by limiting thermal injury. Two methods have attempted to achieve this

goal: 1) *modification of the tip of the delivery system of continuous wave lasers*, and 2) *use of pulsed lasers.*

Hot-tip probes. Sanborn (64) recanalized totally occluded peripheral arteries in human patients using a hot tip probe coupled to a continuous wave argon laser (Fig. 14.10c). Abela et al. (89) used a "hybrid hot tip" system to heat a metal cap and deliver laser energy through the center of the catheter. Histologic sections of vessels subjected to hot tip probes show thermally damaged plaque and media. Fouvier et al. (90) coupled a Nd:YAG laser to a sapphire tip, which diffuses the laser beam over a larger area than that reached by the bare wire (91). Advantages of the hot tip probe include its quickness of action, the creation of a large orifice and a possible reduction in the frequency of vessel perforation. Disadvantages include limitations to its use in small vessels and an associated increased frequency of induction of spasm and thrombosis (65). Radiofrequency energy is an

Figure 14.13. Experimental studies on layers of human cadaver aorta by radiofrequency thermoplasty show tissue fusion ("welding") (**arrow**) of previously separated layers. These results indicate the potential use of thermal angioplasty techniques to "weld" intraluminal flaps from balloon angioplasty.

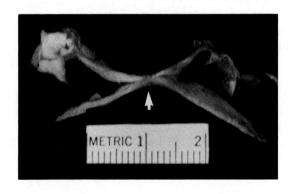

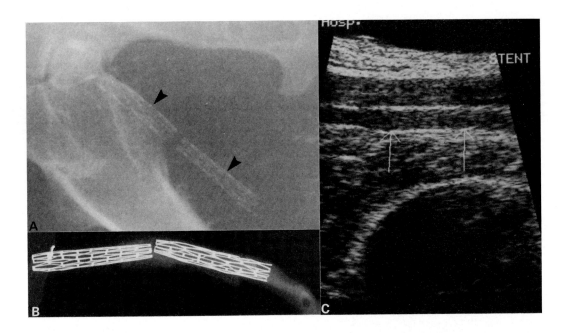

Figure 14.14. Intravascular stents in an experimental model. **A,** Double (tandem) Palmaz stents easily visible radiographically (**arrows**). **B,** Postmortem radiograph of expanded stents located within the vessel seen in **A. C,** Stents can also be recognized with ultrasound (**arrows**). (Courtesy of Dr. Gary Becker, Indiana University.)

alternative power source for thermal probes and has the advantage of being considerably cheaper (20).

Pulsed lasers. Pulsing the laser energy reduces the thermal damage by limiting thermal diffusion (65). Ultraviolet excimer laser light can be transmitted through a fiberoptic bundle with enough pulsed energy to ablate atheroma without a thermal effect. Tissue ablation occurs as a discrete precise event. The mechanism of ablation appears to be disruption of molecular bonds, and no thermal injury occurs because of a very rapid, highly localized heat effect (65). Thus, although it is hypothesized that removing atherosclerotic plaque by laser vaporization may be more effective than balloon angioplasty, the technique has been limited to date by inadequate delivery systems, a high frequency of vessel perforation and thrombosis and the creation of small recanalized channels. Newer systems employing fluorescence spectroscopy will make use of tissue recognition before laser treatment. These "smart" lasers appear to reduce the frequency of vessel perforation.

Atherectomy Devices

Cutting instruments have been developed that can incise obstructing material (Fig. 14.10e and 14.16). A prototype of these devices is the Simpson atherotome, which consists of a circular blade rotating at a high speed and which is pressed against the diseased part of the vessel by an inflated balloon (79,80,91). The procedure can be repeated several times to remove atherosclerotic plaque, thrombus or intimal fibrous hyperplasia of restenosis lesions (79,80). Focal stenoses or short segment total occlusions and ulcerative and calcified lesions can be treated (Fig. 14.16). Atherectomy is an exciting new mechanical technique used in treating restenosis lesions of previous balloon angioplasty. Histologically,

samples of atherosclerotic plaque removed from obstructed coronary arteries show portions of vessel media. Exposure of large segments of medial smooth muscle may predispose atherectomy sites to a frequency of intimal fibrous proliferation similar to or higher than that seen with conventional balloon angioplasty. Other atherectomy devices include the Kinsey catheter, Ritchie rotablater, transluminal extraction catheter and the Wholey reperfusion guidewire.

New Concepts in Atherosclerotic Plaques: Plaque Fissures and Eccentric Lesions

Two new areas in the pathology of atherosclerotic plaque include the concepts of *plaque fissure* and the *eccentric atherosclerotic lesion*. Both concepts will have a major impact on the future pharmacologic and mechanical therapy of patients with coronary artery disease.

Plaque Fissure

The missing link between anatomy, unstable angina pectoris, acute myocardial infarction and sudden coronary death. Disruptions of the atherosclerotic plaque luminal surface have been termed "intimal tears," "surface ulcerations," "plaque ruptures" and, most recently, "plaque fissures" (Fig. 14.17) (92–97). The cause of the disruption is not completely understood, but clinical and homodynamic fac-

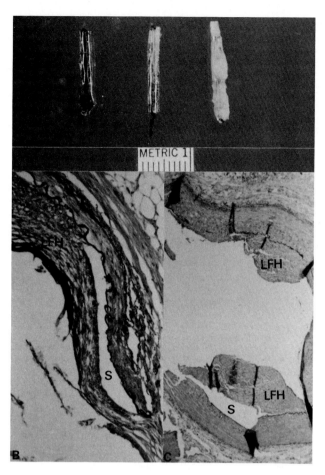

Figure 14.15. Excised vascular stents. **A,** Three excised stents showing progressive fibrosis with advancing age (**left to right**). **B and C,** Histologic studies of peripheral vessel after removal of stent wires (S), showing fibrous hyperplasia (LFH) covering the luminal (L) surface of the stent. Hematoxylin eosin stains; original magnification ×200, reduced by 28%.

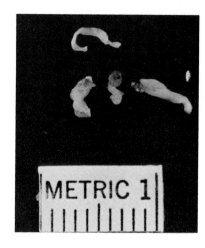

Figure 14.16. Four fragments of human coronary artery atherosclerotic plaque, including portions of vessel media removed by an atherectomy catheter.

tors such as systemic hypertension, smoking, blood lipids and luminal flow characteristics have been implicated. The role of plaque fissuring in the formation of thrombi found in association with fatal *acute myocardial infarction* is well known (93,94). Pathologic studies (92–97), in which coronary artery thrombi found in cases of fatal acute myocardial infarction were reconstructed from serial histologic sections, have shown that nearly all coronary thrombi were related to fissures of the underlying atherosclerotic plaque. Rupture of plaque leads to communication between the lipid content of the plaque and luminal blood products. Fibrin-platelet thrombus covers the fissure site and may or may not propagate (Fig. 14.17). A recent pathologic study (92) found similar plaque fissures and luminal thrombus in 74% of victims of *sudden coronary death*. More recent angiographic-histologic information (98–103) suggests that plaque fissures also occur frequently in patients with *unstable angina pectoris*.

The eccentric coronary lesion with fissuring and thrombus. Coronary artery stenoses characterized by a narrow neck and irregular borders ("type 2 eccentric lesions" [98–100], "T lesion" [101]) were the most common morphologic feature on angiograms from patients with unstable angina pectoris and acute myocardial infarction. The predominance of this angiographic lesion in both unstable angina pectoris and acute myocardial infarction suggests a link between these two conditions. Levin and Fallon (102) reported a valuable study in which postmortem angiography and subsequent histologic sections correlated the irregular luminal borders seen angiographically with histologically "complicated plaques" containing plaque fissures and superimposed partially occluding thrombus. In contrast, the angiographic coronary stenoses with smooth borders were associated with histologically "uncomplicated plaques" having intact intimal surfaces and no thrombus. Thus, fissure of the atherosclerotic plaque with thrombus formation appears to be the "missing link" connecting the acute clinical coronary syndromes of unstable angina pectoris, acute myocardial infarction and sudden coronary death (Fig. 14.18). Several investigators (103–105) recently confirmed these angiographic and necropsy observations in a series of patients undergoing coronary angioscopy. These authors expanded the concept of plaque fissure to the clinical syndromes of stable angina pectoris and accelerated angina pectoris (103). The distinguishing feature among patients with stable angina pectoris and those with accelerated angina or unstable angina pectoris appears to be the presence of the fissured plaques in the latter two groups. These findings have been used in support of thrombolytic and antithrombotic therapy in patients with unstable angina pectoris (106).

Therapeutic implications. The frequent observation of plaque fissures in various coronary syndromes has potential major importance for future treatment programs. Interven-

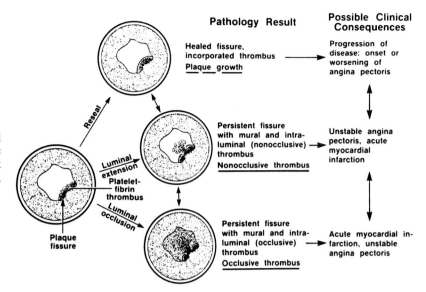

Figure 14.17. Diagram summarizing the clinical and morphologic consequences of atherosclerotic plaque fissures in patients with coronary heart disease. Modified from Davies and Thomas (96), with permission.

tions that *prevent ulceration or plaque fissures, inhibit platelet-fibrin aggregation, lyse superimposed thrombus* and *promote endothelial healing* will be needed to interrupt these clinical events (103). Pharmacologic or mechanical interventions, or both, can inhibit platelet-fibrin aggregation and lyse thrombus, but as yet no interventions are available to promote endothelial healing and prevent plaque fissures (103).

Eccentric Atherosclerotic Plaques

A connecting link between angioplasty restenosis, coronary spasm and angiographic underestimation of disease severity. Variation in the distribution of atherosclerotic plaque along the internal elastic membrane of human coronary arteries results in two major types of cross-sectional luminal shapes: *concentric* and *eccentric* (Fig. 14.19 to 14.21). If the athero-

sclerotic plaque is distributed along the entire circumference of the internal elastic membrane, the resulting vessel lumen is located centrally and is called a *central* or *concentric* type lumen (Fig. 14.20) (36). If the atherosclerotic plaque fails to involve the entire coronary artery circumference, leaving a variable arc of disease-free wall (normal wall), the residual cross-sectional lumen is called *eccentric* (Fig. 14.21) (36). The eccentric lumen has been further subdivided into slit-like, polymorphous or semilunar types (36,37). Although the polymorphous type of eccentric lumen may be observed with variable degrees of obstruction, the slitlike eccentric lumen is always associated with severe (>75%) cross-sectional area narrowing (33).

Frequency. The frequency of concentric and eccentric type lesions has been evaluated by several investigators (33–37). On the basis of examination of 200 atherosclerotic coronary artery sections, Vlodaver and Edwards (36) ob-

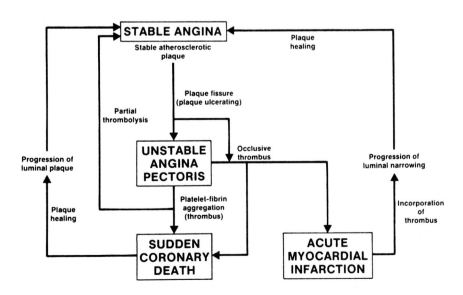

Figure 14.18. Diagram showing that the *plaque fissure* represents the "connecting link" to various clinical syndromes in atherosclerotic coronary heart disease. Modified from Forrester et al. (103), with permission.

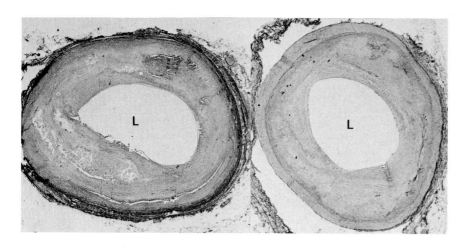

Figure 14.19. Cross sections of human coronary arteries showing the *concentric* form of luminal (L) narrowing by atherosclerotic plaque. Hematoxylin eosin stains; original magnification ×11, reduced by 25%.

served an eccentric (that is, eccentric polymorphous and eccentric slitlike) coronary lumen in 70% of cross sections examined and a concentric coronary lumen in the remaining 30% of sections. Baroldi (37) examined 1,069 sites of severe (>70%) diameter reduction and found that 46% of the coronary lumen shapes were concentric, 24% eccentric (lateral lumen position but still encircled by plaque) and 30% "semilunar" (a variable arc of disease-free wall). We (35) reported histologic observations in 500 coronary artery segments narrowed 76% to 95% in cross-sectional area by

Figure 14.20. Composite of six coronary artery cross sections of the *eccentric* form of luminal (L) narrowing by atherosclerotic plaque. Hematoxylin eosin stains; original magnification ×10 to 12, reduced by 28%. From Waller (35), with permission.

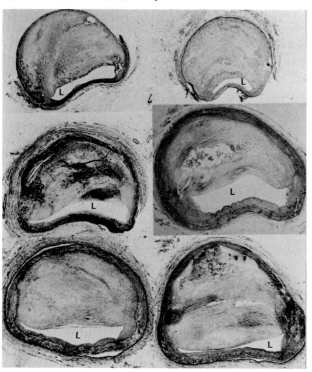

atherosclerotic plaque. Of the 500 segments, 365 (73%) were eccentric and 135 (27%) were concentric. The portion of vessel circumference in the eccentric lesion that is free of disease varies from 17% to 23% (mean 20%) (33) and from 2.3% to 32% (mean 17%) (35). We (35) also compared the thickness of the coronary medial layer in diseased and disease-free portions of the coronary artery segments (Fig. 14.21). The average thickness of the coronary artery media was *thinner* in diseased segments (mean 99.4 μm) compared with disease-free wall segments in the same vessel (mean 202.9 μm).

Role of eccentric plaque in coronary angioplasty and restenosis. Recent interest in eccentric coronary plaque has connected this lesion to mechanisms of coronary artery angioplasty and restenosis (34,35), coronary artery spasm (33,35) and angiographic underestimation of severity of coronary atherosclerosis (Fig. 14.20) (34,35,107).

As described earlier, *stretching* of the plaque-free wall in eccentric atherosclerotic lesions is one of the mechanisms of coronary balloon angioplasty (Fig. 14.5). Morphologic data indicating the high degree of frequency of the eccentric lesion in patients with clinical coronary heart disease suggests that stretching of the plaque-free wall may be a more frequent mechanism than previously thought (35). In addition, dilation of the disease-free arc without damage to plaque on the opposite walls may provide an explanation for *early* (Fig. 14.6b and 14.22) and *late* (Fig. 14.7b and 14.22) "restenosis" after an angiographically successful dilation. Initial stretching of the plaque-free segment may gradually "relax" ("restitution of tone") and decrease the coronary lumen toward its predilation state ("restenosis"). Thermal angioplasty may prove to be an effective way of preventing this elastic recoil of the eccentric lesion (Fig. 14.12).

Role of eccentric plaque and coronary spasm. In addition to stretching, the disease-free wall of the eccentric plaque may be susceptible to *spasm*. The normal or nearly normal arc of coronary wall (normal medial thickness) is capable of "reacting" to various humoral or neurogenic stimuli (Fig. 14.22). The extent to which dynamic augmentation or con-

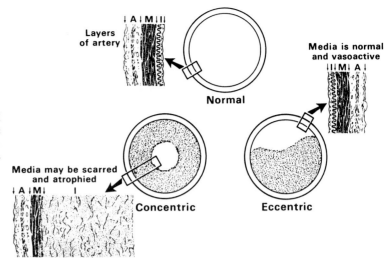

Figure 14.21. Diagram comparing the thickness and structure of coronary artery media (M) in the concentric and eccentric types of atherosclerotic plaque. A = adventitia, I = intima. From Waller (35), with permission.

traction of the coronary wall (that is, *spasm*) is possible appears to be a function of the amount and location of the wall smooth muscle. The potential for dynamic alterations of the coronary lumen (spasm) is less likely to occur along the diseased circumference, but more likely to occur along the disease-free segment of an eccentric coronary lesion. Thermal angioplasty also may be useful in preventing spasm of eccentric plaque by producing injury to the medial smooth muscle cell (Fig. 14.12) (87).

Role in interpreting coronary angiograms. A third role of eccentric plaque occurs in interpreting coronary angiograms. Several necropsy studies (107) indicated some degree of

underestimation of the angiographic assessment of coronary stenosis severity. Variability in coronary lumen shape represents one explanation for this underestimation. The eccentric plaque, and in particular, the slitlike lumen (Fig. 14.20), is most likely to pose a problem for the angiographic assessment of disease. Because the length of the luminal slit approaches the full dimension of the original luminal diameter, the angiographic appearance will be that of a "normal" vessel. The luminal reduction in cross-sectional area is, however, >75%.

Diagnosis. The current development of intravascular ultrasound imaging catheters will aid in the detection of the

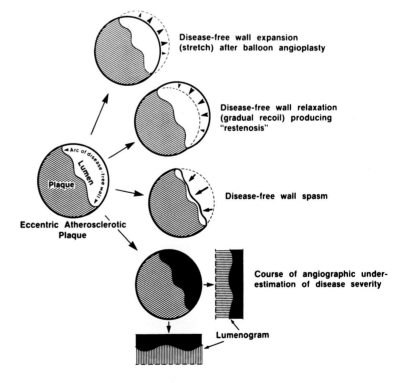

Figure 14.22. Diagram showing the clinical relevance (angioplasty, spasm, angiography) of eccentric atherosclerotic plaque in patients with coronary artery disease.

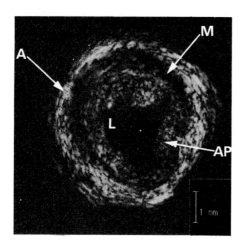

Figure 14.23. Photograph of an in vitro ultrasound image of a diseased human coronary artery, showing the coronary lumen (L), atherosclerotic intima (AP), echo-free media (M) and adventitia (A). (Courtesy of Paul Zalesky, Intertherapy, Inc.)

eccentric coronary lesion. These devices generate highly accurate cross-sectional pictures of the arterial wall showing its three-layered structure and wall composition (Fig. 14.23). From the ultrasound image, it is possible to determine the *presence or absence* of atherosclerotic plaque or thrombus, or both, determine the *integrity of the luminal surface* (that is, detect plaque fissures) and determine the *location, size, type* (that is, concentric versus eccentric) and *composition* (that is, fatty versus fibrous, calcified versus noncalcified) of atherosclerotic plaque (108,109). This new intravascular device represents an exciting and promising potential for visualization of the coronary artery and assessing the results of various new interventional techniques.

Conclusion

Although various public health preventive efforts and prescribed pharmacologic methods will have long-term benefits in the reduction of coronary artery atherosclerosis and subsequent cardiac events, the immediate and short-term future in the treatment of coronary artery disease will be focused on various interventional devices designed to *remodel* or *remove* the causes of acute and chronic coronary artery occlusion.

I acknowledge the artistic talents of George Buckley and the secretarial assistance of Marcy Culp.

References

1. Brensike JF, Kelsey SF, Passamani ER, et al. NHLBI Type II Coronary Intervention study: design, methods, and baseline characteristics. Controlled Clin Trials 1982;3:91–111.
2. Brensike JF, Levy RI, Kelsey SF, et al. Effects of therapy with cholestyramine on progression of coronary atherosclerosis: results of the NHLBI Type II Coronary Intervention study. Circulation 1984;69:313–24.
3. Blankenhorn DH, Nessim SA, Johnson RL, Sanmarco ME, Azen SP, Cashin-Hemphil L. Beneficial effects of combined colestipol-niacin therapy on coronary atherosclerosis and coronary venous bypass grafts. JAMA 1987;257:3233–40.
4. Gruentzig AR, Myler RK, Hanna EH, Turina MI. Coronary transluminal angioplasty (abstr). Circulation 1977;84(suppl II):II-55–II-6.
5. Baim DS (ed). A symposium: interventional cardiology–1987. Am J Cardiol 1988;61:1G–117G.
6. Block PC, Myler RK, Stertzer S, Fallon JT. Morphology after transluminal angioplasty in human beings. N Engl J Med 1981;305:382–5.
7. Essed CD, Brand MVD, Becker AE. Transluminal coronary angioplasty and early restenosis. Br Heart J 1983;49:393–6.
8. Waller BF. Early and late morphologic changes in human coronary arteries after percutaneous transluminal coronary angioplasty. Clin Cardiol 1983;6:363–72.
9. Waller BF, Dillon JC, Cowley MH. Plaque hematoma and coronary dissection with percutaneous transluminal angioplasty (PTCA) of severely stenotic lesions: morphologic coronary observations in 5 men within 30 days of PTCA (abstr). Circulation 1983;68(suppl III):III-144.
10. Waller BF, McManus BM, Gorfinkel HJ, et al. Status of the major coronary arteries 80 to 150 days after percutaneous transluminal coronary angioplasty: analysis of 5 necropsy patients. Am J Cardiol 1983;5:403–21.
11. Saffitz JE, Rose TE, Oaks JB, Roberts WC. Coronary arterial rupture during coronary angioplasty. Am J Cardiol 1983;51:902–4.
12. Mizuno K, Jurita A, Imazeki N. Pathologic findings after percutaneous transluminal coronary angioplasty. Br Heart J 1984;52:588–90.
13. Waller BF, Gorfinkel HJ, Rogers FJ, Kent KM, Roberts WC. Early and late morphologic changes in major epicardial coronary arteries after percutaneous transluminal coronary angioplasty. Am J Cardiol 1984;53:42C–7C.
14. Soward AL, Essed CE, Serruys PW. Coronary arterial findings after accidental death immediately after successful percutaneous transluminal coronary angioplasty. Am J Cardiol 1985;56:794–5.
15. Austin GE, Norman NB, Hollman J, Tabei S, Phillips DF. Intimal proliferation of smooth muscle cells as an explanation for recurrent coronary artery stenosis after percutaneous transluminal coronary angioplasty. J Am Coll Cardiol 1985;6:369–75.
16. Waller BF, Pinkerton CA, Foster LN. Morphologic evidence of accelerated left main coronary artery stenosis: a late complication of percutaneous transluminal balloon angioplasty of the proximal left anterior descending coronary artery. J Am Coll Cardiol 1987;9:1019–23.
17. Waller BF, Rothbaum DA, Pinkerton CA, et al. Status of the myocardium and infarct-related coronary artery in 19 necropsy patients with acute recanalization using pharmacologic, mechanical or combined types of reperfusion therapy. J Am Coll Cardiol 1987;9:785–801.
18. Waller BF. Pathology of transluminal balloon angioplasty used in the treatment of coronary heart disease. Hum Pathol 1987;18:476–84.
19. La Delia V, Rossi PA, Sommers S, Kreps E. Coronary histology after percutaneous transluminal coronary angioplasty. Texas Heart Inst J 1988;15:113–6.
20. Litvack F, Grundfest W, Mohr F, et al. "Hot-tip" angioplasty by a novel radiofrequency catheter (abstr). Circulation 1987;76(suppl IV):IV-47.
21. Sanborn TA, Cumberland, Greenfield AJ, Welsh CA, Guben JK. Percutaneous laser thermal angioplasty: initial results and 1-year followup in 129 femoropopliteal lesions. Radiology 1988;168:121–5.
22. Stroh JA, Sanborn TA, Haudenschild CC. Experimental argon laser thermal angioplasty as an adjunct to balloon angioplasty (abstr). J Am Coll Cardiol 1988;11(suppl A):108A.
23. Sigward U, Puel J, Mirkowitch V, Joffre F, Kappenberger L. Intravascular stents to prevent occlusion and restenosis after transluminal angioplasty. N Engl J Med 1987;316:701–6.
24. Dotter CT, Judkins MP. Transluminal treatment of atherosclerotic obstructions: description of new technic and a preliminary report of its application. Circulation 1964;30:654–70.
25. Gruentzig AR. Transluminal dilatation of coronary artery stenosis. Lancet 1978;1:263–6.

26. Block PC. Histological and ultrastructural studies in animals. In: Proceedings of the Workshop on Percutaneous Transluminal Coronary Angioplasty. DHEW Pub. No. (NIH) 80-2030, 1980:155–9.

27. Block PC, Baughman KL, Pasternak RC, Fallon JT. Transluminal angioplasty: correlation of morphologic and angiographic findings in an experimental model. Circulation 1980;61:778–85.

28. Faxon DP, Weber VJ, Haudenschild C, Gottsman SB, McGovern WA, Ryan TJ. Acute effects of transluminal angioplasty in three experimental models of atherosclerosis. Arteriosclerosis 1982;2:125–33.

29. Baughman KL, Pasternak RC, Fallon JT, Block PC. Transluminal coronary angioplasty of postmortem human hearts. Am J Cardiol 1981; 48:1044–7.

30. Block PC, Fallon JT, Elmer D. Experimental angioplasty: lessons from the laboratory. Am J Radiol 1980;135:907–12.

31. Castaneda-Zuniga WR, Formarek A, Todavarthy M, Edwards JE. The mechanism of balloon angioplasty. Radiology 1980;135:565–9.

32. Levine S, Ewels CJ, Rosing DR, Kent KM. Coronary angioplasty: clinical and angiographic follow-up. Am J Cardiol 1985;55:673–6.

33. Saner HE, Gobel FL, Salomonowitz E, Erlien DA, Edwards JE. The disease-free wall in coronary atherosclerosis: its relation to degree of obstruction. J Am Coll Cardiol 1985;6:1096–9.

34. Waller BF. Coronary luminal shape and the arc of disease-free wall: morphologic observations and clinical relevance. J Am Coll Cardiol 1985;6:1100–1.

35. Waller BF. The eccentric coronary atherosclerotic plaque: morphologic observations and clinical relevance. Clin Cardiol 1989;12:14–20.

36. Vlodaver Z, Edwards JE. Pathology of coronary atherosclerosis. Prog Cardiovasc Dis 1971;14:256–74.

37. Baroldi G. Diseases of the coronary arteries. In: Silver MD, ed. Cardiovascular Pathology. New York: Churchill Livingstone, 1983:341–2.

38. Cowley MJ, Dovros G, Kelsey SF, Van Raden M, Detre KM. Emergency coronary bypass surgery after coronary angioplasty: the National Heart, Lung and Blood Institute's Percutaneous Transluminal Coronary Angioplasty Registry experience. Am J Cardiol 1984;53:22C–6C.

39. Bredlau CE, Roubin GS, Leimgruber PP, Douglas JS Jr, King SB III, Gruentzig AR. In-hospital morbidity and mortality in patients undergoing elective coronary angioplasty. Circulation 1985;72:1044–52.

40. Simpfendorfer C, Belardi J, Bellamy G, Galan K, Franco I, Hollman J. Frequency, management and follow-up of patients with acute coronary occlusions after percutaneous coronary angioplasty. Am J Cardiol 1987;59:267–9.

41. Sinclair IN, McCabe CH, Sipperly ME, Baim DS. Predictors, therapeutic options and long-term outcome of abrupt reclosure. Am J Cardiol 1988;61:615–65.

42. Baim DS, Ignatius EJ. Use of percutaneous transluminal coronary angioplasty: results of a current survey. Am J Cardiol 1988;61:3G–8G.

43. Angelini P, Leachman R, Heibig J. Distal coronary hemoperfusion during balloon angioplasty. Cardiology 1988;5:31–4.

44. Erbel R, Clas W, Busch U, et al. New balloon catheter for prolonged percutaneous transluminal coronary angioplasty and bypass flow in occluded vessels. Cathet Cardiovasc Diagn 1986;12:116–23.

45. Turi ZG, Campbell CA, Gottimukkala MV, Kloner RA. Preservation of distal coronary perfusion during prolonged balloon inflation with an autoperfusion angioplasty catheter. Circulation 1987;75:1273–80.

46. Turi ZG, Rezkalla S, Campbell CA, Kloner RA. Amelioration of ischemia during angioplasty of the left anterior descending coronary artery with an autoperfusion catheter. Am J Cardiol 1988;62:513–7.

47. Baim DS. Interventional catheterization techniques: percutaneous transluminal balloon angioplasty, valvuloplasty, and related procedures. In: Braunwald E, ed. Heart Disease. A Textbook of Cardiovascular Medicine. 3rd ed. Philadelphia: WB Saunders, 1988:1379–94.

48. Ferguson TB Jr, Hinohara T, Simpson J, Stack RS, Wechsler AS. Catheter reperfusion to allow optimal coronary bypass grafting following failed transluminal coronary angioplasty. Ann Thorac Surg 1986;42:399–405.

49. Jenkins RD, Sinclair IN, Leonard BM, Sandor T, Schoen FJ, Spears JR. Laser balloon angioplasty vs balloon angioplasty in normal rabbit iliac arteries (abstr). Circulation 1987;76(suppl IV):IV-47.

50. Sanborn TA, Faxon DP, Haudenschild CC, Ryan TJ. Experimental angioplasty: circumferential distribution of laser thermal energy with a laser probe. J Am Coll Cardiol 1985;5:934–8.

51. Sanborn TA, Cumberland DC, Welsh CL, Greenfield AJ, Guben JK. Laser thermal angioplasty as an adjunct to peripheral balloon angioplasty: one year follow-up results (abstr). Circulation 1987;76(suppl IV):IV-230.

52. White RA, Grundfest WS. Lasers in Cardiovascular Disease. Chicago: Year Book Medical, 1987:1–129.

53. Kaplan J, Barry KJ, Connolly RJ, et al. Thermal angioplasty with a radiofrequency balloon system (abstr). Circulation 1988;78(suppl II):II-503.

54. Serruys DW, Juiliere Y, Bertrand ME, Puel J, Richards AF, Sigwart U. Additional improvement of stenosis geometry in human coronary arteries by stenting after balloon dilatation. Am J Cardiol 1988;61:71G–6G.

55. Palmaz JC, Sibbitt RR, Reuter SR, Tio FO, Rice WJ. Expandable intraluminal graft: a preliminary study. Radiology 1985;156:73–7.

56. Palmaz JC, Sibbitt RR, Tio FO, Reuter SR, Peters JE, Garcia F. Expandable intraluminal vascular graft: a feasibility study. Surgery 1986;99:199–205.

57. Palmaz JC, Windeler SA, Garcia F, Tio FO, Sibbitt RR, Reuter SR. Atherosclerotic rabbit aortas: expandable intraluminal grafting. Radiology 1986;160:723–6.

58. Schatz R, Palmaz J, Garcia F, Tio F, Reuter S. Balloon expandable intracoronary stents in dogs (abstr). Circulation 1986;74(suppl II):II-458.

59. Roubin G, Giaturco C, Brown J, Robinson K, King S. Intracoronary stenting of canine coronary arteries after percutaneous coronary angioplasty (abstr). Circulation 1986;74(suppl II):II-458.

60. Roubin GS, Robinson KA, King SB, et al. Acute and late results of intracoronary arterial stenting after coronary angioplasty in dogs. Circulation 1987;76:891–7.

61. Sanborn TA. Laser thermal angioplasty. In: White RA, Grundfest WS, eds. Lasers in Cardiovascular Disease. Chicago: Year Book Medical, 1987:75–90.

62. Cumberland DC, Sanborn TA, Taylor DI, et al. Percutaneous laser thermal angioplasty—initial clinical results with a laser probe in a total peripheral artery occlusion. Lancet 1986;1:1457–9.

63. Sanborn TA, Haudenschild CC, Faxon DP, Ryan TJ. Angiographic and histologic follow-up of laser angioplasty with a laser probe (abstr). J Am Coll Cardiol 1985;5:408.

64. Sanborn TA. Laser angioplasty. What has been learned from experimental studies and clinical trials? Circulation 1988;78:769–74.

65. Forrester JS, Litvack F, Grundfest W. Vaporization of atheroma in man: the role of lasers in the era of balloon angioplasty. Int J Cardiol 1988;20:1–7.

66. Bertrand ME, LeBranche JM, Thieuleux FA, Fourrier JL, Traisnel G, Asseman P. Comparative results of percutaneous transluminal coronary angioplasty in patients with dynamic versus fixed coronary stenosis. J Am Coll Cardiol 1986;8:504–8.

67. Corcos T, David PR, Val PG, et al. Failure of diltiazem to prevent restenosis after percutaneous transluminal coronary angioplasty. Am Heart J 1985;109:926–31.

68. Holmes DR, Vlietstra RE, Smith HC, et al. Restenosis after percutaneous transluminal coronary angioplasty (PTCA): a report from the PTCA Registry of the National Heart, Lung, and Blood Institute. Am J Cardiol 1984;53:77C–81C.

69. Kaltenback M, Kober G, Scherer D, Vallbracht C. Recurrence rate after successful coronary angioplasty. Eur Heart J 1985;6:276–281.

70. Leimgruber PP, Roubin GS, Hollman J, et al. Restenosis after successful coronary angioplasty in patients with single vessel disease. Circulation 1986;73:710–7.

71. Mabin TA, Holmes DR, Smith HC, et al. Follow-up clinical results in patients undergoing percutaneous transluminal coronary angioplasty. Circulation 1985;71:754–60.

72. Myler RM, Shaw RE, Stertzer SH, Clark DA, Fishman J, Murphy MG. Recurrence after coronary angioplasty. Cathet Cardiovasc Diagn 1987; 13:77–86.

73. Nobuyoski M, Kimura T, Nosaka H, et al. Restenosis after successful percutaneous transluminal coronary angioplasty: serial angiographic followup of 229 patients. J Am Coll Cardiol 1988;12:616–23.

74. Shaw RE, Myler RK, Stertzer SH, Clark DA. Restenosis after coronary angioplasty. Cardiology 1987;4:42–5.

75. Whitworth HB, Roubin GS, Hollman J, et al. Effect of nifedipine on recurrent stenosis after percutaneous transluminal coronary angioplasty. J Am Coll Cardiol 1986;8:1271–6.

76. Fuster V, Adams PC, Badimon JJ, Chesebro JH. Platelet-inhibitor drugs role in coronary artery disease. Prog Cardiovasc Dis 1987;29:325–46.

77. Meier B, King SB, Gruentzig AR, et al. Repeat coronary angioplasty. J Am Coll Cardiol 1984;4:463–6.

78. Castellot JJ, Favreau LV, Karnovsky MJ, Rosenberg RR. Inhibition of vascular smooth muscle cell growth by endothelial cell-derived heparin. J Biol Chem 1982;257:11256–60.

79. Simpson JB, Zimmerman JJ, Selmon MR, et al. Transluminal atherectomy: initial clinical results in 27 patients (abstr). Circulation 1986; 74(suppl II):II-203.

80. Simpson JB, Selmon MR, Robertson GC, et al. Transluminal atherectomy for occlusive peripheral vascular disease. Am J Cardiol 1988;61: 965–1016.

81. Graf RH, Verani MS. Left main coronary artery stenosis: a possible complication of transluminal coronary angioplasty. Cathet Cardiovasc Diagn 1984;10:163–6.

82. Slack JD, Pinkerton CA. Subacute left main coronary stenosis: an unusual but serious complication of percutaneous transluminal angioplasty. Angiology 1985;36:130–6.

83. Spears JR. Percutaneous transluminal coronary angioplasty restenosis: potential prevention with laser balloon angioplasty. Am J Cardiol 1987;60:61B–4B.

84. Jenkins RD, Sinclair IN, Leonard BM, Sandor T, Schoen FJ, Spears JR. Laser balloon angioplasty vs balloon angioplasty in normal iliac arteries (abstr). Circulation 1987;76(suppl IV):IV-47.

85. Sinclair IN. Effect of laser balloon angioplasty on normal dog coronary arteries in vivo (abstr). J Am Coll Cardiol 1988;11:108A.

86. Jenkins RD, Sinclair IN, Anand RK, James LM, Spears JR. Laser balloon angioplasty: effect of exposure duration on shear strength of welded layers of postmortem human aorta (abstr). Circulation 1987; 76(suppl IV):IV-46.

87. Lee BI, Becker GJ, Waller BF, et al. Thermal compression and molding of atherosclerotic vascular tissue with use of radiofrequency energy: implications for radiofrequency balloon angioplasty. J Am Coll Cardiol 1989;13:1167–75.

88. Myler RK, Cumberland DA, Clark DA, Stertzer SH, Tatpati DA, Sarma PK. High and low power thermal laser angioplasty for total occlusions and restenosis in man (abstr). Circulation 1987;76(suppl IV):IV-230.

89. Abela GS, Seeger JM, Barbieri E, Conti CR. Laser angioplasty with angioscopic guidance in humans. J Am Coll Cardiol 1986;8:184–92.

90. Fouvier JL, Marache P, Brunetand JM, Mordon S, Lablanche JM, Bertrand ME. Laser recanalization of peripheral arteries by contact sapphire in man (abstr). Circulation 1986;74(suppl II):II-231.

91. Hofling B, Simpson JB, Remberger K, Lauterjung L, Backa D. Percutaneous atherectomy in iliac, femoral and popliteal arteries. Klin Wochenschr 1987;65:528.

92. Davies MJ, Thomas A. Thrombosis and acute coronary-artery lesions in sudden cardiac ischemic death. N Engl J Med 1984;310:1137–40.

93. Davies MJ, Thomas T. The pathological basis and microanatomy of occlusive thrombus formation in human coronary arteries. Philos Trans R Soc Lond (Biol) 1981;294:225–9.

94. Falk E. Plaque rupture with severe pre-existing stenosis precipitating coronary thrombosis characteristics of coronary atherosclerotic plaques underlying fatal occlusive thrombi. Br Heart J 1983;50:127–34.

95. Friedman M. The coronary thrombus: its origin and fate. Hum Pathol 1971;2:81–128.

96. Davies MJ, Thomas AC. Plaque fissuring—the cause of acute myocardial infarction, sudden ischemic death, and crescendo angina. Br Heart J 1985;53:363–73.

97. Davies MJ, Fulton WFM, Robertson WB. The relation of coronary thrombosis to ischemic myocardial necrosis. J Pathol 1979;127:99–110.

98. Ambrose JA, Winters SL, Arora RR, et al. Coronary angiography morphology in myocardial infarction: a link between the pathogenesis of unstable angina and myocardial infarction. J Am Coll Cardiol 1985;6: 1233–8.

99. Ambrose JA, Winters SL, Arora RR, et al. Angiographic evolution of coronary artery morphology in unstable angina. J Am Coll Cardiol 1986;7:472–8.

100. Ambrose JA, Winters SL, Stern A, et al. Angiographic morphology and the pathogenesis of unstable angina pectoris. J Am Coll Cardiol 1985;5: 609–16.

101. Haft JI, Goldstein JE, Niemiera ML. Coronary arteriographic lesion of unstable angina. Chest 1987;92:609–12.

102. Levin DC, Fallon JT. Significance of the angiographic morphology of localized coronary stenosis: histopathologic correlations. Circulation 1982;66:316–20.

103. Forrester JS, Litvack F, Grundfest W, Hickey A. A perspective of coronary disease seen through the arteries of living man. Circulation 1987;75:505–13.

104. Litvack F, Hickey A, Grundfest W, et al. Angioscopy is superior to angiography for detecting complex atheroma (abstr). Circulation 1986; 74(suppl II):II-362.

105. Sherman CT, Litvack F, Grundfest WS, et al. Demonstration of thrombus and complex atheroma by in-vivo angioscopy in patients with unstable angina pectoris. N Engl J Med 1986;315:913–9.

106. Vetrovec GW, Cowley MJ, Overton H, Richardson DW. Intracoronary thrombus in syndromes of unstable myocardial ischemia. Am Heart J 1981;102:1202–8.

107. Isner JM, Donaldson RF. Coronary angiographic and morphologic correlation. In: Waller BF, ed. Symposium on cardiac morphology. Cardiol Clin 1984;2:571–92.

108. Mallery JA, Tobis JM, Gessert J, et al. Identification of tissue components in human atheroma by an intravascular ultrasound imaging catheter (abstr). Circulation 1988;78(suppl II):II-22.

109. McKay C, Waller BF, Gessert J, et al. Quantitative analysis of coronary artery morphology using intracoronary high frequency ultrasound: validation by histology and quantitative coronary arteriography (abstr). J Am Coll Cardiol 1989;13(suppl A):228A.

◆ CHAPTER 15 ◆

Growth and Development of State of the Art Care for People With Congenital Heart Disease

MARY ALLEN ENGLE, MD

This is a tale of steady progress during the past 40 years in the art and science of care for patients with congenital heart disease. Our story begins over 10 years earlier.

We have done little to prevent congenital heart disease but we have done lots to save lives in the 50 years since Robert Gross successfully tied off a patent ductus arteriosus (1). He did that at the time when diagnostic skills depended on a stethoscope, a three lead electrocardiogram (ECG) and a chest radiograph. Anesthesia was by gas, oxygen and open-drop ether. Recovery took place because of loving care and not with the benefit of antibiotics or even sulfonamides and without any of the accoutrements we associate with intensive care suites.

The beginnings. The state of the art began to flower after 1944 when Helen Taussig and Alfred Blalock teamed up for the first blue baby operation, the subclavian to pulmonary artery anastomosis (2). Sulfa drugs and penicillin were available and the use of unipolar ECGs with limb and precordial leads was just beginning. The excitement that accompanied the miracle of turning a handicapped blue baby or child into an active person with pink color stimulated the development of cardiac catheterization and uniplane, cut film angiocardiography.

The independent reports by Crafoord and Nylin (3) and Gross and Hufnagel (4) of relief of coarctation of the aorta by resection and end to end anastomosis were soon followed by the method of Brock (5) and Sellors (6) for providing transvalvular relief of valvular pulmonary stenosis by insertion of a valvulotome through an incision in the right ventricle. Closed heart surgery thus became established.

Medical management advanced, too: improved treatment of heart failure by use of cardiac glycosides, rather than digitalis leaf, in dosages based on the weight of the infant or child (7); diuretics were chiefly mercurials. This same period saw successful treatment of bacterial endocarditis with a month of penicillin administration and the promotion of the concept of prevention of that complication through prophylactic use of antibiotics at times of high risk such as after dental extractions. The beneficial effect of 10 days of oral penicillin for patients with identified B-hemolytic streptococcal pharyngitis came to be recognized and translated into programs for primary and secondary prevention of rheumatic fever and rheumatic heart disease. Now valvular heart disease is uncommon.

In this country the American College of Cardiology and the American Heart Association were leaders not only in the research and promotion of these programs of treatment and prevention of rheumatic fever, but also in encouraging the development of teams of cardiologists and surgeons dedicated to the common goal of saving the lives of people with congenital heart disease. This became the chief challenge in heart disease of the young as rheumatic fever began to decline.

Developments that made possible today's state of the art care. The 1950s brought diagnosis and treatment to new heights, with Helen Taussig and Alfred Blalock leading the way in the team approach in long-term follow-up and training programs. Diagnostic methodology advanced with biplane cut film angiocardiography, cineangiocardiography (8) and the combination of cardiac catheterization with selective injection of contrast medium, together with techniques for combined left and right heart studies. Miniaturization of sampling techniques and development of soft catheters made it possible to begin to study even the small, sick baby in need of accurate diagnosis and surgical relief.

Not all handicapping anomalies were extracardiac; exploration of how to see and repair conditions such as pulmonary stenosis and atrial septal defect led to the use of hypothermia and inflow occlusion for treatment of these two malformations that could be relieved quickly in the limited time available by this form of circulatory arrest. In Canada, Bigelow and his coworkers (9) led in the next step forward of general hypothermia in surgery for congenital heart disease.

Another approach to salvage of babies was for the common intracardiac anomaly of a large ventricular septal defect, with failure to thrive and with cardiac failure that could not be controlled despite intensive medical management (10). Surgical palliation (pulmonary artery banding) was offered by Muller (surgeon) and Dammann (pediatrician) (11). They created a new lesion, pulmonary stenosis, by banding the pulmonary artery to stem the excessive flow of blood through the defect and into the pulmonary artery.

C. Walton Lillehei (12) pioneered open heart surgery as we know it today with his dramatic use in the mid 1950s, of controlled cross circulation and then the bubble oxygenator to close septal defects and repair tetralogy of Fallot. Kirklin and coworkers (13) adopted the membrane oxygenator of Gibbons et al. (14) to perfect and expand the art and science of surgery for congenital heart disease. These two Minnesota surgeons and their pediatric and medical colleagues were joined by cardiologists and cardiac surgeons around the world in quest of definitive repair of as many complex anomalies as existed in need of repair.

The postoperative complication of postpericardiotomy syndrome was created when intrapericardial surgery for heart disease came into being (15,16). This entity required recognition for what it was and for what it was not (not sepsis, endocarditis or reactivation of rheumatic fever) and for the fact that it was self-limited and usually did not recur. Critical analysis of operative mortality, morbidity and short- as well as long-term results refined the selection of cases and improved the results of cardiac surgery.

Interventional pediatric cardiology. The 1960s witnessed the perfection of catheterization techniques for infants recognized to be critically in need of medical or surgical help, or both. Rashkind (17) became the father of interventional cardiology when he introduced the balloon catheter creation of an atrial septal defect as life-saving palliation for the cyanotic newborn with complete transposition of the great arteries. This accomplishment for such neonates was matched by the effective surgical physiologic repair in children by the venous switch operation of William Mustard (18). This procedure rerouted venous return to the atria to match the transposed great arteries, thereby achieving physiologic blood flow and conversion of a sickly, cyanotic patient to a pink, healthy one.

The 1970s saw two major diagnostic and surgical advances in this leapfrogging of medical and surgical improvements in the care of congenital heart disease. Let us consider the surgical accomplishments first. Since the 1950s, the importance of severe congenital heart disease in young infants had been appreciated, but the risks in efforts at surgical salvage were still high. The sad story was that only half of these critically affected babies reached their first birthday, and that most deaths due to congenital heart disease occurred in the first 3 to 6 months of life. A combination of events in the 1970s changed that: miniaturization of equipment in laboratories and operating rooms, monitoring and ventilatory support in neonatal and pediatric intensive care units and skills in sophisticated anesthesiologic management. Added to these were the surgical techniques of hypothermia combined with cardiopulmonary bypass and the development by Barratt-Boyes and colleagues (19) in New Zealand of the use of profound hypothermia and circulatory arrest.

All of these measures accomplished more saving of lives for babies with cyanotic and acyanotic anomalies. Previously, such children often died before reaching the suitable and safe age of 5 or 6 years for surgery with cardiopulmonary bypass. The door was now open for early repair as the definitive procedure in infancy rather than later repair in childhood after palliation in infancy. Babies born with the common anomalies of large ventricular septal defect or with tetralogy of Fallot benefited especially by this new approach to open repair. In this country, Paul Ebert (20) and Aldo Castaneda (21) and their coworkers led in the excellent results of surgery for infants with severe congenital heart disease.

Advances in the diagnosis of congenital heart disease. The major advance in diagnosis in the 1970s was the advent of echocardiography, at first M-mode and then two-dimensional (22). At the outset, this imaging technique was validated by comparison with the findings at cardiac catheterization with contrast visualization. As credibility was established, echocardiography came to be used increasingly to confirm the clinical diagnosis in mild or moderately severe conditions where cardiac catheterization would not ordinarily be needed, and to be used in serial, noninvasive follow-up of patients with unoperated or postoperative congenital heart disease. Next it began to replace cardiac catheterization as confirmation of diagnosis for patients undergoing cardiac surgery on their malformation (23). This trend increased as Doppler methodology was added in the 1980s.

Recent medical and surgical progress. Other improvements in treatment in the 1970s were both medical and surgical. Management of cardiac failure was helped greatly by the introduction of an effective diuretic, furosemide (24), and by the use, when necessary, of afterload-reducing drugs. New antiarrhythmic agents helped to control difficult problems and new antibiotics were developed that helped cure infections due to resistant organisms.

Pharmacologic manipulations of the ductus arteriosus often accomplished its closure when it was open and physiologically significant in very small premature babies. The agent employed, indomethacin, was a prostaglandin-synthetase inhibitor (25,26). The converse effect involved the use of prostaglandin in newborns to maintain temporary patency of the ductus arteriosus until diagnosis and surgery could be performed. For instance, a baby whose survival depends on patency of the ductus because of severe congenital pulmonary atresia or stenosis needs an open ductus to shunt blood left to right into the pulmonary circuit (27). Alternatively, the infant with severe coarctation of the aorta also needs a patent ductus to permit a right to left shunt from the pulmonary artery to the descending aorta to maintain flow into the descending aorta. The neonate with complete transposition of the great arteries may benefit from a patent ductus to provide bidirectional shunting as a temporary measure. The temporary induction of patency of the ductus in these critically ill newborns permitted stabilization of their condition and the avoidance of middle of the night, high risk cardiac catheterization and emergency surgery.

Surgical inventiveness in the use of external conduits to connect the right ventricle to the pulmonary artery in conditions of truncus arteriosus and pulmonary atresia was led by Dwight McGoon and his coworkers (28). Francis Fontan (29) introduced the revolutionary concept that, in the malformation of tricuspid atresia and rudimentary right ventricle with diminished pulmonary blood flow, the right atrium alone could serve to receive systemic venous return and deliver it to the pulmonary circulation. Fontan, of Bordeaux, France and William Kreutzer (30), of Buenos Aires, Argentina independently demonstrated that this approach afforded a new kind of palliation that separated systemic and pulmonary circulations. Jatene and coworkers (31) introduced the arterial switch operation for transposition of the great arteries. Critical analysis of results modified criteria for selection for surgery and perioperative management so that mortality rates began to decline. Surgical suppression of accessory conduction pathways began to be used to treat people with Wolff-Parkinson-White syndrome and serious arrhythmias refractory to usual drug therapy (32).

The team approach. During the 1960s and 1970s, organized medicine and the health care system articulated and formalized guidelines for centers of excellence in the short- and long-term care of people with congenital heart disease. The Intersociety Commission on Heart Disease Resources, headed by cardiologist Irving Wright, published a series of guidelines for optimal care (33,34). The American College of Cardiology was a participating society. These guidelines emphasized the team approach with trained medical and pediatric cardiologists, cardiac surgeons, anesthesiologists, pathologists, nurses and related professional personnel and social services, all working in coordination and cooperative collaboration in a center well equipped and staffed for diagnosis and medical-surgical care and follow-up.

The 1980s have seen the flowering of the field of echocardiography with Doppler and Doppler color flow mapping studies that not only image defects but also quantitate physiologic events of flow and pressure. In many instances Doppler studies have become the standard, replacing cardiac catheterization as the first confirmation of diagnosis and in follow-up. Radionuclide cineangiocardiography (35) and nuclear magnetic resonance imaging (36) and digital subtraction angiocardiography (37) have enhanced imaging capabilities with minimal or no invasive aspect to the study.

Yet the cardiac catheterization laboratories continue to be busy as they carry out electrophysiologic studies (38) of extraordinary arrhythmias and perform invasive cardiovascular therapy. Jean Kan and coworkers (39) of Johns Hopkins demonstrated the safety and efficacy of balloon dilation of the moderately or severely stenotic pulmonary valve. This is now widely accepted as an alternative to open heart surgery for relief of the obstruction. James Lock and other interventional cardiologists are carefully performing and analyzing other balloon dilations that are not yet so successful and remain investigational, such as dilation of native coarctation (40), congenital valvular aortic stenosis (41) or peripheral pulmonary stenosis (42).

Cardiovascular surgical teams proceed with meticulous care to repair, often in very young infants, even the most complex of anomalies. William Norwood and colleagues (43) accepted the ultimate surgical challenge for salvage of a desperate situation when they carried out the first of several proposed stages of palliation for the usually lethal and all too

common hypoplastic left heart syndrome. Mechanical valves are long lasting, and sometimes the native valve may be rendered functional after surgery. Aortic homografts are more readily available for external conduits than in the past. Pacemakers are sophisticated, miniaturized and longer lasting (44). Heart transplantation is saving lives, even in childhood (45), and heart-lung transplantation offers hope of redemption to some patients with Eisenmenger syndrome.

This recital of developments that took us to where we are today is liberally laced with surgical names, which pays due respect to but unfair emphasis on one important group of the team that brought the care of people with congenital heart disease to this high state of the art. Procedures tend to have names attached, whereas medical diagnosis and care do not. As these surgeons would quickly agree, the success of a surgical technique depends not only on the concept, the research and development and the skill in the operating room. It also requires the correct diagnosis of the patient by the cardiologist, the careful selection for surgery by both partners of the team and preoperative and postoperative team care. Thereafter, their partner in pediatric cardiology carries out long-term postoperative follow-up with analysis of outcome so that results can be continuingly improved. Many giants in the field of pediatric cardiology contributed their skills, talents, research, teaching and warm-hearted care of the patients to this chronicle of the growth and development of high quality care in congenital heart disease. Most people with cardiac birth defects do not require cardiac surgery; they have also been helped by what we have learned from the surgical experience.

The future. What does the future hold? I wouldn't dare to guess! State-of-the-art care as it has developed decade by decade over the past 50 years has without question saved lives and made longer lives healthier. It has accomplished the mission of the American College of Cardiology and American Heart Association by preventing disability and premature death for thousands of people born with cardiovascular malformations.

Future developments will continue to build on past knowledge and will employ the team approach with each member contributing clinical and research abilities and medical, pediatric, surgical, nursing, technical, social, engineering and laboratory skills in centers with up to date facilities for ambulatory and in-patient diagnosis and treatment, both medical and surgical. Early diagnosis and compassionate, long-term, informed care will always be important. During the present and on into the future, just as in the past, we do well to remember that in state of the art care, sympathetic understanding and knowledgeable care are the key.

References

1. Gross RE, Hubbard P. Surgical ligation of patent ductus arteriosus. Report of the first successful case. JAMA 1939;112:729–31.
2. Blalock A, Taussig HB. The surgical treatment of malformations of the

heart in which there is pulmonary stenosis or pulmonary atresia. JAMA 1945;128:189–202.

3. Crafoord C, Nylin G. Congenital coarctation of the aorta and its surgical treatment. J Thorac Surg 1945;14:347–61.

4. Gross RE, Hufnagel CA. Coarctation of the aorta; Experimental studies regarding its surgical correction. N Engl J Med 1945;233:287–93.

5. Brock RC. Pulmonary valvulotomy for the relief of congenital pulmonary stenosis. Report of three cases. Br Med J 1948;1121–6.

6. Sellors TH. Surgery of pulmonary stenosis. A case in which the pulmonary valve was successfully divided. Lancet 1948;1:988–9.

7. Keith JD. Congestive heart failure. Pediatrics 1956;18:491–500.

8. Sones FM. Cine-cardio-angiography. Pediatr Clin North Am 1958;5:945–79.

9. Bigelow WG, Callaghan JC, Hoppo GA. General hypothermia for experimental intracardiac surgery. Ann Surg 1950;132:531–9.

10. Engle MA. Ventricular septal defect in infancy. Pediatrics 1954;14:16–27.

11. Muller WH Jr, Dammann JF Jr. Treatment of certain malformations of the heart by the creation of pulmonary stenosis to reduce pulmonary hypertension and excessive pulmonary blood flow. Surg Gynecol Obstet 1952;95:213–9.

12. Lillehei CW, Cohen M, Warden HE, et al. The direct-vision intracardiac correction of congenital anomalies by controlled cross-circulation: results in 32 patients with ventricular septal defects, tetralogy of Fallot, and atrioventricular communis defects. Surgery 1955;38:11–29.

13. Kirklin JW, DuShane JW, Patrick RT, et al. Intracardiac surgery with the aid of a mechanical pump-oxygenator system (Gibbon type): report of eight cases. Mayo Clin Proc 1955;30:201–6.

14. Gibbons JH Jr, Miller BJ, Fineberg C. An improved mechanical heart and lung apparatus: its use during open cardiotomy in experimental animals. Med Clin North Am 1953;37:1603–24.

15. Ito T, Engle MA, Goldberg HP. Postpericardiotomy syndrome following surgery of nonrheumatic heart disease. Circulation 1958;17:549–56.

16. Engle MA, Ito T. The postpericardiotomy syndrome. Am J Cardiol 1961;7:73–82.

17. Rashkind WJ, Miller WW. Creation of an atrial septal defect without thoracotomy. JAMA 1966;196:991–2.

18. Mustard WT. Successful two-stage correction of transposition of the great vessels. Surgery 1964;55:469–72.

19. Barratt-Boyes BG, Simpson MM, Neutze JM. Intracardiac surgery in neonates and infants using deep hypothermia with surface cooling and limited cardiopulmonary bypass. Circulation 1971;43(suppl I):I-25–30.

20. Ebert PA, Gay WA Jr, Engle MA. Correction of transposition of the great arteries: relationship of the coronary sinus and postoperative arrhythmias. Ann Surg 1974;140:433–8.

21. Castaneda AR, Lamberti J, Sade RM, et al. Open-heart surgery during the first three months of life. J Thorac Cardiovasc Surg 1974;68:719–31.

22. Feigenbaum H. Echocardiography. 4th ed. Philadelphia: Lea & Febiger, 1986.

23. Engle MA. Cardiac surgery without preoperative cardiac catheterization. Pediatr Ann 1987;16:623–8.

24. Engle MA, Lewy JE, Lewy PR, et al. The use of furosemide in infants and children. Pediatrics 1978;62:811–8.

25. Friedman NF, Hirschklau MJ, Printz MP, et al. Pharmacologic closure of patent ductus arteriosus in the premature infant. N Engl J Med 1976;295:526–9.

26. Heymann HM, Rudolph AM, Silverman NH. Closure of the ductus arteriosus in premature infants by inhibition of prostaglandin synthesis. N Engl J Med 1976;295:530–3.

27. Olley PM, Coceani F, Bodach E. E-type prostaglandins. A new emergency therapy for certain cyanotic congenital heart malformations. Circulation 1976;53:728–31.

28. Rastelli GC, Titus JL, McGoon DC. Homograft of ascending aorta and aortic valve as a right ventricular outflow: an experimental approach to the repair of truncus arteriosus. Arch Surg 1967;95:698–708.

29. Fontan F, Baudet E. Surgical repair of tricuspid atresia. Thorax 1971;26:240–8.

30. Kreutzer G, Galindez E, Bono H, et al. An operation for the correction of tricuspid atresia. J Thorac Cardiovasc Surg 1973;66:613–21.

31. Jatene AD, Fontes VF, Paerlista PP, et al. Successful anatomic correction of transposition of the great vessels. A preliminary report. Arq Bras Cardiol 1975;28:461–4.

32. Gallagher JJ, Gilbert M, Svenson RH, et al. WPW syndrome. The problem, evaluation and surgical correction. Circulation 1975;51:767–74.

33. Engle MA, Adams FH, Betson R, et al. Resources for the optimal acute care of patients with congenital heart disease. Circulation 1971;43(suppl A):A-123–33.

34. Engle MA, Adams FH, Betson R, et al. Resources for optimal long-term care of congenital heart disease. Report of Inter-Society Commission for Heart Disease Resources. Circulation 1971;44(suppl A):A-205–19.

35. Treves ST, Newberger J, Hurwitz R. Radionuclide angiography in children. J Am Coll Cardiol 1985;5(suppl):120S–7S.

36. Higgins CB, Lanzer P, Stark D, et al. Assessment of cardiac anatomy using nuclear magnetic resonance imaging. J Am Coll Cardiol 1985;5(suppl):77S–81S.

37. Levin AR, Goldberg HL, Borer JS, et al. Digital angiography in the pediatric patient with congenital heart disease: comparison with standard methods. Circulation 1983;68:374–84.

38. Gillette PC, Garson A Jr. Pediatric Cardiac Dysrhythmias. New York: Grune & Stratton, 1981:474.

39. Kan JS, White RI, Mitchell SE, et al. Percutaneous transluminal balloon valvuloplasty for pulmonary valve stenosis. Circulation 1984;69:554–60.

40. Lock JE, Bass JL, Amplatz K, Fuhrman BP, Castaneda-Zuniga W. Balloon dilation angioplasty of aortic coarctations in infants and children. Circulation 1983;68:109–16.

41. Shaller GF, Keane JF, Sanders SP, et al. Balloon dilation of congenital aortic valve stenosis. Results and influence of technical and morphologic features on outcome. Circulation 1988;78:351–60.

42. Lock JE, Castaneda-Zuniga WR, Fuhrman BP, Bass JL. Balloon dilation angioplasty of hypoplastic and stenotic pulmonary arteries. Circulation 1983;67:962–7.

43. Norwood WS, Kirklin JK, Sanders SP. Hypoplastic left heart syndrome: experience with palliative surgery. Am J Cardiol 1980;45:87–91.

44. Serwer GA, Merick JM, Armstrong BE. Epicardial ventricular pacemaker longevity in children. Am J Cardiol 1988;61:104–6.

45. Rose EA. Cardiac transplantation during childhood. Cardiac transplantation of small children. In: Doyle EF, Engle MA, Gersony NN, Rashkind NJ, Talner NS, eds. Pediatric Cardiology. New York: Springer-Verlag, 1981:676–7.

CHAPTER 16

Genetics and Congenital Heart Disease: Perspectives and Prospects

REED E. PYERITZ, MD, PhD, EDMOND A. MURPHY, MD, ScD

Congenital anomalies of the structure of the heart have been described since the time of Leonardo da Vinci and Morgagni, but it was Maude Abbott (1,2) early in this century who first investigated systematically and rigorously (from 1,000 personal cases) the pathology of such anomalies. Helen Taussig (3) extended this enquiry to the bedside and showed that much pathology could be deduced by clinical examination and the simple tests then available, the electrocardiogram and chest radiograph. Most clinicians, however, dismissed specific diagnosis because they believed that cardiac anomalies ". . . were hopeless finalities in which the function of the physician was limited to matters of general advice and prognosis" (4). Angiocardiography, cardiac catheterization and, more importantly, cardiac surgery rapidly and profoundly changed this sense of futility.

Although the diagnosis and management of congenital heart disease have made impressive progress, understanding etiology and pathogenesis has not. This observation is particularly true for the role of the genome in congenital cardiac anomalies, whose study has never engendered any saltatory advances akin to the first repair of a patent ductus arteriosus or the first palliation of tetrology of Fallot. Indeed, although most embryologists believe that genes are important in the majority of congenital heart defects, and many pathologists and clinicians might concur, no one has yet developed successful ways to render this belief practical. All who deal with patients give counsel as best they can about current and future affected relatives; but, except for the occasional Mendelian disorder, advice is based on an all-purpose empiric recurrence risk estimate of 3 to 5%. This approach has scarcely changed in 3 decades, an embarrassing contrast with developments in cellular, developmental and molecular biology.

Accurate genetic counseling requires not only precision in diagnosis but knowledge of cause. Effective management of disease requires not only understanding of natural history and therapeutics but knowledge of pathogenesis. In most instances of cardiac anomalies, etiology and pathogenesis are unknown; discovering them is the focus of this article. Our goals are to review in brief the methods used to address these issues and the reasons that, at best, they have led to partial answers, to urge the study of pathophysiologic mechanisms in developmental systems subject to evolutionary constraint and to identify directions of research likely to promote clinical effectiveness. We limit ourselves to structural anomalies of the heart evident during embryogenesis and, if compatible with survival, evident at birth. Excluded are disorders of electrophysiology, some of which are clearly genetic, and the many age-dependent heritable disorders that are not congenital, for example, the autosomal dominant hypertrophic and dilated cardiomyopathies, mitral valve prolapse and the Marfan syndrome.

Preliminary Considerations

We well understand the risk of compressing the massive information bearing on the genetics of congenital heart disease. But, because our chief purpose is to place what is known in the perspective of where future investigation might be directed, we state our beliefs with brief support.

First, the embryology of the heart is unquestionably under genetic control. For example, some disorders of ontogeny segregate in families as Mendelian traits. About 11% of autosomal and X-linked disorders that are compatible with survival into adulthood affect the cardiovascular system; the figure is 17% for those Mendelian disorders lethal in the neonatal period (5). Moreover, most phenotypes caused by aneuploidy, including common ones such as the Down and Turner syndromes, lead to major cardiovascular malformations.

Second, how genes exert their effects on organogenesis is not at all clear from simple inspection of the clinical phenotype. In some Mendelian disorders, the cardiovascular manifestations of the phenotype tend to breed true, as in the common atrium of the Ellis-van Creveld syndrome. In the Noonan syndrome, the malformation is quite diverse in detail (septal hypertrophy, pulmonary valve stenosis, pulmonary artery stenosis, aortic valve stenosis), but perhaps somewhat more unified in general (all defects are obstructive). In lesions less clearly Mendelian, in which multiple genes and environmental factors are usually incriminated, relatives of probands, although at increased risk of cardiovascular malformations, often have anatomically disparate lesions. If what is encoded by the genome is the specific *anatomic* structure, these empiric facts are difficult to understand. On the other hand, ready interpretation may prove possible if the genome encodes *mechanisms of development.* For instance, we surmise that genes control both the amounts of factors that govern growth and development of a particular organ as well as whether they are active or inactive. A defect in one developmental gene might have pleiotropic effects not in one organ only but in distant parts of the body as well (6).

Third, a major area of uncertainty relevant to both normal and defective ontogeny is how genetically encoded chemical messages are transformed into processes with spatial orientation, handedness and highly organized timing. That such requirements are reliably met is unequivocal, but details and the way that specialized nuances, such as asymmetries either of structure (for example, the rotation of the heart) or of function (for example, the cerebral hemispheres) are accommodated, remain obscure. Selection pressures require that these developmental demands be met with high reliability; one result is the precise conservation of the d-cardiac loop across diverse taxonomic classes. Reliability would presumably be favored by simple processes rather than complex ones, by properties that are intrinsic (such as the geometric consequences of physical relations) rather than arbitrary (as the genetic codes) and by redundancy rather than uniqueness. We thus begin with strong presumptions in favor of robust processes with rich properties, rather than complicated, fragile and narrowly specific devices.

Fourth, the heart has a vital role at every stage of evolution of higher organisms. Mutation is rare and not at once relevant unless it alters the overt phenotype. In contrast, reproduction, by which mutation is integrated and perpetuated in the human gene pool, is common and efficient. As a result, cardiac defects are heavily penalized in the genetic sense that selection impedes reproduction. For our purposes here the most important implication is that ontogenic mechanisms need not be complex.

Fifth, ontogeny is regulated to some extent by homeostasis or "feedback" (7). Common experience, such as navigating across large distances, shows that provision for reducing cumulative effects of small *initial* errors and their propagation vastly reduces the demands of accuracy of the preliminary course. Hence, there is powerful selective value to feedback control in developmental mechanisms, just as there is for physiologic ones (8,9). However, feedback control is necessarily unbiased and *any such process with a mean effect of zero would not ordinarily be detected by classic quantitative genetics.*

Fundamental Approaches to Congenital Heart Disease

Several academic approaches have helped our understanding of the nature and origin of congenital heart disease: high resolution investigations of molecular and cellular dysfunction, embryology and teratology, careful inspection of clinical phenotypes, formal genetic analysis of empiric data and theoretic modeling. They are most usefully seen as complements rather than as rivals (Fig. 16.1). The genetics of cardiac anomalies cannot be fully understood until the diverse demands of every approach are satisfied. Another, generally tacit, principle is that congenital heart disease will not be grasped until "normal" cardiac development is understood, and vice versa.

Each approach must accommodate certain demands. The functioning heart of a progenitor must be perpetuated by reliable mechanisms in the offspring. These mechanisms must prescribe, at a minimum, a means of encoding in deoxyribonucleic acid (DNA) both the chemical constituents of the cardiovascular system and the ways the chemical messages are to be translated into the phenomena of embryology—how a one-dimensional genetic instruction specifies a three-dimensional structure. It is not enough that the message instructs cells to form diverse tissues: a teratoma does that. There must also exist methods of ensuring both topologic and geometric organization of these tissues to form the heart itself and the spatial orientation of the heart within the body. When the mechanism goes awry, it is not enough to document that the same cardiac lesion recurs in the relatives of probands; one must also explain why there are both a higher risk of disparate cardiovascular lesions in the relatives of probands and structural changes at distant sites, especially the craniofacies and the hand. Moreover, a reliable ontogenic mechanism alone is insufficient; the phylogenetic path by which the mechanism evolved must be deduced and satisfy evolutionary dynamics and conservatism. The latter is exemplified by the use of the same parts and mechanisms repeatedly.

Finally, it is not enough to know in exquisite detail the biochemistry of development, because genetic (and hence evolutionary) selection operates not on these basic mechanisms but on the remote, coarse-grained clinical phenotype, which governs such crass matters as survival, reproduction and death. The demands made by the various constituents of Figure 16.1 may even be in open conflict. The physiologist and embryologist perhaps suppose that mechanisms do not have to be simple, and indeed there is much biochemistry to support grand multiplicity. On the other hand, the evolutionist will seek mechanisms that are simple, robust, pleiotropic and adaptable. We call attention to these clashes, which sober the triumphant accounts of success in many individual, narrow enquiries.

Perspectives on Formal Studies

Population Studies

Epidemiologists typically appeal to the notion that things that are independent in cause will have independent effects, and conversely. This notion is a kind of minimalist logic: it is insensitive, but it is highly secure because the axiom of independence can rarely be challenged. In the present context, this approach has had two areas of application.

First it has shown that certain types of heart defects occur together more often than could be accounted for by chance. Thus arises the notion of the syndrome: the tetralogy of Fallot or the concurrence of lesions of the hand and the heart, as in the Holt-Oram syndrome. Such conjunctions can be studied without any family history at all and do not necessarily imply the interjection of genetic factors.

Second, relatives of probands with congenital heart disease are themselves at higher risk of congenital heart disease than are unselected subjects or their relatives. Many surveys

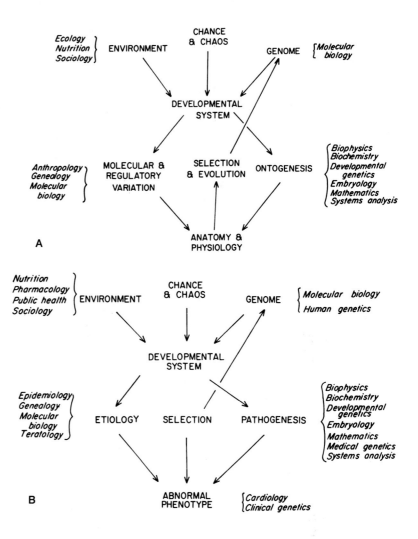

Figure 16.1. Epistemologic linkages in normal and pathologic development. **A,** In normal development, the genome is the primary component of the system that directs development; the macroenvironment (for example, the mother) and the microenvironment (for example, local oxygen tension) as well as stochastic (for example, chance and chaos) factors influence the system but not to the point of disruption. The **arrows** indicate the directions of information flow. Alongside the components of this schema (italics) are the fields of study especially devoted to them. **B,** In pathologic development, the schema is identical to that of **A,** but the components reflect subsets of the former and the fields of study have been modified. Medical genetics subsumes cytogenetics, immunogenetics and biochemical genetics.

of congenital heart disease have been of this kind and have established beyond doubt that there is "familial aggregation" (10–12). Furthermore, relatives of probands are also at added risk of cardiac lesions other than those in the probands (11,13,14). These findings alone do not prove a genetic cause because relatives tend to share similar habits, diet, social status, infections, any of which might be culpable. Nevertheless, it is at least suggestive evidence. Few epidemiologists go beyond this minimalist logic of independence and, with some justification, need to be taken to task for their neglect of genetic factors (15–17). The impact of the closeness of relation between affected individuals on etiology has been examined to some extent; unfortunately, nebulous terms such as "first degree" relatives have too often been used, ignoring the fact that sibling-sibling, mother-son, mother-daughter, father-son and father-daughter are all first degree relations but with quite different implications under any rational genetic model. There has also been little concern with false paternity, birth order (with the impact of sensitizing pregnancies) and parental age, matters that a geneticist would automatically address. Some recent explor-

atory studies (12,18) have dealt with these issues much more clearly.

Genealogic Studies

The geneticist generally insists on rather more structure than does the epidemiologist. The most important addition is detailed study of the pedigree. Epidemiologic minimalism would not, for instance, ordinarily distinguish between a population in which all subjects were at 10% risk of a defect and one in which 10% of the population are at 100% risk. To the geneticist, the distinction would be vital.

Five classic approaches may be mentioned.

Chromosomal approach. For some 70 years it has been known that genetic information is contained in the chromosomes. Even in disorders that are genetically lethal (that is, preclude reproduction) or nearly so, such as the Turner and Down syndromes, the occurrence of heart defects in the phenotype is taken to be evidence of a genetic etiology on grounds of karyotype, not of genealogic pattern.

Mendelian approach. More than a dozen congenital disorders of cardiac structure show evidence of being caused by a defect at a single genetic locus and occur often enough to be familiar to most clinicians. A far greater number of "private" syndromes, occurring in apparent Mendelian pattern in one or a few families, have been described; however, few meet the most stringent standards of proof. Many pseudomendelian disorders are known in animals in which extended breeding studies have shown that a trait is due to a tight cluster of genes rather than one locus. In humans, such deception would show up in an extensive pedigree, as genes in a cluster eventually segregate; however, because of a trend to smaller families and of reproductive disability, a given rare phenotype commonly is not transmitted, or, if it is, rapidly dies out and so deprives us of the critical evidence. For this reason, Mendelian inheritance is, paradoxically, more readily demonstrated for recessive traits, such as the Ellis-van Creveld syndrome, than for the more conspicuous dominant disorders.

Galtonian approach. Certain traits are evidently under the control of multiple loci, all more or less equally important and with additive effects. Fisher (19) showed that, when measurable, such traits tend to follow the Gaussian ("normal") distribution, and the degree of similarity among relatives can be adequately expressed—as Galton had expressed it 40 years previously—by regression and correlation coefficients. A thriving field of quantitative genetics has resulted. We mention four shortcomings of this model (20). First, the "democratic" assumption that the genes are many and have comparable impacts on the phenotype. The model does not, for instance, account for a phenotype *partly* determined by a major single locus. Second, to require additivity limits the area of applicability. Many well established examples violate this assumption, for example, chemical interactions subject to the law of mass action. Third, the model is not concerned with what the components are and hence (especially in view of the "democratic" assumption) has no heuristic value; indeed, it is a dead end inquiry. Fourth, in the present context, congenital cardiovascular defects are not matters of measurable changes but *quantal* phenotypes; that is, the person concerned either exhibits the trait or not—there is no intermediate state. (To anticipate, we may point out that modern trends in noninvasive high resolution phenotyping will shift inquiry toward quantitation of structural distortions, such as that which occurs in the Ebstein heart, the size of septal defects and subclinical manifestations of any malformation.)

Threshold approach. Although widely used in analysis of hypercholesterolemias, blood pressure and allied topics, classic Galton-Fisher analysis has shed little light on cardiac malformations. However, a modification derived from the work of Pearson (21) is the threshold model. It is based on the idea that a measurable trait may itself exhibit continuous variation, but only those values above a threshold lead to overt disease. A classic illustration is that blood pressure

may vary continuously, but there is an abrupt change in the clinical picture when at some critical pressure a berry aneurysm ruptures. The cardiologist (dealing with the blood pressure) and the neurologist (dealing with subarachnoid hemorrhage) may see the disorder quite differently. Pearson used his threshold model in two distinguishable models: where there is a measurable trait underlying the dichotomy (the analogue of the blood pressure in the hemorrhage) and, somewhat more cautiously, where the measurable trait is unidentified and indeed quite conjectural. The principal proponents of this threshold model in congenital heart disease have been the Noras (22,23) and Sanchez-Cascos (11). There has been neither a claim that the hypothetical "measurable" trait has been identified nor, so far, much attempt to find it. But Nora and Nora (23) have found in extensive family data that the recurrence rate in relatives corresponds to the expected (average) rate predicted from Pearson's method by Edwards' approximation (24). We stress that Edwards predicted the *average* rate, not the *probability* of being affected; and the Noras (22,23) have been in some difficulties in applying their results to the probability of recurrence when more than one relative is already affected. Nor is this surprising, because the mathematics is laborious even with the computer program of Curnow (25) and Smith (26). We may add that as it stands, this model sheds no light on the increased risk of discordant lesions in relatives.

Our intent is not to belittle these studies: in genetic analysis of such traits they represent the highest level of achievement so far, and perhaps nothing more sophisticated is practicable. In the last 15 years, no better analysis has been put forward.

Logistic regression approaches. This method of dealing with quantal characters has achieved some popularity in recent years. It has a long history of use in bioassay; and generalization of it to deal with cardiovascular traits due to multiple measurable causal factors has been elaborated (27,28). It is especially valuable in dealing with several causal factors, some discrete and some continuous. It is not expressly Galtonian in logic except that any measurable trait may be seen as the resultant of several additive effects. On the other hand, it much more readily accommodates explicit Mendelian structure than do other quantitative epidemiologic models, and it has been applied recently to familial aggregation of congenital heart disease (12,29).

Etiology and Pathogenesis

The approaches so far have been directed to finding the causes of congenital cardiac malformations. However, it is necessary to make a distinction that to medical readers will be obvious but to many nonmedical geneticists may seem very subtle. The notion of the cause of a disease comprises two features: etiology and pathogenesis. They deal as it were with the ingredients and the recipe, respectively. To quote a familiar genetic example, the etiology of sickle cell disease is perhaps better known than that for any other disease; yet the pathogenesis of the sickle cell crisis, or growth retardation, or arterial occlusions is still mysterious. Yet it is of these crass complications that the patient dies, and that Darwinian selection takes its toll, rather than the anomalous biochemistry in the beta chain of hemoglobin. In no sense can the genetics of the disorder be said to be understood until all the links from mutation to the "bottom line" phenotype have been made clear. Structural cardiovascular defects are presumably the end point of a disorder in the process by which the heart and vessels develop. To deepen our understanding of it, we must turn to a study of normal development.

Embryology

We consider this vast subject not only in the terms in which it has been formulated by most embryologists but also in its relation to fields to which it is ordinarily a stranger. What are the genetic factors involved in embryology, and are the appropriate methods qualitative or quantitative? How far are the studies directed to grappling with, not anatomy alone or biochemistry alone, but with the *explicit* operation of the mechanism connecting the two? Can the data of experimental and descriptive embryology on genesis and pathogenesis be cast in terms that can be usefully explored in humans?

In the century since Born's pioneering studies (30) on human cardiogenesis, much descriptive research has appeared and been critically reviewed (31–33). Not surprisingly, controversy persists about aspects of normal human cardiac development, and the major impediment of access to specimens cannot be totally circumvented by examination of animals, even other mammals. Extrapolations to human organogenesis from structures observed in other higher organisms are hazardous and not supportable solely on the basis of striking similarities of macromolecules across species. Species should be expected to differ in how they regulate complex processes such as embryogenesis, and little variation in control is required to produce major alterations in the finished product. As Jacob (34) has put it, evolution ". . . is always a matter of tinkering."

Morphogenetic processes in embryogenesis. Impressive gains in the understanding of the cellular and molecular biology of human fetal development in general (35–37) and of the human heart specifically (38,39) have far outstripped more classic embryologic morphology. One widely held schema explains embryogenesis by the six morphogenetic processes listed in Table 16.1. Much current basic research focuses on the molecular bases for these processes, their regulation and their coordination (36,40–42).

The Role of Classification

In clinical medicine as in all other fields, the prime requisite for any classification is utility. Inevitably, a variety of classifications for the same group of disorders emerges

and reflects a diversity of interests. For congenital heart disease, a clinical classification based on the presence or absence of cyanosis, shunts, abnormal pulmonary blood flow and so forth has ready application in bedside diagnosis, but with no evident or accepted relevance to etiology or pathogenesis. This common, if unobstrusive, clash between the goal of the clinician to cater to individual needs and that of the scientist to seek sound generalities (43) exists in medical genetics as well. Classic human genetics appealed to the existence of homogeneous classes, so that the findings in unrelated families could be generalized. Only thus has it been possible to understand concepts like mutation rate, paternal age effect and selection. In major ways, modern molecular biology has undermined this premise, and for the population survey, we find substituted exquisitely detailed studies on one family, one individual or perhaps a single cell line.

Classification of congenital malfunctions based on pathogenetic mechanisms. It is unclear how best to adapt the burgeoning molecular understanding of normal and abnormal development for the epidemiologist, the genetic statistician or the clinician interested in malformations of the cardiovascular system. A key issue is whether the classification of cardiovascular malformations is cast in the right terms. Utility of the threshold model, beyond simple predictions of recurrence risks in populations, has not blossomed because it has been used without any attempt to identify the characteristic on which the threshold was predicated.

If, as we surmised in the previous section, the real importance of genes in congenital heart disease resides in perturbations of mechanisms, then both theoretic modeling and a search for empiric validation must be based on a classification of defects rooted in ontogeny. We find the scheme proposed by Clark [(44) and personal communication 1989] appealing (Table 16.2). The first four of his six pathogenetic classes are supported by experimental evidence, mostly in animals. An ongoing, prospective investigation of congenital heart disease, with reasonable attention to both genetics and epidemiology, has utilized this classification to stratify data analysis (12,45,46), with results somewhat different from other recent work (13,23,47).

Classification based on embryonic hemodynamics. Table 16.3 expands on the class of anomalies due to abnormal embryonic blood flow patterns; some defects are caused by decreased flow in the right heart chambers and others caused by decreased flow in the left. The probands in the Baltimore-Washington Infant Study (12) were partitioned by this classification and the familial prevalence of cardiovascular malformations was determined by history. In relatives of the 363 patients with flow lesions (29% of all probands), 37 first degree relatives were affected (45,48). Further partitioning probands by defect and race and employing regressive logistic models produced strong evidence for etiologic heterogeneity in familial aggregation. Relatives of black probands with perimembranous ventricular septal defects and

Table 16.1. Fundamental Processes of Morphogenesis

Cell proliferation
Migration of cells
Migration of sheets of cells
Cell death
Cell differentiation
Pattern formation

Table 16.2. Classification of Congenital Cardiovascular Malformations Based on Pathogenetic Mechanism*

Mechanistic Group	Example of Malformation
Mesenchymal tissue migration errors	Tetralogy of Fallot
Intracardiac blood flow defects	Coarctation of the aorta
Extracellular matrix abnormalities	Endocardial cushion defect
Abnormal cellular death	Ebstein anomaly
Looping and situs abnormalities†	L-transposition of the great arteries
Abnormal targeted growth†	Total anomalous pulmonary venous return

*Classification scheme after Clark (44,45); †these groups are hypothesized and not substantiated by experiment.

relatives of white probands with right heart defects were both at increased risk of some cardiovascular malformation. The data are still insufficient to ask whether the heterogeneity is due solely to race (an imprecise descriptor in genetic terms) or to additional genetic factors. For one flow-associated defect, hypoplastic left heart, the collaborators in this study performed echocardiography on the first degree relatives of probands in 14 families (49), five relatives with previously undetected and one with known bicuspid aortic valve (another flow-associated defect) were found, a frequency of 12.5% which was considerably greater than the estimated population prevalence of about 1%. Affected relatives clustered in families in which probands had no extracardiac malformations.

Prospects for Improved Understanding of the Genetics of Congenital Heart Disease

Little further is to be gained, we believe, by refinements of classification or family studies based on coarse, clinical phenotypes. The mechanistic system proposed by Clark (44) seems useful, at least provisionally, for the immediate future in guiding studies of pathogenesis. A system in generalities and specifics based on etiology will emerge only when a great deal more work is performed, perhaps along the lines we suggest in this section. Descriptions of familial occurrences, even novel ones, of cardiovascular anomalies are unlikely to prove useful beyond counseling of individual

families. More bird watching is passé; the ornithologist must reign henceforth.

Classic Genetics

One should not infer from the foregoing that family studies will be unprofitable. At least two applications of pedigree analysis need to be capitalized on.

Linkage analysis. For cardiovascular malformations that behave as Mendelian traits, their segregation within a pedigree can be compared with segregation of cloned DNA probes that contain restriction fragment length polymorphisms (RFLPs) (50–53). If a given RFLP tends to occur in affected, but not in unaffected, relatives, the DNA probe may be close to a gene that causes the malformation. With a large enough family and a probe sufficiently close to the true mutant locus, the human gene map location of the defect can be narrowed considerably. As the human genome becomes saturated with anonymous DNA probes, mapping a Mendelian disorder will become trivial. For the next few years, yield will be highest when a DNA probe from a gene of known function shows total linkage (that is, *no* recombination) with a cardiac phenotype; for the families showing no

Table 16.3. Congenital Cardiovascular Defects Associated With Altered Embryonic Hemodynamics

Timing of Alteration	Type of Alteration	Resultant Defect	Percent of Flow Defects*
Before ventricular septation	Increased left heart flow	Perimembranous ventricular septal defect	30.8
After ventricular septation	Decreased left heart flow	Hypoplastic left heart, mitral or aortic atresia	10.7
		Aortic valve stenosis	13.5
		Bicuspid aortic valve	n.d.
		Patent ductus arteriosus	5.5
	Increased right heart flow	Hypoplastic right heart, tricuspid/pulmonary atresia	4.4
		Pulmonary valve stenosis	14.9
		Secundum atrial septal defect	11.0
Independent of ventricular septation	Abnormal direction of ductus arteriosus blood flow	Interruption of the aortic arch, type A and aortic coarctation	9.1

*Adapted from ref. 48 on the basis of 363 probands with a congenital cardiovascular malformation classified as due to abnormalities of hemodynamics out of a total of 570 cases ascertained. n.d. = not determined.

recombination between a candidate gene and the disorder, the product of that gene, or one very close to it, is part of the cause. This approach has shown the cause of some forms of osteogenesis imperfecta to be mutations in either the pro α 1 or pro α 2 genes of type I collagen (54,55), and the cause of the Stickler syndrome in some families to be the pro α 1 gene of type II collagen (56). Demonstrating nonlinkage is also useful; the cause of the Marfan syndrome is not any of the common fibrillar collagens, elastin or the core protein of proteoglycan (57,58).

Reverse genetics. Demonstrating close linkage (that is, occasional recombination) with an anonymous DNA probe only narrows the map location to a few million base pairs. Considerable work remains to "walk" or "jump" along the chromosome to identify the gene sequence in which the mutation resides and then to determine the product of that gene (59). This process, termed "reverse genetics," has demonstrated that, in Duchenne muscular dystrophy, a protein called dystrophin is defective (60) and that, in chronic granulomatous disease, one of the two polypeptides comprising cytochrome b is defective (61). But a great many more apparently Mendelian disorders, including familial polyposis coli, Huntington disease, myotonic dystrophy and cystic fibrosis have been mapped, although their loci remain unidentified or even conjectural (53). Several Mendelian cardiovascular disorders, especially Marfan syndrome and hypertrophic and dilated cardiomyopathies, will likely be mapped and their biochemical defects identified or verified by reverse genetics.

These and other technical capabilities for asking and answering questions engendered by molecular biology will have a major impact on cardiovascular diseases and the practice of cardiology. However, two caveats bear mentioning. *First, at present, gene mapping and reverse genetics are applicable only to those congenital malformations clearly caused by mutation at a single locus.* The next step will be to explain in molecular terms how the presence of one too few or too many alleles at a particular locus, as occurs in chromosome aneuploidy such as the Down syndrome, predisposes to cardiac anomalies. The final stages—explaining the cause and pathogenesis of the majority of congenital heart diseases—is the subject of the latter part of this section.

The second caveat pertains to the highly visible, national and international effort to sequence the entire human genome. Once this sequence is accomplished, and it surely will be in a decade or two, the job of understanding the molecular basis of common and multifactorial diseases will not be finished—just starting. Indeed, the tasks of deducing how the 3 billion-nucleotide linear sequence is organized into genes, what these 50,000 or so genes produce and what regulatory elements lie in and around each gene will appear trivial (though they are far from it) compared with the task of deducing how these genes function in systems. An alphabet of 26 letters gives no hint of the richness and complexity of

the language. Similarly, to a naive observer enquiring about the diversity of immunoglobulin specificities, being presented with tandem arrays of slightly different nucleotide sequences would provide scant clue; only in light of the system of combinatorial joining, flexible joining and somatic point mutation does the solution emerge.

Segregation analysis of subclinical phenotypes. Mendelian disorders, especially dominant ones, show considerable intrafamilial variability. If some aspect of a mechanism of morphogenesis or of a homeostatic system were controlled by a single gene, and that gene were mutant in some members of a family, the phenotype might vary widely among them. If some of these affected relatives had an obvious congenital cardiovascular anomaly, others with the same mutation might have a subclinical anomaly that could remain undetected by insensitive methods of detection such as auscultation, electrocardiogram or chest radiograph. More sensitive, yet noninvasive, techniques are now available for detecting subtle variations in structure; cross-sectional echocardiography, Doppler color echocardiography and, especially, nuclear magnetic resonance imaging may well detect relatives who have a clinically silent cardiovascular anomaly and, hence, are presumptively heterozygous for the same mutant gene as their more flagrantly affected family members. There will be at least two beneficial applications. First, with appropriate hypotheses and controls, segregation analysis and linkage analysis can be improved considerably. Second, pathogenetic mechanisms will be unraveled and major gene effects supported if a spectrum of ontogenetically related defects is found segregating in a family (14,48).

Embryologic Modeling

Changes in topology and geometry. In a recent book, Arthur (62) notes that attempts to recast natural selection in genetic terms (known as neo-Darwinism) have been feasible only because genetics had a well established, general abstract theory. In stark contrast, such a *general* and *abstract* theory does not exist for embryology, despite much descriptive and experimental work and even a few attempts at modeling. In the absence of such a theory, entente between embryology and neo-Darwinism is unlikely, and serious study of the genetics of congenital heart disease is seriously impaired. At the same time, it is hard to say what the exact form of this theory of morphogenesis would be. It seems clear that it must be concerned with *topology*, that is, those properties that are unchanged by bending and stretching. For instance, at birth the geometry of the lungs is changed by aeration, but the topology is unchanged. In distinction, closures of the ductus arteriosus and the foramen ovale change the topology of the cardiovascular system. In addition, cardiac morphogenesis must deal with *geometry*; for instance, a hypoplastic left heart is topologically intact but functionally inadequate. Indeed, because the embryonic heart supports the developing embryo as the heart itself is developing, its geometry, topology and function are intricately related.

Mathematical models of growth. A number of topics in pure mathematics—catastrophe theory (63), chaos theory (64,65), fractal sets (66–68)—have been cultivated with some thought of their biologic implications. Progress has languished in part because of their difficulty and chilly abstractness. Nonetheless, some results demonstrate both how worthwhile additional investigations might prove and how difficult it is for intuition, examining the empirical facts alone, to discern the level of complexity of the causal mechanisms. We have found in our own studies in dynamic systems as applied to the regulation of growth that a wide range of apparently quite different and disparate forms—the circle, spiral, dome, membranous sheet, torus and digitations—may result from a single model with only two arbitrary specifications (69,70). In other words, the notion that so complex a task as generating the geometry (as distinct from the fine structure) of the heart requires the instructions from a very large number of genetic loci may be misleading. For instance, a rough approximation to the hand can be achieved by five instructions (Fig. 16.2); and the same five instructions specify mechanisms that conceivably account for much of the anatomy of the heart.

Another fresh approach is a stochastic (probabilistic) single gene model of mammalian malformations (71). Introduction of chance in addition to genes and environment has also been suggested as a refinement of multifactorial models (71).

Embryologic Research

Further detailed descriptive investigation of human cardiogenesis will be hampered by ethical and political impediments to fetal research. Reexamination of fetal specimens that were preserved years ago will contribute some insight (72,73). Experiments in animals will continue to suggest ontogenetic mechanisms that may be generalizable (74) but difficult to test in humans.

Molecular biologic approaches to embryogenesis. We do expect, however, major progress in molecular embryology in the near future. In particular, intriguing results are emerging on the roles of three classes of genes and their products: oncogenes (75) and growth factors (76–78), cell surface molecules such as integrins (79,80) and homeotic genes (37,81). Cardiovascular abnormalities, although not necessarily congenital ones, are well known accompaniments of heritable defects of the extracellular matrix, such as the mucopolysaccharidoses and the Marfan syndrome. The importance of connective tissue to the structural stability of differentiated tissues is incontrovertible (82–84). Less well appreciated, however, is the crucial role of the extracellular matrix during embryogenesis and organogenesis (85–87). A

subtle, genetically specified variation in one macromolecule of connective tissue markedly affects not only that molecule but also the myriad of other components of the matrix (88). These alterations, in turn, can affect any of the fundamental processes of embryogenesis (Table 16.1). If the genetic change either was inherited from a parent similarly affected or arose in an egg or sperm that underwent a spontaneous mutation, then the entire embryo will be affected and widespread pleiotropic effects may appear (6). Alternatively, the genetic change in connective tissue may arise in a single cell of the early embryo and produce somatic mosaicism in which only the clonal descendants of the mutant cell will be abnormal. The resultant phenotype and its transmission will depend on where those mutant cells migrate in the embryo, how widely the extracellular matrix they produce encounters nonmutant embryonic cells and other factors yet to be identified (89).

Somatic mutation: etiology of cardiac malformations. Somatic mutation is much more common than was thought even 5 years ago, and it is quite obviously not limited to connective tissue. The phenomenon may prove to be extremely important in the etiology of many congenital malformations. One special class of somatic mutation is that which occurs in a gonad and produces germinal mosaicism. The individual who is a germinal mosaic for a mutation that causes a dominant phenotype (as many congenital malformations may be) will be clinically normal, but all offspring will have a risk of being affected in proportion to the number of mutant germ cells. This nuance, among others, will increasingly complicate genetic counseling in the future.

Genetic Regulation of Complex Systems

The molecular biology of gene regulation will hold our interest for years to come. It will become clearer that the same signal (often a polypeptide such as a hormone receptor or a product of a homeotic gene) can induce one gene, repress another and render a third sensitive to regulation by *another* signal such as a hormone. We will begin to understand how environmental factors such as pressure and temperature modulate gene expression and, thereby, developmental and compensatory alterations of cardiovascular structure and function.

Investigations of the genetic regulation of developmental processes other than organogenesis may well shed light on congenital malformations. Even a thorough understanding of how genes control physiologic homeostasis, such as blood glucose levels (9), may generate practical solutions to more complex cybernetic systems.

Fields as diverse as fundamental mathematics, fluid dynamics and cellular automata (90,91) may ultimately be applicable to understanding congenital cardiovascular defects. Already the chaos theory is finding wide attention in

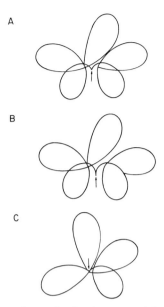

Figure 16.2. The *anlage* of a hand generated by a model of a dynamic system. In each diagram, the same two paths are involved, generating the right two digits and the others, respectively. The lobes are unlike adult fingers but resemble their precursors, the primitive buds in the limb disk. The grouping of the fingers corresponds to innervation. Each group is defined by the path of a dynamic process whereby growth is directed by pre-axial and post-axial centers (technically called *targets*). Two variables (measures of the strength and proportions of each adjustment) control each path and a fifth variable specifies the angle between the branches of the cusp (**arrow**). The tracings show a progressive increase in the lengths of the digits toward the middle. Changes of the cusp angle alone produce patterns characteristic of the hand deformities seen in the polydactylies, Holt-Oram syndrome and various clefting malformations (lobster claw and so forth). The paths start from a common cusp (**arrow**). **A** (normal), the thumb lies at the bottom left, the little finger at bottom right. **B**, The paths start somewhat earlier and a deep cleft forms between the third and fourth fingers as in the so called "absence" deformities. **C**, The left path starts late and no thumb forms, as in the Holt-Oram syndrome.

population dynamics; extending its precepts to cellular dynamics is not unrealistic.

Conclusion

Substantial progress toward understanding how genes are involved in etiology and pathogenesis of congenital heart disease is likely in the next decade. Indeed, this progress will only be part of a much more complete picture of human ontogeny. Achieving this progress will involve vastly more than molecular biology, although that field will have a preeminent technical contribution. The major obstacle will be fundamental investigations of highly complex, interactive systems; both the theory and empiric studies are in their infancy.

We end with the optimistic projection that before many more years pass, simple reliance on a stock "3% to 5%"

recurrence risk for anxious parents will prove not only inappropriate but inaccurate. The burden on the clinician to understand the affected child's congenital defect, its etiology and pathogenesis and the likely contribution of the parents' genes will increase, but the reward in more informed counseling will be even greater.

References

1. Abbott M. Congenital cardiac disease. In: Osler W, McCrae T, eds. Osler's Modern Medicine. Philadelphia: Lea & Febiger, 1908:323–425.
2. Abbott M. Atlas of Congenital Cardiac Disease. New York: American Heart Association, 1936.
3. Taussig HB. Congenital Malformations of the Heart. New York: Commonwealth Fund, 1947.
4. Park EA. Foreword. In: Ref 3, page vii–ix.
5. Costa T, Scriver CR, Childs B. The effect of Mendelian disease on human health: a measurement. Am J Med Genet 1985;21:231–42.
6. Pyeritz RE. Pleiotropy revisited: molecular explanations of a classic concept. Am J Med Genet 1989;34:124–34.
7. Waddington CH. The Strategy of the Genes. London: Allen & Unwin, 1957:41.
8. Murphy EA, Trojak JE. The dynamics of quantifiable homeostasis. 1. The individual. Am J Med Genet 1983;15:275–90.
9. Murphy EA, Pyeritz RE. Homeostasis. VII. A conspectus. Am J Med Genet 1986;24:735–51.
10. McKeown T, MacMahon B, Parsons CG. The family incidence of congenital malformations of the heart. Br Heart J 1953;15:273–7.
11. Sanchez-Cascos A. The recurrence risk in congenital heart disease. Eur J Cardiol 1978;7:197–210.
12. Boughman JA, Berg KA, Astemborski JA, et al. Familial risks of congenital heart defect assessed in a population-based epidemiologic study. Am J Med Genet 1987;26:839–49.
13. Rose V, Gold RJM, Lindsay G, Allen M. A possible increase in the incidence of congenital heart defects among the offspring of affected parents. J Am Coll Cardiol 1985;6:376–82.
14. Pierpont MEM, Gobel JW, Moller JH, Edwards JE. Cardiac malformations in relatives of children with truncus arteriosus or interruption of the aortic arch. Am J Cardiol 1988;61:423–7.
15. Khoury MJ, Adams MJ Jr, Flanders WD. An epidemiologic approach to ecogenetics. Am J Hum Genet 1988;42:89–95.
16. Murphy EA. The basis for interpreting family history. Am J Epidemiol 1989;129:19–22.
17. Susser E, Susser M. Familial aggregation studies: a note on their epidemiologic properties. Am J Epidemiol 1989;129:23–30.
18. Ferencz C, Rubin JD, McCarter RJ, et al. Congenital heart disease: prevalence at birth. The Baltimore-Washington Infant Study. Am J Epidemiol 1985;121:31–6.
19. Fisher RA. The correlation between relatives on the supposition of Mendelian inheritance. Trans R Soc (Edinburgh) 1918;52:399–433.
20. Murphy EA. Quantitative genetics: a critique. Soc Biol 1979;26:126–41.
21. Pearson K. On the generalized theory of alternative inheritance with special references to Mendel's law. Philos Trans R Soc Lond (Biol) 1904;203:53–86.
22. Nora JJ, Nora AH. The evolution of specific genetic and environmental counseling in congenital heart disease. Circulation 1978;57:205–13.
23. Nora JJ, Nora AH. Genetic epidemiology of congenital heart disease. In: Steinberg AG, Bearn AG, Motulsky AG, Childs V, eds. Progress in Human Genetics. Philadelphia: WB Saunders, 1983;5:91–137.
24. Edwards JH. The simulation of Mendelism. Acta Genet Stat Med 1960;10:63–70.
25. Curnow RN. The multifactorial model for the inheritance of liability to disease and its implications for relatives at risk. Biometrics 1972;28:931–46.
26. Smith C. Recurrence risks for multifactorial inheritance. Am J Hum Genet 1971;23:578–88.

27. Cornfield J, Gordon T, Smith WW. Quantal response curves for experimentally uncontrolled variables. Bull Inst Int Statist 1961;38:97–115.

28. Walker SH, Duncan DB. Estimation of the probability of an event as a function of several independent variables. Biometrika 1967;54:167–79.

29. Rubin JD, Ferencz C, McCarter RJ, et al. Congenital cardiovascular malformations in the Baltimore-Washington area. Md Med J 1985;34:1079–83.

30. Born G. Beiträge zur Entwicklungsgeschichte der Säugetierherzen. Arch Mikrosk Anat 1889;33:284–378.

31. O'Rahilly R. The timing and sequence of events in human cardiogenesis. Acta Anat 1971;79:70–5.

32. Steding G, Seidl W. Contribution to the development of the heart. Part I. Normal development. Thorac Cardiovasc Surg 1980;28:386–409.

33. Zak R, ed. Growth of the Heart in Health and Disease. New York: Raven Press, 1984.

34. Jacob F. Evolution and tinkering. Science 1977;196:1161–6.

35. Cooke J. The early embryo and the formation of body pattern. Am Sci 1988;76:35–41.

36. Edelman GM. Topobiology. An Introduction to Molecular Embryology. New York: Basic Books, 1988.

37. Gehring WJ. Homeotic genes, the homeo box, and the genetic control of development. Cold Spring Harb Symp Quant Biol 1985;50:243–51.

38. Breitbart RE, Nguyen HT, Medford RM, Destree AT, Mahdavi V, Nadal-Ginard B. Intricate combinatorial patterns of exon splicing generate multiple regulated troponin T isoforms from a single gene. Cell 1985;41:67–82.

39. Mar JH, Antin PB, Cooper TA, Ordahl CP. Analysis of the upstream regions governing expression of the chicken cardiac troponin T gene in embryonic cardiac and skeletal muscle cells. J Cell Biol 1988;107:573–85.

40. Gurdon JB. Embryonic induction—molecular prospects. Development 1987;99:285–306.

41. Ingham PW. The molecular genetics of embryonic pattern formation in Drosophila. Nature 1988;335:25–34.

42. Wieczorek DF, Smith CW, Nadal-Ginard B. The rat alpha-tropomyosin gene generates a minimum of six different mRNAs coding for striated, smooth, and nonmuscle isoforms by alternative splicing. Mol Cell Biol 1988;8:679–94.

43. Murphy EA. Public and private hypotheses. J Clin Epidemiol 1989;42:79–84.

44. Clark EB. Mechanisms in the pathogenesis of congenital cardiac malformations. In: Pierpont MEM, Moller JH, eds. Genetics of Cardiovascular Disease. Boston: Martinus Nijhoff, 1987:3–12.

45. Maestri N. Familial Aggregation of Congenital Cardiovascular Malformations (Dissertation). Baltimore: Johns Hopkins University School of Hygiene and Public Health, 1989.

46. Boughman JA. Familial risks of congenital heart defects. Am J Med Genet 1988;29:233.

47. Nora JJ, Nora AH. Familial risk of congenital heart defect. Am J Med Genet 1988;29:231.

48. Maestri NE, Beaty TH, Liang K-Y, Boughman JA, Ferencz C. Assessing familial aggregation of congenital cardiovascular malformations in case-control studies. Genet Epidemiol 1988;5:343–54.

49. Brenner JI, Berg KA, Schneider DS, Clark EB, Boughman JA. Congenital cardiovascular malformations in first degree relatives of infants with hypoplastic left heart syndrome. Am J Dis Child 1989;143:1492–94.

50. Francomano CA, Kazazian HH Jr. DNA analysis in genetic disorders. Ann Rev Med 1986;37:377–95.

51. Gusella JF. Recombinant DNA techniques in the diagnosis of inherited disorders. J Clin Invest 1986;77:1723–6.

52. Shapiro LJ, Comings DE, Jones OW, Rimoin DL. New frontiers in genetic medicine. Ann Int Med 1986;104:527–39.

53. Antonarakis SE. Diagnosis of genetic disorders at the DNA level. N Engl J Med 1989;320:153–63.

54. Sykes BC, Ogilvie D, Wordsworth P, Anderson J, Jones N. Osteogenesis imperfecta is linked to both type I collagen structural genes. Lancet 1986;2:69–72.

55. Byers PH. Inherited disorders of collagen gene structure and expression. Am J Med Genet 1989;34:72–80.

56. Francomano CA, Liberfarb RM, Hirose T, et al. The Stickler syndrome: evidence for close linkage to the structural gene for type II collagen. Genomics 1987;1:293–6.

57. Ogilvie DJ, Wordsworth BP, Priestley LM, et al. Segregation of all four major fibrillar collagen genes in the Marfan syndrome. Am J Hum Genet 1987;41:1071–2.

58. Francomano CA, Streeten EA, Meyers DA, Pyeritz RE. Exclusion of fibrillar procollagens as causes of the Marfan syndrome. Am J Med Genet 1988;29:457–62.

59. Orkin SH. Reverse genetics and human disease. Cell 1986;47:845–50.

60. Hoffman EP, Brown RH Jr, Kunkel LM. The protein product of the Duchenne muscular dystrophy locus. Cell 1987;51:919–28.

61. Royer-Pakora B, Kunkel LM, Monaco AP, et al. Cloning the gene for an inherited human disorder—chronic granulomatous disease—on the basis of its chromosomal location. Nature 1986;322:32–8.

62. Arthur W. A Theory of the Evolution of Development. New York: John Wiley & Sons, 1988.

63. Thom R. Stabilité structurelle et morphogénèse: Essai d'une théorie générale des modèles. In: Foweler DH, English translation. Structural Stability and Morphogenesis: An Outline of a General Theory of Models. Reading, MA: WA Benjamin, 1975.

64. May RM. Simple mathematical models with very complicated dynamics. Nature 1976;261:459–67.

65. Gleick J. Chaos. New York: Viking-Penguin, 1987:279–84.

66. Mandelbrot BB. The Fractal Geometry of Nature. New York: Freeman, 1977.

67. Falconer JJ. The Geometry of Fractal Sets. Cambridge: Cambridge University Press, 1986.

68. Goldberger AL. Nonlinear dynamics, fractals, cardiac physiology, and sudden death. In: Rensing L, An der Heiden U, Mackey M, eds. Temporal Disorder in Human Oscillatory Systems. New York: Springer-Verlag, 1987:137–54.

69. Sagawa Y, Berger KR, Trojak JE, Brown KL, Murphy EA. Angular homeostasis. II. Pursuit of a moving target in a plane and some implications for teratology. Am J Med Genet 1988;31:395–405.

70. Murphy EA, Berger KR, Trojak JE, Sagawa Y. Angular homeostasis. 5. Some issues in genetics, ontogeny, and evolution. Am J Med Genet 1988;31:963–79.

71. Kurnit DM, Layton WM, Matthysse S. Genetics, chance and morphogenesis. Am J Hum Genet 1987;41:979–95.

72. Ursell PC, Byrne JM, Strobino BA. Significant cardiac defects in the developing fetus: a study of spontaneous abortions. Circulation 1985;72:1232–6.

73. Hutchins GM, Kessler-Hanna A, Moore GW. Development of the coronary arteries in the embryonic human heart. Circulation 1988;77:1250–7.

74. Langdon TJ, Boerboom LE, Olinger GN, Rodriguez ER, Ferrans VJ. Rheologic genesis of aortic coarctation in a canine model. Am Heart J 1988;115:489–92.

75. Adamson ED. Oncogenes in development. Development 1987;99:449–71.

76. Mercola M, Stiles CD. Growth factor superfamilies and mammalian embryogenesis. Development 1988;102:451–60.

77. Rizzino A. Transforming growth factor-R: multiple effects on cell differentiation and extracellular matrices. Dev Biol 1988;130:411–22.

78. Sporn MB, Roberts AB. Peptide growth factors are multifunctional. Nature 1988;332:217–9.

79. Edelman GM. Cell adhesion and morphogenesis: the regulator hypothesis. Proc Natl Acad Sci USA 1984;81:1460–4.

80. Rutishauser U, Acheson A, Hall AK, Mann DM, Sunshine J. The neural cell adhesion molecule (NCAM) as a regulator of cell-cell interactions. Science 1988;240:53–7.

81. Bender W. Homeotic gene products as growth factors. Cell 1985;43:559–60.

82. Pyeritz RE. Cardiovascular manifestations of heritable disorders of connective tissue. In: Motulsky AG, Bearn AG, Motulsky AG, Childs V, eds. Progress in Medical Genetics. Philadelphia: WB Saunders, 1983;5:191–302.

83. Pyeritz RE. Heritable disorders of connective tissue. In: Pierpont MEM, Moller JH, eds. The Genetics of Cardiovascular Disease. Boston: Martinus Nijhoff, 1986:265–303.

84. Pyeritz RE. Heritable defects in connective tissue. Hosp Pract 1987;22:153–68.

85. Kurnit DM, Aldridge JF, Matsuoka R, Maathysse S. Increased adhesiveness of trisomy 21 cells and atrioventricular canal malformations in Down syndrome: a stochastic model. Am J Med Genet 1985;20:385–99.

86. Hay E. The extracellular matrix, cell skeletons, and embryonic development. Am J Med Genet 1989;34:14–29.

87. Solursh M. The extracellular matrix and cell surface as determinants of connective tissue differentiation. Am J Med Genet 1989;34:30–34.

88. Holbrook KA, Byers PH. Skin is a window on heritable disorders of connective tissue. Am J Med Genet 1989;34:105–21.

89. Hall JG. Somatic mosaicism: observations related to clinical genetics. Am J Hum Genet 1988;43:355–63.

90. Farmer D, Toffoli T, Wolfram S, eds. Cellular Automata. New York: Elsevier North-Holland, 1984.

91. Wolfram S. Cellular automata as models of complexity. Nature 1984;311:419–24.

◆ CHAPTER 17 ◆

Primary Pulmonary Hypertension: A Look at the Future

JOHN H. NEWMAN, MD, JOSEPH C. ROSS, MD

Historical Background

Primary pulmonary hypertension was first described as a distinct clinical entity by Dresdale et al. in 1951 (1). They defined a disease, primarily of young women, in whom pulmonary artery pressure was markedly elevated for no apparent reason, resulting in cor pulmonale and death. The crucial features that distinguished this illness from other causes of pulmonary hypertension were that cardiac disorders and alveolar hypoventilation could be excluded, and some patients transiently responded to a vasodilator. Over the next 30 years, until the establishment of the National Institutes of Health Registry for Primary Pulmonary Hypertension (2), the major effort with regard to understanding primary pulmonary hypertension involved simply the collection of small series of patients to establish the clinical and demographic features of the illness (3,4). It was discovered that patients presented late in the illness, usually after a short symptomatic period, and survival time in the majority of patients was brief, averaging 2 to 5 years. Because the disease is rare, most reports were limited to a few patients each and therapeutic approaches were a matter of guesswork. Despite this limitation, enough cases were reported to establish reasonably well that treatment with oxygen and antiinflammatory drugs, such as corticosteroids, has had no beneficial effect and there has been no marked response to anticoagulants, but some patients have responded to one of a variety of vasodilator drugs (4).

Pathogenesis

The pathogenesis of primary pulmonary hypertension is unknown. Clinicians and scientists alike have expressed fascination with this dramatic and rare illness. Postmortem examination of the lungs reveals a normal lung parenchyma with disease peculiarly limited to the small muscular pulmonary arteries (5,6). The pathologic lesions are characteristic, but they are not pathognomonic because they can be found in other conditions such as scleroderma and Eisenmenger's syndrome (7). Theories of pathogenesis are scarce; the most prevalent theory has focused on vasoconstriction, but there has been little supporting clinical evidence. Little information exists on the inciting mechanism, susceptibility to the illness or ongoing mechanisms of cellular and humoral pathogenesis. Until recently, fundamental knowledge of vascular biology has simply not been available, and the vocabulary to describe the pathogenesis of vascular lesions

is just now being developed. Currently there is a rapid growth in the available information about the determinants of vascular behavior and on injury and repair in both systemic and pulmonary vessels. It appears that the groundwork finally exists to allow us to begin to understand this rare disease.

Current State of the Art

Clinical features. The clinical description of primary pulmonary hypertension seems relatively complete. The initial publication from the National Institutes of Health Registry (2), which describes the clinical characteristics of 187 patients, seems to agree with previous reviews on the features of this illness (3,4). Primary pulmonary hypertension is a disease affecting women over men in a 1.7:1 ratio; 5% to 10% of cases are familial with exactly the same clinical features as those seen in sporadic cases. Genetic transmission in familial disease appears to be autosomal dominant with highly variable expression of disease among different families (8). The mean age at the time of diagnosis of sporadic primary pulmonary hypertension is approximately 36 years (range of 1 to 80). The time from onset of symptoms to diagnosis is approximately 2 years, and the time of survival after diagnosis is approximately 2 to 5 years. There have also been cases of exceptional longevity, exceeding 20 years.

Most patients present with shortness of breath (>90%) and loss of energy (>75%). Some patients have cough, hemoptysis, peripheral cyanosis, and they may have chest pain, probably due to ischemia of the right ventricle. At cardiac catheterization mean pulmonary artery pressure is usually about 60 mm Hg, and it is not clear that the level of pulmonary hypertension pressure correlates well with survival. The pressures and flows that correlate best with a short survival time are elevated right atrial pressure (>11 mm Hg), a function of right ventricular performance, and low cardiac output (cardiac index <2.1).

Approximately 30% of patients respond to vasodilator drugs and these patients tend to have a longer survival time. Although every known vasodilator drug has been reported to have beneficial effects in isolated patients (1,9–12), the calcium channel blockers seem to have the greatest likelihood of efficacy. Continuous infusion of prostacyclin may also confer lasting benefit, although it is technically demanding (13). Whether the beneficial effects of calcium channel blockers occur primarily or fully through vasodilation is not clear, but in recent studies (14) it appears that high dose calcium channel blockade can cause dramatic unequivocal vasodilation in some patients. Daily doses in such cases may consist of up to 240 mg of nifedipine and up to 720 mg of diltiazem.

Pathologic features. The pathologic lesions of primary pulmonary hypertension are well described but poorly understood. Controversy exists whether there is one origin of primary pulmonary hypertension that exhibits multiple pathologic features, or whether there are two or more separate origins that lead to the same clinical syndrome (15–17). The most frequently encountered pathologic features in primary pulmonary hypertension are those of "plexogenic arteriopathy" in which there is concentric intimal fibroelastosis of small arteries, complex lesions called plexiform lesions and associated small vascular dilations. Some patients have no plexiform lesions or concentric intimal fibrosis but manifest what appear to be recanalized thrombotic lesions in small pulmonary arteries. In the lesion called "eccentric intimal fibrosis," the fibroelastosis is not concentric but bulges asymmetrically from one portion of the vascular lumen. This lesion has been strongly thought by some pathologists (18) to be related to small vessel thrombosis with recanalization.

Loyd et al. (16) recently made a careful morphometric analysis of pathologic specimens from patients with familial primary pulmonary hypertension, in whom the pathogenesis of disease should be the same. They found an unpredicted coexistence of eccentric intimal fibrosis, isolated medial hypertrophy, concentric intimal fibrosis and plexiform lesions within and among families. The correlation of the pattern and frequency of these lesions in families was weak and there was a great deal of variability within individuals among families. These data raise serious questions about the previous belief that the presence of eccentric intimal fibrosis points to a separate origin of microthrombotic or microembolic pulmonary hypertension. The possibility that the pathogenesis of primary pulmonary hypertension involves coagulation at the endothelial surface or secondary thrombosis in situ as a result of low flow is not questioned. It appears to us that the etiology or etiologies of primary pulmonary hypertension will not be revealed from discussions based on our current understanding of pathologic presentations. The pathobiology of the vascular wall is where understanding of this disease is likely to emerge.

Pathogenesis

Vasoconstriction. Current theories of the pathogenesis of primary pulmonary hypertension are few and unsupported by hard data. For many years *vasoconstriction* was viewed as the primary mechanism of disease. The reason is not clear because another disease of vasoconstriction, hypoxic pulmonary hypertension of high altitude, is not associated with intimal fibrosis and vascular obstruction but merely with medial hypertrophy (19). On the other hand, the lesions in

primary pulmonary hypertension do resemble the end stage vascular lesions of systemic hypertension. The reactivity of the pulmonary vascular bed to hypoxia in patients with primary pulmonary hypertension appears to be blunted, but recent studies showing unequivocal vasodilation in response to calcium channel blockers certainly implicate vasoconstriction in the end stage of this illness. Ten percent of female patients with primary pulmonary hypertension have Raynaud's syndrome, an illness of vasoconstriction (14,20).

Excessive flow and pressure. Because Eisenmenger's syndrome, most often associated with patent ductus arteriosus or ventricular septal defect, is associated with irreversible pulmonary hypertension and the same plexiform lesions seen in primary pulmonary hypertension, it is appealing to speculate that excessive *flow and pressure* in the pulmonary circulation cause the pathologic response. It has been difficult to create good animal models of pulmonary overflow, although models made by implantation of a systemic artery into the pulmonary artery have been attempted with variable success. One difficulty in the study of primary pulmonary hypertension is that there is no good animal model, a deficiency that desperately needs to be corrected. Studies examining the effect of pressure and shear stress on vascular endothelium are likely to yield important insights; this is a new and exciting area of investigation (21).

Catecholamine-induced injury. The aminorex epidemic (9) and isolated cases of primary pulmonary hypertension related to catecholamine-like drugs (22) permit the speculation that the pathogenesis of primary pulmonary hypertension is related to *susceptibility of the vasculature to catecholamine agents* (23). How this association may occur is unknown. We recently made a preliminary examination of the pulmonary arteries from autopsy specimens of patients whose death resulted from pheochromocytoma and found what appears to be mild medial hypertrophy and endothelial hyperplasia (unpublished observations). Patients with primary pulmonary hypertension may have some unusual susceptibility to catecholamine-induced injury, and perhaps these patients also have increased susceptibility to shear stress in the pulmonary circulation. The association of liver cirrhosis and primary pulmonary hypertension may be due to catecholamines (24). Systemic vasodilation, increased cardiac output and wide pulse pressure are catecholamine-like features of severe cirrhosis.

Coagulation at the endothelial surface. This is a current theory about the origin of primary pulmonary hypertension. The evidence is scant and inferential but intriguing (25). Thromboxane B_2 was found to be elevated in the plasma of a patient with primary pulmonary hypertension (26). Activated platelet aggregates and increased circulating beta-thromboglobulin have been found in patients with systemic sclerosis and pulmonary vascular disease (27). Data from one study (28) suggest that anticoagulation may benefit patients with primary pulmonary hypertension. Defective fibrinolysis has been found in one family with primary pulmonary hypertension (28). Finally, primary pulmonary hypertension was recently reported (29) in five hemophiliacs in whom factor VIII therapy was a mainstay of existence. Surely the surface of the endothelium and its interaction with the humoral and cellular elements of blood will yield answers about the mechanism of this illness, and it seems likely that the coagulation cascade will be involved in some way.

New Developments in Vascular Biology

Aided by molecular techniques, advances in vascular biology are occurring in so many areas that insights into primary pulmonary hypertension will soon emerge. As yet, there are no known direct links between these new lines of research and the pathogenesis of primary pulmonary hypertension. What follows will be a brief survey of the areas of current development.

Proliferative lesions: role of platelet-endothelial interactions. The proliferative lesions in systemic arteries resulting in atherosclerosis should serve as a model for the study of the pulmonary circulation (30). The similarities between atherosclerotic lesions and the lesions of primary pulmonary hypertension are numerous; these include smooth muscle hypertrophy and phenotypic conversion of smooth muscle cells, resulting in secretion of elastin and other fibrous elements, and hyperplasia of the intima. A great deal of insight related to angiogenic factors, especially platelet-derived growth factor and macrophage-derived factors, supports the possibility that platelet-endothelial interactions or other interactions between endothelium and circulating cells may initiate the proliferative response seen in primary pulmonary hypertension (31).

The differences between atherosclerosis in systemic arteries and the obliterative lesion in the pulmonary circulation are certainly significant. The pulmonary circulation does not develop atherosclerotic lesions as such, although hypertensive main pulmonary arteries may eventually develop sclerotic plaques. Why the pulmonary circulation, even at systemic levels of pressure, does not develop atherosclerotic lesions is surely an important clue. The one constant difference between the pulmonary circulation and the systemic circulation is the partial pressure of oxygen of the perfusing blood. The systemic arterial bed is highly oxygenated, whereas the pulmonary artery bed is hypoxic. Perhaps atherosclerosis in systemic vessels is enhanced by toxic oxygen radicals whose concentration is less in the pulmonary circulation.

Cytokines: peptide factors. Peptide growth factors (32,33) are likely to be involved in the intimal hyperplasia, medial hypertrophy and angioid lesions of primary pulmonary hypertension. As yet, none of these peptides has been directly linked to primary pulmonary hypertension, although transforming growth factor-alpha release has been found recently in an animal model of chronic pulmonary hypertension induced by air emboli (34). Multiple growth factors have been identified, but they surely represent only a partial list of the true number (33). These factors are involved in direct target cell activation (such as endothelium), cell to cell interactions and modulation of inflammation and growth. A cytokine may stimulate or inhibit growth, depending on the conditions of the microenvironment. This is an explosive area of research where important insights into the pathogenesis of primary pulmonary hypertension will emerge.

Role of heparin-heparan and heparanase enzymes in the control of pulmonary vascular morphology. This is a fascinating area. Heparin, in addition to having anticoagulant properties, is one of the most anionic biologic substances known. It is responsible in part for the negatively charged domains on the endothelial surface. Charge-related lung microvascular injury by endogenous polycationic substances is an area worthy of attention in regard to primary pulmonary hypertension (35). Heparin has an additional attribute of inhibiting smooth muscle proliferation and can inhibit the vascular remodeling associated with chronic hypoxic exposure (36). Heparanase enzymes secreted by activated macrophages and T lymphocytes may be involved in the atherosclerotic process in systemic arteries by changing surface charge or the inhibitory effects of heparin (37). It is unknown whether similar events may occur in the pulmonary circulation during the development of primary pulmonary hypertension. The interaction of the endothelium and its underlying smooth muscle involves communication directing either vasoconstriction or vasodilation, as in the case of endothelial-derived relaxation factor, angiogenin and certainly other mediators as yet undiscovered. Elastogenic and other proliferative factors secreted from hypoxic pulmonary arteries have been found (38), and the nature and communication between cells by way of these mediators must influence the hypertrophic response to inciting stimuli.

Abnormal cell adhesion: adhesive proteins. Rapid progress has been made in understanding the interactions between certain proteoglycans and cell surface receptors that result in cell adhesion (39). Abnormal cell adhesion is potentially an important problem in primary pulmonary hypertension because migrating cells in the media and intima may have altered adhesiveness to the underlying basement membrane or in cell/cell interactions. Adhesive proteins are present both in the extracellular matrix and in the blood. These adhesive proteins, called integrins, include thrombospondin, fibronectin, fibrinogen, von Willebrand's factor and others. Each of these proteoglycans has an arginine-glycine-aspartic acid sequence called RGD as its recognition site for cell receptors (40). It is clear from preliminary work that the interactions of cells with integrins influence vascular behavior including anchorage of cells, traction for cell migration across cells and clues for cell position and polarity. It is also likely that these adhesion proteins help control cell and tissue growth. It is conceivable that primary pulmonary hypertension involves an abnormality of the receptor sites of the cells of the vascular wall to integrins.

Studies of endothelial and smooth muscle cells in culture taken from the lungs of patients with primary pulmonary hypertension undergoing transplantation will be of interest. Characterization of the behavior of these cells both by standard cell techniques and by measuring molecular signals such as the messenger ribonucleic acid (RNA) of proliferative substances is likely to give insight into the mechanisms of the vascular abnormality seen in primary pulmonary hypertension.

Primary Pulmonary Hypertension: The Future

In this brief overview, we have tried to outline the current state of knowledge with regard to primary pulmonary hypertension and to highlight a few exciting developments in vascular biology that might pertain to primary pulmonary hypertension. Because patients with this disease usually present near the end stage of their disease, it will be most useful if some agent of reversibility can be identified to benefit them. Otherwise, the present unsatisfactory clinical status quo will continue. Currently we are able to improve the quality of life in a minority of patients and perhaps increase their survival time. Organ transplantation for primary pulmonary hypertension remains a dramatic therapy for a few patients, but the complications of lung rejection versus life-threatening infections, particularly with cytomegalovirus, make heart-lung transplantation a choice of last resort.

Early detection of primary pulmonary hypertension would be highly desirable. Recent developments in two-dimensional echocardiography with Doppler techniques to measure pulmonary artery pressure noninvasively are encouraging (41). The logistic problem is that primary pulmonary hypertension is a rare disease, and it is not feasible to screen an entire population to detect a disease that occurs in 1 in 1 million patients. Thus, in the short run, we will continue to identify these patients late in their disease and will be able to offer them only the best palliative care that can be developed by clinical trials. Nonetheless, it seems certain that over the next few decades primary pulmonary hypertension will be understood at the cellular and molecular level. We can, therefore, be optimistic about the future.

References

1. Dresdale DT, Schultz M, Michtom RJ. Primary pulmonary hypertension. Am J Med 1951;11:686–705.
2. Rich S, Dantzker DR, Ayres SM, et al. Primary pulmonary hypertension: a national prospective study. Ann Intern Med 1987;107:216–23.
3. Hughes JD, Rubin LJ. Primary pulmonary hypertension: an analysis of 28 cases and a review of the literature. Medicine 1986;65:56–72.
4. Voelkel N, Reeves JT. Primary pulmonary hypertension. In: Moser K, ed. Lung Biology in Health & Disease, Vol. 14. New York, Marcel Dekker 1979:573–628.
5. Heath D, Smith P, Dalenz JR, Williams D, Harris P. Small pulmonary arteries in some natives of La Paz, Bolivia. Thorax 1981;36:599–604.
6. Wagenvoort CA, Wagenvoort N. Primary pulmonary hypertension: a pathologic study of the lung vessels in 156 clinically diagnosed cases. Circulation 1970;42:1163–84.
7. Heath D, Edwards JE. The pathology of hypertensive pulmonary vascular disease: a description of six grades of structural changes in the pulmonary arteries with special reference to congenital cardiac septal defects. Circulation 1958;18:533–47.
8. Loyd LE, Primm RK, Newman JH. Familial primary pulmonary hypertension: clinical patterns 1,2. Am Rev Respir Dis 1984;129:194–7.
9. Rubin LJ, Rubin LS, Peter RH. Oral hydralazine therapy for primary pulmonary hypertension. N Engl J Med 1980;302:69–73.
10. Cha SD, Kirschbaum M, Maranhao V, Paine E, Gooch AS. Phentolamine for primary pulmonary hypertension. Ann Intern Med 1979;91:927–8.
11. Daoud FS, Reeves JT, Kelly DB. Isoproterenol as a potential pulmonary vasodilator in primary pulmonary hypertension. Am J Cardiol 1978;42:817–22.
12. Halpern SM, Shah PK, Lehrman S, Goldberg HS, Jasper AC, Koerner SK. Prostaglandin E1 as a screening vasodilator in primary pulmonary hypertension. Chest 1987;92:686–91.
13. Higenbottam T, Wheeldon D, Wells F, Wallwork J. Long-term treatment of primary pulmonary hypertension with continuous intravenous epoprostenol (prostacyclin). Lancet 1984;1:1046–7.
14. Rich S, Brundage BH. High-dose calcium channel-blocking therapy for primary pulmonary hypertension: evidence for long-term reduction in pulmonary arterial pressure and regression of right ventricular hypertrophy. Circulation 1987;76:135–41.
15. Pietra GG, Rattner JR. Specificity of pulmonary vascular lesions in primary pulmonary hypertension. Respiration 1987;52:81–5.
16. Loyd JE, Atkinson JB, Pietra GG, Virmani R, Newman JH. Heterogeneity of pathologic lesions in familial primary pulmonary hypertension. Am Rev Respir Dis 1988;138:952–7.
17. Weir EK, Archer SL, Edwards JE. Chronic primary and secondary thromboembolic pulmonary hypertension. Chest 1988;93:149S–154S.
18. Edwards WD, Edwards JE. Clinical primary pulmonary hypertension: three pathologic types. Circulation 1977;56:884–8.
19. Heath D, Whitaker W. Hypertensive pulmonary vascular disease. Circulation 1956;XIV:323–43.
20. DeFeyter PJ, Kerkkamp HJJ, deJong JP. Sustained beneficial effect of nifedipine in primary pulmonary hypertension. Am Heart J 1983;105:333–4.
21. Davies PF. How do vascular endothelial cells respond to flow? NIPS 1989;4:22–5.
22. Douglas JG, Munro JF, Kitchin AH, Muir AL, Proudfoot AT. Pulmonary hypertension and fenfluramine. Br Med J 1981;283:881–3.
23. Guazzi MD, Alimeato M, Fiorentini C, Pepi M, Polese A. Hypersensitivity of lung vessels to catecholamines in systemic hypertension. Br Med J 1986;293:291–4.
24. Edwards BS, Weir EK, Edwards WD, Ludwig J, Dykoski RK, Edwards JE. Coexistent pulmonary and portal hypertension: morphologic and clinical features. J Am Coll Cardiol 1987;10:1233–8.
25. Eisenberg PR, Rich S, Kaufmann L, Jaffe AS. Evidence for increased thrombin activity in patients with primary pulmonary hypertension (abstr). Circulation 1987;(suppl IV):IV-49.
26. Barst RJ, Stalcup SA, Steeg CN, et al. Relation of arachidonate metabolites to abnormal control of the pulmonary circulation in a child. Am Rev Respir Dis 1985;131:171–7.
27. Kahaleh MB, Osborn I, LeRoy EC. Increased factor VIII/von Willebrand factor antigen and von Willebrand factor activity in scleroderma and in Raynaud's phenomenon. Ann Intern Med 1981;94(Part 1):482–4.
28. Cohen M, Edwards WD, Fuster V. Regression in thromboembolic type of primary pulmonary hypertension during 2½ years of antithrombotic therapy. J Am Coll Cardiol 1986;7:172–5.
29. Franz RC, Ziady F, Coetzee WJC, Hugo N. A possible causal relationship between defective fibrinolysis and pulmonary hypertension. S Afr Med J 1979;55:170–3.

30. Goldsmith GH, Baily RG, Brettler DB, et al. Primary pulmonary hypertension in patients with classic hemophilia. Ann Intern Med 1988;108: 797–9.

31. Ross R. The pathogenesis of atherosclerosis. In: Braunwald E, ed. Heart Disease: A Textbook of Cardiovascular Medicine. Philadelphia: WB Saunders, 1988:1135–52.

32. Devel TF. Polypeptide growth factors: roles in normal and abnormal cell growth. Ann Rev Cell Biol 1987;3:443–92.

33. Kelly J. Cytokines of the lung. Am Rev Respir Dis 1990;141:765–88.

34. Perkett EA, Lyons RM, Moses HL, Brigham KL, Meyrick BO. Transforming growth factor-α in sheep lung lymph: changes during the development of chronic pulmonary hypertension. J Clin Invest 1990;86:1459–64.

35. Folkman J, Klagsbrun M. Angiogenic factors. Science 1987;235:442–7.

36. Chang SW, Voelkel NF. Charge-related lung microvascular injury. Am Rev Respir Dis 1989;139:534–45.

37. Hales CA, Kradin RL, Brandstetter RD, Zhu Y. Impairment of hypoxic pulmonary artery remodeling by heparin in mice. Am Rev Respir Dis 1983;128:747–51.

38. Campbell JH, Campbell GR. Potential role of heparanase in atherosclerosis. NIPS 1989;4:9–12.

39. Mecham RP, Whitehouse LA, Wrenn DS, et al. Smooth muscle-mediated connective tissue remodeling in pulmonary hypertension. Science 1987; 237:423–6.

40. Ruoslahti E, Pierschbacher MD. New perspectives in cell adhesion: RGD and integrins. Science 1987;238:491–7.

41. Nishimura RA, Miller FA, Callahan MJ, Benassi RC, Seward JB, Tajik J. Doppler echocardiography: theory, instrumentation, technique, and application. Mayo Clin Proc 1985;60:321–43.

CHAPTER 18

Pulmonary Hypertension: A Cellular Basis for Understanding the Pathophysiology and Treatment

STUART RICH, MD, BRUCE H. BRUNDAGE, MD

Pulmonary hypertension is a relatively common sequela of a variety of cardiac and lung diseases. Interest in pulmonary hypertension has more recently been stimulated by identification of the rare disease known as "primary pulmonary hypertension" in which high pulmonary artery pressure and pulmonary vascular resistance from unknown causes produce chronic right heart failure and lead to death (1). Physicians have extrapolated from observations regarding primary pulmonary hypertension to pulmonary hypertensive conditions in general, with respect to both pathophysiologic mechanisms and effective treatments. This review will highlight new data that suggest a need to refocus our understanding of the etiology of pulmonary hypertensive states and the basis of our therapeutic efforts.

Primary Pulmonary Hypertension: A Human Disease Model

Primary pulmonary hypertension serves as a clinical model of "pure" pulmonary hypertension without an obvious secondary cause. Although primary pulmonary hypertension was originally described by Dresdale et al. (2) in 1951, the most widely publicized description of the condition came from a World Health Organization symposium on the disease in Geneva in 1973 (3). At that time, three subtypes of primary pulmonary hypertension were described: plexogenic pulmonary arteriopathy, recurrent pulmonary thromboembolism and pulmonary venoocclusive disease. Little is known about pulmonary venoocclusive disease, as it is clearly the most rare form of primary pulmonary hypertension, occurring in approximately 5% of all cases of primary pulmonary hypertension (4). The other two histologic subtypes are more common and occur in both primary and secondary forms of pulmonary hypertension.

Plexogenic Pulmonary Arteriopathy

Etiology. The histologic features of plexogenic pulmonary arteriopathy are medial hypertrophy, intimal proliferation and plexiform lesions involving the pulmonary arterioles that are believed to be a result of intense vasoconstriction (3,5,6). Autopsy findings in patients with primary pulmonary hypertension vary from medial hypertrophy with intimal proliferation to the entire spectrum of these histologic changes. These findings suggest that medial hypertrophy is the earliest lesion, thus supporting the notion that primary

vasoconstriction is the mechanism for plexogenic pulmonary arteriopathy (7). Reports that agents of the vasodilator type reduce pulmonary vascular resistance strengthened the concept that vasoconstriction was the underlying mechanism (8–10). It is important to recognize that plexogenic pulmonary arteriopathy is not pathognomonic for primary pulmonary hypertension, but exists in other forms of pulmonary hypertension, suggesting that vasoconstriction is occurring in secondary forms of pulmonary hypertension as well (5,7). Therefore, pulmonary hypertension arising from post-tricuspid left to right intracardiac shunts (e.g., ventricular septal defect, patent ductus arteriosus) suggests that reactive pulmonary vasoconstriction is a response to increased pulmonary blood flow (11).

The observation that collagen vascular diseases are associated with plexogenic pulmonary arteriopathy in the absence of significant parenchymal lung disease suggests that some autoimmune mechanism may be stimulating pulmonary vascular smooth muscle (12–14). Liver cirrhosis of any etiology has also been associated with plexogenic pulmonary arteriopathy, leading to speculation that unmetabolized vasoactive compounds pass through the liver to the lung and produce pulmonary vasoconstriction, although these compounds have never been identified (15,16). Finally, aminorex fumarate, an appetite suppressant drug with sympathomimetic properties introduced in Europe in the 1960s, was shown to induce a dietary form of pulmonary hypertension, and it was presumed that aminorex produced pulmonary vasoconstriction (17).

Hypothesis: plexogenic pulmonary arteriopathy is a result of endothelial cell injury that affects endothelial derived mediators of smooth muscle. A closer look at the data on the mechanisms of the secondary forms of plexogenic pulmonary arteriopathy does not implicate pulmonary vascular smooth muscle as the culprit, but rather points toward the pulmonary vascular endothelium. With the recent discovery that endothelial derived mediators are the primary determinants of vascular smooth muscle tone, it is interesting to speculate that abnormalities of endothelial cell function may lead to pulmonary vasoconstriction (18). It is well established that the pulmonary vascular bed is a low resistance circuit, suggesting that the endothelium maintains a state of chronic smooth muscle relaxation, probably through the release of endothelial derived relaxing factors (19–21). Clinical data demonstrating that acetylcholine, which stimulates the release of endothelial derived relaxing factors, is often an effective pulmonary vasodilator in primary pulmonary hypertension suggests impaired function of the pulmonary vascular endothelial cell in these patients (22). The fact that other vasodilators that work directly on vascular smooth muscle are also effective in the same patients is consistent with a state of increased pulmonary vascular tone as a result of abnormal endothelial cell mediation (22).

Pulmonary hypertension in congenital heart disease. Histologic studies in patients with pulmonary hypertension associated with congenital heart defects have revealed ultrastructural abnormalities in the endothelial cells that suggest heightened metabolic function (23). Recently, higher levels of von Willebrand factor antigenic activity were described in these patients (24), further implicating abnormal endothelial cell function in congenital heart disease with pulmonary hypertension. The fact that these abnormalities are present in patients irrespective of the severity of the pulmonary vascular disease, but not in patients with congenital heart disease without pulmonary hypertension, suggests that it may be an early feature in the development of the pulmonary hypertensive disease state. Because increased shear stress has been shown to be a mechanical factor that can cause endothelial cell disruption (25), it is now understandable why shunts appearing after development of the tricuspid valve commonly produce pulmonary hypertension, whereas shunts appearing before development of the tricuspid valve (such as atrial septal defect and anomalous pulmonary venous drainage) with similar magnitudes of left to right shunting are much less likely (11).

Aminorex-associated pulmonary hypertension. This condition is an interesting syndrome that resulted from the introduction of this appetite suppressant drug in Western Europe in the late 1960s (17). The incidence of patients who developed pulmonary hypertension after drug ingestion was approximately 1 in 1,000, suggesting that some underlying predisposition was also necessary. In addition, when the offending agent was withdrawn, although the condition of some patients improved, it remained the same in others and continued to worsen in many others. No animal model for aminorex-induced pulmonary hypertension has been produced, possibly because some type of genetic susceptibility is also necessary. However, dietary pulmonary hypertension has been induced in animals after the ingestion of crotolaria, an herbal plant found in tropical areas (26). Rats fed crotolaria develop acute pulmonary hypertension within several weeks (27). Studies on the activity of the pulmonary endothelium and vascular smooth muscle in these animals (28) show that the initial effect of crotolaria is to cause acute endothelial cell injury that is followed by endothelial cell proliferation and several weeks later by an increase in vascular smooth muscle cells. Therefore, the basis of this form of dietary pulmonary hypertension that results in plexogenic arteriopathy also appears to be endothelial cell damage followed by smooth muscle cell proliferation.

Collagen vascular disease. Although collagen vascular disease can cause plexogenic pulmonary arteriopathy, there has been no pathologic confirmation that acute cellular infiltration of the vascular smooth muscle is the earliest lesion (7). Rather, immune mediated injury of the endothelium is more likely. Patients with primary pulmonary hypertension have been shown to have high levels of antinuclear antibodies with a prevalence rate of approximately 40% (29). This prevalence rate puts primary pulmonary hypertension between rheumatoid arthritis and scleroderma with respect to the frequency of antinuclear antibodies in the spectrum of collagen vascular syndromes. Indeed, it does appear that some patients with primary pulmonary hypertension may have a forme fruste of collagen vascular disease confined to the lung.

Role of pulmonary endothelial injury. Each of the secondary causes of plexogenic pulmonary arteriopathy implicates pulmonary endothelial cell injury as the event that leads to abnormal pulmonary vascular smooth muscle constriction and long-standing pulmonary hypertension. This finding lends support to the hypothesis that in primary pulmonary hypertension, plexogenic pulmonary arteriopathy is a result of pulmonary endothelial injury.

Recurrent Pulmonary Thromboembolism

Etiology. Recurrent pulmonary thromboembolism is the histologic subtype that accounts for most of the remaining patients with primary pulmonary hypertension (3). The pathologic features include miliary embolization or thrombosis in situ, followed by eccentric intimal proliferation and obliteration of the pulmonary vascular bed with the histologic demonstration of intravascular fibrous webs as evidence for either embolization or thrombosis in situ (30). The fact that pulmonary hypertension can be created in animals by the embolization of a variety of substances, with the amount of pulmonary hypertension related to the degree of embolization, supported the notion that recurrent microemboli might be a mechanism for this disease (31). The observation that some patients with recurrent pulmonary thromboembolism have pulmonary hypertension is consistent with this concept (32).

It has only recently been appreciated that, in addition to primary pulmonary hypertension, "thromboembolic" pulmonary hypertension may occur in patients with pretricuspid left to right congenital shunts, primarily atrial septal defects (33). Why an atrial septal defect would produce miliary embolization in the lung has never been adequately addressed. In actuality, the data show that recurrent microembolization is highly unlikely to be the cause of primary or secondary pulmonary hypertension for several reasons. First, the number of emboli required to create severe pulmonary hypertension in vessels at the arteriolar level is enormous. In the dog, the number of emboli that would be needed to measure the pulmonary artery pressure by 5 to 10 mm Hg is between 90,000 and 22 million, which implies that a constant showering of emboli must be occurring (34). However, no source for miliary embolization has been documented in studies of patients with primary pulmonary hypertension (35). The histologic findings in patients with primary pulmonary hypertension with the ''recurrent thromboembolism'' pattern are also inconsistent with recurrent embolization, as the predominant finding in these patients is widespread severe eccentric intimal fibrosis (36). Although evidence for small vessel thrombosis exists, it is apparent in only approximately 10% of the vessels, clearly not enough to cause severe pulmonary hypertension (unpublished observations).

Hypothesis: thrombotic pulmonary arteriopathy is a result of endothelial injury that produces a procoagulant environment in the pulmonary vascular bed. Because there are no data supporting the concept of recurrent embolization as the cause of this syndrome, a more appropriate name would be ''thrombotic pulmonary arteriopathy.'' It has now been shown (37) that damage to vascular endothelium will result in an alteration of the environment for circulating platelets and thrombotic blood components rendering it susceptible to vascular thrombosis. Diffuse eccentric intimal proliferation, as a result of endothelial cell damage, with subsequent thrombosis as a result rather than a cause, would be a more logical pathophysiologic mechanism for thrombotic pulmonary arteriopathy. Patients with thrombotic pulmonary arteriopathy have an intimal pattern that appears distinct from plexogenic arteriopathy, in which the predominant lesion is concentric laminar intimal fibrosis (30). In congenital heart disease, it is probable that high pulmonary blood flow and pressure over time, associated with high shear stress, results in one type of endothelial injury (i.e., ventricular septal defect and plexogenic arteriopathy), whereas high pulmonary blood flow without increased pressure and shear stress produces a different endothelial response (atrial septal defect and thrombotic arteriopathy). The fact that pulmonary hypertension develops in only approximately 6% of patients with an atrial septal defect again suggests that some genetic predisposition is necessary (38).

Types of pulmonary perfusion patterns. It would be helpful to be able to determine the histologic subtype of primary pulmonary hypertension from clinical findings. We recently studied patterns of perfusion lung scans in patients with primary pulmonary hypertension (39) and were able to distinguish two types of perfusion patterns: 1) normal, and 2) diffuse patchy perfusion abnormalities. Although it was originally thought that the latter represented a more severe form of vascular disease, the patterns appear to be distinct because the patients who have normal lung scans apparently never develop the patchy pattern as their pulmonary hypertension progresses. In this radiographic-pathologic study, we demonstrated that the patchy lung scan pattern, in association with a normal chest X-ray film, correlates with the thrombotic arteriopathic pattern and can be distin-

guished from findings in patients with the plexogenic arteriopathic pattern, who have a normal chest X-ray film and lung scan. With use of these clinical criteria, it appears that plexogenic arteriopathy is more likely to occur in young women, whereas thrombotic arteriopathy seems to have a similar prevalence in men and women of a slightly older age.

Thrombosis in situ. That thrombosis in situ is occurring has now been confirmed. We recently studied (40) the sera of 31 patients with primary pulmonary hypertension for the presence of fibrinopeptide A, a small peptide that is released by the action of thrombin with fibrinogen. We found a wide spectrum of values of fibrinopeptide A in our patients; in the majority, values were elevated several times above the normal value, suggesting an intense thrombotic state, with the highest levels in patients with the abnormal patchy lung scans. Fibrinopeptide A levels were brought toward normal after the administration of intravenous heparin, confirming that this is a biologically active peptide in these patients. The fact that they also had elevated levels of plasminogen activator inhibitor-1 activity, but normal levels of cross-linked fibrin degradation products, suggests some type of acquired fibrolytic defect. Therefore, endothelial cell injury causing diffuse eccentric intimal proliferation and thrombosis in situ would seem to be the most scientifically sound explanation for this form of pulmonary hypertension. Data underscoring the importance of thrombosis was provided by Fuster et al. (41), who observed a salutary effect of warfarin anticoagulants on survival in a large number of patients with primary pulmonary hypertension studied retrospectively.

From these observations, one could conclude that primary pulmonary hypertension results from pulmonary endothelial injury, which leads either to intimal proliferation with smooth muscle hypertrophy (plexogenic pulmonary arteriopathy) or to intimal proliferation with intravascular thrombosis (thrombotic pulmonary arteriopathy). In primary pulmonary hypertension, as in other diseases, the histologic distinction between these two may not always be pure, and some overlap may exist.

Pulmonary hypertension due to toxic oil ingestion. Recently, an epidemic of pulmonary hypertension due to toxic oil ingestion has been reported (42). After the ingestion of contaminated rapeseed oil in Spain in 1981, there was an outbreak of pulmonary hypertension that affected approximately 1 in 1,000 exposed patients (once again raising the specter of an underlying genetic predisposition). Recent pathologic studies have shown that plexogenic pulmonary arteriopathy was the histologic finding in most patients, although some patients had coexisting thrombotic lesions and some had thrombotic pulmonary arteriopathy (43). The toxic oil syndrome is another clinical example of how an agent that produces acute pulmonary endothelial damage can result in plexogenic or thrombotic pulmonary arteriopathy (perhaps dose related) or an overlap of the two.

Therapeutic interventions. This unitarian hypothesis on the pathogenesis of primary pulmonary hypertension provides a clearer understanding of the limited success of therapeutic interventions. Warfarin anticoagulant therapy has been shown to be of probable benefit in some patients (41), whereas vasodilator drugs, primarily the calcium channel blockers at high doses, appear to cause regression of right ventricular hypertrophy and possibly prolong survival in some patients (44). Although not yet demonstrated, it is reasonable to expect that the success of a particular form of therapy may correlate with the histologic subtype, anticoagulants for thrombotic arteriopathy and vasodilators for plexogenic arteriopathy. This would apply not only to primary pulmonary hypertension, also to secondary forms of pulmonary hypertension that cause similar endothelial reactions. Nevertheless, the most common forms of secondary pulmonary hypertension, those caused by lung disease and left heart failure, do not appear to respond to vasodilators or anticoagulant therapy. They also do not appear to be associated with endothelial injury. They do seem to be quite treatable and even reversible.

Pulmonary Venous Hypertension

Mechanism. The histopathology of pulmonary venous hypertension shows primarily arterialization of the pulmonary venous bed, with secondary medial hypertrophy of the pulmonary arterioles and is only infrequently associated with concentric or eccentric intimal lesions (45). A classic example of this form of pulmonary hypertension is mitral stenosis. The observation has been made that pulmonary hypertension from mitral stenosis is reversible after mitral valve replacement, irrespective of the preoperative level of the pulmonary hypertension or elevation in pulmonary vascular resistance (46). Thus, by directing treatment toward the underlying mechanism, and in the absence of severe pulmonary endothelial damage, pulmonary venous hypertension is reversible.

Therapy. Histologic examination of the lungs in patients with pulmonary hypertension from chronic obstructive pulmonary disease reveals the muscular arteries to have largely normal media and occasional eccentric intimal fibrosis. The predominant lesion is in the small arterioles, with severe medial hypertrophy and longitudinal proliferation of muscle cells that can infiltrate into the intima (45). Vasodilators appear to be ineffective in humans with hypoxic lung disease, even though hypoxia seems to be one of the most potent stimuli for smooth muscle hypertrophy and vasoconstriction in the pulmonary vascular bed (47). Long-term oxygen therapy, in contrast, has been associated with improved survival and modest improvement in pulmonary hemodynamics (48). Thus, this other common form of secondary pulmonary hypertension, also without evidence of extensive endothelial cell injury, seems to be treatable by reversing the offending etiologic agent.

Conclusions

Given these observations, we can propose a more sensible approach toward our understanding of the origin of primary and secondary forms of pulmonary hypertension based on the nature of the pulmonary vascular damage, which may form the basis for developing more effective therapeutic regimens. The fact that vasodilators are not uniformly successful in primary or secondary pulmonary hypertension should not be considered as disappointing, but expected, given the heterogeneous nature of the diseases. The precise etiologic agents causing the endothelial cell damage in primary pulmonary hypertension have yet to be identified. However, as our understanding of the role of the endothelial cell in arterial vascular disease increases, more focused and effective treatments of pulmonary hypertensive states should be forthcoming.

References

1. Rich S. Primary pulmonary hypertension. Prog Cardiovasc Dis 1988;3:205–38.
2. Dresdale DT, Schultz M, Michtom RJ. Primary pulmonary hypertension. 1. Clinical and hemodynamic study. Am J Med 1951;11:686–705.
3. World Health Organization. Hatano S, Strasser T, eds. Primary Pulmonary Hypertension. Geneva: World Health Organization, 1975:7–45.
4. Wagenvoort CA, Wagenvoort N, Takahashi T. Pulmonary venoocclusive disease: involvement of the pulmonary arteries and review of the literature. Hum Pathol 1985;16:1033–41.
5. Lockhart A, Reeves JT. Plexogenic pulmonary hypertension of unknown origin: what's new? Clin Sci 1984;67:1–5.
6. Yamaki S, Wagenvoort CA. Plexogenic pulmonary arteriopathy: significance of medial thickness with respect to advanced pulmonary vascular lesions. Am J Pathol 1981;105:70–5.
7. Wagenvoort CA, Wagenvoort N. Primary pulmonary hypertension: a pathologic study of the lung vessels in 156 clinically diagnosed cases. Circulation 1970;42:1163–84.
8. Dresdale PT, Michtom RJ, Schultz M. Recent studies in primary pulmonary hypertension including pharmacodynamic observation on pulmonary vascular resistance. Bull NY Acad Med 1954;30:195–207.
9. Daoud FS, Reeves JT, Kelly DB. Isoproterenol as a potential pulmonary vasodilator in primary pulmonary hypertension. Am J Cardiol 1978;42:817–22.
10. Wood P. Pulmonary hypertension with special reference to the vasoconstrictive factor. Br Heart J 1958;20:557–70.
11. Hoffman JIE, Rudolph AM, Heymann MA. Pulmonary vascular disease with congenital heart lesions: pathologic features and causes. Circulation 1981;64:873–7.
12. Wakaki K, Koizumi F, Fukase M. Vascular lesions in systemic lupus erythematosus (SLE) with pulmonary hypertension. Acta Pathol Jpn 1984;34:593–604.
13. Sullivan WD, Hurst DJ, Harmon CE, et al. A prospective evaluation emphasizing pulmonary involvement in patients with mixed connective tissue disease. Medicine 1984;63:92–107.
14. Salerni R, Rodnan GP, Leon DF, et al. Pulmonary hypertension in the CREST syndrome variant of progressive systemic sclerosis (scleroderma). Arch Intern Med 1977;86:394–9.
15. McDonnell PJ, Toye PA, Hutchins GM. Primary pulmonary hypertension and cirrhosis: are they related? Am Rev Respir Dis 1983;127:437–41.
16. Bernthal AC, Eybel CE, Payne JA. Primary pulmonary hypertension after portacaval shunt. J Clin Gastroenterol 1983;5:363–6.
17. Gurtner HP. Aminorex and pulmonary hypertension. Cor Vasa 1985;27:160–71.
18. Vanhoutte PM. The endothelium-modulator of vascular smooth-muscle tone. N Engl J Med 1988;319:512–3.

19. Furchgott RF. Role of the endothelium in responses of vascular smooth muscle. Circ Res 1983;53:557–73.
20. DeMey JG, Gray SD. Endothelium-dependent reactivity in resistance vessels. Prog Appl Microcirculation 1988;88:181–7.
21. Peach MJ, Loeb AL, Singer HA, Saye J. Endothelium-derived vascular relaxing factor. Hypertension 1985;7(suppl I):I-94–I-100.
22. Furchgott RF. The requirement for endothelial cells in the relaxation of arteries by acetylcholine and some other vasodilators. Trends Pharmacol Sci 1981;2:173–6.
23. Rabinovitch M, Bothwell T, Hayakawa BN, et al. Pulmonary artery endothelial abnormalities in patients with congenital heart defects and pulmonary hypertension. Lab Invest 1986;55:632–53.
24. Rabinovitch M, Andrew M, Thom H, et al. Abnormal endothelial factor VIII associated with pulmonary hypertension and congenital heart defects. Circulation 1987;76:1043–52.
25. Miller VM, Aarhus LL, Vanhoutte PM. Modulation of endothelium-dependent responses by chronic alterations of blood flow. Am J Physiol 1986;251:H520–H7.
26. Hislop A, Reid L. Arterial changes in Crotalaria Spectabilis-induced pulmonary hypertension in rats. Br J Exp Pathol 1974;55:153–7.
27. Meyrick B, Gamble W, Reid L. Development of Crotalaria pulmonary hypertension: hemodynamic and structural study. Am J Physiol 1980;239:H692–9.
28. Meyrick B, Reid L. Development of pulmonary arterial changes in rats fed Crotalaria Spectabilis. Am J Pathol 1979;94:37–48.
29. Rich S, Kieras K, Hart K, et al. Antinuclear antibodies in primary pulmonary hypertension. J Am Coll Cardiol 1986;8:1307–11.
30. Bjornsson J, Edwards WD. Primary pulmonary hypertension: a histopathologic study of 80 cases. Mayo Clin Proc 1985;60:16–25.
31. Malik AB. Pulmonary microembolism. Physiol Rev 1983;63:1114–92.
32. Sharma GV, McIntyre KM, Sharma S, Sasahara AA. Clinical and hemodynamic correlates in pulmonary embolism. Clin Chest Med 1984;5:421–37.
33. Yamaki S, Horiuchi T, Miura M, et al. Pulmonary vascular disease in secundum atrial septal defect with pulmonary hypertension. Chest 1986;5:694–8.
34. Dexter L, Smith GT. Quantitative studies of pulmonary embolism. Am J Med Sci 1964;247:641–8.
35. Rich S, Levitsky S, Brundage BH. Pulmonary hypertension from chronic pulmonary thromboembolism. Ann Intern Med 1988;108:425–34.
36. Edwards W. Pathology of pulmonary hypertension. Cardiovasc Clin 1988;18:321–59.
37. Ryan US. The endothelial surface and responses to injury. Fed Proc 1986;45:101–8.
38. Steele PM, Fuster V, Cohen M, et al. Isolated atrial septal defect with pulmonary vascular obstructive disease—long-term follow-up and prediction of outcome after surgical correction. Circulation 1987;76:1037–42.
39. Rich S, Pietra GG, Kieras K, et al. Primary pulmonary hypertension: radiographic and scintigraphic patterns of histologic subtypes. Ann Intern Med 1986;105:499–502.
40. Eisenberg PR, Rich S, Kaufmann L, et al. Evidence for increased thrombin activity in patients with primary pulmonary hypertension (abstr). Circulation 1987;76(suppl IV):IV-1246.
41. Fuster V, Steele PM, Edwards WD, et al. Primary pulmonary hypertension: natural history and the importance of thrombosis. Circulation 1984;70:580–5.
42. Tabuenca JM. Toxic-allergic syndrome caused by ingestion of rapeseed oil denatured with aniline. Lancet 1981;2:567–8.
43. Gomez-Sanchez MA, Mestre de Juan M, Gomez-Pajuelo C, et al. Pulmonary hypertension due to toxic oil syndrome. Chest 1989;95:325–31.
44. Rich S, Brundage BH. High dose calcium blocking therapy for primary pulmonary hypertension: evidence for long-term reduction in pulmonary arterial pressure and regression of right ventricular hypertrophy. Circulation 1987;76:135–41.
45. Wagenvoort CA, Wagenvoort N. Pathology of Pulmonary Hypertension. New York: John Wiley & Sons, 1977:1–290.
46. Zener JC, Hancock EW, Shumway NE, et al. Regression of extreme pulmonary hypertension and mitral valve surgery. Am J Cardiol 1972;30:820–6.
47. Fishman AP. Chronic cor pulmonale. Am Rev Respir Dis 1976;114:775–9.
48. Timms RM, Khaja FU, Williams GW, et al. Hemodynamic response to oxygen therapy in chronic obstructive pulmonary disease. Ann Intern Med 1985;103:29–36.

CHAPTER 19

Current Status of Cardiac Surgery: A 40 Year Review

WAYNE E. RICHENBACHER, MD, JOHN L. MYERS, MD,
JOHN A. WALDHAUSEN, MD,

Coronary Artery Disease

Coronary bypass surgery. Surgical management of atherosclerotic coronary artery disease began in the mid 1950s with the introduction of coronary endarterectomy by Bailey (1) and Longmire (2) and their co-workers. These procedures were performed on the beating heart without cardiopulmonary bypass. In 1961, Goetz et al. (3) performed a nonsuture anastomosis over a tantalum ring between the right internal mammary artery and the right coronary artery. The first reversed saphenous vein bypass graft was performed by Garrett in 1964 (4). In 1968, Favaloro (5) reported his landmark series of 15 patients who underwent reversed saphenous vein bypass of segmentally occluded right dominant coronary arteries. These bypass procedures were also performed on a beating heart with intermittent anoxic arrest.

Anoxic arrest, with or without hypothermia, resulted in a 9% to 20% intraoperative or early postoperative myocardial infarction rate (6). Early results of coronary artery bypass improved with the introduction of hypothermia and induced ventricular fibrillation without anoxic arrest (7). A desire to reduce the metabolic demands of ischemic myocardium led Melrose et al. (8) to develop cold, hypertonic potassium citrate blood cardioplegia in 1955. The recognition that this procedure was associated with irreversible postoperative left ventricular injury led to its subsequent abandonment (9). Interest in cardioplegic arrest was rekindled when Gay and Ebert (10) documented a fourfold reduction in myocardial oxygen consumption in hearts preserved with high potassium cardioplegia as compared with the beating and nonworking, paced or fibrillating heart.

Twenty-four thousand coronary bypass operations were performed in the United States in 1971; by 1980 that number exceeded 125,000 (11). Current indications for aortocoronary bypass grafting include class III angina that is unresponsive to medical therapy, unstable angina, left main coronary artery stenosis and symptomatic status triple vessel disease (11). Percutaneous transluminal coronary angioplasty, introduced into the clinical arena by Gruentzig in 1979 (12), is ideally reserved for the coronary bypass surgery candidate who has one or two noncalcified, high grade stenoses of the proximal left anterior descending, right or left circumflex coronary artery.

Surgery after myocardial infarction. Traditional teaching states that myocardial revascularization should either be undertaken within 4 to 6 h of the onset of an acute myocardial infarction or be delayed in an effort to avoid reperfusion injury. Katz et al. (13) evaluated 145 patients who underwent coronary artery bypass surgery within 4 weeks of an acute myocardial infarction. Postoperative heart failure was a strong predictor of mortality and was related to the presence of preoperative heart failure, ischemia and a low ejection fraction. Their study indicated that, whereas ischemia and congestive failure did influence mortality, the time after infarction did not, thus suggesting that myocardial revascularization should proceed without delay in the presence of ongoing ischemia or life-threatening coronary anatomy.

Effect of coronary angioplasty on surgical revascularization. Coronary angioplasty has had a significant effect on coronary bypass surgery in that angioplasty removes low risk patients from the surgical candidate pool. The number of operative risk factors, including advanced age, female gender, severity of angina, triple vessel disease and left ventricular dysfunction, has increased among patients currently undergoing coronary artery bypass surgery (14–16). Naunheim et al. (15) reported an increase from 3% to 7% in operative mortality for coronary bypass procedures during the past 10 years due, in part, to the inclusion of more high risk patients in the surgically treated population. These authors point out, however, that the clinical profile of current angioplasty patients closely resembles that of the coronary artery bypass patients of 1975. Other studies (16) have demonstrated that, despite an increase in risk factors, operative mortality can be maintained at a low rate. Two reports (17,18) have shown that coronary artery bypass surgery can be offered to patients in their 8th or 9th decade of life with acceptable results.

Failed coronary angioplasty procedures also contribute to the group of patients requiring emergency myocardial revascularization. Patients who require an emergency operation after unsuccessful angioplasty have a higher mortality rate and greater incidence of postoperative hemorrhage, cardiac tamponade, myocardial infarction and length of hospitalization than do patients who undergo elective coronary artery bypass surgery (19). Ferguson et al. (20) concur but have shown that mortality and nonhemorrhagic complication rates among patients who undergo coronary artery bypass surgery after failed elective coronary angioplasty are comparable with those in patients who undergo coronary artery bypass after failed emergency angioplasty.

Surgery in acute myocardial infarction. Patients with an acute myocardial infarction who undergo thrombolysis may subsequently require emergency bypass surgery or coronary angioplasty. Bypass grafting yields excellent long-term results, especially in patients with an ischemic interval of <3 h (21). Results with either method of primary revascularization are comparable, although mortality remains highest in patients who have had unsuccessful angioplasty and require an emergency operation (22).

Results of surgery versus angioplasty. The efficacy of coronary artery bypass surgery and coronary angioplasty in selected patients with one and two vessel coronary artery disease is well established. Gruentzig et al. (23) reported on 169 patients who were followed up for 5 to 8 years after coronary angioplasty. They noted that, in their initial experience, angioplasty was successful in 79% of cases, while 30% of patients developed recurrent stenoses within 6 months. As more recent randomized, prospective follow-up studies are reported, Daily (24) notes that the results of coronary angioplasty should be comparable with the results of bypass surgery in the pre-angioplasty era (similar risk groups). His benchmark for coronary angioplasty includes a complete revascularization rate of 99.8%, a hospital mortality rate of 0.2%, a perioperative myocardial infarction rate of 2.2%, a 5 year survival rate of 89.8% and freedom from reintervention at 5 years of 97.7%.

Internal mammary artery grafts. The internal mammary artery remains the coronary bypass graft of choice (25). Zeff et al. (26) followed up 80 patients with a left anterior descending coronary artery bypass graft (41 patients with a saphenous vein graft, 39 with a left internal mammary artery graft) for 10 years and reported a lower mortality and higher patency rate in the patients with an internal mammary artery graft. In an effort to maximize the number of distal internal mammary artery anastomoses, sequential (27), bilateral and free internal mammary artery grafts have been employed. Bilateral internal mammary artery grafts provide excellent conduits with which to revascularize the left anterior descending, left anterior descending diagonal and marginal coronary arteries (28). Ten year follow-up studies show significantly greater freedom from reoperation and infarction and significantly lower rates of recurrent angina in the patients with internal mammary artery grafts than in those with saphenous vein grafts (28). Furthermore, the use of bilateral internal mammary artery grafts does not increase patient mortality or morbidity, with the exception of a slight increase in mean transfusion requirement, over that of patients with saphenous vein grafts (29). The posterior and diaphragmatic surfaces of the heart, inaccessible to in situ internal mammary artery grafts, can be bypassed with free internal mammary artery grafts. Concern that division of the internal mammary artery pedicle would result in reduced long-term graft patency and patient survival appears to be unfounded (30,31). Passage of the right internal mammary artery through the transverse sinus (27) and use of the distal internal mammary artery as a retrograde mammary bypass graft (32) are not recommended. Internal mammary artery

grafts can be used in patients with smaller body habitus (33), and vasoactive drugs do not appear to reduce internal mammary artery flow (34).

Transfusion requirements and precautions. Transfusion-related infectious disease has been featured prominently in the lay press because of increased public concern over acquired immunodeficiency syndrome. Approximately 2% of acquired immunodeficiency syndrome cases in the United States have resulted from transfusion of blood or blood products (35). As a large number of transfusion-related acquired immunodeficiency syndrome infections occur after cardiac operations (36), attention has recently been directed to perioperative blood conservation. Both intraoperative autotransfusion of washed red blood cells (37) and postoperative reinfusion of shed mediastinal blood (38) decrease the need for homologous transfusion. Transfusion requirements can also be reduced by the avoidance of aspirin preoperatively (39) and the perioperative administration of dipyridamole (40). In the event nonsurgical postoperative bleeding occurs, the transfusion of 1 U of fresh whole blood has a hemostatic effect equal, if not superior, to that of 10 U of platelets (41). Moreover, the number of donors is minimized, thereby reducing the risk of exposure to blood-borne viruses.

Acquired Valvular Disease

Mitral Valve Disease

Mitral stenosis. The first valve operations attempted to correct rheumatic mitral stenosis without the use of cardiopulmonary bypass. Closed mitral commissurotomy was accomplished by transatrial digital dilation (42), transapical partial valvulectomy (43) and transventricular mechanical dilation (44). The introduction of cardiopulmonary bypass made possible mitral valve replacement. The first mitral valve prosthesis, constructed of woven Teflon fabric, was implanted by Kay et al. (45) in 1960. The Starr-Edwards ball-valve (Baxter Healthcare Corporation), the first true mechanical valve prosthesis, was implanted in the mitral position in 1961 (46).

Despite 30 years of experimental and clinical experience, the ideal prosthetic valve has yet to be manufactured. The 70° convexo-concave Björk-Shiley valve (Shiley Inc.) has an increased incidence of outlet strut fractures (47) and is no longer commercially available. The 7 year actuarial incidence of mechanical failure in the 29 to 31 mm, 70° convexo-concave Björk-Shiley valve is 12.5%, regardless of whether the valve is placed in the aortic or mitral position (48). Björk and coworkers (48) have recently recommended that selected patients with an early production valve of this type be considered for re-replacement. A newer, more durable, monostrut Björk-Shiley valve has been implanted in 486 patients (537 prostheses) with no structural failures noted at an average follow-up interval of 33 months (49).

The Edwards-Duromedics bileaflet valve (Baxter Healthcare Corporation) has developed mechanical failure due to fatigue-related leaflet fractures and is also no longer commercially available (50). At present, patients with this valve require careful long-term follow-up, but prophylactic rereplacement has not been recommended.

The Starr-Edwards prosthesis remains the standard against which other mechanical and tissue valves must be compared. Starr et al. (51) reported on 707 patients with a Starr-Edwards valve with follow-up extending beyond 20 years (mean 5.2). Valve-related mortality at 20 years is 13% with a 3.3% incidence of thromboembolism per year. There was no incidence of structural deterioration.

Magovern et al. (52) have reviewed the status of 130 patients who underwent mitral valve replacement with or without concomitant coronary artery bypass grafting. Overall mortality was 9.2%, whereas the subgroup with mitral regurgitation and coronary artery disease had the highest mortality rate (21.7%). Factors associated with death were preoperative functional class IV or cardiogenic shock, age >60 years or a left ventricular end-diastolic pressure of 15 mm Hg.

Mitral regurgitation. The majority of patients with mitral regurgitation can be successfully treated by mitral valve repair rather than replacement. Although Carpentier (53) remains the international authority on mitral valve repair, the techniques of mitral annular plication, annuloplasty ring insertion and repair of chordae tendineae rupture were well described by Kay et al. (45) in 1960. Repair of the mitral valve is preferred as it is associated with a lower actuarial probability of anticoagulation hemorrhage and higher actuarial incidence of freedom from thromboembolism when compared with prosthetic replacement of the mitral valve (54). In patients with ischemic mitral regurgitation, mitral valve repair results in improved operative survival when compared with mitral valve replacement (55).

A variety of new and innovative techniques for repairing regurgitant mitral valves have been described. Major anterior leaflet prolapse can be dealt with by chordal transposition from the posterior leaflet (56) or creation of a neochorda with use of a strip of tissue from the anterior leaflet itself (57). In the event the mitral valve must be replaced, it is thought that preservation of the posterior leaflet and subvalvular apparatus (58,59) and even the chordae tendineae to the anterior leaflet (60) will enhance postoperative left ventricular performance and reduce operative mortality.

Aortic Valve Disease

Aortic valve replacement. The origins of aortic valve surgery date back to 1954, when Hufnagel et al. (61) successfully introduced a ball-valve chamber into the cross-clamped descending thoracic aorta in patients with aortic insufficiency. Again, the introduction of cardiopulmonary bypass permitted subcoronary aortic valve replacement. A mechanical prosthesis was first inserted in the aortic position

by Harken et al. (62) in 1960, whereas Ross (63) implanted the first aortic homograft in 1962.

Magovern et al. (64) reviewed results in 259 patients who underwent aortic valve replacement with or without concomitant coronary artery bypass grafting. Operative mortality was highest in patients undergoing aortic valve replacement and coronary artery bypass grafting (13.5% versus 3.5%). The strongest predictors of operative death were emergency operation and patient age over 70 years. Factors associated with late death were preoperative age, male gender, left ventricular end-diastolic pressure, cardiac index and functional class.

Aortic stenosis: balloon valvuloplasty. Aortic stenosis in elderly, high risk patients has most recently been managed by balloon valvuloplasty. It appears that this procedure may produce suboptimal results (65) and can potentially lead to annular disruption (66). It is unlikely that results with this method should be much different from those of the closed methods described in the 1950s by Bailey et al. (67) and long since abandoned as ineffective and dangerous. The high risk patient population may be smaller than anticipated in that at least two recent reports (68,69) document the safety of aortic valve replacement in the elderly.

Congenital Cardiac Disease

Coarctation of aorta. Twenty-five years ago it was generally agreed that aortic coarctation should be repaired when diagnosed in children and adults. At that time, however, there was considerable disagreement regarding optimal management of infants with coarctation (70). Surgical repair in this age group was most readily accomplished by resection of the coarctation and end to end anastomosis (71), but the mortality rate was high (43%) (70) and recoarctation was common (72). The introduction of the subclavian flap procedure by Waldhausen and Nahrwold (73) obviated this problem to a large degree. The current standard of care in the treatment of neonates and infants with coarctation of the aorta is to initially stabilize the decompensated heart of the neonate by infusing prostaglandin E_1 to maintain ductal patency, which allows perfusion of the distal aorta from the patent ductus. Early subclavian flap repair using absorbable suture (74) can be accomplished with an operative mortality rate of 3.5% and a negligible recurrence rate (75).

Atrial septal defect. This is one of the most common congenital cardiac lesions, accounting for 10% to 15% of patients with congenital heart disease. This was the first defect successfully corrected with use of cardiopulmonary bypass, a feat accomplished by Gibbon (76) in 1953. The surgical management of uncomplicated atrial septal defects has changed little during the past 35 years, with most centers reporting operative mortality rates for elective closure of <1% (77).

Ventricular septal defect. This is the most common of all congenital cardiac lesions, accounting for 25% of all congenital heart defects. Before the advent of cardiopulmonary bypass, patients with ventricular septal defect and high pulmonary flow were managed with a pulmonary artery band (78). Subsequent intracardiac repair was accomplished with minimal morbidity and mortality (79); however, pulmonary artery reconstruction is frequently required after removal of the band. Currently, primary repair of a ventricular septal defect can routinely be accomplished in symptomatic infants using cardiopulmonary bypass, deep hypothermia and total circulatory arrest (80). Pulmonary artery banding is now reserved for symptomatic infants with multiple muscular septal defects in whom the risk of early primary intracardiac repair remains significant (81).

Atrioventricular (AV) canal. Before 1969, infants with an AV canal defect were primarily managed with a pulmonary artery band (82). Palliation was preferred as the results of corrective operation were less than encouraging. The first large series of patients who had undergone complete surgical repair of an endocardial cushion defect was reported by Ellis et al. (83) in 1960. The average age of these 66 patients was 8 to 12 years and the hospital mortality rate was 21% (67% among patients undergoing repair of complete AV canal). A better understanding of the anatomic details of endocardial cushion defects, based on Rastelli's classification (84), led to improved operative results (85) and the application of corrective surgery to infants with a complete AV canal (86). Currently, corrective surgery is recommended in older patients with a complete AV canal who have not developed pulmonary vascular obstructive disease, whereas the use of cardiopulmonary bypass and hypothermic circulatory arrest permits early repair in symptomatic infants with acceptable results (87).

Tetralogy of Fallot. This was the first complex congenital heart defect to be palliated with a systemic to pulmonary artery shunt. The Blalock-Taussig shunt was first performed on a 16 month old girl with tetralogy of Fallot in November 1944 (88). This complex congenital cardiac anomaly was also the first to be totally corrected, in an operation performed by Scott et al. (89) in 1954, using hypothermia and circulatory arrest. Lillehei et al. (90) performed a successful intracardiac repair using cross-circulation in 1955, whereas Kirklin et al. (91) performed the first complete repair using cardiopulmonary bypass. Gustafson et al. (92) recently reported on the early intracardiac repair of tetralogy of Fallot in 40 infants. A right ventricular outflow tract patch was utilized in 34 patients (85%), of whom the youngest was 7 weeks old. Follow-up extended from 2 to 37 months, at which time no residual ventricular septal defect and only one moderate right ventricular outflow tract gradient was observed. The authors state that the only infants undergoing a shunt procedure initially were those with pulmonary atresia, complete AV canal or coronary anomalies. Kirklin et al. (93), however, believe that a two stage approach is still indicated in infants under 6 months of age.

Transposition of great arteries. In 1959 Senning (94) described a technique for the atrial repair of transposition of the great arteries. By 1970, Waldhausen et al. (95) reported a series of 12 patients with simple transposition in whom a second type of atrial baffle, the Mustard procedure (96), was performed with no mortality. Senning's original report (94) also described the steps that would be required for surgical correction of the arterial side of transposition of the great arteries. The latter procedure involved suturing the ventricular septum to the right of the aortic valve, and the proximal pulmonary artery, with its valve, to the right ventricular free wall. Although Senning's arterial repair never achieved the popularity of his atrial baffle, a single stage arterial repair is now possible using the arterial switch operation described by Jatene et al. (97).

Currently, simple transposition of the great arteries can be managed by either an atrial baffle or an arterial switch operation. A 20 center cooperative study (98) that randomized infants to each of three surgical management strategies (Mustard, Senning or arterial switch operation) showed the survival and incidence of the need for reoperation to be similar among all groups. On the basis of a series of 23 infants with transposition of the great arteries and an intact ventricular septum who underwent an arterial switch procedure in the 1st month of life, Idriss et al. (99) proposed that the atrial baffle be reserved for patients with anatomic or functional left ventricular inadequacy. Idriss (100) and Norwood (101) and their co-workers also demonstrated the efficacy of the arterial switch operation in patients with transposition of the great arteries and a ventricular septal defect. It appears that early anatomic repair results in good preservation of right and left ventricular function, avoiding the need for additional palliative procedures (102). In addition, the socioeconomic advantages of performing a definitive repair in the 1st weeks of life demand consideration.

Complex anomalies. The modified Fontan procedure has now been applied to lesions other than classic tricuspid atresia. Infants with a single ventricle heart or double outlet right ventricle and noncommitted ventricular septal defect can undergo an early modified Fontan procedure with right atrial to pulmonary artery anastomosis with minimal mortality (103). Total cavopulmonary connection has similar clinical applicability for the Fontan procedure and is associated with a reduced risk of postoperative arrhythmias and atrial thrombosis (104).

Hypoplastic left heart syndrome. Before the development of the Norwood procedure (105) in 1981, infants with the hypoplastic left heart syndrome uniformly died within the 1st week of life. Recently, Norwood et al. (106) reviewed the status of 104 infants who underwent palliative reconstruction for hypoplastic left heart syndrome. They noted no contraindication to palliation. Lessons learned in this large series include the need for wide excision of the septum primum to avoid late pulmonary venous obstruction, patch closure of the main pulmonary artery to avoid loss of continuity between the right and left pulmonary arteries and the advantage of a central shunt that avoids relative hypoplasia of the left pulmonary artery associated with a modified right Blalock-Taussig shunt.

Congenital aortic stenosis. This is one of the more common cardiac anomalies, but results of operative intervention in the neonate with critical aortic stenosis remain poor. Brown et al. (107) described 257 patients with aortic stenosis and noted that the operative mortality rate in infants older than 6 months of age was 4%, whereas neonates with critical aortic stenosis had a 60% mortality rate. More recently, Turley et al. (108) reported on 33 patients who underwent either open valvotomy (25 patients) or transventricular dilation (8 patients). The hospital survival rate was 85% with no significant difference between methods. Our most recent experience also shows that a simple transventricular dilation of the stenotic valve in neonates gives excellent results with a very low mortality.

Patients with supravalvular or subvalvular aortic stenosis and those undergoing aortic valve replacement had a reduction or elimination of associated aortic insufficiency. Conversely, patients requiring valvotomy for valvular aortic stenosis developed a significant increase in the degree of aortic insufficiency (107). Infants with multilevel lesions required a complex repair with an attendant increase in mortality. Hammon et al. (109) studied a series of infants <6 months of age who presented with critical valvular aortic stenosis and concluded that a small left ventricular dimension and elevated pulmonary artery pressure were predictive of a poor outcome.

Aortic valve replacement. Children who require aortic valve replacement often have a small aortic anulus. Fleming and Sarafian (110) performed an aortic valve replacement and Konno ventriculoplasty in 16 patients aged 2 to 23 years. Eighty-one percent of patients received a valve ≥25 mm. There was one operative death; postoperatively, all patients remain in New York Heart Association class I. Cardiac valve replacement in children is technically feasible, but the management of postoperative anticoagulation remains problematic. Bioprostheses are to be avoided because of early leaflet calcification and valve failure. Sade et al. (111) previously reported the use of the St. Jude valve in children without anticoagulation, but recently withdrew this recommendation when a number of patients in their cohort developed thromboembolic complications. Robbins et al. (112) observed a similar high incidence of thromboembolic complications in patients with a mechanical valve and no anticoagulation. They concluded from their study of 94 children with a prosthetic cardiac valve that anticoagulation with warfarin could be safely employed.

Cardiac Transplantation

Human cardiac transplantation began in 1964 when Hardy et al. (113) transplanted a chimpanzee heart into a 68 year old man. The patient survived for 1 h after the termination of cardiopulmonary bypass. Cardiac allotransplantation was first performed by Barnard (114) in 1967. The patient survived for 18 days but ultimately died of pneumonia. A number of centers developed cardiac transplant programs (115), and early results indicated that the principal determinant of long-term survival was the successful management of acute rejection. In the early 1970s immunosuppression was based on the administration of prednisone, azathioprine and anti-human thymocyte globulin. Results with this triple drug regimen were less than satisfactory, as the 1 year survival rate in 1971 was 50% (115).

Immunosuppressive therapy. Interest in cardiac transplantation waned in the subsequent decade but was renewed with the introduction of cyclosporin A (116). The effect of using cyclosporin A in combination with azathioprine and steroids is reflected in data reported by the International Society for Heart Transplantation (117), which indicate that 5 year survival after cardiac transplantation now approaches 80%.

Political versus medical aspects of cardiac transplantation. The most revealing aspect of a recent literature review is the disturbingly large number of studies that deal with the "political" as opposed to "medical" aspects of cardiac transplantation. Limited donor organ availability has resulted in the adoption of a "routine inquiry" law in the majority of states (118). This law requires that hospital administrators or their designees advise families of deceased patients that their organs can be made available for transplantation. Even so, the rapid increase in the number of cardiac transplant centers has reduced the relative number of donor organs available to any institution. An attempt to expand the donor pool by harvesting organs from anencephalic infants has generated considerable controversy (119). Xenogeneic transplants, although technically feasible, remain experimental (120). The most ominous development is the decision by the state of Oregon to limit funding available for organ transplantation (121).

Recent experience. Bolman et al. (122) reviewed the transplantation experience at The Washington University during the past 2 years (59 patients, 62 heart transplants) and observed a number of well recognized trends. Low priority status patients usually experience a prolonged preoperative waiting period. Critically ill patients, requiring cardiotonic, ventilatory or mechanical circulatory support undergo transplantation more expeditiously, with reasonable results. With use of the combined immunosuppressive regimen of cyclosporin, azathioprine and prednisone, 50% of patients were rejection free and 56% were infection free at 12 months.

Role of patient age. Cardiac transplantation is now being offered to both infants (123) and patients >60 years of age (124). Problems encountered in the pediatric population include the need for on-site donor harvesting because of intolerance of the neonatal heart to prolonged ischemia, as well as an inability to definitively diagnose rejection (123). In the series of Frazier et al. (124) of 28 patients >60 years of age who underwent cardiac transplantation, the 1 year actuarial survival rate was 83%. Renlund et al. (125) propose that there may actually be an age-associated decline in cardiac allograft rejection due to a decrease in T effector cell-mediated immunity.

Myocardial Preservation

Crystalloid versus blood cardioplegia. The ideal constituents and route of administration of cardioplegic solutions have yet to be determined. A rekindled interest in retrograde perfusion of the coronary sinus shows this technique to be efficacious in aortic valve replacement, elective myocardial revascularization (126) and repeat coronary artery bypass procedures (127). Standard anterograde perfusion of the aortic root with crystalloid and blood cardioplegic solutions has failed to demonstrate a distinct advantage to the use of either perfusate. One experimental study employing crystalloid cardioplegia suggests that the volume of cardioplegic solution infused and the duration of infusion are the most significant determinants of the degree of myocardial protection (128). Oxygenation of crystalloid cardioplegic perfusate (129,130) and hypothermia to <20°C in either blood or crystalloid cardioplegia (131) also appear to result in a greater degree of myocardial preservation. Warner et al. (132), in an experimental study, found that intermittent administration of blood cardioplegia resulted in a lower myocardial pH and hydrogen ion concentration when compared with crystalloid cardioplegia (132). Khuri et al. (133) described a clinical series in which blood cardioplegia was administered continuously while the aorta was cross-clamped. When compared with crystalloid or intermittent blood cardioplegia, continuous blood cardioplegia led to a marked reduction in myocardial acidosis and hydrogen ion concentration.

Mechanical Circulatory Assistance

Ventricular assist devices. The indications for use, technique of implantation and principles of postoperative care in patients on a mechanical blood pump are well described. Ventricular assist devices are employed in patients with postcardiotomy cardiogenic shock and as a bridge to cardiac transplantation. Among patients with postcardiotomy ventricular failure, 41% to 50% can be weaned from their device, and 29% to 40% are discharged from the hospital (134, 135,136). At an average follow-up interval of 29 months, 16 of 23 survivors of mechanical ventricular assistance were either attending school or gainfully employed, whereas only 4 patients had evidence of cardiac disability (New York Heart Association functional class III or IV) (137). Pae et al. (138) followed up nine ventricular assist pump survivors for an average of 31 months. All nine patients were in functional class IV preoperatively, whereas eight of nine were in

functional class I or II after surgery. At least 50% of patients with end-stage cardiomyopathy who are supported with a ventricular assist device are able to undergo subsequent cardiac transplantation (139).

Artificial heart. The pneumatically powered total artificial heart is used primarily as a bridge to cardiac transplantation. A total of 41% to 88% of patients receive a cardiac allograft, whereas hospital discharge rates vary from 25% to 50% (140,141). Sepsis precludes transplantation in many patients receiving mechanical circulatory support and limits long-term survival in patients who undergo cardiac transplantation (140,142).

We gratefully acknowledge the assistance of Cynthia A. Miller in the preparation of the manuscript.

References

1. Bailey CP, May A, Lemmon WM. Survival after coronary endarterectomy in man. JAMA 1957;164:641–6.
2. Longmire WP Jr, Cannon JA, Kattus AA. Direct-vision coronary endarterectomy for angina pectoris. N Engl J Med 1958;259:993–9.
3. Goetz RH, Rohman M, Haller JD, Dee R, Rosenak SS. Internal mammary-coronary artery anastomosis. J Thorac Cardiovasc Surg 1961;41:378–86.
4. Reul GJ, Morris GC Jr, Howell JF, Crawford ES, Stetler WJ. Current concepts in coronary artery surgery. Ann Thorac Surg 1972;14:243–59.
5. Favaloro RG. Saphenous vein autograft replacement of severe segmental coronary artery occlusion. Ann Thorac Surg 1968;5:334–9.
6. Hultgren HN, Miyagawa M, Buck W, Angell WW. Ischemic myocardial injury during coronary artery surgery. Am Heart J 1971;82:624–31.
7. Wilson HE, Dalton ML, Kiphart RJ, Allison WM. Increased safety of aorto-coronary artery bypass surgery with induced ventricular fibrillation to avoid anoxia. J Thorac Cardiovasc Surg 1972;64:193–292.
8. Melrose DG, Dreyer B, Bentall HH, Baker JBE. Elective cardiac arrest. Lancet 1955;2:21–2.
9. Waldhausen JA, Braunwald NS, Bloodwell RD, Cornell WP, Morrow AG. Left ventricular function following elective cardiac arrest. J Thorac Cardiovasc Surg 1960;39:799–807.
10. Gay WA Jr, Ebert PA. Functional, metabolic, and morphologic effects of potassium-induced cardioplegia. Surgery 1973;74:284–90.
11. Cohen LS. Coronary artery revascularization: indications for surgery and results. In: Glenn WWL, Baue AE, Geha AS, Hammond GL, Laks H, eds. Thoracic and Cardiovascular Surgery. 4th ed. Norwolk, CT: Appleton-Century-Crofts, 1983:1418–27.
12. Gruentzig AR, Senning A, Siegenthaler WE. Nonoperative dilation of coronary-artery stenosis. N Engl J Med 1979;301:61–8.
13. Katz NM, Kubanick TE, Ahmed SW, et al. Determinants of cardiac failure after coronary bypass surgery within 30 days of acute myocardial infarction. Ann Thorac Surg 1986;42:658–63.
14. Arcidi JM, Powelson SW, King SB, et al. Trends in invasive treatment of single-vessel and double-vessel coronary disease. J Thorac Cardiovasc Surg 1988;95:773–81.
15. Naunheim KS, Fiore AC, Wadley JJ, et al. The changing mortality of myocardial revascularization: coronary artery bypass and angioplasty. Ann Thorac Surg 1988;46:666–74.
16. Davis PK, Parascondola SA, Miller CA, et al. Mortality of coronary artery bypass grafting before and after the advent of angioplasty. Ann Thorac Surg 1989;47:493–8.
17. Naunheim KS, Kern MJ, McBride LR, et al. Coronary artery bypass surgery in patients aged 80 years or older. Am J Cardiol 1987;59:804–7.
18. Rich MW, Keller AJ, Schectman KB, Marshall WG Jr, Kouchoukos NT. Morbidity and mortality of coronary bypass surgery in patients 75 years of age or older. Ann Thorac Surg 1988;46:638–44.

19. Parsonnet V, Fisch D, Gielchinsky I, et al. Emergency operation after failed angioplasty. J Thorac Cardiovasc Surg 1988;96:198–203.

20. Ferguson TB, Muhlbaier LH, Salai DL, Wechsler AS. Coronary bypass grafting after failed elective and failed emergent percutaneous angioplasty. J Thorac Cardiovasc Surg 1988;95:761–72.

21. Messmer BJ, Uebis R, Rieger C, Minale C, Hofstadter F, Effert S. Late results after intracoronary thrombolysis and early bypass grafting for acute myocardial infarction. J Thorac Cardiovasc Surg 1989;97:10–8.

22. Petrovich JA, Wellons HA Jr, Schneider JA, Kauten JR, Mikell FL, Taylor GJ. Revascularization after thrombolytic therapy for acute myocardial infarction: an analysis of 573 patients. Ann Thorac Surg 1988;46:163–6.

23. Gruentzig AR, King SB, Schlumpf M, Siegenthaler W. Long-term follow-up after percutaneous transluminal coronary angioplasty. N Engl J Med 1987;316:1127–32.

24. Daily PO. Early and five-year results for coronary artery bypass grafting. J Thorac Cardiovasc Surg 1989;97:67–77.

25. Ivert T, Huttunen K, Landou C, Björk VO. Angiographic studies of internal mammary artery grafts 11 years after coronary artery bypass grafting. J Thorac Cardiovasc Surg 1988;96:1–12.

26. Zeff RH, Kongtahworn C, Iannone LA, et al. Internal mammary artery versus saphenous vein graft to the left anterior descending coronary artery: prospective randomized study with 10-year follow-up. Ann Thorac Surg 1988;45:533–6.

27. Rankin JS, Newman GE, Bashore TM, et al. Clinical and angiographic assessment of complex mammary artery bypass grafting. J Thorac Cardiovasc Surg 1986;92:832–46.

28. Geha AS, Hammond GL, Stephan RN, Kleiger RK, Krone RJ. Long-term outcome of revascularization of the anterior coronary arteries with crossed double internal mammary versus saphenous vein grafts. Surgery 1987;102:667–73.

29. Cosgrove DM, Lytle BW, Loop FD, et al. Does bilateral internal mammary artery grafting increase surgical risk? J Thorac Cardiovasc Surg 1988;95:850–6.

30. Loop FD, Lytle BW, Cosgrove DM, Golding LAR, Taylor PC, Stewart RW. Free (aorta-coronary) internal mammary artery graft: late results. J Thorac Cardiovasc Surg 1986;92:827–31.

31. Daly RC, McCarthy PM, Orszulak TA, Schaff HV, Edwards WD. Histologic comparison of experimental coronary artery bypass grafts. J Thorac Cardiovasc Surg 1988;96:19–29.

32. Cohen AJ, Ameika JA, Briggs RA, Grishkin BA, Helsel RA. Retrograde flow in the internal mammary artery. Ann Thorac Surg 1988;45:48–9.

33. Suma H, Takeuchi A, Kondo K, et al. Internal mammary artery grafting in patients with smaller body structure. J Thorac Cardiovasc Surg 1988;96:393–9.

34. Beavis RE, Mullany CJ, Cronin KD, et al. An experimental in vivo study of the canine internal mammary artery and its response to vasoactive drugs. J Thorac Cardiovasc Surg 1988;95:1059–66.

35. Centers for Disease Control. Human immunodeficiency virus infection in transfusion recipients and their family members. MMWR 1987;36:137–40.

36. Schiff M, Katz A, Farber B, Kaplan M. Acquired immunodeficiency syndrome, a complication of cardiothoracic surgery. J Thorac Cardiovasc Surg 1989;97:126–9.

37. Giordano GF, Goldman DS, Mammana RB, et al. Intraoperative autotransfusion in cardiac operations. J Thorac Cardiovasc Surg 1988;96:382–6.

38. Hartz RS, Smith JA, Green D. Autotransfusion after cardiac operation. J Thorac Cardiovasc Surg 1988;96:178–82.

39. Ferraris VA, Ferraris SP, Lough FC, Berry WR. Preoperative aspirin ingestion increases operative blood loss after coronary artery bypass grafting. Ann Thorac Surg 1988;45:71–4.

40. Teoh KH, Christakis GT, Weisel RD, et al. Dipyridamole preserved platelets and reduced blood loss after cardiopulmonary bypass. J Thorac Cardiovasc Surg 1988;96:332–41.

41. Mohr R, Martinowitz U, Lavee J, Amroch D, Ramot B, Goor DA. The hemostatic effect of transfusing fresh whole blood versus platelet concentrates after cardiac operations. J Thorac Cardiovasc Surg 1988;96:530–4.

42. Souttar HS. The surgical treatment of mitral stenosis. Br Med J 1975;2:603–6.

43. Cutler EC, Levine SA, Beck CS. The surgical treatment of mitral stenosis: experimental and clinical studies. Arch Surg 1924;9:689–821.

44. Logan A, Turner R. Surgical treatment of mitral stenosis. Lancet 1959;2:874–80.

45. Kay EB, Nogueira C, Zimmerman HA. Correction of mitral insufficiency under direct vision. Circulation 1960;21:568–77.

46. Starr A, Edwards ML. Mitral replacement: clinical experience with a ball-valve prosthesis. Ann Surg 1961;154:726–40.

47. Lindblom D, Bjork VO, Semb BKH. Mechanical failure of the Bjork-Shiley valve: incidence, clinical presentation, and management. J Thorac Cardiovasc Surg 1986;92:894–907.

48. Lindblom D, Rodriguez L, Bjork VO. Mechanical failure of the Bjork-Shiley valve. J Thorac Cardiovasc Surg 1989;97:95–7.

49. Thulin LI, Bain WH, Huysmans HH, et al. Heart valve replacement with the Bjork-Shiley monostrut valve: early results of a multicenter clinical investigation. Ann Thorac Surg 1988;45:164–70.

50. Klepetko W, Moritz A, Mlczoch J, Schurawitzki H, Domanig E, Wolner E. Leaflet fracture in Edwards-Duromedics bileaflet valves. J Thorac Cardiovasc Surg 1989;97:90–4.

51. Cobanoglu A, Fessler CL, Guvendik L, Grunkemeier G, Starr A. Aortic valve replacement with the Starr-Edwards prosthesis: a comparison of the first and second decades of follow-up. Ann Thorac Surg 1988;45:248–52.

52. Magovern JA, Pennock JL, Campbell DB, Pierce WS, Waldhausen JA. Risks of mitral valve replacement and mitral valve replacement with coronary artery bypass. Ann Thorac Surg 1985;39:346–52.

53. Carpentier A. Cardiac valve surgery—the "French correction." J Thorac Cardiovasc Surg 1983;86:323–37.

54. Cohn LH, Kowalker W, Bhatia S, et al. Comparative morbidity of mitral valve repair versus replacement for mitral regurgitation with and without coronary artery disease. Ann Thorac Surg 1988;45:284–90.

55. Rankin JS, Feneley MP, Hickey MStJ, et al. A clinical comparison of mitral valve repair versus valve replacement in ischemic mitral regurgitation. J Thorac Cardiovasc Surg 1988;95:165–77.

56. Lessana A, Romano M, Lutfalla G, et al. Treatment of ruptured or elongated anterior mitral valve chordae by partial transposition of the posterior leaflet: experience with 29 patients. Ann Thorac Surg 1988;45:404–8.

57. Gregory F Jr, Takeda R, Silva S, Facanha L, Meier MA. A new technique for repair of mitral insufficiency caused by ruptured chordae of the anterior leaflet. J Thorac Cardiovasc Surg 1988;96:765–8.

58. Goor DA, Mohr R, Lavee J, Serraf A, Smolinsky A. Preservation of the posterior leaflet during mechanical valve replacement for ischemic mitral regurgitation and complete myocardial revascularization. J Thorac Cardiovasc Surg 1988;96:253–60.

59. Sarris GE, Cahill PD, Hansen DE, Derby GC, Miller DC. Restoration of left ventricular systolic performance after reattachment of the mitral chordae tendineae. J Thorac Cardiovasc Surg 1988;95:969–79.

60. Miki S, Kusuhara K, Ueda Y, Komeda M, Ohkita Y, Tahata T. Mitral valve replacement with preservation of chordae tendineae and papillary muscles. Ann Thorac Surg 1988;45:28–34.

61. Hufnagel CA, Harvey WP, Rabil PJ, McDermott TF. Surgical correction of aortic insufficiency. Surgery 1954;35:673–83.

62. Harken DE, Soroff HS, Taylor WJ, Lefemine AA, Gupta SK, Lunzer S. Partial and complete prostheses in aortic insufficiency. J Thorac Cardiovasc Surg 1960;40:744–62.

63. Ross DN. Homograft replacement of the aortic valve. Lancet 1962;2:487.

64. Magovern JA, Pennock JL, Campbell DB, et al. Aortic valve replacement and combined aortic valve replacement and coronary artery bypass grafting: predicting high risk groups. J Am Coll Cardiol 1987;9:38–43.

65. Robicsek F, Harbold NB Jr, Daugherty HK, et al. Balloon valvuloplasty in calcified aortic stenosis: a cause for caution and alarm. Ann Thorac Surg 1988;45:515–25.

66. Seifert PE, Auer JE. Surgical repair of annular disruption following percutaneous balloon aortic valvuloplasty. Ann Thorac Surg 1988;46:242–3.

67. Bailey CP, Bolton HE, Jamison WL, Nichols HT. Commissurotomy for rheumatic aortic stenosis. I. Surgery. Circulation 1954;9:22–31.

68. Bessone LN, Pupello DF, Hiro SP, Lopez-Cuenca E, Glatterer MS Jr, Ebra G. Surgical management of aortic valve disease in the elderly: a longitudinal analysis. Ann Thorac Surg 1988;46:264–9.

69. Borkon AM, Soule LM, Baughman KL, et al. Aortic valve selection in the elderly patient. Ann Thorac Surg 1988;46:270–7.

70. Waldhausen JA, King H, Nahrwold DL, Lurie PR, Shumaker HB. Management of coarctation in infancy. JAMA 1964;187:270–5.

71. Schuster SR, Gross RE. Surgery for coarctation of the aorta. J Thorac Cardiovasc Surg 1962;43:54–70.

72. Eshaghpour E, Olley PM. Recoarctation of the aorta following coarctectomy in the first year of life. J Pediatr 1972;80:809–14.

73. Waldhausen JA, Nahrwold DL. Repair of coarctation of the aorta with a subclavian flap. J Thorac Cardiovasc Surg 1966;51:532–3.

74. Myers JL, Campbell DB, Waldhausen JA. The use of absorbable monofilament polydioxanone suture in pediatric cardiovascular operations. J Thorac Cardiovasc Surg 1986;92:771–5.

75. Campbell DB, Pae WE Jr, Waldhausen JA. Coarctation of the aorta: current surgical management. World J Surg 1985;9:543–9.

76. Gibbon JH Jr. Application of a mechanical heart and lung apparatus to cardiac surgery. Minn Med 1954;37:171–85.

77. Stansel HC Jr, Talner NS, Deren MM, Heeckeren DV, Glenn WWL. Surgical treatment of atrial septal defect. Am J Surg 1971;121:485–9.

78. Muller WH, Dammann JF Jr. The treatment of certain congenital malformations of the heart by the creation of pulmonic stenosis to reduce pulmonary hypertension and excessive pulmonary blood flow. Surg Gynecol Obstet 1952;95:213–9.

79. Kirklin JW, Harshbarger HG, Donald DE, Edwards JE. Surgical correction of ventricular septal defect: anatomic and technical considerations. J Thorac Cardiovasc Surg 1957;33:45–59.

80. Barratt-Boyes BG, Neutze JM, Clarkson PM, Shardey GC, Brandt PWT. Repair of ventricular septal defect in the first two years of life using profound hypothermia-circulatory arrest techniques. Ann Surg 1976;184:376–90.

81. Arciniegas E. Ventricular septal defect. In Ref 11:745–56.

82. Boruchow I, Waldhausen JA, Miller WW, Rashkind WJ, Friedman S. Pulmonary artery hypertension in infants with congenital heart disease: palliative management by pulmonary artery binding. Arch Surg 1969;99:716–22.

83. Ellis FH, McGoon DC, Kirklin JW. Surgical management of persistent common atrioventricular canal. Am J Cardiol 1960;6:598–604.

84. Rastelli GC, Kirklin JR, Titus JL. Anatomic observations on complete form of persistent common atrioventricular canal with special reference to atrioventricular valves. Mayo Clin Proc 1966;41:296–308.

85. McMullan MH, Wallace RB, Weidman WH, McGoon DC. Surgical treatment of complete atrioventricular canal. Surgery 1972;72:905–12.

86. McGoon DC, McMullan MH, Mair DD, Danielson GK. Correction of complete atrioventricular canals in infants. Mayo Clin Proc 1973;48:769–72.

87. Norwood WI, Castaneda AR. Atrio-ventricular canal defects: partial, intermediate, and complete. In Ref 11:757–69.

88. Blalock A, Taussig HB. The surgical treatment of malformations of the heart in which there is pulmonary stenosis or pulmonary atresia. JAMA 1945;128:189–202.

89. Scott HW Jr, Collins HA, Foster JH. Hypothermia as an adjuvant in cardiovascular surgery: experimental and clinical observations. Am Surg 1954;20:799–812.

90. Lillehei CW, Cohen M, Warden HE, et al. Direct vision intracardiac surgical correction of the tetralogy of Fallot, pentalogy of Fallot, and pulmonary atresia defects. Ann Surg 1955;142:418–45.

91. Kirklin JW, Ellis FH Jr, McGoon DC, DuShane JW, Swan HJC. Surgical treatment for the tetralogy of Fallot by open intracardiac repair. J Thorac Surg 1959;37:22–51.

92. Gustafson RA, Murray GF, Warden HE, Hill RC, Rozar GE Jr. Early primary repair of tetralogy of Fallot. Ann Thorac Surg 1988;45:235–41.

93. Kirklin JW, Blackstone EH, Pacifico AD, Brown RN, Bargeron LM Jr. Routine primary repair vs. two-stage repair of tetralogy of Fallot. Circulation 1979;60:373–86.

94. Senning A. Surgical correction of transposition of the great vessels. Surgery 1959;45:966–80.

95. Waldhausen JA, Pierce WS, Rashkind WJ, Miller WW, Friedman S. Total correction of transposition of the great arteries following balloon atrioseptostomy. Circulation 1970;41(suppl II):II-123–9.

96. Mustard WT, Keith JD, Trusler GA, Fowler R, Kidd L. The surgical management of transposition of the great vessels. J Thorac Cardiovasc Surg 1964;48:953–8.

97. Jatene AD, Fontes VF, Paulista PP, et al. Anatomic correction of transposition of the great vessels. J Thorac Cardiovasc Surg 1976;72:364–70.

98. Castaneda AR, Trusler GA, Paul MH, Blackstone EH, Kirklin JW. The early results of treatment of simple transposition in the current era. J Thorac Cardiovasc Surg 1988;95:14–28.

99. Idriss FS, Ilbawi MN, DeLeon SY, et al. Transposition of the great arteries with intact ventricular septum. J Thorac Cardiovasc Surg 1988;95:255–62.

100. Idriss FS, Ilbawi MN, DeLeon SY, et al. Arterial switch in simple and complex transposition of the great arteries. J Thorac Cardiovasc Surg 1988;95:29–36.

101. Norwood WI, Dobell AR, Freed MD, Kirklin JW, Blackstone EH. Intermediate results of the arterial switch repair. J Thorac Cardiovasc Surg 1988;96:854–63.

102. Quaegebeur JM, Rohmer J, Ottenkamp J, et al. The arterial switch operation. J Thorac Cardiovasc Surg 1986;92:361–84.

103. Stellin G, Mazzucco A, Bortolotti U, et al. Tricuspid atresia versus other complex lesions. J Thorac Cardiovasc Surg 1988;96:204–11.

104. de Leval MR, Kilner P, Gewillig M, Bull C. Total cavopulmonary connection: a logical alternative to atriopulmonary connection for complex Fontan operations. J Thorac Cardiovasc Surg 1988;96:682–95.

105. Norwood WI, Lang P, Castaneda AR, Campbell DN. Experience with operations for hypoplastic left heart syndrome. J Thorac Cardiovasc Surg 1981;82:511–9.

106. Pigott JD, Murphy JD, Barber G, Norwood WI. Palliative reconstructive surgery for hypoplastic left heart syndrome. Ann Thorac Surg 1988;45:122–8.

107. Brown JW, Stevens LS, Holly S, et al. Surgical spectrum of aortic stenosis in children: a thirty-year experience with 257 children. Ann Thorac Surg 1988;45:393–403.

108. Turley K, Bove EL, Amato JJ, Iannettoni M, Yeh J. Neonatal aortic stenosis (abstr). Am Assoc Thorac Surg 1989:98.

109. Hammon JW Jr, Lupinetti FM, Maples MD, et al. Predictors of operative mortality in critical valvular aortic stenosis presenting in infancy. Ann Thorac Surg 1988;45:537–40.

110. Fleming WH, Sarafian LB. Aortic valve replacement with concomitant aortoventriculoplasty in children and young adults: long-term follow-up. Ann Thorac Surg 1987;43:575–8.

111. Sade RM, Crawford FA Jr, Fyfe DA, Stroud MR. Valve prostheses in children: a reassessment of anticoagulation. J Thorac Cardiovasc Surg 1988;95:553–61.

112. Robbins RC, Bowman FO Jr, Malm JR. Cardiac valve replacement in children: a twenty-year series. Ann Thorac Surg 1988;45:56–61.

113. Hardy JD, Chavez CM, Kurrus FD, et al. Heart transplantation in man. JAMA 1964;188:1132–40.

114. Barnard CN. The operation: a human cardiac transplant. S African Med J 1967;41:1271–4.

115. Caves PK, Stinson EB, Griepp RB, Rider AK, Dong E Jr, Shumway NE. Results of 54 cardiac transplants. Surgery 1973;74:307–14.

116. Jamieson SW, Burton NA, Bieber CP, et al. Cardiac-allograft survival in primates treated with cyclosporin A. Lancet 1979;1:545.

117. Fragomeni LS, Kaye MP. The Registry of the International Society for Heart Transplantation: fifth official report—1988. J Heart Transplant 1988;7:249–53.

118. Cosimi AB. What's new in surgery for 1989: transplantation. ACS Bulletin 1989;74:41–7.

119. Arras JD, Shinnar S. Anencephalic newborns as organ donors: a critique. JAMA 1988;259:2284–5.

120. Auchincloss H. Xenogeneic transplantation: a review. Transplantation 1988;46:1–15.

121. Welch HG, Larson EB. Dealing with limited resources: the Oregon decision to curtail funding for organ transplantation. N Engl J Med 1988;319:171–3.

122. Bolman RM, Cance C, Spray T, et al. The changing face of cardiac transplantation: the Washington University program, 1985–1987. Ann Thorac Surg 1988;45:192–7.

123. Mavroudis C, Harrison H, Klein JB, et al. Infant orthotopic cardiac transplantation. J Thorac Cardiovasc Surg 1988;96:912–24.

124. Frazier OH, Macris MP, Duncan JM, Van Buren CT, Cooley DA. Cardiac transplantation in patients over 60 years of age. Ann Thorac Surg 1988;45:129–32.

125. Renlund DG, Gilbert EM, O'Connell JB, et al. Age-associated decline in cardiac allograft rejection. Am J Med 1987;83:391–8.

126. Diehl JT, Eichhorn EJ, Konstam MA, et al. Efficacy of retrograde coronary sinus cardioplegia in patients undergoing myocardial revascularization: a prospective randomized trial. Ann Thorac Surg 1988;45: 595–602.

127. Snyder HE, Smithwick W, Wingard JT, Agnew RC. Retrograde coronary sinus perfusion. Ann Thorac Surg 1988;46:389–90.

128. Takahashi A, Chambers DJ, Braimbridge MV, Hearse DJ. Optimal myocardial protection during crystalloid cardioplegia. J Thorac Cardiovasc Surg 1988;96:730–40.

129. Ledingham SJM, Braimbridge MV, Hearse DJ. Improved myocardial protection by oxygenation of the St. Thomas' Hospital cardioplegic solutions. J Thorac Cardiovasc Surg 1988;95:103–11.

130. Tabayashi K, McKeown PP, Miyamoto M, et al. Ischemic myocardial protection. J Thorac Cardiovasc Surg 1988;95:239–46.

131. Rousou JA, Engleman RM, Breyer RH, Otani H, Lemeshow S, Das DK. The effect of temperature and hematocrit level on oxygenated cardioplegic solutions on myocardial preservation. J Thorac Cardiovasc Surg 1988;95:625–30.

132. Warner KG, Josa M, Butler MD, et al. Regional changes in myocardial acid production during ischemic arrest: a comparison of sanguineous and asanguineous cardioplegia. Ann Thorac Surg 1988;45:75–81.

133. Khuri SF, Warner KG, Josa M, et al. The superiority of continuous cold blood cardioplegia in the metabolic protection of the hypertrophied human heart. J Thorac Cardiovasc Surg 1988;95:442–54.

134. Rose DM, Connolly M, Cunningham JN Jr, Spencer FC. Technique and results with a roller pump left and right heart assist device. Ann Thorac Surg 1989;47:124–9.

135. Pennington DG, McBride LR, Swartz MT, et al. Use of the Pierce-Donachy assist device in patients with cardiogenic shock after cardiac operations. Ann Thorac Surg 1989;47:130–5.

136. Richenbacher WE, Pae WE Jr, Rosenberg G, Pennock JL, Pierce WS. Experimental and clinical experience with the Pennsylvania State University pneumatic ventricular assist device and total artificial heart. Eur Rev Biomed Tech 1987;9:31–4.

137. Kanter KR, Ruzevich SA, Pennington DG, McBride LR, Swartz MT, Willman VL. Follow-up of survivors of mechanical circulatory support. J Thorac Cardiovasc Surg 1988;96:72–80.

138. Pae WE Jr, Pierce WS, Pennock JL, Campbell DB, Waldhausen JA. Long-term results of ventricular assist pumping in postcardiotomy cardiogenic shock. J Thorac Cardiovasc Surg 1987;93:434–41.

139. Kanter KR, McBride LT, Pennington DG, et al. Bridging to cardiac transplantation with pulsatile ventricular assist devices. Ann Thorac Surg 1988;46:134–40.

140. Muneretto C, Solis E, Pavie A, et al. Total artificial heart: survival and complications. Ann Thorac Surg 1989;47:151–7.

141. Griffith BP. Interim use of the Jarvik-7 artificial heart: lessons learned at Presbyterian-University Hospital of Pittsburgh. Ann Thorac Surg 1989; 47:158–66.

142. Griffith BP, Kormos RL, Hardesty RL, Armitage JM, Dummer JS. The artificial heart: infection-related morbidity and its effect on transplantation. Ann Thorac Surg 1988;45:409–14.

◆ CHAPTER 20 ◆

Cardiac Surgery: A Glimpse Into the Future

WILLIAM S. PIERCE, MD, WALTER E. PAE, MD, JOHN L. MYERS, MD, JOHN A. WALDHAUSEN, MD

The progress that has occurred in medicine during our lifetimes has been unparalleled. Forty years ago, rheumatic fever was widespread, mitral valvulotomy had not been successfully performed, the heart-lung machine had not been applied to humans and intensive care meant that the physician sat at the patient's bedside. Today, rheumatic fever has been all but eliminated, valvular heart surgery is commonplace with an operative mortality of <4%, the heart-lung machine is used in over one quarter of a million patients each year and our intensive care units, with their sophisticated monitoring apparatus, are showplaces of modern technology as applied to medicine. Although day to day progress by medical scientists occurred slowly, the overall effect produced by our unique blend of academic medicine, industry and the practitioner has resulted in a level of progress that no Solomon could have predicted.

Advances in cardiac surgery have occurred through so many routes that future directions are very difficult to predict. The dedicated clinician-scientist tackles a recognized problem, a surgeon changes the format of an operation, an industrial laboratory focuses money and personnel; each approach appears to have an even chance of advancing our field. The most we can accomplish in our review is to indicate areas in which research effort is being expended and areas in which advances in our abilities would have a favorable impact on patient care.

Vascular Surgery

Prosthetic grafts. The recognition that inert fabric tubes could serve as blood vessel substitutes provided a range of therapeutic options for patients with vascular disease (1). The use of prosthetic grafts evolved along with the specialty of vascular surgery. Modifications to encourage uniform tissue ingrowth, low initial porosity and external supports to prevent buckling have been secondary improvements that have been readily incorporated into clinical surgery.

When fabric grafts are used in vessel sizes of <10 mm in diameter the patency rate decreases to unacceptable values when compared with the rate obtained with the use of the reversed autogenous saphenous vein. A variety of treated biologic vessels have been used but, thus far, initial enthusiasm has been counteracted by premature degeneration. The development of microporous polytetrafluoroethylene (PTFE) grafts has resulted in an off the shelf prosthesis that provides acceptable results in the 6 to 10 mm range when autogenous vein is not available or its use is inadvisable (2).

The need for a small vessel prosthesis (<6 mm in diameter) has been recognized for ≥2 decades. Although there is no shortage of scientific articles indicating the accomplishment of this task, no small vessel prosthesis is available when a graft is required for a specific clinical application (3–4). Despite the general recognition that the availability of a small vessel prosthesis would have a major clinical impact and that fortunes are to be made from the development of such a graft, no satisfactory prosthesis is forthcoming. A better understanding of the phenomena that occur at the anastomotic sites, new knowledge regarding the relative advantages and disadvantages of a porous versus a nonporous prosthesis wall and, possibly, improved materials will play a role in this development. Although the saphenous vein is a "friend" of the vascular surgeon, there are many instances in which it is not available or should be left alone, an autogenous artery is not sufficient and a commercial prosthesis, sized for the task at hand, should be used.

Techniques for blood vessel anastomosis. The potential usefulness of rapid techniques for blood vessel anastomoses have been recognized for decades. The Soviet blood vessel stapling device rekindled an interest in non-suture techniques (5). Vascular staplers work satisfactorily if there is reasonable access to the vessels, adequate cuff lengths and minimal atherosclerosis. When these criteria are not met, most surgeons find it quicker to perform a conventional suture anastomosis. However, the successful application of the sutureless blood vessel connector has been very helpful in simplifying the repair of aneurysms of the thoracic aorta (6). Similar techniques will be applied to other blood vessels with advantage. Other options of rapid blood vessel anastomoses that have promise include the use of tissue adhesives and laser welding (7,8).

Laser techniques. The availability of laser techniques will increase the therapeutic options in vascular surgery (8). Laser angioscopy will allow visualization of stenotic lesions and will permit the surgeon to decide on the pros and cons of angioplasty techniques (dilation versus laser ablation) versus direct surgical approaches. Blind vascular procedures will no longer be performed. Moreover, for vessels in which direct dilation is the treatment of choice, but in which restenosis is a distinct possibility, a thin-walled, mesh type, metal stent will be inserted intravascularly to obviate this possibility (9).

Cardiopulmonary Bypass

Heparin anticoagulation. The availability of heparin was crucial to the development of the heart-lung machine. Commercial heparin remains a complex biologic chemical, extracted from slaughterhouse animals and composed of a mixture of mucopolysaccharides of varying anticoagulant. A single compound having uniform activity, no antigenicity and no effect on platelets will improve our ability to achieve anticoagulation during cardiopulmonary bypass and then completely reverse the effect of the drug (10). Of possibly greater importance will be the availability of a heparin antagonist that does not have the allergenic effects or the cardiovascular effects of biologically derived protamine (11).

Modern membrane oxygenators without heparin. The ability to perform cardiopulmonary bypass without heparin would simplify certain open heart operations, decrease operating time and reduce blood loss and transfusion requirements. At present, the thoracic aorta can be bypassed with use of left atrial to aortic pumping without heparin (12). Shed blood is heparinized as it is sucked from the operative field. The advantages of such a system are clear. The major element in a pump oxygenator, in which clotting occurs if inadequate heparin is present, is the oxygenator. Modern membrane oxygenators are now making their mark in cardiac surgery; their modification to prevent activation of coagulation without the use of systemic heparin will represent another major advance.

Agents to prevent platelet sequestration and activation. Platelets are sequestered in the liver during cardiopulmonary bypass and those that are available after bypass may not be capable of participating in the formation of platelet plugs. Congeners of prostacycline are now being studied that may significantly reduce sequestration and activation of the platelet during cardiopulmonary bypass (13). Again, the appropriate use of such pharmacologic agents will result in the reestablishment of normal coagulation mechanisms immediately after the completion of cardiopulmonary bypass.

Percutaneous cardiopulmonary bypass. The availability of percutaneous techniques to initiate cardiopulmonary bypass will mean that such bypass will be used to advantage as a resuscitation tool, with strict guidelines regarding indications for use, and as a circulatory support tool for patients undergoing intracardiac (valvular) or coronary artery manipulation (14,15). In the emergency situation, the benefit of the prompt institution of percutaneous cardiopulmonary support will be as apparent as are the advantages of the percutaneous intraaortic balloon.

Congenital Heart Disease

Advances in membrane oxygenation, myocardial protection and ventricular assist pumps. Over the past 2 decades, the thrust toward primary definitive repair early in life has required increasing sophistication in anesthetic management, cardiopulmonary bypass and circulatory arrest techniques and postoperative intensive care. Further advances with more efficient membrane oxygenation requiring smaller priming volume are still needed and are currently in development. Myocardial protection in the neonate has been shown to be quite different from that in the mature myocardium (16). Although basically more resistant to ischemia, neonatal myocardium is not protected by multidose cardioplegia with use of St. Thomas Hospital solution as is the adult heart (17). This metabolic riddle, possibly related to calcium flux, will be resolved, providing improved myocardial protection allowing longer aortic cross-clamp times and thus more time for intracardiac repair of complex defects. The use of extracorporeal membrane oxygenation for complete cardiopulmonary support has been successful in neonates with reversible lung disease and in pediatric patients with acute cardiorespiratory failure after repair of cardiac defects (18). Ventricular assist pumps for infants and children are under development and should be ready for clinical trials within the next 2 years. This pump will be of great benefit not only in the management of postoperative low cardiac output but as a bridge to transplantation in infants requiring cardiac substitution. These ventricular assist pumps may also be of immense help in the management of postoperative right ventricular failure so common after repair of congenital cardiac lesions.

Tetralogy of Fallot repair. Although some advocate complete repair of tetralogy of Fallot in neonates (19), most recommend a modified Blalock-Taussig shunt in the first 6 months of life in view of the higher mortality for the single stage approach (20). With surgical experience, improved cardiopulmonary bypass and other support techniques, neonatal repair will become more universal.

The arterial switch operation for transposition of the great arteries in neonates. This operation has shown great promise and the operative mortality has continued to decrease (21). Shortly, the mortality rate will undoubtedly fall to the 2 to 3% level now associated with the overall less satisfactory atrial redirection operation, which in long-term follow-up has been associated with arrhythmia and right ventricular dysfunction.

Atrioventricular septal defects and pulmonary hypertension. Results of operations for complete atrioventricular septal defect have vastly improved as we have gained a better understanding of the cardiac anatomy of this complex defect (22). Further understanding of the complexities of the pathophysiology of pulmonary hypertension in these babies is, however, required to master the problems associated with repair of atrioventricular septal defects and other intracardiac lesions. Repair earlier in infancy eliminates some of the problems with long-standing pulmonary artery hypertension. In addition, improved ventilators and drugs specifically acting on the pulmonary circulation will be developed.

Tricuspid atresia and univentricular and hypoplastic heart syndrome. The dramatic results achieved with the modified Fontan procedure now allow not only excellent palliation in tricuspid atresia but many other complex lesions such as univentricle (double inlet right ventricle, double inlet left ventricle) heterotaxy syndrome and even the hypoplastic left heart syndrome (23). Further refinements in preoperative assessment, surgical techniques and support systems will enhance the results in the repair of these lesions (24–27).

The argument for cardiac transplantation in the hypoplastic left heart syndrome is a persuasive one: 19 of 22 infants have survived (28). However, the lack of donors and the high attrition rate of these infants while awaiting a suitable donor result in a final overall outcome not unlike that for the two stage Norwood procedure (29).

Coarctation of the aorta. Repair of coarctation of the aorta in the future will be done during the 1st year of life even in asymptomatic infants to avoid the serious late sequelae so common after repair in older children. The use of absorbable sutures and the subclavian flap procedure in infants provide immediate postoperative results almost comparable with those in older children (30,31). Further refinement in techniques will eliminate the small number of recurrences (3%). Repair of the associated intracardiac defects has been a major challenge but, as the repair of these defects without coarctation improves, a similar improvement will be seen when they are associated with coarctation.

Interrupted aortic arch remains a challenge. Better support techniques will make a one stage repair of the arch, as well as closure of the ventricular septal defect, the operation of choice with good immediate and long-term results (32).

Therefore, the number of congenital cardiac lesions not amenable to operative repair has rapidly declined to a point where almost all lesions can be either repaired or palliated. The future will bring greatly improved immediate and long-term results.

Cardiac Valve Prostheses

Mechanical versus biologic prosthesis. The first cardiac valve to be successfully implanted in a patient was of the ball-in-cage type (33). Valves of this type, albeit with minor but important changes, are being used today as state-of-the-art mechanical prostheses. Several types of tilting disc valves which have certain advantages over the ball-in-cage prosthesis, are also available. In some valves, inert, highly polished pyrolytic carbon has replaced inert, highly polished

metal. All mechanical valves now available have excellent durability, but the patients require continuous anticoagulant therapy with warfarin to minimize thromboembolism. The balance between bleeding and thrombus formation is a delicate one and requires periodic prothrombin time determinations for the life of the patient. The use of glutaraldehyde-fixed biologic valves brought the hope that the incidence of valve-related thromboembolism would be reduced and that, at least in certain instances, anticoagulant therapy would no longer be required. As these hopes have materialized, gradual, progressive valve degeneration has occurred (34). Deterioration results in a need to replace a bioprosthesis, frequently in elderly patients, and has led surgeons to reevaluate their use of fixed tissue valves. Accordingly the pendulum is currently swinging toward the use of mechanical prosthetic valves in most patients, even those into their 70s, a group for whom tissue valves were previously reserved.

Unfortunately, research activity to develop improved heart valves in the United States has declined to new lows because of a scarcity of really good, new ideas, the tremendous costs, the long time frame associated with obtaining Food and Drug Administration approval and concern for the potential liability associated with any maloccurrence.

Aortic valve homografts. The use of stored aortic valve homografts has offered some hope and, if reported results indicating good, long-functioning life are confirmed, many more of these valves will be used in the future in the aortic location (35). The logistics of obtaining sterile cadaver valves and the additional complexity of insertion mean that the homograft valve will not qualify as the elusive ideal valvular prosthesis.

Polyurethane trileaflet valve prosthesis. Manufactured frame-mounted trileaflet valves have many desirable features, but the material design combinations evaluated thus far have not resulted in a clinically useful prosthesis (36,37). It is hoped that a better understanding of the valve mechanics, improved design using sewing rings that become incorporated into the valve annulus and the use of thin, inert, flexible polymer leaflets will result in a manufactured valve, suitable for any location, that does not require anticoagulant therapy and has a functional lifetime measured in decades.

Coronary Artery Surgery

Internal mammary artery versus saphenous vein grafts. Few areas in contemporary medicine have been the subject of as much debate as the role of surgery in the treatment of coronary artery disease. As coronary artery surgery enters its 3rd decade, there continues to be more frequent use of both internal mammary arteries, thereby reducing the need to use the saphenous vein for coronary artery grafting (38,39). The superior long-term patency of the internal mammary artery when compared with saphenous vein graft will provide improved survival, reduced cardiac-related morbidity and a decreased need for reoperation (40–42).

Changing characteristics of surgical candidates. Unfortunately, operative mortality and morbidity rates for coronary artery bypass grafting are likely to increase. This increase is and will be related to major changes in the baseline characteristics of patients undergoing the operation. Clearly, the surgical population will continue to consist of a subset with a high incidence of advanced age, severe coronary artery disease, left ventricular dysfunction and multiple concomitant medical problems (43). Additionally, urgent procedures will probably continue to increase in frequency, in many cases after other therapeutic interventions, such as thrombolysis and percutaneous transluminal angioplasty have been performed (44–47). In contrast, exciting new developments in myocardial protection and salvage and the use of devices designed for intra-arterial application will help the surgeon improve the aspects of coronary artery surgery not related to the surgeon's patient selection. This future use of improved myocardial protection and high technology, including lasers and angioscopes, may allow the surgeon to deal more effectively with severe, diffuse coronary artery disease and with patients who have impaired ventricular function.

Coronary angioscopy. Direct visual examination of the interior surface of intact human coronary arteries is now a reality (48,49). Certainly, it will prove to be a valuable research application in characterizing the atherosclerotic process. However, the most important future surgical application lies in its potential use as an adjunct to intraoperative angioplasty, thus allowing more suitable revascularization in patients with diffuse coronary artery disease. Additionally, technical anastomotic misadventures may be visualized and corrected, leading to improved graft patency (50).

Laser ablation of atherosclerotic plaques. Manual coronary endarterectomy to deal with diffuse coronary artery disease has not gained widespread acceptance in the United States because its safety and durability have been questioned (51). The laser can vaporize calcific plaques in a partially or totally obstructed artery making it a potentially useful tool to treat totally occluded as well as diffusely narrowed vessels (52). Apparently, laser surgery of normal and atherosclerotic arteries results in a scar that heals quickly with a new endothelial covering (53). For laser systems to become useful for ablation of atherosclerotic plaque, they must have little effect on normal tissue to minimize risk of perforation. At present "hot tip" (argon or YAG), excimer or "cold" and carbon dioxide lasers are under investigation. With each, the investigator must find the proper power and time of exposure to allow selective ablation without perforation or damage to normal structures. Advances and development of exogenous chromophores to detect fluorescent plaque will enable the laser system to spectroscopically recognize and distinguish atheroma and normal arterial wall and may assist in preventing perforation or vessel damage (54,55).

In the operating room, open laser endarterectomy may provide precise control over the plane of dissection. Heat sealing the surface and end points of dissection may be a potential improvement over the conventional manual surgical techniques (56). Eventually, these techniques may be possible percutaneously. Laser welding of small vessel anastomoses in which low-laser energy is applied to opposed vessel edges may prove quicker and superior to conventional suturing techniques (57). These anastomoses show no suture foreign body reaction, and neointimal hyperplasia may be reduced (58). These characteristics may enhance the patency of these small vessel anastomoses.

Myocardial Protection and Salvage

Newer techniques to preserve myocardial structure and prevent ischemic damage. The quest for the optimal alchemy of cardioplegic solutions will continue. As the mechanism of reperfusion injury is unlocked, appropriate pharmacologic additives will scavenge or inhibit production of oxygen free radicals, block intracellular calcium influx, favorably change the balance between prostacylin and thromboxane and inhibit lipolysis to afford additional myocardial protection and limit ischemic damage (59). Other changes in the composition of the reperfusate in an effort to provide substrate for adenosine triphosphate (ATP) production may prove pivotal in preserving myocardial structure and function after periods of ischemia (60). Further insights into the conditions of reperfusion are certain to evolve as laboratory findings, indicating the critical importance of decompressing the left ventricle and gentle reperfusion, are applied in clinical trials and compared with current techniques of thrombolytic therapy with or without angioplasty in the acute setting of ischemia (61,62).

Retrograde coronary sinus infusion. Obviously, myocardial protection cannot be separated from its methodology. The role of retrograde infusion of cardioplegia through the coronary sinus as well as other coronary sinus interventions will unravel (63,64). This complex area of myocardial protection will continue to be an area of fruitful investigation, and certainly methodology first applied in the operating room will be found useful in the percutaneous route to assist the invasive cardiologist in certain acute ischemic settings.

Arrhythmia Surgery

Cardiac pacemakers. More than 50 years ago, an artificial external pacemaker and bipolar leads were designed and used successfully in patients. From these crude beginnings, change in the field of cardiac stimulation has been so rapid that the future becomes the past. Soon, most pacemakers will be dual chamber devices as small as, if not smaller than, present day single chamber units and will have similar longevity and programmable features. A single implantable unit will have a multiplicity of antitachycardia modes and even permit automatic defibrillation. It is conceivable that units designed for defibrillation will no longer require thoracotomy for defibrillator lead placement (65). Physiologic sensors will be developed to permit autoregulation of the pacemaker to maintain optimal hemodynamics. Transtelephonic monitoring systems will be developed to fully interrogate and even reprogram devices. These pacemakers will be capable of data acquisition and storage and allow serial electrophysiologic testing to assess a given therapeutic regimen (66). The technologic advances in this area appear limited only by our investigative and capital resources.

Direct arrhythmia surgery. Such surgery is now entering its 3rd decade and is well established for certain patients with refractory supraventricular and ventricular arrhythmias. Surgical division of accessory pathways in the Wolff-Parkinson-White syndrome is associated with minimal risk and excellent results (67). Clinical trials in the future will define the superiority or equality of endocardial versus epicardial closed heart approaches.

Supraventricular tachyarrhythmias. Although atrioventricular (AV) node reentrant tachycardia has been approached in a variety of ways, most entailed His bundle ablation coupled with permanent pacer implantation. Recent experience (68) indicates that this syndrome may be effectively treated by discrete cryosurgical lesions placed about the borders of the AV node. Future clinical experience may allow a closed heart technique and ultimately even a percutaneous technique. Although computerized mapping techniques are not necessary to obtain optimal results in the previously discussed conditions, mapping originally developed for use in ventricular tachycardia surgery may allow detailed electrophysiologic study of the atrium during automatic atrial tachycardias as well as atrial fibrillation and flutter. If the arrhythmia can be mapped, then a surgical technique to ablate it can be developed. Already, left and right atrial isolation procedures as well as local procedures for refractory atrial tachycardias have been employed successfully (69–71). Certainly, with future understanding and technical developments, wider applications will result. We have previously ignored the potential role of surgery in the most common of supraventricular tachyarrhythmias, atrial fibrillation. This rhythm, which causes 10% of all strokes (~50,000/year) will certainly come under surgical scrutiny (72). Surgical techniques will develop to nullify both the embolic potential and the hemodynamic consequences of atrial fibrillation by preserving a normal sinus mechanism.

Ventricular tachyarrhythmias. Direct surgical techniques for the therapy of medically refractory ischemic ventricular tachycardia have been in clinical use for a decade. However, this cumulative experience would indicate high operative mortalities as well as high postoperative rates of reinducibility (73–79). These experiences would suggest that properly performed procedures to exercise or exclude a focus guided by proper intraoperative mapping reduces a postoperative reinducibility (80,81). With the future development of intraoperative mapping systems that can simultaneously record endocardial data from multiple sites without opening the ventricle, many of the current difficulties will be overcome and results will surely improve (82,83). Great advances in computer technology will allow the manufacture and widespread availability of such a system at reasonable cost. Nonetheless, patient selection will need to improve to exclude those patients with concomitant disease or poor left ventricular function. With the expected improvement in automatic internal cardiodefibrillators (AICD), ventricular tachycardia surgery will be performed in appropriately selected patients, achieving cure, and AICDs will be implanted for palliation in the others. The role of additional protection of concomitant AICD implantation after directed surgery will surely be defined more clearly (84). Additional advances in the conduct of these direct surgical therapies will combine excision with laser or cryoablative techniques, or both (85,86).

Transplantation

Donor heart availability and preservation. Cardiac transplantation will continue to be an important therapeutic modality for patients with end-stage heart disease. Because the profession and the lay public will be better informed regarding the usefulness of donor organs, fewer potential donor organs will be wasted. However, enforced occupational and vehicular safety rules will further limit the number of trauma deaths and thus the availability of donor organs. The need for donor organs will exceed the availability by a factor of 10. Because permanent support devices and artificial hearts will be shelf items, triage will occur with the younger, better risk patients having the transplant and the older patient having the mechanical device.

Techniques for long-term (i.e., >24 h) preservation of the heart will allow the transplant to be performed in a more efficient manner and will allow country-wide and even worldwide organ sharing (87). These techniques will also be helpful in increasing the number of available donor organs. The idea of using animal hearts to replace the deceased human heart is not new; major advances in immunology will be required and would have major implications throughout the field of transplantation.

Lung transplantation. Unilateral and bilateral lung transplantation will be useful therapeutic techniques because of a better understanding of anastomotic techniques and the

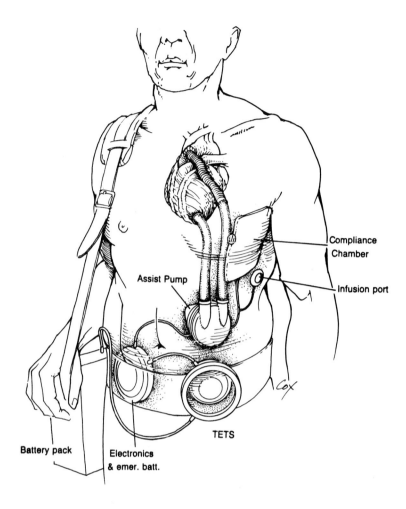

Figure 20.1. Proposed placement of the permanent left ventricular assist pump. The pump is positioned in the preperitoneal space in the abdomen, fills from the left ventricular apex and ejects into the ascending aorta. The energy is provided by a battery pack and is transmitted through the skin by a transcutaneous energy transmission system (TETS). The electronic control system, emergency battery (emer. batt.) pack and air system (infusion port and compliance chamber) are necessary components.

availability of improved immunosuppressive therapy (88). Improved preservation techniques will allow distant organ procurement and organ storage and, accordingly, will in-

crease the availability of lungs suitable for transplantation. The use of combined heart-lung transplantation will seldom be required.

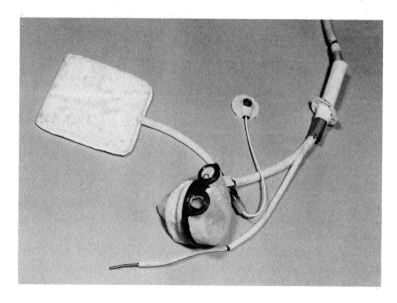

Figure 20.2. Prototype of the permanent left ventricular assist system that is being developed at The Pennsylvania State University. The miniature blood pump with Björk-Shiley valves is seen in the center of the photograph. Currently, this pump is energized by wires crossing the chest wall (**right**). Other components include an infusion port (**top, center**), a compliance chamber (**left**) and a thermistor probe (**lower left**). Left ventricular assist pumps have been used in animal studies for >6 month periods.

Mechanical Circulatory Support and the Artificial Heart

The end result of a variety of forms of heart disease is irreversible left ventricle muscle damage. No currently known technique can restore contractile force. Cardiac transplantation offers the only available hope but is not readily available; it is costly and the long-term results are a compromise. The use of skeletal muscle to replace areas of cardiac muscle or support devices or the use of blood pumps powered by such muscle or by conventional power provides potential alternatives.

Skeletal muscle cardiomyoplasty. After the development of techniques to make skeletal muscle fatigue resistant, many investigations have begun to develop and evaluate techniques to wrap or incorporate skeletal muscle strips into the damaged left ventricle (90). Alternatively, some type of counterpulsation apparatus or blood pump can be powered by such a preconditioned muscle (91,92). The use of skeletal muscle to provide augmentation of the cardiac muscle has a definite advantage over the mechanical cardiac assist devices currently under development in that no external power source is required, although the energy available through muscle contraction is limited. Therefore, major circulatory support by such a biologic system seems unlikely. Accordingly, patients who require a 15% to 20% augmentation in cardiac output may benefit from some variant of cardiomyoplasty, whereas patients who require a greater degree of support or who require exercise ability will be candidates for transplantation or an implanted blood pump.

Ventricular assist devices. Within the next several years, implantable left ventricular assist pumps for permanent circulatory support will undergo clinical trials (Fig. 20.1) (93,94). These blood pumps will be used in patients who are not eligible for cardiac transplantation by virtue of age, contraindication to transplantation (insulin-dependent diabetes, for example) or lack of availability of a donor heart at the time of need. Permanent left ventricular assist pump system features include an implantable, valved, pulsatile pump and a miniature, electrically powered prime mover in the form of a rotary solenoid or brushless direct current motor (Fig. 20.2). The electrical energy required (12 to 18 W) will be provided by conventional house supply or by a rechargeable battery pack that can be carried and will be transmitted across the chest wall by inductive coupling (transformer principle) techniques, obviating the need for a wire or tube to cross the chest wall and reducing the risk of infection associated with percutaneous access sites. Patients with these blood pumps will require anticoagulant therapy and will have the added inconvenience of the external electrical source.

The original design features for an implantable ventricular assist pump incorporated an implantable thermal energy source (plutonium-238) and a compact external combustion (Stirling cycle) engine (95). However, the high cost of the

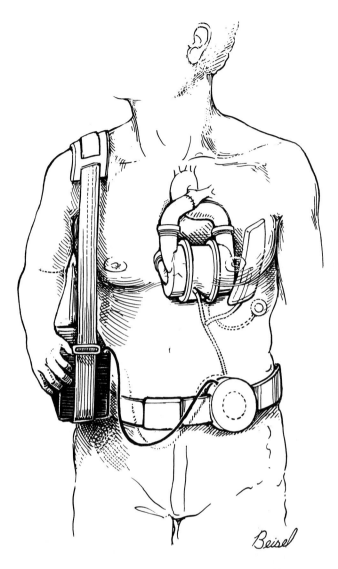

Figure 20.3. Proposed placement of an electric artificial heart within the thorax. To obviate the problems of percutaneous tubes, the design will employ a transcutaneous energy transmission system with the primary coil positioned with use of a belt. The patient will carry a case containing chargeable batteries.

Organ selection. Immunosuppressive drug programs will be organ selective, donor antigen specific, and, accordingly, will minimize systemic side effects such as Cushing's syndrome and bulemia. The need for donor organ biopsy to define rejection and to monitor immunotherapy limits the organ recipient to living near medical centers and adds to the medical costs. Better techniques will be identified that will decrease or eliminate the need for organ biopsy and permit patient follow-up without necessitating hospitalization. Current candidate studies include echocardiography, nuclear magnetic resonance spectroscopy, detection of characteristics of circulating white cells or detection of changes in antibody levels in peripheral blood (89). Clearly, this is a current topic of great interest and importance.

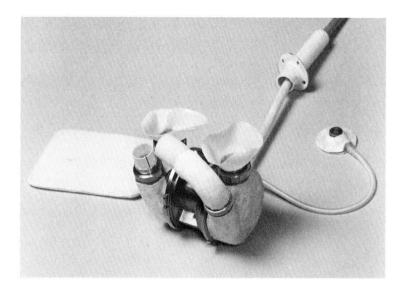

Figure 20.4. Prototype of the electric artificial heart. The two valved ventricles are positioned at the end of the electric motor-motion translator unit. Also shown is the percutaneous wire and the air system (compliance chamber and air port). A heart of this type has been used for >7 months in an experimental animal.

plutonium and the risks associated with the radionuclide (two major nuclear reactor accidents have occurred in the 1980s) have led to a virtual standstill in this design. Alternatively, the major advances in permanent magnets and in the availability of microprocessors have made the completely electrical system even more practical.

Implantable artificial heart. An implantable artificial heart will be available for patients with biventricular failure in whom a transplant cannot be performed and in those in whom univentricular support is inappropriate (Fig. 20.3). The artificial heart that will be available at the turn of the century will have a distinct advantage over the pneumatic devices used for Dr. Barney Clark (96). The electrical devices under development obviate the need for percutaneous pneumatic power lines and, in place of the bulky pneumatic power unit, have a highly portable battery pack (Fig. 20.4) (97,98). Again the electrical energy will be transmitted across the skin with use of wireless techniques. At present, prototype systems are designed, suitable control techniques are available and animal implant studies are in progress. One animal has been supported for 7 months with an artificial heart of this type (although hard wire electrical transmission was used) (99).

Although these implanted pumps will be designated as permanent devices, they will have a definite functional life, analogous to that of a pacemaker. The first implantable pumps will have a proved functional life from 1 to 2 years. Periodic noninvasive parameter checks will indicate impending device failure (increased power consumption, abnormal noise, for example) and the need for device replacement. Premature failure may also occur. In the patient with the implanted assist device, such a failure will not be catastrophic because the patient's own heart will be capable of some degree of circulatory support. Although safety circuits will be included in the implantable artificial hearts, complete backup systems will not be available because of the limited

space within the chest. However, because the artificial heart will come to clinical use after the assist device, many of the premature failure modes will have been studied and eliminated.

References

1. Creech O Jr, Deterling RA Jr, Edwards S, Julian O, Linton R, Shumacker H. Report of committee for study of vascular prostheses of the Society for Vascular Surgery. Surgery 1957;41:62–80.
2. Campbell CD, Brooks DH, Webster MW, Bahnson HT. The use of expanded microporous polytetrafluoroethylene for limb salvage: a preliminary report. Surgery 1976;79:485–93.
3. Lyman DJ, Albo D Jr, Jackson R, Knutson K. Development of small diameter vascular prostheses. Trans Am Soc Artif Intern Organs 1977;13:253–61.
4. Sparks CH. Development of a successful silicone rubber arterial graft. Ann Thorac Surg 1966;2:585.
5. Steichen FM, Ravitch MM. History of mechanical devices and instruments for suturing. Curr Probl Surg 1982;19:1–52.
6. Ablaza SGG, Ghosh SC, Grana VP. Use of a ringed intraluminal graft in the surgical treatment of dissecting aneurysms of the thoracic aorta. J Thorac Cardiovasc Surg 1978;76:390–6.
7. Cooper CN, Falb RD. Surgical adhesives. Ann NY Acad Sci 1968;146:214–24.
8. White RA, Kopchok G, Donayre C, et al. Argon laser-welded arteriovenous anastomoses. J Vasc Surg 1987;6:447–53.
9. Sugita Y, Shimomitsu T, Oku T, et al. Nonsurgical implantation of a vascular ring prosthesis using thermal shape-memory Ti/Ni alloy (Nitinol wire). Trans Am Soc Artif Intern Organs 1986;32:30–4.
10. Henny CP, Cate HT, Cate JWT, et al. A randomized blind study comparing standard heparin and a new low molecular weight heparinoid in cardiopulmonary bypass surgery in dogs. J Lab Clin Med 1985;106:187–95.
11. Horrow JC. Protamine: a review of its toxicity. Anesth Analg 1985;64:348–61.
12. Olivier HF Jr, Maher TD, Liebler GA, Park SB, Burkholder JA, Magovern GJ. Use of the Biomedicus centrifugal pump in traumatic tears of the thoracic aorta. Ann Thorac Surg 1984;38:586–91.
13. Addonizio VP Jr, Fisher CA, Jenkin BK, Strauss JF III, Musial JF, Edmunds LH Jr. Iloprost (ZK36374), a stable analogue of prostacyclin, preserves platelets during simulated extracorporeal circulation. J Thorac Cardiovasc Surg 1985;89:926–33.

14. Reichman RT, Joyo CI, Dembitsky WP, Griffith LD, Adamson RM, Daily PO. Improved patient survival after cardiac arrest using a cardiopulmonary support system. Soc Thor Surg Abstract Book, 24th Annual Meeting, 1988:93.

15. Riley JB, Litzie AK, Overlie PA, et al. Supported angioplasty: a new contribution for extra-corporeal circulation technology. J Extra-Corp Techn 1988;20:134–7.

16. Magovern JA, Pae WE, Miller CA, Waldhausen JA. The immature and the mature myocardium. J Thorac Cardiovasc Surg 1988;95:618–24.

17. Magovern JA, Pae WE, Waldhausen JA. Protection of the immature myocardium. J Thorac Cardiovasc Surg 1988;96:408–13.

18. Toomasian JM, Sandy M, Cornell RG, Cilley RE, Bartlett RH. National experience with extracorporeal membrane oxygenation for newborn respiratory failure. Trans Am Soc Artif Intern Organs 1988;32:140–7.

19. Castaneda AR, Freed MD, Williams RG, Norwood WI. Repair of tetralogy of Fallot in infancy. J Thorac Cardiovasc Surg 1977;74:372–81.

20. Arciniegas E, Blackstone EH, Pacifico AD, Kirklin JW. Classic shunting operations as part of two-stage repair for tetralogy of Fallot. Ann Thorac Surg 1979;27:514–8.

21. Norwood WI, Dobell AR, Freed MD, Kirklin JW, Blackstone EH. Intermediate results of the arterial switch repair. J Thorac Cardiovasc Surg 1988;96:854–63.

22. Chin AJ, Keane JF, Norwood WI, Castaneda AR. Repair of complete common atrioventricular canal in infancy. J Thorac Cardiovasc Surg 1982;84:437–45.

23. Humes RA, Porter CJ, Mair DD, et al. Intermediate follow-up and predicted survival after the modified Fontan procedure for tricuspid atresia and double-inlet ventricle. Circulation 1987;76(suppl III):III-67–71.

24. Kirklin JK, Blackstone EH, Kirklin JW, Pacifico AD, Bargeron LM. The Fontan operation. J Thorac Cardiovasc Surg 1986;92:1049–64.

25. deLeval MR, Kilner P, Gewillig M, Bull C. Total cavopulmonary connection: a logical alternative to atriopulmonary connection for complex Fontan operations. J Thorac Cardiovasc Surg 1988;96:682–95.

26. Mayer JE, Helgason H, Jonas RA, et al. Extending the limits for modified Fontan procedures. J Thorac Cardiovasc Surg 1986;92:1021–8.

27. Pasque MK. Fontan hemodynamics. J Cardiac Surg 1988;3:45–52.

28. Bailey LL, Nehlsen-Cannarella SL, Doroshow RW. Cardiac allotransplantation in newborns as therapy for hypoplastic left heart syndrome. N Engl J Med 1986;315:949–51.

29. Pigott JD, Murphy JD, Barber G, Norwood WI. Palliative reconstructive surgery for hypoplastic left heart syndrome. Ann Thorac Surg 1988;45:122–8.

30. Myers JL, Waldhausen JA. Subclavian flap angioplasty: the optimal repair for coarctation of the aorta in infants. In: Proceedings of the First World Congress of Pediatric Cardiac Surgery. Futura Publishers (in press).

31. Myers JL, Campbell DB, Waldhausen JA. The use of absorbable monofilament polydioxanone suture in pediatric cardiovascular operations. J Thorac Cardiovasc Surg 1986;92:771–5.

32. Sell JE, Jonas RA, Mayer JE, Blackstone EH, Kirklin JW, Castaneda AR. The results of a surgical program for interrupted aortic arch. J Thorac Cardiovasc Surg 1988;96:864–77.

33. Starr A, Edwards ML. Mitral replacement: clinical experience with a ball valve prosthesis. Ann Thorac Surg 1961;154:726.

34. Barnhart GR, Jones M, Ishihara T, Chavez AM, Rose DM, Ferrans VJ. Bioprosthetic valve failure: clinical and pathological observations in an experimental animal model. J Thorac Cardiovasc Surg 1982;83:618–31.

35. Matsuki O, Robles A, Gibbs S, et al. Long-term performance of 555 aortic homografts in the aortic position. Ann Thorac Surg 1988;46:187–91.

36. Wisman CB, Pierce WS, Donachy JH, Pae WE, Myers JL, Prophet GA. A polyurethane trileaflet cardiac valve prosthesis: in vivo and in vitro studies. Trans Am Soc Artif Intern Organs 1982;28:164–8.

37. Hilbert SL, Ferrans VJ, Tomita Y, Eidbo EE, Jones M. Evaluation of explanted polyurethane trileaflet cardiac valve prostheses. J Thorac Cardiovasc Surg 1987;94:419–29.

38. Sauvage LR, Hong-DE W, Kowalsky TE, et al. Healing basis and surgical techniques for complete revascularization of the left ventricle using only the internal mammary arteries. Ann Thorac Surg 1986;42:449–65.

39. Russo P, Orszulak TA, Schaff H, Holmes DR. Use of internal mammary artery grafts for multiple coronary bypasses. Circulation 1986;74(suppl III):III-48–52.

40. Loop FD, Lytle BW, Cosgrove DM, et al. Influence of the internal mammary artery graft on 10-year survival and other cardiac events. N Engl J Med 1986;314:1–6.

41. Cameron A, Kemp HG, Green GE. Bypass surgery with the internal mammary graft: 15 year follow-up. Circulation 1986;74(suppl III):III-30–6.

42. Cameron A, Davis KB, Green GE, Myers WO, Pettinger M. Clinical implications of internal mammary bypass grafts: the Coronary Artery Surgery Study experience. Circulation 1988;77:815–9.

43. Naunheim KS, Fiore AC, Wadley JJ, et al. The changing profile of the patient undergoing coronary artery bypass surgery. J Am Coll Cardiol 1988;11:494–8.

44. Davis PK, Parascandola SA, Miller CA, et al. Mortality of coronary artery bypass grafting before and after the advent of angioplasty. Ann Thorac Surg 1989;47:493–8.

45. Naunheim KS, Fiore AC, Walden JJ, et al. The changing mortality of myocardial revascularization of coronary artery bypass and angioplasty. Ann Thorac Surg 1988;46:666–74.

46. Petrovich JA, Wellons HA, Schneider JA, Kauten JR, Mikell FL, Taylor GL. Revascularization after thrombolytic therapy for acute myocardial infarction: an analysis of 573 patients. Ann Thorac Surg 1988;46:163–6.

47. Lee FK, Mandell J, Rankin JS, Muhlbaier LH, Wechsler AS. Immediate versus delayed coronary grafting after streptokinase treatment: postoperative blood loss and clinical results. J Thorac Cardiovasc Surg 1988;95:216–22.

48. Grundfest WS, Litvack F, Sherman T, et al. Delineation of peripheral and coronary detail by intraoperative angioscopy. Ann Surg 1985;202:394–400.

49. Crew J. Intraoperative coronary angioscopy: clinical application. In: White GH, White RA, eds. Angioscopy: Vascular and Coronary Applications. Boca Raton, FL: Year Book Medical Publishers, 1989:157–60.

50. Sanborn TA, Rygaard JA, Westbrook BM, Lazar HL, McCormick JR, Roberts AJ. Intraoperative angioscopy of saphenous vein and coronary arteries. J Thorac Cardiovasc Surg 1986;91:339–43.

51. Kay PH, Brooks N, Magee P, Sturidge MF, Walesby RK, Wright JEC. Bypass grafting to the right coronary artery with and without endarterectomy: patency at one year. Br Heart J 1985;54:489–94.

52. Abela GS, Vincent MG. Cardiovascular applications of lasers. In: Dixon JA, ed. Surgical Application of Lasers. Boca Raton, FL: Year Book Medical Publishers, 1987:255–74.

53. Abela GS, Crea F, Seeger JE, et al. The healing process in normal canine arteries and in atherosclerotic monkey arteries after transluminal laser irradiation. Am J Cardiol 1985;56:983–8.

54. Geschwind HJ, Dubois-Rande JL, Bonner FR, Boussignac G, Prevosti LG, Leon MB. Percutaneous pulsed laser angioplasty with atheroma detection in humans (abstr). J Am Coll Cardiol 1988;11:107A.

55. Leon MB, Almagor Y, Baztarelli AL, et al. Fluorescence-guided laser angioplasty in patients with femoropopliteal occlusions (abstr). Circulation 1988;78(suppl II):II-1173.

56. Eugene J, McColgan SJ, Hammer-Wilson M, et al. Laser endarterectomy. Lasers Surg Med 1985;5:265–74.

57. White RA, White GH. The current and future use of lasers in vascular surgery. Perspect Vasc Surg 1988;1:1–20.

58. Frazier OH, Painvin GA, Morris JR, Thomsen S, Neblett CR. Laser-associated microvascular anastomosis: angiographic and anatomopathologic studies on growing microvascular anastomosis: preliminary report. Surgery 1985;97:585–90.

59. Kouchoukos NT. Cardiac Surgery. ACS Bulletin 1987;72:9–12.

60. Buckberg GD. Studies of controlled reperfusion after ischemia. I. When is cardiac muscle damaged irreversibly? J Thorac Cardiovasc Surg 1986;92(suppl):483–7.

61. Allen BS, Okamoto F, Buckberg GD, Bugyi H, Leaf J. Studies of controlled reperfusion after ischemia. XIII. Reperfusion conditions: critical importance of total ventricular decompression during regional reperfusion. J Thorac Cardiovasc Surg 1986;92(suppl):605–12.

62. Okamoto F, Allen BS, Buckberg GD, Bugyi B, Leaf JL. Studies of controlled reperfusion after ischemia. XIV. Reperfusion conditions: im-

portance of ensuring gentle versus sudden reperfusion during relief of coronary occlusion. J Thorac Cardiovasc Surg 1986;92(suppl):613–20.

63. Gundry SR, Kirsch MM. A comparison of retrograde versus antegrade cardioplegia in the presence of coronary artery obstruction. Ann Thorac Surg 1984;38:124–7.

64. Mohl W, Roberts AJ. Coronary sinus retroperfusion and pressure-controlled intermittent coronary sinus occlusion (PISCO) for myocardial protection. Surg Clin North Am 1985;65:477–95.

65. Bardy GH, Allen MD, Mehra R, Johnson G, Green HL, Ivey TD. A flexible and effective 3 electrode non-thoracotomy defibrillation system in man (abstr). J Am Coll Cardiol 1989;13:65A.

66. Levine PA. Cardiac pacing: past, present, and future. In: Roberts AL, Conti CR, eds. Current Surgery of the Heart. Philadelphia: JB Lippincott, 1987:257–74.

67. Cox JL, Gallagher JJ, Cain ME. Experience with 118 consecutive patients undergoing surgery for the Wolff-Parkinson-White syndrome. J Thorac Cardiovasc Surg 1985;90:490–501.

68. Cox JL, Holman WL, Cain ME. Cryosurgical treatment of atrioventricular node reentry tachycardia. Circulation 1987;76:1329–36.

69. Williams JM, Ungerleider RM, Lofland GK, Cox JL. Left atrial isolation: new technique for the treatment of supraventricular arrhythmias. J Thorac Cardiovasc Surg 1980;80:373–80.

70. Seals AA, Lawrie GM, Magro S, et al. Surgical treatment of right atrial focal tachycardia in adults. J Am Coll Cardiol 1988;11:1111–7.

71. Harada A, D'Agostino HJ, Schuessler RB, Boineau JP, Cox JL. Right atrial isolation: a new surgical treatment for supraventricular tachycardia. I. Surgical technique and electrophysiologic effects. J Thorac Cardiovasc Surg 1988;95:643–50.

72. Fisher CM. Embolism in atrial fibrillation. In: Kulbertus HE, Olsson SB, Schlepper M, eds. Atrial Fibrillation. Molndel, Sweden: AB Hassle Publishing, 1982:192–207.

73. Moran JM, Kehoe RF, Loeb JM, Lichtenthal PR, Sanders JH Jr, Michaelis LL. Extended endocardial resection for the treatment of ventricular tachycardia and ventricular fibrillation. Ann Thorac Surg 1982;34:538–52.

74. Ostermeyer J, Borggrefe M, Breithardt G, et al. Direct operations for the management of life-threatening ischemic ventricular tachycardia. J Thorac Cardiovasc Surg 1987;94:848–65.

75. Bolooki H, Palatianos GM, Zaman L, Thurer RJ, Luceri RM, Myerburg RJ. Surgical management of post-myocardial infarction ventricular tachyarrhythmia by myocardial debulking, septal isolation, and myocardial revascularization. J Thorac Cardiovasc Surg 1986;92:716–25.

76. Ivey TD, Brady GH, Misbach GA, Greene HL. Surgical management of refractory ventricular arrhythmias in patients with prior inferior myocardial infarction. J Thorac Cardiovasc Surg 1985;89:369–77.

77. Brodman R, Fisher JD, Johnston DR, et al. Results of electrophysiologically guided operations for drug-resistant recurrent ventricular tachycardia and ventricular fibrillation due to coronary artery disease. J Thorac Cardiovasc Surg 1984;87:431–8.

78. Kron IL, Lerman BB, Nolan SP, Flanagan TL, Haies DE, DiMarco JP. Sequential endocardial resection for the surgical treatment of refractory ventricular tachycardia. J Thorac Cardiovasc Surg 1987;94:843–7.

79. Yee ES, Scheinman MM, Griffin JC, Ebert PA. Surgical options for treating ventricular tachyarrhythmia and sudden death. J Thorac Cardiovasc Surg 1987;94:866–73.

80. Krafchek J, Lawrei GM, Roberts R, Magro SA, Wyndham CR. Surgical ablation of ventricular tachycardia: improved results with a map-directed regional approach. Circulation 1986;73:1239–47.

81. Svenson RH, Gallagher JJ, Selle JG, Zimmern SH, Fedor JM, Robicsek R. Neodymium: YAG laser photocoagulation: a successful new map-guided technique for the intraoperative ablation of ventricular tachycardia. Circulation 1987;76:1319–28.

82. Mickleborough LL, Harris L, Downar E, Parson I, Gay G. A new intraoperative approach for endocardial mapping of ventricular tachycardia. J Thorac Cardiovasc Surg 1988;95:271–80.

83. Ideker RE, Smith WM, Wallace AG, et al. A computerized method for the rapid display of ventricular activation during the intraoperative study of arrhythmias. Circulation 1979;59:449–58.

84. Platia EV, Griffith LSC, Watkins L, et al. Treatment of malignant ventricular arrhythmias with endocardial resection and implantation of the automatic cardioverter-defibrillator. N Engl J Med 1986;314:213–6.

85. Selle JG, Svenson RH, Sealy WC, et al. Successful clinical laser ablation of ventricular tachycardia: a promising new therapeutic method. Ann Thorac Surg 1986;42:380–4.

86. Holman WL, Ikeshita M, Douglas JM, Smith PK, Lofland GK, Cox JL. Ventricular cryosurgery: short-term effects on intramural electrophysiology. Ann Thorac Surg 1983;35:386–93.

87. Solis E, Tyce GM, Bianco R, Mahoney J, Kaye MP. High energy phosphates and catecholamine stores after prolonged ex vivo heart preservation. J Heart Transplant 1986;5:444–9.

88. Patterson GA, Cooper JD, Goldman B, et al. Technique of successful clinical double-lung transplantation. Ann Thorac Surg 1988;45:626–33.

89. Hall TS, Baumgartner WA, Borkon AM, et al. Diagnosis of acute cardiac rejection with antimyosin monoclonal antibody, phosphorous nuclear magnetic resonance imaging, two-dimensional echocardiography, and endocardial biopsy. J Heart Transplant 1986;5:419–24.

90. Magovern GJ, Heckler FR, Park SB, et al. Paced skeletal muscle for dynamic cardiomyoplasty. Ann Thorac Surg 1988;45:614–9.

91. Kochamba G, Desrosiers C, Dewar M, et al. The muscle-powered dual-chamber counterpulsator: rheologically superior implantable cardiac assist device. Ann Thorac Surg 1988;45:620–5.

92. Acker MA, Anderson WA, Hammond RL, et al. Skeletal muscle ventricles in circulation. J Thorac Cardiovasc Surg 1987;94:163–74.

93. Jassawalla JS, Daniel MA, Chen H, et al. In vitro and in vivo testing of a totally implantable left ventricular assist system. Trans Am Soc Artif Intern Organs 1988;34:470–5.

94. Richenbacher WE, Pae WE Jr, Magovern JA, Rosenberg G, Snyder AJ, Pierce WS. Roller screw electric motor ventricular assist device. Trans Am Soc Artif Intern Organs 1986;32:46–8.

95. Pierce WS, Myers JL, Donachy JH, et al. Approaches to the artificial heart. Surgery 1981;90:137–48.

96. DeVries WC. The permanent artificial heart: four case reports. JAMA 1988;259:849–59.

97. Pierce WS. The artificial heart—1986: partial fulfillment of a promise. Trans Am Soc Artif Intern Organs 1986;32:5–73.

98. Jarvik RK, Smith LM, Lawson JH, et al. Comparison of pneumatic and electrically powered total artificial hearts in vivo. Trans Am Soc Artif Intern Organs 1978;24:581–4.

99. Rosenberg G, Snyder AJ, Landis DL, Geselowitz DB, Doanchy JH, Pierce WS. An electric motor-driven total artificial heart: seven months' survival in the calf. Trans Am Soc Artif Intern Organs 1984;30:69–73.

CHAPTER 21

Ventricular Arrhythmias: Why Is It So Difficult to Find a Pharmacologic Cure?

BORYS SURAWICZ, MD

Ventricular arrhythmias encompass a wide spectrum of rhythm disturbances, ranging from occasional premature ventricular complexes to ventricular fibrillation. The abnormal site of origin and the abnormal impulse propagation result in characteristic and readily recognizable electrocardiographic (ECG) patterns of ectopic ventricular activity. On those rare occasions when the surface ECG fails to resolve the differential diagnosis of ventricular ectopic activity from supraventricular rhythms conducted with aberration or from ventricular pre-excitation, intracardiac recording may be needed to make the correct diagnosis.

The relative facility of establishing the diagnosis contrasts with the difficult dilemmas in the prevention and treatment of ventricular arrhythmias. A consensus on therapeutic guidelines exists only at the two extremes of the arrhythmia spectrum (that is, the most harmless and the most dangerous types). In the first case, there is probably agreement that antiarrhythmic drugs need not be used in asymptomatic subjects with infrequent premature ventricular complexes in the absence of heart disease. Similarly, agreement prevails that life-threatening ventricular tachyarrhythmias causing hemodynamic compromise must be emergently terminated. However, there are no uniformly accepted guidelines for handling problems such as treatment of nonlife-threatening symptoms, treatment of "complex" but asymptomatic arrhythmias and prevention of serious life-threatening arrhythmias.

This absence of uniform policies in the management of most patients with ventricular arrhythmias can be traced to two fundamental problems: uncertainty of therapeutic goals and deficiencies in the available therapeutic armamentarium. The purpose of this review is to examine the relation between therapeutic goals and the available means of therapy within the framework of accumulated knowledge about the epidemiology, mechanisms and treatment of ventricular arrhythmias.

Defining the Goals

Prevalence

Role of aging. Ventricular premature complexes seldom occur in healthy children, but from adolescence on, they begin to increase in frequency with advancing age (1). In 23 to 27 year old medical students, ambulatory monitoring revealed at least one premature ventricular complex in 50% of the subjects (2). From their survey of the literature, Sherman et al. (3) concluded that the increase in ventricular arrhythmias in males from 16 to 74 years of age was exponential. In keeping with this, the incidence of ventricular arrhythmias was 62% in men whose average age was 55 years (4) and 69% to 100% in seven studies (5–11) encompassing 609 healthy individuals aged ≥60 years.

The "complexity" of ventricular arrhythmias also increases with age. For instance, in one representative study from this country (8), 57% of 147 healthy and active persons >65 years of age had >1,000 premature ventricular complexes/24 h, multiform premature ventricular complexes or ventricular tachycardia. In another study (6) of 98 asymptomatic subjects aged 60 to 85 years, 36% had >30 premature ventricular complexes/h, 35% had multiform premature ventricular complexes, 11% had couplets and 4% had ventricular tachycardia. Similar findings were reported in healthy old persons in England (5), France (7) and Germany (11). Nonsustained ventricular tachycardia, which is rarely present in healthy young adults, was recorded in 2.0% to 9.7% (average 5%) of healthy and active old persons enrolled in six studies (5–9,11) encompassing 603 subjects. Nonsustained ventricular tachycardia was present in 3 of 10 apparently healthy centenarians (12).

Role of underlying heart disease. The results of extensive ambulatory monitoring (1) suggest that the presence of heart disease contributes to increased frequency of ventricular premature complexes and increased occurrence of couplets and short runs of nonsustained ventricular tachycardia even when cardiac function remains normal or minimally impaired. An even greater increase in frequency and complexity of ventricular arrhythmias tends to accompany the impairment of ventricular function and development of congestive heart failure in a variety of heart diseases, ranging from congenital to ischemic and idiopathic cardiomyopathy.

Role of impaired ventricular function. The reported results of ambulatory monitoring suggest that frequent and complex ventricular arrhythmias, including nonsustained ventricular tachycardia, are present in the majority of patients with congestive heart failure in New York Heart Association functional classes III and IV. For instance, in eight studies of such patients that I reviewed (1), the incidence of nonsustained ventricular tachycardia ranged from 49% to 100% (average 65%).

Table 21.1. The Lown and Wolf Grading System

Lown Grade	Definition
0	No VPDs
1	<30 VPDs/h
2	≥30 VPDs/h
3	Multiform VPDs
4a	Paired VPDs
4b	Ventricular tachycardia
5	R on T VPDs

Reproduced with permission from Lown and Wolf (14). VPDs = ventricular premature depolarizations.

Comment: importance of establishing norms. It appears that each of the three factors (that is, advancing age, presence of heart disease and impairment of ventricular function) contributes to an increasing incidence of premature ventricular complexes and facilitates the formation of repetitive forms. Available information from widespread use of ambulatory ECG monitoring can be used to establish age-dependent ranges of normal distribution of various types of ventricular arrhythmias in different groups of individuals with and without heart disease. One such study (13) in a sample of healthy men and women was recently reported. The availability of "norms" would be helpful in defining the therapeutic objectives, in particular in asymptomatic individuals. For example, a finding of a three to five beat ventricular tachycardia at a rate of 120 to 180 beats/min may be "within normal limits" for a 70 year old patient in functional class III or IV and, therefore, should be perceived as would any other manifestation peculiar to this stage of heart disease. However, the low probability of a similar arrhythmia in a 25 year old subject without evidence of manifest heart disease should lead to an intensive search for incipient heart disease. The establishment of norms will be particularly useful in geriatric practice, where ventricular arrhythmias appear to represent no more than a sign of physiologic aging that is comparable with the age-dependent decline in the maximal heart rate during exercise, or the leftward shift of the mean QRS axis in the frontal plane on the ECG.

Classification

The grading system with respect to the frequency and complexity of ectopic beats. The two commonly used criteria in classifying ventricular arrhythmias in clinical practice are the frequency of ectopic complexes and the "complexity" of ventricular arrhythmias. The most popular system proposed by Lown and Wolf (14) (Table 21.1) is the hierarchy of mutually exclusive grades. The hierarchic classification of ventricular arrhythmias can be useful because it facilitates communication among observers in describing findings and reporting outcomes of therapy. However, the hierarchy in the classification of Lown and Wolf (14) bears no relation to the severity of the disease, the degree of impairment or the prognosis. This can be best illustrated by contrasting this classification with that of the New York Heart Association, in which assignment to one of the four classes implies clearly defined clinical, prognostic and therapeutic data. However, assignment to any of the grades of ventricular arrhythmias (with the possible exception of sustained ventricular tachycardia or ventricular fibrillation) provides no information as to whether the patient has heart disease, whether the arrhythmia is symptomatic, has prognostic significance or needs to be treated and whether a repeat examination on a different day will show the same grade of arrhythmia. This means that no useful clinical information can be derived from grading arrhythmias with respect to frequency or "complexity" of ventricular premature complexes. Moreover, the spontaneous variability of the frequency and complexity of ventricular arrhythmias in the absence of treatment (15–17) can change the grade without any detectable change in the patient's condition.

The R on T phenomenon. An additional shortcoming of the grading system proposed by Lown and Wolf (14) is the designation of the R on T phenomenon as the most advanced form of ventricular arrhythmias. There is little doubt that an R on T complex frequently initiates ventricular fibrillation in the prehospital and early hospital phase of acute myocardial infarction. Also, it not infrequently initiates torsade de pointes in the setting of hypokalemia or long QT interval of various origins. However, under all other circumstances, an R on T complex is no more dangerous than any other ventricular premature complex (18), and perhaps less dangerous than a late premature ventricular complex because ventricular tachycardia tends to occur more often after a late than after an early premature ventricular complex (19,20).

The infrequent occurrence of repetitive rhythms after an R on T premature complex is not surprising. It is known that stimuli from an implanted pacemaker cause no electrical accidents when the inhibiting function is removed by the magnet applied over the chest. Also, single stimuli of 2 ms duration and twice diastolic threshold strength applied during the T wave in the course of the measurements of the refractory period in humans cause no repetitive rhythms in the absence of heart disease and very seldom induce such rhythms in patients with a history of spontaneous ventricular tachycardia and syncope. Therefore, the evaluation of coupling intervals and prematurity indexes of the ventricular ectopic complexes has not influenced the approach to ventricular arrhythmias in clinical practice.

Grading by nonlife-threatening versus life-threatening and fatal arrhythmias. Another classification of ventricular arrhythmias proposed by Myerburg et al. (21) does not include the R on T phenomenon as a separate category and permits the assignment of arrhythmias simultaneously to two categories based on the parallel hierarchies of frequency and form. A classification that I consider useful for prognostic purposes is shown in Table 21.2. I categorize ventricular

Table 21.2. Nonhierarchial Classification of Ventricular Arrhythmias

Rare, Frequent, "Complex" VPC; Asymptomatic Nonsustained VT	Sustained Symptomatic VT	Ventricular Fibrillation
Increases with age and severity of heart disease	Usually a marker of severe heart disease and not a result of preexisting "complex" ventricular arrhythmias	Usually an electrical accident unrelated to preexisting ventricular arrhythmias, although it may emerge from an episode of sustained VT
No independent prognostic implications, but may be an early manifestation of heart disease		

VPC = ventricular premature complex; VT = ventricular tachycardia.

arrhythmias as: 1) nonlife-threatening arrhythmias that cause no appreciable hemodynamic compromise, 2) life-threatening arrhythmias that precipitate significant hemodynamic compromise, and 3) fatal electrical accidents.

The overwhelming majority of ventricular arrhythmias fall into category 1, which encompasses single, multiple, uniform and multiform premature ventricular complexes, couplets or triplets and most episodes of brief nonsustained ventricular tachycardia. These arrhythmias cause either no symptoms or only mild to moderate discomfort. The distinction between an asymptomatic and mildly symptomatic arrhythmia is largely a matter of subjective perception and is not a matter of the severity or characteristics of each. The subjective awareness of arrhythmias and the degree of discomfort bear no relation to the frequency or complexity of ventricular arrhythmias.

Category 2—life-threatening arrhythmias—consists mainly of sustained ventricular tachycardia that frequently precipitates serious hemodynamic deterioration requiring emergency treatment. Nonsustained ventricular tachycardia may also precipitate hemodynamic deterioration, particularly at rapid heart rates and in patients with marked diastolic or systolic dysfunction. However, most nonsustained ventricular tachycardias are asymptomatic, probably because the episodes are of short duration and the rate of the arrhythmia seldom exceeds the individual maximal sinus rate.

Both nonsustained and sustained ventricular tachycardia occur most frequently in patients with advanced heart disease and severe ventricular dysfunction—the category of patients with a high incidence of nonlife-threatening arrhythmias—so they often coexist in the same patient. However, coexistence does not necessarily mean that the arrhythmias share the same mechanism or have a common substrate. It has been shown (22) that in patients harboring both forms of arrhythmia, the configuration and rate of nonsustained ventricular tachycardia are not predictive of the occurrence and characteristics of subsequent sustained ventricular tachycardia. This suggests that sustained ventricular tachycardia repesents an independent event rather than a failed termination of the preexisting nonsustained ventricular tachycardia.

Category 3—ventricular arrhythmias that cause sudden

death—includes "primary" ventricular fibrillation, polymorphic ventricular tachycardia known as torsade de pointes and sustained ventricular tachycardia degenerating into ventricular fibrillation. Primary ventricular fibrillation associated with myocardial ischemia is the principal cause of sudden cardiac death at the onset of myocardial infarction. The numerically much less frequent torsade de pointes is usually associated with a long QT interval, hypokalemia and treatment with class IA and class III antiarrhythmic drugs. In a number of studies (23), the most common mechanism of sudden cardiac death affecting patients in functional classes III and IV was ventricular tachycardia degenerating into ventricular fibrillation.

Comment. The origin of the hierarchic classification of ventricular arrhythmias and the ventricular premature complex hypothesis of sudden cardiac death (14) can be traced historically to the era when ECG monitoring was carried out predominantly in coronary care units. In these patients, ventricular tachycardia and ventricular fibrillation were frequently preceded by "high density" ventricular premature complexes, and the onset of ventricular fibrillation was precipitated by R on T phenomenon. These events occurred frequently in the setting of acute ischemia manifested by ST segment deviation from baseline values. I recall a statement by a coronary care nurse instructed in the use of defibrillators: "When I see the ST segment going up, I grease the paddles." Indeed, monitoring the ECG in the early days of coronary care units established a strong link between acute myocardial ischemia, ventricular arrhythmias and sudden cardiac death. In addition, the ventricular premature complex hypothesis of sudden cardiac death derived some support from the apparent efficacy of intravenously administered lidocaine in the suppression of all types of ventricular arrhythmias and assumed prevention of ventricular tachyarrhythmias. In retrospect, the therapeutic efficacy of intravenously administered lidocaine might have been exaggerated because of the inadequately understood natural history of rapidly diminishing severity of ventricular arrhythmias during the first few days after myocardial infarction.

When ambulatory ECG monitoring became available in a large number of inpatient and outpatient groups with and

Table 21.3. Causes of Electrical Accidents Resulting in Ventricular Fibrillation

Preexcitation
Electrocution
Hypokalemia
Digitalis
Antiarrhythmic drugs
Extrastimulation
Long QT syndrome
Myocardial ischemia

without heart disease and in a setting other than acute myocardial infarction, it became necessary to revise the concepts relating ventricular arrhythmias to sudden death. However, despite vanishing usefulness, the ventricular premature complex hypothesis of sudden cardiac death has continued to play an important role in both the clinical investigation of antiarrhythmic drugs and the treatment of arrhythmias in practice.

Because no drug can consistently eliminate all ventricular ectopic complexes, it is customary to express the success of antiarrhythmic therapy in terms of near suppression of the more "complex" forms and appreciable reduction in frequency of the less "complex" forms of ventricular arrhythmias. However, the benefit of a successful transition from a higher to a lower grade of ventricular arrhythmia or of a declining frequency of ventricular premature complexes is difficult to assess. Although the improvement of symptoms related to arrhythmias represents a therapeutic goal that is important to a relatively small proportion of patients with arrhythmias, it is the only recognizably rewarding outcome of therapy. Other potential benefits such as amelioration of myocardial ischemia or improved hemodynamics are more elusive, so that in the majority of patients treated for asymptomatic or mildly symptomatic ventricular arrhythmias, the benefit of therapy remains unknown. The preoccupation with achieving a lower grade of ventricular arrhythmias does not fulfill any valid therapeutic objective, but all too often has the deplorable effect of shifting the focus of interest from the patient with arrhythmia to the arrhythmia itself.

Prognosis

Normal subjects and patients with preserved ventricular function. In the absence of heart disease or in the presence of heart disease with well preserved ventricular function, sustained ventricular tachycardia seldom occurs. In these patients, arrhythmias assigned to category I in Table 21.3 have no independent prognostic significance for either sudden or nonsudden cardiac death unless the arrhythmia is an early manifestation of incipient organic heart disease.

Patients with severely impaired ventricular function and heart failure. It is well known that patients with severely impaired ventricular function and congestive heart failure

are at high risk for sudden cardiac death. However, in this group of patients, an independent relation of ventricular arrhythmias to death has been difficult to determine because ventricular arrhythmias are so strongly related to left ventricular dysfunction (24). Sudden death is equally distributed between patients with ischemic and idiopathic cardiomyopathy (24). A review of published reports (1) suggests that the prognosis is similar in patients with severe heart disease who suffer predominantly from congestive heart failure and those with the chief complaint of recurrent symptomatic ventricular tachyarrhythmia. In both, the recorded incidence of sudden cardiac death is about 15% to 20% per year.

Ventricular arrhythmias and sudden death. In 9 of 13 studies that considered the relation between ventricular arrhythmia and death, sudden cardiac death was unrelated to nonsustained ventricular tachycardia (1). In the studies previously reviewed (1) in which ventricular arrhythmia had an independent prognostic significance, the correlation was not strong. More recent studies (25–31) showed similar results. In one study (25) of 50 patients with chronic ischemic heart disease and heart failure, the 2 year mortality rate was 62%. In this group, left ventricular ejection fraction, ventricular arrhythmia and pulmonary capillary wedge pressure differed significantly between survivors and patients who died. However, there were no differences in any of the variables between those who died suddenly and those who did not. In another study (26) of 755 patients, ventricular tachycardia was present in 115 (15%) but had only a borderline association with sudden cardiac death, whereas congestive heart failure was the strongest predictor of sudden cardiac death.

In a German study (31) of 73 patients with idiopathic dilated cardiomyopathy observed for >3 years, the mortality rate was 38% and 50% of deaths were sudden. Ventricular tachycardia was a frequent finding, but the characteristics of arrhythmias did not distinguish between patients who died of pump failure and those who died of arrhythmia, and ventricular arrhythmia was not a major independent risk factor for sudden cardiac death. In a British study (30) of 84 patients with severe chronic heart failure, the frequency of ventricular extrasystoles was an important predictor of death, but ventricular tachycardia was not. However, ventricular arrhythmia was related to severity of left ventricular dysfunction and exercise intolerance.

Comment. *Treatment of ventricular arrhythmias to prevent life-threatening symptoms or sudden cardiac death* is justified only if there is evidence that the arrhythmia in question represents an independent risk factor for these events. The prophylactic therapy of ventricular arrhythmias has been studied most intensively in the survivors of myocardial infarction. In nine previous trials (32–34) of antiarrhythmic drugs encompassing 2,899 patients, the results failed to achieve statistical significance. The available evidence (1) suggests that within a large pool of survivors of myocardial infarction, the correlation between ventricular arrhythmia and sudden cardiac death is either weak or absent. This in turn means that in the absence of uniformly effective and nontoxic drugs (see later), the trials of antiarrhythmic drugs for the prevention of death should be limited to those groups of patients in whom ventricular arrhythmias may be expected to represent a strong independent risk factor for arrhythmic sudden cardiac death.

One such group consists of patients discharged from the hospital after a non-Q wave infarction (35). However, many of these patients may have unstable angina pectoris and require treatment of myocardial ischemia. Another group in whom ventricular arrhythmia appears to be a moderately strong predictor of sudden cardiac death includes patients with obstructive cardiomyopathy (36,37) and nonsustained ventricular tachycardia. Although further attempts to identify similar subsets of patients are in order, this may be a difficult task because, in patients with adequate ventricular function, the low incidence of sudden cardiac death makes it difficult to recruit a sufficiently large sample to establish the benefit. Conversely, in patients with severely impaired ventricular function in whom the incidence of sudden cardiac death is high, the arrhythmias are more difficult to suppress, the proarrhythmic effects are more common and the negative inotropic effects of the antiarrhythmic drugs are more dangerous.

Gaining Insight

Factors Responsible for the Age- and Heart Disease-Dependent Increase in Ventricular Arrhythmias

Role of increasing age. Ambulatory ECG monitoring of patients with ventricular arrhythmias disclosed new targets of potential investigation. Among these, of great interest is the elucidation of factors responsible for the increasing incidence of ventricular arrhythmias with increasing age. One difficulty in studying this problem is the unknown mechanism of the single ventricular premature complex in any age group. Also, no systematic studies are available about the effect of age on the response to antiarrhythmic therapy and the response of arrhythmia to exercise, changes in heart rate, autonomic influences or circadian rhythm. This means that it is not known whether the process of aging creates new age-specific mechanisms or, alternatively, facilitates the operation of mechanisms operating at a younger age.

Aging is associated with a variety of anatomic and physiologic alterations that may increase the propensity to both automatic and reentrant ventricular arrhythmias. Among these are an increase in left ventricular wall thickness, slower isometric relaxation, reduced filling rate and impaired ventricular compliance (38). Some of the morphologic changes consist of lipofuscin accumulation at the poles of the nuclei, basophilic degeneration within the sarcoplasmic reticulum, deposition of amyloid and adipose tissue between muscle cells and an increase in elastic and collagenous tissue surrounding the conducting system (38).

Morphologic, functional and electrophysiologic correlations. It is possible that an increased understanding of the causes and mechanisms of age-related arrhythmias will emerge from correlations between morphology, mechanical function and electrophysiologic properties of cardiac tissue during the aging process studied either longitudinally or by comparing age-matched groups of subjects differing in the incidence of ventricular arrhythmias. Studies (39) of human atrial tissue removed during operation have shown that, with advancing age, there is uncoupling of side to side electrical connections between parallel-oriented cardiac fibers, a process attributed to separation of the fibers by collagenous septa.

Continuing investigations of this type, both in vivo and in vitro, may elucidate the characteristics of the arrhythmogenic electrophysiologic milieu in the absence of the complicating influences of dilation, excessive stretch, diseased or scarred tissue and defective perfusion. Similar information may be forthcoming from studies of ventricular arrhythmias in subjects with heart disease but normal ventricular function (for example, early stages of valvular disease or coronary artery disease without ischemia).

Electrical Accidents

Electrical accidents represent serious and often lethal ventricular tachyarrhythmias precipitated by an abrupt onset of an electrophysiologic dysfunction. Electrophysiologic accidents have an unpredictable pattern of recurrence. Their natural history has become more evident since the introduction of the automatic troubleshooting cardioverters and defibrillators (40). Studies (41) of patients equipped with these devices have shown that in 42% of the survivors of a nearly fatal electrical accident, these events did not recur during a follow-up period of up to 7 years.

Ventricular fibrillation. Sudden cardiac death precipitated by the ventricular tachyarrhythmias may be caused by either ventricular fibrillation or ventricular tachycardia, which may or may not degenerate into ventricular fibrillation. Ventricular fibrillation is the most common cause of electrical accidents occurring in a structurally undamaged heart. Table 21.3 lists some of the electrical accidents resulting in ventricular fibrillation. Because the electrophysiologic disturbances listed in Table 21.3 are capable of disrupting electrical activity in a normal heart, the mechanisms of most of these disturbances can be studied in the models of normal cardiac tissue both in vivo and in vitro.

Ventricular fibrillation can be induced in the laboratory by a series of successive premature impulses or by rapid pacing. A similar event can occur spontaneously in patients with atrial flutter or fibrillation when the rapid atrial impulses reach the ventricles by means of an atrioventricular (AV) bypass tract with a short refractory period. Such electrical accidents demonstrate the physiologic importance of the AV node, which protects the ventricles from critical acceleration of atrial rate and subsequent depolarization of the ventricles before the recovery of normal excitability.

The mechanism of ventricular fibrillation caused by electrocution can be simulated by the application of direct or alternating currents of moderate strength. These procedures result in depolarization and automatic activity arising in the depolarized myocardium (42). Digitalis poisoning can disrupt electrical activity by increased automaticity due to enhanced phase 4 depolarization or the induction of delayed depolarizations generated by the transient inward current in the calcium-overloaded fibers (43).

Hypokalemia. Hypokalemia prolongs the relative refractory period, increases automaticity and facilitates the appearance of early afterdepolarizations that are caused by low potassium conductance (44). Such afterdepolarizations can also occur when the action potential duration is prolonged by antiarrhythmic drugs that block the repolarizing potassium current or currents. Various procedures that decrease potassium conductance and prolong action potential duration cause polymorphic ventricular tachycardia or ventricular fibrillation in the appropriate animal models (44).

Prolonged QT intervals. Ventricular tachyarrhythmias seldom occur when the duration of action potential is uniformly prolonged (for example, in the presence of hypocalcemia or steady state hypothermia). This suggests that ventricular tachycardia and ventricular fibrillation occurring in patients with congenital or acquired long QT syndromes may be facilitated by an increased dispersion of refractoriness that is present in such patients (44).

Acute myocardial ischemia. By far the most common and clinically most important cause of ventricular fibrillation in a structurally intact heart is myocardial ischemia in the prehospital or early hospital phase of acute myocardial infarction. The corresponding animal model of coronary ligation (45,46) shows that the onset of ventricular fibrillation is preceded by a regional increase in interstitial potassium concentration, regional acidosis, uneven polarization and displacement of the QT segment. Characteristically, ventricular fibrillation occurs more frequently either shortly after ligation of the coronary artery (occlusion arrhythmia) or on release (reperfusion arrhythmia) than during sustained occlusion. This suggests that fibrillation is generated or facilitated by nonhomogeneous depolarization. In contrast to the destabilizing effects of local depolarization, generalized depolarization results in uniform slowing of conduction without increasing the propensity to arrhythmia (47).

Destabilizing electrophysiologic properties leading to serious ventricular arrhythmias. Figure 21.1 illustrates the abnormalities assumed to be responsible for the disturbances of conduction and refractoriness resulting in electrical accidents in the nondamaged heart. The normally absent destabilizing electrophysiologic features in the diagram from top to bottom are: 1) long relative refractory period produced by

hypokalemia and certain antiarrhythmic drugs; 2) nonuniform membrane potential at rest and action potential amplitude in the presence of acute myocardial ischemia; 3) afterdepolarizations in the nonpacemaker fibers resulting from calcium overload (as during digitalis poisoning) and diastolic depolarizations in the presence of low potassium conductance (for example, during hypokalemia); 4) marked dispersion of repolarization that may be present in patients with the long QT syndrome; and 5) an imbalance between slow conductance and short refractoriness induced by rapid pacing. It can be seen that the two prevailing disturbances resulting in the electrical accidents are nonuniform depolarization and nonuniform refractoriness.

Diseased myocardium may become victim of the same accidents as those affecting structurally intact myocardium. However, diseased myocardium may also harbor substrates responsible for the perpetuation of ventricular tachycardia. In this setting, fatal electrical accidents may result from the inability to preserve adequate hemodynamic function or from transition of ventricular tachycardia into ventricular flutter or fibrillation.

Nonsustained Ventricular Tachycardia

This arrhythmia seldom appears in the absence of single ventricular premature complexes and couplets. Most subjects with hundreds or thousands of single premature complexes during a 24 h monitoring period have fewer than tens of couplets and one or few episodes of nonsustained ventricular tachycardia that rarely consists of >10 ventricular ectopic complexes.

Mechanisms. The great predominance of single ventricular premature complexes compared with the less frequently occurring couplets and the rare episodes of nonsustained ventricular tachycardia suggest the existence of mechanisms that prevent the perpetuation of repetitive ventricular ectopic activity. Understanding such putative mechanisms that abort the repetitive activity may be helpful in explaining their failure. Nonsustained ventricular tachycardia is frequently irregular and polymorphic and its rate often varies in the same individual. These features suggest the existence of mechanisms that oppose smooth perpetuation of repetitive activity. The understanding of mechanisms responsible for such behavior may be helpful in designing approaches to the prevention and treatment of tachyarrhythmias.

Sustained Ventricular Tachycardia

Electrophysiologic and pharmacologic studies during the past two decades have increased the understanding of the mechanisms of ventricular tachycardias both in the clinical setting and in experimental animal models. Increased normal automaticity or triggered automaticity in the Purkinje fibers appears to operate in a relatively small number of patients with ventricular tachycardias. In these, ventricular arrhyth-

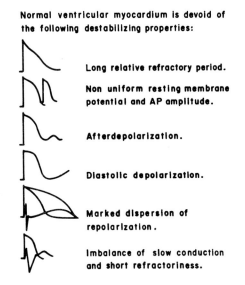

Normal ventricular myocardium is devoid of the following destabilizing properties:

Long relative refractory period.

Non uniform resting membrane potential and AP amplitude.

Afterdepolarization.

Diastolic depolarization.

Marked dispersion of repolarization.

Imbalance of slow conduction and short refractoriness.

Figure 21.1. Diagram of putative destabilizing electrophysiologic properties in the ventricular myocardium known to contribute to serious ventricular arrhythmias. Ventricular action potential (AP) and the electrocardiogram are superimposed in the two lowest tracings. See text. Reproduced with permission from Surawicz B. Contributions of cellular electrophysiology to the understanding of the electrocardiogram. Experientia 1987;43:1061–8.

mia is precipitated by beta-adrenergic stimulation or exercise and is suppressed by beta-adrenergic blockade and the calcium channel blocker verapamil (48–50).

Reentry. The prevailing evidence suggests that the most common cause of tachyarrhythmia is reentry, a process requiring the presence of a reentrant pathway, unidirectional block and slow conduction. In a small number of patients, usually those with dilated cardiomyopathy, the long reentrant loop involves the His bundle and both bundle branches (51), but in the majority of patients with sustained ventricular tachycardia, the His-Purkinje system is not necessary for perpetuation of reentry (52). The intramyocardial reentrant circuit is frequently small, relatively "protected" (52) and at least in part anatomically determined (53). Phenomena favoring reentry include 1) reproducible initiation and termination by one or more extrastimuli; 2) inverse relation between the coupling interval of the premature complex initiating ventricular tachycardia and the interval from the initiating complex to the first complex of ventricular tachycardia; 3) resetting or entrainment (continuous resetting) with single or multiple extrastimuli; and 4) interruption by incision in the region of slow conduction (52–55). Intraoperative mapping using a large array of endocardial electrodes and high gain recording (56) showed that initiation of induced ventricular tachycardia was dependent on a microreentrant loop, the first part of which was formed by critically delayed potentials in response to premature stimuli.

The reentrant mechanism has been documented in a number of studies of sustained ventricular tachycardia in-

duced in dogs within 1 day to about 3 weeks after experimental myocardial infarction. In these preparations, the arrhythmias frequently originate in the surviving subendocardial Purkinje fibers (57,58), and the reentrant activity develops mainly in the surviving epicardial fibers or the intramural layers, or both (59–65). The site of undirectional block in these models may be a region of impaired conduction, prolonged refractory period (64,66) or depressed excitability. These abnormalities frequently coexist.

It was recently shown (67,68) that reentrant tachycardia was associated with slow conduction caused by impulse propagation that was not parallel but perpendicular to fiber orientation. Such anisotropic conduction probably results from the presence of structural barriers in the damaged myocardium (39). The possible role of anisotropic conduction in the reentrant arrhythmias in humans is under investigation (69). If anisotropic conduction is proved to be of importance, it will be necessary to reassess the mechanisms of drugs acting on such substrate (70–72).

Prediction of sustained ventricular tachycardia. The occurrence of sustained ventricular tachycardia is believed to require the presence of two factors: an appropriate substrate and a releasing trigger such as a ventricular premature complex. Assessment of the frequency and complexity of ventricular ectopic activity by ambulatory monitoring has failed to predict sustained ventricular tachycardia or sudden cardiac death in patients with ischemic (73) or dilated (74) cardiomyopathy. Similarly, exercise testing is seldom helpful in detecting these life-threatening arrhythmias.

Two procedures that may detect the arrhythmic substrate are programmed electrical stimulation and signal-averaged ECG. Programmed electrical stimulation is a provocative test that elicits nonsustained or sustained ventricular tachycardia or ventricular fibrillation in the presence of an appropriate substrate, depending on the method of stimulation. The main strength of this procedure is reproducible initiation of sustained ventricular tachycardia in most patients with chronic ischemic heart disease and a history of that arrhythmia (75). The procedure is less successful in initiating sustained ventricular tachycardia in patients with congestive cardiomyopathy and a history of the arrhythmia and in initiation of ventricular fibrillation in patients with a history of ventricular fibrillation that is not followed by acute myocardial infarction. The value of programmed electrical stimulation as a predictor of sustained ventricular tachycardia or ventricular fibrillation in patients without a history of these arrhythmias is uncertain (74–76).

The signal-averaged ECG detects high frequency, low amplitude potentials at the end of the QRS complex and during the ST segment (77). This noninvasive test appears to be a moderately sensitive predictor of both spontaneous and inducible sustained ventricular tachycardia in patients with chronic ischemic heart disease. A normal test result also reliably predicts a low risk of developing sustained ventricular tachycardia during the follow-up period. However, there is no rigid demarcation between normal and abnormal durations and voltages of the detected signals. Therefore, arbitrarily set criteria for abnormality represent the best trade-off between sensitivity and specificity; the two are inversely related to each other.

Comment. Important advances in basic and applied cardiac electrophysiology have contributed to better understanding of the mechanism of ventricular arrhythmias. The electrical accidents can be prevented more effectively by an improved knowledge of the precipitating factors (for example, myocardial ischemia, hypokalemia or drug toxicity). Localization of the arrhythmia site by mapping has made it possible to develop various surgical and nonsurgical ablative therapies. The successful application of pacing and defibrillating devices is a direct extension of the fundamentals of cardiac electrophysiology. However, the recognition of reentry as the most likely and the most prevalent mechanism of ventricular tachycardia has not yet importantly benefited the practical approaches to the pharmacologic treatment of ventricular arrhythmias. The stumbling block is the inability to investigate the electrophysiologic interaction of the drug with cellular or tissue elements responsible for the origin and perpetuation of arrhythmias. This translates into ignorance of both the desired site of drug action and the mechanism of action at the desired site.

It is doubtful whether an immediate solution to this problem can be expected using available techniques. However, several important questions contributing to a more rational use of the drugs can be answered more easily. Some of these include better understanding of factors allowing reentry to perpetuate, those allowing the drug to terminate reentry, the control of ventricular tachycardia rate and the factors contributing to the degeneration of ventricular tachycardia into ventricular fibrillation.

Limitations of Antiarrhythmic Drug Therapy

Antiarrhythmic Drug Action

Calcium channel blockers. Of the several drug classes used in the treatment of ventricular arrhythmias, calcium channel blockers play the smallest role. Verapamil suppresses certain exercise-induced and a few other rare types of ventricular tachycardia (49,50,78) attributed to triggered automaticity (50), but rarely affects other types of ventricular arrhythmia even when the impulse propagation is very slow (79). This suggests an absence of slow channel-dependent automaticity or conduction within the substrate of reentrant ventricular arrhythmias.

Beta-adrenergic blockers. These agents may be expected to suppress automatic activity in the Purkinje fibers. They appear to be useful in the treatment of ventricular tachycardia induced by increased sympathetic stimulation or isoproterenol (48). Other types of ventricular arrhythmias can be influenced indirectly by the decrease in heart rate and other effects of beta-adrenergic blockade. High concentrations of propranolol (80) and other beta-adrenergic blockers have sodium channel blocking properties, but the significance of such action at the clinical level is uncertain. One of the most effective antiarrhythmic drugs among the beta-adrenergic blockers is sotalol (81). However, its effectiveness does not depend on the beta-adrenergic properties, but on the prolongation of action potential duration (82) attributed to the suppression of the time-dependent potassium current (83). Because therapeutic sotalol concentrations do not block the sodium current, the action of sotalol demonstrates that suppression of arrhythmias can take place by lengthening the refractoriness without a direct effect on conduction.

Sodium channel blockers (class I drugs). Most drugs used in the treatment of ventricular arrhythmias slow conduction by blocking the sodium channel. During each action potential, the sodium channel undergoes transformation from the open to the inactivated to the closed state. Sodium channel blockers differ in their kinetics of binding to and unbinding from the channel at each of the three states of the channel (84,85). When the drug is bound to the receptor within the channel, sodium entry during depolarization is assumed to be blocked and conduction velocity decreases. The blocking effect is usually enhanced by depolarization and rapid heart rate (voltage- and use-dependent drug properties, respectively).

Sodium channel blockers can be characterized as fast, intermediate and slow, depending on the kinetics of the recovery from block (86). The recovery kinetics of the class IB (lidocaine-like) drugs are fast and, therefore, the blocking effects of the drug at normal resting potential are limited to short time intervals after depolarization (that is, early extrasystoles and very rapid heart rates). The recovery kinetics of most class IA and IC drugs are intermediate or slow, and the blocking effects on conduction are manifest within a wide range of coupling intervals and heart rates. Class IA (quinidine-like) drugs prolong action potential duration in both Purkinje and ventricular muscle fibers (87), an effect attributed to the block of time-independent potassium current (88), whereas class IC (flecainide-like) drugs shorten action potential duration in Purkinje fibers, but have no appreciable effect on the duration of action potential in ventricular fibers (87).

The diversity of antiarrhythmic drug action on depolarization and repolarization of ventricular muscle fibers is detectable in the ECG QRS complex as follows: 1) lengthening of the QT complex without change in the QRS duration (for example, sotalol); 2) lengthening of the QRS complex and JT interval (for example, quinidine); 3) lengthening of the QRS complex without change of JT interval (for example, flecainide); and 4) no QRS or JT duration change (for example, mexiletine).

Drug selection for long-term treatment. It seems remarkable that despite the large diversity of electrophysiologic actions, we use each of these drugs for the identical purpose, namely, suppression of ventricular ectopic activity. Our drug selection for long-term treatment is not determined by the specific electrophysiologic or ECG effects, but by the preliminary results obtained by trial and error, ambulatory ECG monitoring, exercise testing or electrophysiologic studies. Although the potency of each drug is dose dependent, the dosing is usually dictated by the considerations of cardiac and extracardiac toxicity (see later).

Programmed electrical stimulation. The impact of programmed electrical stimulation on the selection of drugs for treatment of life-threatening ventricular tachyarrhythmias is controversial. Arrhythmias are rendered noninducible by a class I drug or amiodarone in 15% to 30% of patients. It appears that patients in whom drugs prevent inducibility of ventricular tachycardia have a less complex or anatomically smaller substrate because they tend to have less impaired ventricular function and less pronounced fractionated activity as detected by the signal-averaged ECG.

Unfortunately, the programmed electrical stimulation procedure does not escape empiricism, for on any single hospital admission, a patient can undergo only a limited number of trials with only a few drugs or combinations of drugs selected from a vast array of possibilities. Therefore, the selection of drugs tends to be arbitrary. A number of earlier studies (75,89) suggested that failure to induce sustained ventricular tachycardia in the presence of a drug predicts a better prognosis. However, it is not certain whether treatment guided by programmed electrical stimulation improves the outcome or merely selects patients with a better prognosis.

Some of the more recent studies (76,90–92) have cast doubt on the ability of programmed electrical stimulation to predict the results of antiarrhythmic therapy, in particular when using amiodarone. It also is not certain that programmed stimulation-guided therapy is superior to treatment with beta-adrenergic blockers. In a study (93) of 166 patients with sustained ventricular tachycardia, ventricular fibrillation or syncope, the incidence of recurrence of arrhythmias and sudden cardiac death was equal in patients treated with drugs selected by means of programmed electric stimulation and those treated with metoprolol without drug testing. Also, it has been reported (94) that there was no difference in the outcome of treatment in patients with ventricular tachycardia or ventricular fibrillation followed up for 24 months when treatment was designed empirically or when drugs were selected by means of serial testing. In a recent editorial, Lehman et al. (95) pointed out that favorable results of programmed electrical stimulation leave a considerable segment of patients at risk of sudden cardiac death, which averages 13% a year in patients with noninducible ventricular tachycardia and 11% during a follow-up period of 18 to 26 months in patients in whom inducibility was suppressed by drugs.

Long-term results. Sodium channel blockers suppress most ventricular arrhythmias in category I (nonlife-threatening with no hemodynamic compromise) in >80% of pa-

tients who tolerate the drug (34,96), but are less successful in prevention and treatment of ventricular tachyarrhythmias in categories II and III (life-threatening with hemodynamic compromise and fatal electrical accidents). In theory, each of the available sodium channel blockers used in sufficient doses is probably capable of eradicating reentrant ventricular arrhythmia by an appropriate slowing of conduction or lengthening of refractoriness, or both. This hypothesis finds support in previous experience with the Sokolow method (97) used for conversion of atrial fibrillation to sinus rhythm. This method (97) consisted of a gradual increase in daily quinidine doses up to 3.2 g/day. Action of quinidine transformed atrial fibrillation into a slow and regular atrial rhythm known as quinidine flutter; afterward, sinus rhythm resumed in about 75% of trials. Thus, the fibrillatory activity in the atria can be eliminated by slowing conduction or prolonging refractoriness, or both.

In the ventricles, drugs cannot be used to stop fibrillation, but they can be employed to prevent recurrent fibrillatory activity (98), terminate ventricular tachycardia or transform a rapid tachycardia into a slower and better tolerated ventricular rhythm. Recent studies (99,99a) have shown that the cycle length of ventricular tachycardia can be calculated from the drug's effect on ventricular conduction or refractoriness, or both.

Unfortunately, satisfactory long-term therapeutic results can be obtained only in a minority of patients with life-threatening ventricular tachyarrhythmias. Conceivably, a drug's inefficacy may be caused by an inadequate perfusion, resulting in delayed or inadequate delivery to the site of arrhythmia genesis (100). However, there are no clinical studies to support or refute such a phenomenon. In the majority, the drugs fail because they must be discontinued before maximal drug efficacy can be achieved as a result of one or more intervening toxic manifestations that may include negative inotropic, hypotensive, proarrhythmic or extracardiac side effects.

Negative Inotropic Effects

All beta-adrenergic, calcium channel and sodium channel blockers depress contractility. The negative inotropic effect most adversely affects patients with impaired ventricular function and reduced mass of the viable myocardium.

Sodium channel blockers (class I drugs). The negative inotropic effect of the sodium channel blockers is attributed to the decreased intracellular sodium activity. It has been shown (101) that lidocaine, encainide, high propranolol doses and tetradotoxin produced concomitant reduction of intracellular sodium activity and depression of contractile force in sheep Purkinje strands. The depressed contractility was attributed to the decreased intracellular sodium activity resulting from the operation of the sodium-calcium exchange (102). This means that the electrochemical sodium gradient determines the electrochemical calcium gradient, and suggests that the negative inotropic effect is an unavoidable consequence of the drug-induced reduction of intracellular sodium activity.

Lidocaine and other class IB drugs. The negative inotropic effect of lidocaine in Purkinje fibers has been attributed to shortening of the action potential, which could result in decreased calcium influx through the slow channel (103). However, sodium channel blockers that do not change or prolong action potential duration also depress contractility.

Clinical impressions and experimental observations (104) suggest that lidocaine and other class IB drugs produce a less pronounced negative inotropic effect than do the other two classes of sodium channel blockers. If these assertions are valid, one can speculate that the lesser negative inotropic effect is related to the faster recovery of the sodium channel from the block (86). A faster recovery may be expected to lessen the reduction of both intracellular sodium and calcium activity. This hypothesis needs to be tested.

The hypotensive and vasodilating effects of sodium channel blockers are not always deleterious and may be beneficial when the vasodilation results in decreased afterload. Also, vasoconstricting effects of certain antiarrhythmic drugs have been reported (104).

Proarrhythmic Effects

Categories of proarrhythmic effects. Each drug capable of arrhythmia suppression is also capable of arrhythmia aggravation. Brugada and Wellens (105) divided the proarrhythmic effects into categories of true arrhythmogenesis, facilitation and unmasking of a new substrate. True arrhythmogenesis means creation of a new arrhythmia form (for example, torsade de pointes after administration of quinidine or other drugs that prolong the QT interval). The other two categories of arrhythmia aggravation may result from critical changes in conduction or refractoriness, or both, within a preexisting substrate of arrhythmia. This may lead to either facilitation (that is, worsening of spontaneously occurring arrhythmias) or a new type of arrhythmia created by unmasking a "latent" substrate. In the case of true arrhythmogenesis, the offending agent must be eliminated, whereas in the other categories, dose adjustment may be possible in some cases.

In one study (106), the aggravation was defined as a 4-fold increase in the frequency of ventricular premature complexes, a 10-fold increase in repetitive forms or the first emergence of sustained ventricular tachycardia (107). The frequency of aggravation for nine tested drugs ranged from 5.9% to 15.8%. According to Hondeghem (107), drugs with slow recovery kinetics from sodium channel block (for example, class IC drugs) may be expected to have a more pronounced proarrhythmic effect.

Serious proarrhythmic effects. Of greatest concern is the drug-induced provocation of life-threatening ventricular tachyarrhythmias. The incidence of these events varies in different studies. For instance, in one representative flecainide study (108), the incidence of serious proarrhythmias was 4.5%, and in another (109), it was 13%. Similarly, in one encainide study (110), the incidence of serious proarrhythmia was 7% and in another (111), it was 15%. Such differences can be attributed to variety in the dosages, duration of follow-up and, more importantly, the characteristics of the studied patients.

Serious proarrhythmic effects occur more frequently in patients with impaired ventricular function (112,113) and more serious arrhythmias (113). For instance, in one study (113), encainide induced ventricular tachyarrhythmia in 11% of 90 patients receiving the drug for recurrent ventricular tachycardia and ventricular fibrillation and in only 2.2% of patients receiving the drug for "chronic complex ventricular ectopic activity." In another study (114) of 1,330 patients treated with flecainide, nonlethal proarrhythmic effects occurred in 6.6% of patients with sustained ventricular tachycardia, 0.9% of those with nonsustained ventricular tachycardia and in no patients with ventricular premature complexes. In a large moricizine study (115), no proarrhythmic effects occurred in patients with "benign" ventricular arrhythmias as opposed to a 3.7% incidence rate of such effects in patients with "potentially lethal" and "lethal" ventricular arrhythmias.

Diagnosis by ECG or drug interaction. Because the electrophysiologic drug properties that contribute to the antiarrhythmic and proarrhythmic actions are basically the same, it is seldom possible to recognize the impending proarrhythmic effect on the ECG. Monitoring drug concentrations in blood may not be helpful because the proarrhythmic effects are not consistently associated with any particular drug doses or blood drug concentrations. For instance, reentry within the His-Purkinje system in humans was facilitated by an infusion of 500 mg of procainamide (116), but was suppressed by an infusion of 700 mg of procainamide (117).

Diagnosis by electrophysiologic study. It has been shown that in some survivors of out of hospital cardiac arrest during treatment with a class IA antiarrhythmic drug, ventricular tachycardia was not inducible in the absence of drugs, but became inducible after rechallenging with the offending drug (118). Although such demonstration is conclusive proof of proarrhythmias, the procedure is not practical for wide clinical application. Aggravation of arrhythmias during programmed stimulation occurred in 18% of drug tests (113). Drugs that aggravate arrhythmias during programmed stimulation are usually considered to be unsafe. However, the reduction of the number of extrastimuli required to induce tachycardia is not a reliable prognostic indicator of proarrhythmia (119).

Diagnosis by signal-averaged ECG. Drug-induced changes in the late components of local intracardiac electrograms have been reported (99a,120). This suggests that the signal-averaged ECG may be potentially useful in the evaluation of antiarrhythmic and proarrhythmic drug action. However, in some studies (121,122), the effects of antiarrhythmic drugs on the signal-averaged ECG lacked consistency. The proposed practical approaches (112,123,124) to the prevention of proarrhythmias consist of avoiding arrhythmia-precipitating factors (such as hypokalemia) and monitoring the initiation of therapy in the hospital in selected patient groups.

Noncardiac Adverse Drug Effects

Antiarrhythmic drugs share with various other chemical substances the ability to induce idiosyncratic, allergic and immunologic reactions in susceptible individuals. Of these, the most important clinically is the induction of a lupus-like syndrome produced by procainamide (125).

Neurologic side effects. Each class of antiarrhythmic drugs can be expected to exert the systemic effects inherent to their basic action; hence, the systemic beta-adrenergic blocking effect of the beta-adrenergic blockers and the systemic calcium channel blocking effect of the calcium channel blockers. The sodium channel blocking drugs can be expected to interfere with the function of all organs in which conduction or impulse transmission occurs (that is, the central and peripheral nervous systems, autonomic ganglia, neuromuscular junction and all types of muscle fibers) (126). The local anesthetic action of sodium channel blocking drugs causes an initial stimulation of the central nervous system (126), which is an important side effect of lidocaine-like drugs.

The high incidence of neurologic disturbances produced by lidocaine and the structurally similar mexiletine and tocainide may be attributed to their high lipid solubility and low molecular weight (84,86), enabling them to cross the blood-brain barrier easily. However, all other sodium channel blockers produce neurologic side effects. Most sodium channel blockers also produce disturbances of gastrointestinal tract and variable changes in the function of the autonomic nervous system.

Frequency of side effects. In one study (127) of 123 consecutive patients with a history of sustained ventricular tachycardia or ventricular fibrillation, 48% of patients had one or more adverse reactions and 29% had a major reaction requiring discontinuation of drug therapy. Side effects were no more common in patients with a left ventricular ejection fraction <40% than in those with an ejection fraction >40%. Significant adverse effects occurred in 19%, 24%, 49%, and 44% of patients treated with quinidine, procainamide, mexiletine and amiodarone, respectively. No less common are side effects in patients treated with sotalol (124), encainide (110) or flecainide (108). Some of the more common side effects such as the anticholinergic action of disopyramide or the effect of quinidine on the bowel function tend to occur shortly after the onset of therapy, but various other side effects may appear later in the course of therapy.

Although antiarrhythmic drugs are important contributors to iatrogenic morbidity, most side effects are reversible after discontinuation of therapy. The potentially lethal extracardiac effects are limited to bone marrow depression attributed to several of the drugs and to pulmonary toxicity of amiodarone.

Expected Progress in Therapy

Goals and tasks. Progress in pharmacologic therapy of ventricular arrhythmias must be directed toward the following goals: 1) definition of the benefits of therapy in different patient categories, 2) localization of the anatomic arrhythmia substrate, 3) identification of the electrophysiologic disturbances responsible for the perpetuation of arrhythmia, and 4) development of drugs capable of counteracting the arrhythmogenic disturbance without producing negative inotropic, hypotensive, proarrhythmic and systemic side effects.

These four tasks are not interdependent. Accurate assessment of the benefits of therapy can be accomplished without the understanding of the arrhythmia mechanism and the antiarrhythmic drug action. It is conceivable that an effective and nontoxic drug can be developed without the precise understanding of its interaction with arrhythmia substrate. However, in the past, little progress has been made by introducing large numbers of new drugs untested for their action on the arrhythmia substrate in humans. More likely, advances will depend on the progress of continued research in both the arrhythmia mechanism and the mechanism of drug action on the arrhythmia substrate.

Development of new drugs free of side effects. The task that may be most difficult to accomplish is the development of new drugs devoid of serious unwanted effects. Two categories of drugs have been used predominantly for the suppression of serious ventricular tachyarrhythmias (that is, sodium channel blockers and drugs that prolong action potential duration, which is designated as a class III action). Drugs in these two categories have produced serious proarrhythmic effects. If we assume that the electrophysiologic changes responsible for the proarrhythmic and antiarrhythmic effects are closely related, it may be difficult to separate these two effects without improved understanding of how the drug interacts with the arrhythmia substrate. In practice, propensity to proarrhythmia may be reduced by closer monitoring of the ECG and the electrophysiologic drug effects during therapy.

The negative and perhaps hypotensive drug effects appear to be linked to the processes responsible for the antiarrhythmic drug action. Better understanding of the mechanism of these actions may lead to successful counteraction of these effects or to development of drugs with lesser negative inotropic action. Equally difficult is the task of eliminating the extracardiac side effects. When these are dose dependent, combining smaller doses of two or more drugs with similar action may achieve the desired antiarrhythmic effect without toxic side effects (128–130). The combination of two drugs may also favorably affect the combined electrophysiologic profile of antiarrhythmic action (131). Extracardiac toxic drug effects will be eliminated if the future progress in basic electrophysiology leads to the development of heart-specific sodium channel blockers devoid of action on the nervous system and smooth muscle.

Amiodarone. The development of new antiarrhythmic drugs may be aided by better understanding of the therapeutic and toxic actions of amiodarone. Of all available antiarrhythmic drugs, amiodarone appears to be most effective in suppression of life-threatening ventricular tachyarrhythmias. In one of the largest studies (92) of patients treated with amiodarone for sustained ventricular tachycardia or cardiac arrest not responding to other antiarrhythmic drugs, the incidence of sudden cardiac death was 7% during the first 6 months and 9% during the first year and it increased by 3% a year during the subsequent 4 years. There were no sudden cardiac deaths during the first 2 years in patients with a left ventricular ejection fraction >40%. However, treatment with amiodarone was associated with a very high level of extracardiac toxicity (that is, in 45% after 1 year and in 86% after 5 years). Serious side effects necessitated discontinuation of treatment in 14% of patients after 1 year and in 37% after 5 years.

The reported high early mortality rate in patients treated with amiodarone cannot be viewed necessarily as drug failure without taking into account the state of left ventricular function. For comparison, one can cite the 24% incidence of sudden cardiac death at 6 months in a recent study (132) of 72 patients with severe heart failure and left ventricular ejection fraction averaging 18%; all of these patients were receiving antiarrhythmic drugs. It has been shown (133) that when the survival curves are adjusted for baseline prognostic characteristics, amiodarone has no deleterious effect on survival in patients with life-threatening ventricular tachyarrhythmias. Herre et al. (92) commented that the incidence of sudden cardiac death after the first year in their study compared favorably with the results of treatment with automatic implantable cardioverter-defibrillators.

Unique features of amiodarone. Amiodarone exemplifies a combination of uniquely superior therapeutic efficacy with uniquely severe extracardiac toxicity. Detailed discussion of amiodarone's properties is beyond the scope of this review. However, several unique distinctive features of this drug will be mentioned. For instance, unlike other sodium channel blockers, amiodarone combines a lidocaine-like effect on the recovery from sodium channel block (134) with disopyramide-like effect on action potential duration and refractoriness in ventricular muscle fibers (135,136). Several additional potential antiarrhythmic properties include the effect on the calcium channel (137); noncompetitive inhibition of beta-adrenergic and muscarinic receptors; a decrease in space constant, contributing to slower conduction (138); and inhibition of thyroxine synthesis (137). The latter effect is attributed to the presence of iodide, which appears to be essential to the antiarrhythmic action of amiodarone. The unusual pharmacokinetic properties of amiodarone suggest the importance of extensive accumulation in the tissue. The unusual toxic effects include oxidant lung injury (139) and inhibition of phospholipase associated with the formation of inclusion bodies in various cells and development of widespread phospholipidosis (137).

Clues for future drug development. The complex and unusual features of amiodarone may contain important clues for potential drug developers. It may be possible to identify beneficial and toxic properties of amiodarone more accurately in order to separate these two actions and create a safer amiodarone-like drug (137). Other new approaches to drug development will undoubtedly emerge as science continues to bring new understanding of arrhythmias and antiarrhythmic drugs and as human ingenuity continues to meet the challenges of yet unresolved medical problems.

The references that follow represent but a small fraction of important original contributions to the variety of subjects touched upon in this review. The selection of these references was arbitrary, mostly from memory, rather than as a result of a thorough bibliographic search. Hence, I owe an apology to many authors whose work was inadvertently omitted, whose concepts were left out and whose priorities were not acknowledged.

References

1. Surawicz B. Prognosis of ventricular arrhythmias in relation to sudden cardiac death: therapeutic implications. J Am Coll Cardiol 1987;10:435–47.
2. Brodsky M, Wu D, Denes P, Kanakis C, Rosen KM. Arrhythmias documented by 24-hour continuous electrocardiographic monitoring in 50 male medical students without apparent heart disease. Am J Cardiol 1977;39:390–4.
3. Sherman H, Sandberg S, Fineberg HV. Exponential increase in age-specific prevalence of ventricular dysrhythmias among males. J Chronic Dis 1982;35:743–50.
4. Hinkle LE, Carver ST, Stevens M. The frequency of asymptomatic disturbances of cardiac rhythm and conduction in middle-aged men. Am J Cardiol 1969;24:629–50.
5. Camm AJ, Evans KE, Ward DE, Martin A. The rhythms of the heart in active elderly subjects. Am Heart J 1980;99:598–604.
6. Fleg JL, Kennedy HL. Cardiac arrhythmias in a healthy elderly population. Chest 1982;81:302–7.
7. Kantelip JP, Sage E, Duchene-Marallaz P. Findings on ambulatory electrocardiographic monitoring in subjects older than 80 years. Am J Cardiol 1986;57:398–401.
8. Chandra VS, Purday JP, Macmillan NC, Taylor DJ. Rhythm disorders in healthy elderly people. Ger Cardiovasc Med 1988;1:263–6.
9. Bjerregaard P. Mean 24 hour heart rate, minimal heart rate and pauses in healthy subjects 40–79 years of age. Eur Heart J 1983;4:44–51.
10. Clee MD, Smith N, McNeill GP, Wright DS. Dysrhythmias in apparently healthy subjects. Age Ageing 1979;8:173–6.
11. Dietz A, Walter J, Bracharz H, Bracharz M, Unkelbach S, Franke H. Herzrhythmusstörungen bei rüstigen älteren Personen—Altersabhängigkeit von Herzfrequenz und Arrhythmien. Z Kardiol 1987;76:86–94.
12. Callaham P, Kinzel T, Kuo CS, Wekstein D, DeMaria A. Electrophysiologic characteristics of centenarians: evaluation by resting and ambulatory ECG (abstr). J Am Coll Cardiol 1986;7:52A.
13. Takada H, Mikawa T, Murayama M, Surgai J, Yamamura Y. Range of ventricular ectopic complexes in healthy subjects studied with repeated ambulatory electrocardiographic recordings. Am J Cardiol 1989;63:184–6.

14. Lown B, Wolf M. Approaches to sudden death from coronary heart disease. Circulation 1971;44:130–42.

15. Winkle RA, Gradman AH, Fitzgerald JW, Bell PA. Antiarrhythmic drug effect assessed from ventricular arrhythmia reduction in the ambulatory electrocardiogram and treadmill test: comparison of propranolol, procainamide and quinidine. Am J Cardiol 1978;42:473–80.

16. Pratt CM, Slymen DJ, Wierman AM, et al. Analysis of the spontaneous variability of ventricular arrhythmias: consecutive ambulatory electrocardiographic recordings of ventricular tachycardia. Am J Cardiol 1985; 56:67–72.

17. Anastasiou-Nana MI, Menlove RL, Nanas JN, Anderson JL. Changes in spontaneous variability of ventricular ectopic activity as a function of time in patients with chronic arrhythmias. Circulation 1988;78:286–95.

18. Surawicz B. R on T phenomenon: dangerous and harmless. J Appl Cardiol 1986;1:39–61.

19. Qi WH, Fineberg NS, Surawicz B. The timing of ventricular premature complexes initiating chronic ventricular tachycardia. J Electrocardiol 1984;17:377–84.

20. Berger MD, Waxman HL, Buxton AE, Marchlinski FE, Josephson ME. Spontaneous compared with induced onset of sustained ventricular tachycardia. Circulation 1988;78:885–92.

21. Myerburg RJ, Kessler KM, Luceri RM, et al. Classification of ventricular arrhythmias based on parallel hierarchies of frequency and form. Am J Cardiol 1984;54:1355–7.

22. Kim SG, Mercando AD, Fisher JD. Comparison of the characteristics of nonsustained ventricular tachycardia on Holter monitoring and sustained ventricular tachycardia observed spontaneously or induced by programmed stimulation. Am J Cardiol 1987;60:288–92.

23. Bayes de Luna A, Coumel P, Leclercq JF. Ambulatory sudden cardiac death: mechanisms of production of fatal arrhythmia on the basis of data from 157 cases. Am Heart J 1989;1:151–9.

24. Francis GS. Development of arrhythmias in the patient with congestive heart failure: pathophysiology, prevalence, and prognosis. Am J Cardiol 1986;57:3B–7B.

25. Glover DR, Littler WA. Factors influencing survival and mode of death in severe chronic ischaemic cardiac failure. Br Heart J 1987;57:125–32.

26. Rocco MB, Sherman H, Cook EF, Weisberg M, Flatley M, Goldman L. Correlates of cardiac and sudden death after ambulatory monitoring in a community hospital: importance of clinical characteristics, congestive heart failure and tachyarrhythmias. J Chronic Dis 1987;40:977–84.

27. Willens HJ, Blevins RD, Wrisley D, Antonishen D, Reinstein D, Rubenfire M. The prognostic value of functional capacity in patients with mild to moderate heart failure. Am Heart J 1987;114:377–82.

28. Olmsted WL, Groden DL, Silverman ME. Prognosis in survivors of acute myocardial infarction occurring at age 70 years or older. Am J Cardiol 1987;60:971–5.

29. Ritchie JL, Hallstrom AP, Troubaugh GB, Caldwell JH, Cobb LA. Out-of-hospital sudden coronary death: rest and exercise radionuclide left ventricular function in survivors. Am J Cardiol 1985;55:645–51.

30. Dargie HJ, Cleland JG, Leckie BJ, Inglis CG, East BW, Ford I. Relation of arrhythmias and electrolyte abnormalities to survival in patients with severe chronic heart failure. Circulation 1987;75(suppl IV):IV-98–107.

31. Olshausen KV, Stienen U, Math D, Schwarz F, Kubler W, Meyer J. Long-term prognostic significance of ventricular arrhythmias in idiopathic dilated cardiomyopathy. Am J Cardiol 1988;61:146–51.

32. Furberg CD, May GS. Effect of long-term prophylactic treatment on survival after myocardial infarction. Am J Med 1984;76:76–83.

33. Gottlieb SH, Achuff SC, Mellits D, et al. Prophylactic antiarrhythmic therapy of high-risk survivors of myocardial infarction: lower mortality at 1 month but not at 1 year. Circulation 1987;75:792–9.

34. The Cardiac Arrhythmia Pilot Study (CAPS) Investigators. Effects of encainide, flecainide, imipramine and moricizine on ventricular arrhythmias during the year after acute myocardial infarction: the CAPS. Am J Cardiol 1988;61:501–9.

35. Maisel AS, Scott N, Gilpin E, et al. Complex ventricular arrhythmias in patients with Q wave versus non-Q wave myocardial infarction. Circulation 1985;72:963–70.

36. Maron BJ, Savage DD, Wolfson JK, Epstein SE. Prognostic significance of 24 hour ambulatory electrocardiographic monitoring in patients with hypertrophic cardiomyopathy: a prospective study. Am J Cardiol 1981; 48:252–7.

37. McKenna WJ, England D, Doi YL, et al. Arrhythmia in hypertrophic cardiomyopathy: influence on prognosis. Br Heart J 1981;46:168–72.

38. Fleg JL, Gerstenblith G, Lakatta EG. Pathophysiology of the aging heart. In: Messerli FH, ed. Cardiovascular Disease in the Elderly. Boston, The Hague, Dordrecht, Lancaster: Martinus Nijhoff, 1984:11–34.

39. Spach MS, Dolber PC. Relating extracellular potentials and their derivatives to anisotropic propagation at a microscopic level in human cardiac muscle. Circ Res 1986;58:356–71.

40. Mirowski M, Reid PR, Winkle RA, et al. Mortality in patients with implanted automatic defibrillators. Ann Intern Med 1983;98:585–8.

41. Winkle RA, Mead RH, Ruder MA, et al. Long-term outcome with the automatic implantable cardioverter-defibrillator. J Am Coll Cardiol 1989;13:1353–61.

42. Antoni H. Unterschiedliche Wirkungsmechanismen der elektrischen Beeinflussung des Herzens in verschiedenen Stromstarkebereichen. Beitr. z. ersten Hilfe und Behandlung von Unfallen durch elektrischen Strom 1971;6:3–19.

43. Ferrier GR, Saunders JH, Mendez C. A cellular mechanism for the generation of ventricular arrhythmias by acetylstrophanthidin. Circ Res 1973;32:600–9.

44. Surawicz B. Electrophysiologic substrate of torsade de pointes: dispersion of repolarization or early afterdepolarizations? J Am Coll Cardiol 1989;14:172–84.

45. Kléber AG, Janse MJ, VanCapelle FJL, Durrer D. Mechanisms and time course of S-T and T-Q segment changes during acute regional myocardial ischemia in the pig heart determined by extracellular and intracellular recording. Circ Res 1978;42:603–13.

46. Hill JL, Gettes LS. Effect of acute coronary artery occlusion on local myocardial extracellular K^+ activity in swine. Circulation 1980;61:768–77.

47. Surawicz B, Chlebus H, Mazzoleni A. Hemodynamic and electrocardiographic effects of hyperpotassemia. Am Heart J 1967;73:647–64.

48. Woelfel A, Foster JR, McAllister RG Jr, Simpson RJ Jr, Gettes LS. Efficacy of verapamil in exercise-induced ventricular tachycardia. Am J Cardiol 1985;56:292–7.

49. Woelfel A, Foster JR, Simpson RJ Jr, Gettes LS. Reproducibility and treatment of exercise-induced ventricular tachycardia. Am J Cardiol 1984;53:751–6.

50. Lerman BB, Belardinelli L, West AL, Berne RM, DiMarco JP. Adenosine-sensitive ventricular tachycardia: evidence suggesting cyclic AMP-mediated triggered activity. Circulation 1986;74:270–80.

51. Caceres J, Jazayeri M, McKinnie J, et al. Sustained bundle branch reentry as a mechanism of clinical tachycardia. Circulation 1989;79:256–70.

52. Josephson ME, Horowitz LN, Farshidi A, Spielman SR, Michelson JEL, Greenspan AM. Sustained ventricular tachycardia: evidence for protected localized reentry. Am J Cardiol 1978;42:416–24.

53. Almendral JM, Stamato NJ, Rosenthal ME, Marchlinski FE, Miller JM, Josephson ME. Resetting response patterns during sustained ventricular tachycardia: relationship to the excitable gap. Circulation 1986;74:722–30.

54. Okumura K, Olshansky B, Henthorn RW, Epstein AE, Plump VJ, Waldo AL. Demonstration of the presence of slow conduction during sustained ventricular tachycardia in man: use of transient entrainment of the tachycardia. Circulation 1987;75:369–78.

55. Rosenthal ME, Stamato NJ, Almendral JM, Gottlieb CD, Josephson ME. Resetting of ventricular tachycardia with electrocardiographic fusion: incidence and significance. Circulation 1988;77:581–8.

56. Downar E, Harris L, Michleborough LL, Shaikh N, Parson ID. Endocardial mapping of ventricular tachycardia in the intact human ventricle: evidence for reentrant mechanisms. J Am Coll Cardiol 1988;11:783–91.

57. Friedman PL, Stewart JR, Wit AL. Spontaneous and induced cardiac arrhythmias in subendocardial Purkinje fibers surviving extensive myocardial infarction in dogs. Circ Res 1973;33:612–26.

58. Karagueuzian HS, Fenoglio JJ, Weiss MB, Wit AL. Protracted ventricular tachycardia induced by premature stimulation of the canine heart

after coronary artery occlusion and reperfusion. Circ Res 1979;44:833–46.

59. Wit AL, Allessie M, Bonke FIM, Lammers W, Smeets J, Fenoglio JJ. Electrophysiologic mapping to determine the mechanism of experimental ventricular tachycardia initiated by premature impulses: experimental approach and initial results demonstrating reentrant excitation. Am J Cardiol 1982;49:166–85.

60. El-Sherif N, Mehra R, Gough WB, Zeiler RH. Ventricular activation of spontaneous and induced ventricular rhythms in canine one-day-old myocardial infarction. Circ Res 1982;51:152–66.

61. Gessman LJ, Agarawal JB, Endo T, Helfant RH. Localization and mechanism of ventricular tachycardia by ice mapping 1 week after the onset of myocardial infarction in dogs. Circulation 1983;68:657–66.

62. Cardinal R, Savard P, Carson DL, Perry JB, Page P. Mapping of ventricular tachycardia induced by programmed stimulation in canine preparations of myocardial infarction. Circulation 1984;70:136–48.

63. Kramer JB, Saffitz JE, Witkowski FX, Corr PB. Intramural reentry as a mechanism of ventricular tachycardia during evolving canine myocardial infarction. Circ Res 1985;56:736–54.

64. Gough WB, Mehra R, Restivo M, Zeiler RH, El-Sherif N. Reentrant ventricular arrhythmias in the late myocardial infarction period in the dog. 13. Correlation of activation and refractory maps. Circ Res 1985;57:432–42.

65. Garan H, Fallon JT, Rosenthal S, Ruskin JN. Endocardial, intramural, and epicardial activation patterns during sustained monomorphic ventricular tachycardia in late canine myocardial infarction. Circ Res 1987;60:879–96.

66. Restivo M, Gough WB, El-Sherif N. Reentrant ventricular rhythms in the late myocardial infarction period: prevention of reentry by dual stimulation during basic rhythm. Circulation 1988;77:429–44.

67. Gardner PI, Ursell PC, Fenoglio JJ Jr, et al. Electrophysiologic and anatomic basis for fractionated electrograms recorded from healed myocardial infarcts. Circulation 1985;72:596–611.

68. Dillon SM, Alessie MA, Ursell PC, Wit AL. Influences of anisotropic tissue structure on reentrant circuits in the epicardial border zone of subacute canine infarcts. Circ Res 1988;63:182–206.

69. DeBakker JMT, VanCapelle FJL, Janse MJ, et al. Reentry as a cause of ventricular tachycardia in patients with chronic ischemic heart disease: electrophysiologic and anatomic correlation. Circulation 1988;77:589–606.

70. Kadish AH, Spear JF, Levine JH, Moore EN. The effects of procainamide on conduction in anisotropic canine ventricular myocardium. Circulation 1986;74:616–25.

71. Bajaj AK, Kopelman HA, Wikswo JP, Cassidy F, Woosley RL, Roden DM. Frequency- and orientation-dependent effects of mexiletine and quinidine on conduction in the intact dog heart. Circulation 1987;75:1065–73.

72. Spach MS, Dolber PC, Heidlage JF. Influence of the passive anisotropic properties on directional differences in propagation following modification of the sodium conductance in human atrial muscle. Circ Res 1988;62:811–32.

73. Follansbee WP, Michelson EL, Morganroth J. Nonsustained ventricular tachycardia in ambulatory patients: characteristics and association with sudden cardiac death. Ann Intern Med 1980;92:741–7.

74. Stamato NK, O'Connell JB, Murdock DK, et al. The response of patients with complex ventricular arrhythmias secondary to dilated cardiomyopathy to programmed electrical stimulation. Am Heart J 1986;112:505–8.

75. Rahimtoola SH, Zipes DP, Akhtar M, et al. Consensus statement of the conference on the state of the art of electrophysiologic testing in the diagnosis and treatment of patients with cardiac arrhythmias. Circulation 1987;75(suppl III):III-3–11.

76. Roy D, Marchand E, Theroux P, Waters DD, Pelletier GB, Bourassa MG. Programmed ventricular stimulation in survivors of an acute myocardial infarction. Circulation 1985;72:487–94.

77. Simson MB, Untereker WJ, Spielman SR, et al. Relation between late potentials on the body surface and directly recorded fragmented electrograms in patients with ventricular tachycardia. Am J Cardiol 1983;51:105–12.

78. Belhassen B, Shapira I, Pelleg A, Copperman I, Kauli N, Laniado S. Idiopathic recurrent sustained ventricular tachycardia responsive to verapamil: an ECG-electrophysiologic entity. Am Heart J 1984;108:1034–7.

79. Reddy CP, Kuo CS, Atarashi H, Surawicz B, McAllister RG Jr. Absence of slow channel-dependent conduction within the His-Purkinje (bundle branch) reentrant circuit: a clinical and experimental study of the effects of verapamil. Am J Cardiol 1982;49:724–32.

80. Davis LD, Temte JV. Effects of propranolol on the transmembrane potentials of ventricular muscle and Purkinje fibers of the dog. Circ Res 1968;22:661–77.

81. Anderson JL, Askins JC, Gilbert EM, et al. Multicenter trial of sotalol for suppression of frequent, complex ventricular arrhythmias: double-blind, randomized, placebo-controlled evaluation of two doses. J Am Coll Cardiol 1986;8:752–62.

82. McComb JM, McGovern B, McGowan BJ, Ruskin JN, Garan H. Electrophysiologic effects of d-sotalol in humans. J Am Coll Cardiol 1987;10:211–7.

83. Carmeliet E. Electrophysiologic and voltage clamp analysis of the effects of sotalol on isolated cardiac muscle and Purkinje fibers. J Pharmacol Exp Ther 1984;232:817–25.

84. Hondeghem LM, Katzung BG. Time- and voltage-dependent interactions of antiarrhythmic drugs with cardiac sodium channels. Biochem Biophys Acta 1977;472:373–98.

85. Grant AO, Starmer F, Strauss HC. Antiarrhythmic drug action: blockade of the inward sodium current. Circ Res 1984;55:427–39.

86. Varro A, Elharrar V, Surawicz B. Frequency-dependent effects of several class I antiarrhythmic drugs on Vmax of action potential upstroke in canine cardiac Purkinje fibers. J Cardiovasc Pharmacol 1985;7:482–92.

87. Varro A, Nakaya Y, Elharrar V, Surawicz B. Effect of antiarrhythmic drugs on the cycle length-dependent action potential duration in dog Purkinje and ventricular muscle fibers. J Cardiovasc Pharmacol 1986;8:178–85.

88. Salata JJ, Wasserstrom JA. Effects of quinidine on action potentials and ionic currents in isolated canine ventricular myocytes. Circ Res 1988;62:324–37.

89. Horowitz LN, Borggrefe M. Many things are not found in books or journals . . . but some things are!; value of electrophysiologic testing in patients with malignant ventricular arrhythmias. Am J Cardiol 1988;62:1292–4.

90. Brugada P. Should electrophysiologic studies be performed to assess drug efficacy in patients receiving amiodarone? Am J Cardiol 1987;59:1415–6.

91. Kim SG, Felder SD, Figura I, Johnston DR, Mercando AD, Fisher JD. The prognostic value of the changes in the mode of ventricular tachycardia induction noted during therapy with amiodarone or amiodarone and a class Ia antiarrhythmic agent. Am J Cardiol 1987;59:1314–8.

92. Herre JM, Sauve MJ, Malone P, et al. Long-term results of amiodarone therapy in patients with recurrent sustained ventricular tachycardia or ventricular fibrillation. J Am Coll Cardiol 1989;13:442–9.

93. Steinbeck G, Andresen D, Leitner ER. Sind Antiarrhythmika einem Betablocker ueberlegen in der Behandlung lebensbedrohlicher ventrikularer Rhythmus-storungen? Vorläufige Ergebnisse einer kontrollierten Studie. Z Kardiol 1986;75:47–55.

94. Rodriguez LM, Brugada P, Waleffe A, et al. Outcome of empirical antiarrhythmic drug therapy in matched cohorts of patients with ventricular arrhythmias after myocardial infarction (abstr). J Am Coll Cardiol 1989;13:173A.

95. Lehman MH, Steinman RT, Schuger CD, Jackson K. The automatic implantable cardioverter-defibrillator as antiarrhythmic treatment modality of choice for survivors of cardiac arrest unrelated to acute myocardial infarction (editorial). Am J Cardiol 1988;62:803–5.

96. The Flecainide-Quinidine Research Group. Flecainide versus quinidine for treatment of chronic ventricular arrhythmias: a multicenter clinical trial. Circulation 1983;67:1117–23.

97. Sokolow M. Some quantitative aspects of treatment with quinidine. Ann Intern Med 1956;45:582–6.

98. Helmy I, Herre JM, Gee G, et al. Use of intravenous amiodarone for emergency treatment of life-threatening ventricular arrhythmias. J Am Coll Cardiol 1988;12:1015–22.

99. Marchlinski FE, Buxton AE, Kindwall E, et al. Comparison of individual and combined effects of procainamide and amiodarone in patients with sustained ventricular tachyarrhythmias. Circulation 1988;78:583–91.

99a. Schmitt C, Kadish AH, Balke WC, et al. Cycle length-dependent effects on normal and abnormal intraventricular electrograms: effect of procainamide. J Am Coll Cardiol 1988;12:395–403.

100. Wenger TL, Browning DJ, Masterson CE, et al. Procainamide delivery to ischemic canine myocardium following rapid intravenous administration. Circ Res 1980;46:789–95.

101. Fozzard HA, Wasserstrom JA. Voltage dependence of intracellular sodium and control of contraction. In: Zipes DP, Jalife J, eds. Cardiac Electrophysiology and Arrhythmias. Orlando, San Diego, New York: Grune & Stratton, 1985:51–7.

102. Blaustein MP. The interrelationship between sodium and calcium fluxes across cell membranes. Rev Physiol Biochem Pharmacol 1974;70:33–82.

103. Sheu S, Lederer WJ. Lidocaine's negative inotropic and antiarrhythmic actions: dependence on shortening of action potential duration and reduction of intracellular sodium activity. Circ Res 1985;57:578–90.

104. Beltrame J, Aylward PE, McRitchie RJ, Chalmers JP. Comparative haemodynamic effects of lidocaine, mexiletine, and disopyramide. J Cardiovasc Pharmacol 1984;6:483–90.

105. Brugada P, Wellens HJJ. Arrhythmogenesis of antiarrhythmic drugs. Am J Cardiol 1988;61:1108–11.

106. Velebit V, Podrid P, Lown B, Cohen BH, Graboys TB. Aggravation and provocation of ventricular arrhythmias by antiarrhythmic drugs. Circulation 1982;65:886–94.

107. Hondeghem LM. Antiarrhythmic agents: modulated receptor applications. Circulation 1987;75:514–20.

108. Nathan AW, Hellestrand KJ, Beston RS, Banim SO, Spurrell RAJ, Camm AJ. Proarrhythmic effects of the new antiarrhythmic agent flecainide acetate. Am Heart J 1984;107:222–8.

109. Anastasiou-Nana MI, Anderson JL, Stewart JR, et al. Occurrence of exercise-induced and spontaneous wide complex tachycardia during therapy with flecainide for complex ventricular arrhythmias: a probable proarrhythmic effect. Am Heart J 1987;113:1071–7.

110. The Encainide-Ventricular Tachycardia Study Group. Treatment of life-threatening ventricular tachycardia with encainide hydrochloride in patients with left ventricular dysfunction. Am J Cardiol 1988;62:571–5.

111. DiBianco R, Fletcher RD, Cohen AI, et al. Treatment of frequent ventricular arrhythmia with encainide assessment using serial ambulatory electrocardiograms, intracardiac electrophysiologic studies, treadmill exercise tests, and radionuclide cineangiographic studies. Circulation 1982;65:1134–47.

112. Minardo JD, Heger JJ, Miles WM, Zipes DP, Prystowsky EN. Clinical characteristics of patients with ventricular fibrillation during antiarrhythmic drug therapy. N Engl J Med 1988;319:257–62.

113. Podrid PJ, Lampert S, Graboys TB, Blatt CM, Lown B. Aggravation of arrhythmia by antiarrhythmic drugs: incidence and predictors. Am J Cardiol 1987;59:38E–44E.

114. Morganroth J, Anderson JL, Gentzkow GD. Classification by type of ventricular arrhythmia predicts fequency of adverse cardiac events from flecainide. J Am Coll Cardiol 1986;8:607–15.

115. Morganroth J, Pratt CM. Prevalence and characteristics of proarrhythmia from moricizine (ethmozine). Am J Cardiol 1989;63:172–6.

116. Reddy CP, Damato AN, Akhtar M, Dhatt MS, Gomes MAC, Calon AH. Effect of procainamide on reentry within the His-Purkinje system in man. Am J Cardiol 1977;40:957–64.

117. Reddy CP, Lynch M. Abolition and modification of reentry within the His-Purkinje system by procainamide in man. Circulation 1978;58:1010–22.

118. Ruskin JN, McGovern B, Garan H, Dimarco JP, Kelly E. Antiarrhythmic drugs: a possible cause of out-of-hospital cardiac arrest. N Engl J Med 1983;309:1302–6.

119. Rae AP, Kay KR, Horowitz LN, Spielman SR, Greenspan AM. Proarrhythmic effects of antiarrhythmic drugs in patients with malignant ventricular arrhythmias evaluated by electrophysiologic testing. J Am Coll Cardiol 1988;12:131–9.

120. Gallagher JD, Fernandez J, Maranhao V, Gessman LJ. Simultaneous appearance of endocardial late potentials and ability to induce sustained ventricular tachycardia after procainamide administration. J Electrocardiol 1986;19:197–202.

121. Denniss AR, Ross DL, Richards DA, et al. Effect of antiarrhythmic therapy on delayed potentials detected by the signal-averaged electrocardiogram in patients with ventricular tachycardia after acute myocardial infarction. Am J Cardiol 1986;58:261–5.

122. Borbola J, Denes P. Oral amiodarone loading therapy. I. The effect on serial signal-averaged electrocardiographic recordings and the QT_c in patients with ventricular tachyarrhythmias. Am Heart J 1988;115:1202–8.

123. Winkle RA, Mason JW, Griffin JC, Ross D. Malignant ventricular tachyarrhythmias associated with the use of encainide. Am Heart J 1981;102:857–64.

124. Ruder MA, Ellis T, Lebsac C, Mead RH, Smith NA, Winkle RA. Clinical experience with sotalol in patients with drug-refractory ventricular arrhythmias. J Am Coll Cardiol 1989;13:145–52.

125. Dubois EL. Procainamide induction of a systemic lupus erythematosus-like syndrome: presentation of six cases, review of the literature, and analysis and followup of reported cases. Medicine 1969;48:217–27.

126. Ritchie MY, Greene NM. Local anesthetics. In: Gilman AG, Goodman LS, Roll TW, Murad F, eds. Goodman and Gilman's The Pharmacologic Basis of Therapeutics. 7th ed. New York: Macmillan, 1985:302–21.

127. Nygaard TW, Sellers D, Cook TS, DiMarco JP. Adverse reactions to antiarrhythmic drugs during therapy for ventricular arrhythmias. JAMA 1986;256:55–7.

128. Kim SG, Seiden SW, Matos JA, Waspe LE, Fisher JD. Combination of procainamide and quinidine for better tolerance and additive effects for ventricular arrhythmias. Am J Cardiol 1985;56:84–8.

129. Kim SG, Mercando AD, Fisher JD. Combination of tocainide and quinidine for better tolerance and additive effects in patients with coronary artery disease. J Am Coll Cardiol 1987;9:1369–74.

130. Duff HJ, Roden D, Primm RK, Oates JA, Woosley RL. Mexiletine in the treatment of resistant ventricular arrhythmias: enhancement of efficacy and reduction of dose-related side effects by combination with quinidine. Circulation 1983;67:1124–8.

131. Duff HJ, Mitchell B, Manyari D, Wyse DG. Mexiletine-quinidine combination: electrophysiologic correlates of a favorable antiarrhythmic interaction in humans. J Am Coll Cardiol 1987;10:1149–56.

132. Stevenson WG, Stevenson LW, Weiss J, Tillisch JH. Inducible ventricular arrhythmias and sudden death during vasodilator therapy of severe heart failure. Am Heart J 1988;116:1447–54.

133. Kay GN, Pryor DB, Lee KL, et al. Comparison of survival of amiodarone-treated patients with coronary artery disease and malignant ventricular arrhythmias with that of a control group with coronary artery disease. J Am Coll Cardiol 1987;9:877–81.

134. Varro A, Nakaya Y, Elharrar V, Surawicz B. Use-dependent effect of amiodarone on Vmax in cardiac Purkinje and ventricular muscle fibers. Eur J Pharmacol 1985;112:419–22.

135. Varro A, Nakaya Y, Elharrar V, Surawicz B. The effects of amiodarone on repolarization and refractoriness of cardiac fibers. Eur J Pharmacol 1988;154:11–8.

136. Nakaya Y, Elharrar V, Surawicz B. Effect of mexiletine, amiodarone and disopyramide on the excitability and refractoriness of canine cardiac fibers: possible relation to antiarrhythmic drug action and classification. Cardiovasc Drug Ther 1987;1:141–53.

137. Mason JW. Amiodarone. N Engl J Med 1987;316:457–66.

138. Levine JH, Moore EN, Kadish AH, et al. Mechanisms of depressed conduction from long-term amiodarone therapy in canine myocardium. Circulation 1988;78:684–91.

139. Kennedy TP, Gordon GB, Paky A, et al. Amiodarone causes acute oxidant lung injury in ventilated and perfused rabbit lungs. J Cardiovasc Pharmacol 1988;12:23–36.

CHAPTER 22

Treatment of Cardiac Arrhythmias: When, How, and Where?

HEIN J. J. WELLENS, MD, PEDRO BRUGADA, MD

Cardiac "arrhythmology" has seen major changes during the last 40 years. The introduction of several new techniques has contributed to better understanding of the mechanism, site of origin, prognosis and treatment of arrhythmias. These developments have improved the care of patients, but the wide range of possible diagnostic techniques and treatment modes has increased the risk of overtreatment or even maltreatment and unnecessary cost. What, then, is needed to know when, how and where to treat an arrhythmia successfully, safely and cost effectively? We have listed those requirements in Table 22.1 and will discuss these in more detail in this review.

Relation Between Pump Function, Blood Supply, Neurocontrol and Cardiac Rhythm

It is a mistake to prescribe antiarrhythmic medication without realizing that abnormalities of pump function, blood supply or neurocontrol of the heart may be totally or partially responsible for a cardiac arrhythmia. Most physicians know that atrial fibrillation is a rare arrhythmia in the healthy heart and that proper treatment requires a careful evaluation to identify, and when possible correct, causes like cardiac muscle stretch, ischemia, inflammation, fibrosis, infiltration, intoxication or abnormalities in neurocontrol of the atria. In principle, the same holds for any type of supraventricular or ventricular arrhythmia.

Clinical factors. Figure 22.1 illustrates the many factors that play a role in the occurrence of an arrhythmia and how they are interrelated. Some of these factors are present over a long period of time—for example, the degree of vessel narrowing in chronic coronary artery disease or an increased or decreased amount of heart muscle as in ventricular hypertrophy or after an old myocardial infarction. Other factors are dynamic—for example, changes in platelet function, degree of ischemia, the neurophysiologic system and so forth.

The finding of a cardiac arrhythmia should always be a stimulus for careful history taking and an appropriate physical examination. These should be followed by suitable noninvasive and invasive studies in search of indications for heart disease. The discovery of ventricular premature beats in a patient after a myocardial infarction should first be a stimulus to rule out (and when present, treat!) ischemia outside the infarcted area and disturbances of pump function rather than a cue to prescribe antiarrhythmic medication.

A good arrhythmologist should first be a good clinician!

He or she should not only identify (and possibly correct) static contributing factors but also control (as far as possible) dynamic changes.

Different Types of Cardiac Arrhythmias, Their Site of Origin, Electrocardiographic Diagnosis, Mechanism and the Importance of Their Etiology

Observations in the tissue bath, the isolated and intact animal heart and the human heart have resulted in a better understanding of the possible mechanisms of cardiac arrhythmias (1–6). Programmed electrical stimulation of the heart combined with the recordings of local endocardial and epicardial electrical activity frequently allows us to localize the site of origin or pathway of the arrhythmia in the intact human heart (7–11). Careful evaluation of the 12 lead electrocardiogram (ECG) during the arrhythmia at the time of programmed electrical stimulation and cardiac activation mapping has resulted in the recognition of specific ECG patterns. This has made it possible to distinguish among the different types of supraventricular tachycardia, to locate the site of atrioventricular (AV) block, the site of origin of a ventricular tachycardia and the ventricular and atrial end of an accessory AV pathway and to differentiate between a supraventricular and a ventricular origin of a wide QRS tachycardia (12–26). A review of these advances has recently been published elsewhere (27).

Mechanism of reentry. The observation that most clinically occurring regular sustained tachycardias can reproducibly be initiated and terminated by timed extrastimuli during programmed electrical stimulation suggests that reentry is the most common mechanism of these arrhythmias. However, proof that reentry is the tachycardia mechanism can only be provided by delineating the pathway and demonstrating that the arrhythmia can be terminated temporarily by creating refractoriness in a part of the circuit and definitively by (surgical, electrical or chemical) ablation of part of the pathway.

Other arrhythmogenic mechanisms: early and late afterdepolarizations. In recent years, increasing attention has been given to other arrhythmogenic mechanisms that may play a role in clinically occurring arrhythmias. In isolated tissue, early and late afterdepolarizations have been shown to lead to arrhythmias (6). Early afterdepolarizations, which can be produced experimentally by barium, hypoxia, high concentration of catecholamines, sotalol, N-acetyl procainamide

Table 22.1. Requirements for the Cardiologist Treating
Arrhythmias

1. Understanding of the relation between pump function, blood supply,
   neurocontrol and rhythm of the heart.
2. Knowledge of the different types of cardiac arrhythmias, their site of
   origin, electrocardiographic diagnosis, mechanism and importance of
   their etiology.
3. Knowledge of when to treat and understanding of the value and
   limitations of the different diagnostic techniques.
4. Understanding risk stratification of arrhythmias.
5. Knowledge of the value, limitations and costs of the different
   therapeutic options.

and cesium (6), have been suggested as a cause of torsade de
pointes in patients with the congenital or acquired long QT
syndrome (28,29). Late afterdepolarizations can be induced
experimentally by digitalis and seem to be responsible for
some clinical arrhythmias occurring in digitalis intoxication
(30). Arrhythmogenic mechanisms based on afterdepolarizations and their possible clinical implications were recently
discussed by Zipes (2). Unfortunately, intracellular recordings are not possible in the intact human heart, making the
study of the relevance of these mechanisms to human
arrhythmias extremely difficult. A possible solution might be
the development of drugs specifically counteracting early or
delayed afterdepolarizations (31) or the use of special electrode catheters that record a monophasic action potential
resembling an intracellular recording (32).

*It is important to recognize not only the type, site of
origin and mechanism of the arrhythmia but also its etiology.* As shown in Table 22.2, the value of ventricular
tachycardia/fibrillation as a prognostic indicator for cardiac
death in patients with an old myocardial infarction is totally
different from the value in patients who have arrhythmogenic right ventricular dysplasia or are without heart
disease (so called idiopathic ventricular tachycardia or ventricular fibrillation). Similarly, the prognostic importance of

advanced forms of ventricular arrhythmias has been well
documented in ventricular hypertrophy (of all causes) and
cardiomyopathy (33–35).

Value and Limitations of Different Diagnostic Techniques

Ambulatory electrocardiographic recordings. Several
noninvasive and invasive tests are currently used in patients
suffering from arrhythmias. The type, incidence, etiology
and significance of an arrhythmia determine which diagnostic test or tests should be performed. That choice is also
influenced by the preferred treatment (drugs, surgery, electrical ablation, pacing, and so forth). As pointed out by
several investigators, frequently occurring arrhythmias can
best be studied by 24 h ECG ambulatory (Holter) recordings.
Such recordings can also give information about the role of
the autonomic nervous system and the effect of therapeutic
interventions (36). Unfortunately, however, 35% to 50% of
patients with documented sustained ventricular tachycardia
or ventricular fibrillation do not show complex arrhythmias
on Holter monitoring (37).

Invasive electrophysiologic study. Such a study is usually
selected when the arrhythmia occurs infrequently and the
somatic or psychologic consequences, or both, require information as to the site of origin and the best therapeutic
approach. An electrophysiologic study not only identifies the
site of origin of the arrhythmia, which is essential when
surgical, electrical or chemical ablative therapy is considered, but also allows the evaluation of the effect of pharmacologic or nonpharmacologic therapy (38).

Holter versus electrophysiologic study. An important
question is which of the two methods (ambulatory ECG
recording or an electrophysiologic study) provides the most
accurate prediction of antiarrhythmic drug efficacy. The only
available randomized comparison of the two methods (39)
suggests that electrophysiologic study is better than Holter

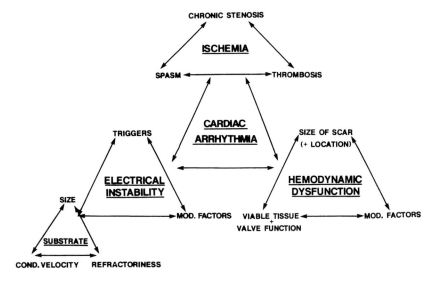

Figure 22.1. Model showing the factors that
play a role in cardiac arrhythmias. The basic
triangle consists of electrical instability, hemodynamic dysfunction and ischemia. Each of
these three cornerstones has static and dynamic
components. Modulating (MOD.) factors include the autonomic nervous system, electrolytes, hormones and drugs. COND. = conduction.

Table 22.2. Relation Between Etiology of Ventricular Tachycardia/Ventricular Fibrillation (VT/VF) and Arrhythmia Recurrence and Death During Follow-Up

	Old MI	RVD		Idiopathic	
	SMVT	VF	SMVT	SMVT	VF
Total no. of patients	79	37	11	52	6
Total deaths	15 (19%)	13 (35%)	1 (19%)	1* (2%)	0
Sudden cardiac deaths	5 (6%)	5 (14%)	0	0	0
No. of patients with VT/VF recurrence	24 (30%)	7 (19%)	6 (67%)	15 (28%)	2 (33%)
Length of follow-up (mo)	26	22	39	86	39

*Patient died of cancer. MI = myocardial infarction; RVD = right ventricular dysplasia; SMVT = sustained monomorphic ventricular tachycardia.

monitoring in predicting success of therapy. Limitations of this investigation include the small number of patients studied and the use of nonstandardized drug therapy. A multicenter study (the Electrophysiologic Study Versus Electrocardiographic Monitoring [ESVEM] trial) (40) involving a much larger number of patients is currently addressing this problem. It should be realized, however, that Holter monitoring primarily registers the effect of an intervention on spontaneously occurring arrhythmias whereas the electrophysiologic study gives information on the effect on the substrate of the arrhythmia. Information from both tests is therefore frequently required to obtain optimal information on the response to therapy.

Signal-averaged electrocardiogram. This recording usually shows late potentials in patients having a myocardial area of slow conduction as the basis for their reentrant ventricular tachycardia (41). The finding of late potentials does not establish the presence of a reentrant circuit but may only indicate an area of delayed activation. The prognostic significance of a ventricular late potential on the signal-averaged surface ECG as a marker for an increased incidence of life-threatening ventricular arrhythmias and sudden death is currently being investigated (42). It is less commonly found in patients with spontaneous ventricular fibrillation than in patients with spontaneous ventricular tachycardia (43). Controversies exist about the signal-processing techniques for detecting ventricular late potentials (44–46). We believe that more follow-up studies are needed to establish the true value (alone or in combination with other techniques, like the left ventricular ejection fraction) of the signal-averaged ECG to identify patients at high risk for the spontaneous occurrence of sustained ventricular tachycardia.

Role of exercise testing. Exercise testing should not only be performed in patients with a history of exercise-related arrhythmias or to identify ischemia in a patient with an arrhythmia but also because induction of a sustained ventricular arrhythmia by exercise carries a poor prognosis. Exercise testing should always be performed when a patient is placed on an antiarrhythmic drug regimen because drugs, especially those slowing intraventricular conduction, may promote the occurrence of ventricular tachycardia during exercise (47,48). Exercise testing is therefore an essential investigation to identify a possible proarrhythmic effect of a drug (49).

Risk Stratification of Arrhythmias

As already discussed (Table 22.2) etiology plays an important role in the prognostic significance of an arrhythmia. But even within a seemingly homogeneous group such as that of patients developing monomorphic ventricular tachycardia or ventricular fibrillation outside the acute phase of myocardial infarction, marked differences in risk can be (and have to be) recognized.

Risk factors for cardiac death. Figures 22.2 and 22.3 present four questions related to the clinical history that can be of great help in assessing risk for nonsudden and sudden cardiac death in these patients (50). These questions are: 1) What is the New York Heart Association functional classification exclusive of the arrhythmia? 2) Did the patient lose

Figure 22.2. Estimation of risk of sudden death based on the four clinical variables discussed in the text. As shown in this group of 200 consecutive patients with a previous myocardial infarction (MI) developing ventricular tachycardia (VT) or ventricular fibrillation (VF), there was a 6% incidence of dying suddenly within 2 years. NYHA = New York Heart Association classification for dyspnea.

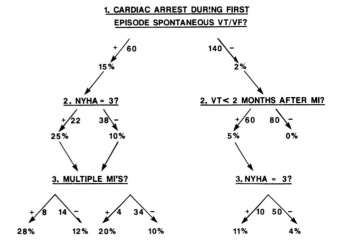

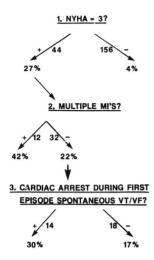

Figure 22.3. Estimation of risk of nonsudden cardiac death in the same patients as in Figure 22.2. The overall incidence of nonsudden cardiac death at 2 years was 9%. Abbreviations as in Figure 22.2.

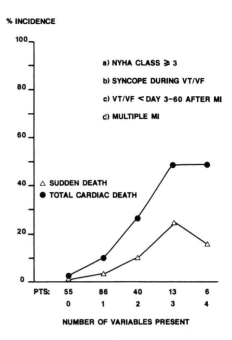

Figure 22.4. Incidence of total cardiac death (●) and sudden cardiac death (△) in relation to the total score of four clinical variables in 200 patients (pts) with ventricular tachycardia (169 patients) or ventricular fibrillation (VF) (31 patients) after myocardial infarction (MI). The four clinical variables are listed in the upper right corner of the figure. As shown, depending on the number of variables present, marked differences exist in sudden and total cardiac death after 2 years of follow-up.

consciousness during the arrhythmia? 3) Did the first episode of ventricular tachycardia or ventricular fibrillation occur between day 3 to day 60 after myocardial infarction, or later? 4) Has the patient had more than one prior myocardial infarction?

We found in 200 consecutive patients with ventricular tachycardia or fibrillation after a myocardial infarction (Fig. 22.2) that with these questions we could recognize patients with a very low chance of dying suddenly (those not losing consciousness during the first episode of their spontaneous ventricular tachycardia or fibrillation and having the arrhythmia >2 months after their myocardial infarction). In contrast, the question also identified patients who had a 25% chance of sudden cardiac death within 2 years (Fig. 22.2).

Figure 22.3 shows that pump function is the most important discriminator for risk of nonsudden cardiac death in patients with ventricular tachycardia and ventricular fibrillation after a myocardial infarction. Figure 22.4 indicates how the total score of the four variables from the clinical history influences the risk for sudden and total cardiac death in the first 2 years in patients whose first episode of ventricular tachyarrhythmia occurs >3 days after a myocardial infarction. Figure 22.5 shows (using the same variables as in Figures 22.2 to 22.4) that, in contrast to survival, recurrences of ventricular tachycardia are not related to the score of the four questions from the clinical history.

Risk of fatal arrhythmia after infarction without spontaneous arrhythmia. All patients shown in Figures 22.2 to 22.5 entered the study after they had had a spontaneous episode of ventricular tachycardia and ventricular fibrillation after a myocardial infarction. A much more difficult problem is to estimate risk of dying from an arrhythmia in the survivor of a myocardial infarction without a spontaneously occurring life-threatening ventricular arrhythmia. It has been recog-

nized that the finding of complex forms of ventricular arrhythmia, primarily runs of nonsustained ventricular tachycardia on ambulatory ECG monitoring, is associated with an increased risk of sudden cardiac death (51–54). Similar observations have been made in patients with hypertrophic or dilated cardiomyopathy (55–57). Additional impairment of left ventricular function leads to an exponential increase in incidence of sudden death (58).

Apart from information about spontaneous ventricular arrhythmias on ambulatory ECG monitoring, pump function (usually obtained by measuring left ventricular ejection fraction) and reversible myocardial ischemia at exercise testing, the use of other techniques has been suggested to improve stratification of risk for a life-threatening arrhythmia after a myocardial infarction. Richards et al. (59) indicated that induction of a "slow" ventricular tachycardia (shortly after myocardial infarction, cycle length ≥230 ms) by programmed stimulation of the heart was a strong predictor of sudden death or spontaneous ventricular tachycardia in the first year after a myocardial infarction. This finding was independent of left ventricular ejection fraction and was of more value than the signal-averaged ECG. There is discussion, however, about the value of programmed electrical stimulation in risk stratification after myocardial infarction (60–63). This factor and the risks and costs of the test do

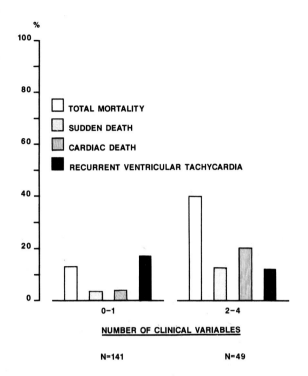

Figure 22.5. Risk of dying suddenly and nonsuddenly and of recurrent episodes of ventricular tachycardia in relation to the presence of the same four variables shown in Figure 22.4. Recurrences of ventricular tachycardia were at least as common in patients with no or one variable as in patients having two to four variables.

not support its use for routine risk stratification of patients recovering from an acute myocardial infarction.

Value, Limitations and Costs of the Different Therapeutic Options

Table 22.3 shows the different therapeutic modes currently available in relation to their effect on the arrhythmia substrate, costs, required expertise, long-term efficacy and side effects.

Antiarrhythmic Drugs

Currently available antiarrhythmic drugs do not destroy the substrate of the arrhythmia. They may change the electrophysiologic properties like conduction velocity or refractory period duration within the substrate or may prevent the trigger of arrhythmia-like ventricular premature beats or sudden changes in heart rate. In Europe, approximately 50 different antiarrhythmic drugs are available. All of these drugs differ in their effects—their half-life (Fig. 22.6), resorption, breakdown, excretion, active metabolites, side effects, and so forth. To make the situation even more complicated, their electrophysiologic effects may be related to heart rate and may be different in healthy and diseased cardiac tissue.

The CAST study: role of class Ic drugs. The interim results of the Cardiac Arrhythmia Suppression Trial (CAST) study (64) highlight some of the problems with antiarrhythmic drug therapy. The intention of the CAST study was to answer the question: Does suppression of ventricular ectopic activity after a myocardial infarction result in better outcome? The CAST study was based on the evidence (51–54) that ventricular ectopic activity after myocardial infarction worsens prognosis. Previous studies (65–67) have failed to show benefit of treatment by antiarrhythmic drugs, with the exception of beta-adrenergic blocking agents, but in those studies patients were not selected after it had been shown that the antiarrhythmic drug was able to markedly reduce ventricular ectopic activity.

Although complete data are not available, preliminary results indicate that administration of flecainide and encainide (after having been shown to suppress ventricular ectopic activity) resulted in a higher arrhythmic death rate than that of patients receiving placebo. What caused this unfavorable effect? A few possible mechanisms have to be considered. First, some patients, after administration of a class Ic drug, show widening of the QRS complex on exercise, indicating slowing in intraventricular conduction with increasing heart rate. This event may have favored the induction of ventricular tachycardia (48,49). Second, Nattel et al. (68) observed some years ago in dogs, that pretreatment with an antiarrhythmic drug slowing conduction (aprindine) followed by coronary artery occlusion resulted in a much higher incidence of life-threatening ventricular arrhythmias than that of dogs having coronary obstruction without previous antiarrhythmic drug treatment. The investigators found marked slowing in conduction in the ischemic area in the dogs pretreated with aprindine. These observations suggest the possibility that, during an ischemic episode the occurrence of ventricular arrhythmias is facilitated in patients with coronary artery disease treated with an antiarrhythmic drug that slows conduction.

Third, class Ic drugs (like flecainide and encainide) slow conduction velocity without affecting the duration of the refractory period of myocardial tissue. Figure 22.7, which is based on observations by Brugada et al. (69) in an animal model of ventricular tachycardia, shows that, depending on the length of the reentrant circuit, slowing in conduction velocity without lengthening of the refractory period may result in the situation that two (instead of one) circulating impulses can fit within one reentrant circuit. A possible clinical example is given in Figure 22.8. Theoretically, therefore, after administration of a class Ic drug, acceleration of a ventricular ectopic rhythm (possibly leading to sudden death) may occur if a ventricular reentrant circuit is present after myocardial infarction.

Our group (62) has demonstrated that ventricular reentrant circuits are present in about 40% of patients studied by programmed stimulation of the heart shortly after myocardial infarction. The incidence of such a circuit did not differ

Table 22.3. Current Modes of Therapy of Arrhythmias in Relation to Effect on Arrhythmia Substrate, Costs, Required Expertise, Long-Term Efficacy and Side Effects

	Drugs	Surgery	Electrical Ablation	Chemical Ablation	Pacing Dev/Defib
Arrhythmia substrate removed	No	Yes	Yes	Yes	No
Costs	Low	High	Moderate	Moderate	Moderately high
Specialized center	?	Required	Required	Required	Required
Long-term efficacy	Yes	Yes	?	?	Yes
Side effects	Yes	10 to 15% operative mortality in VT	Myocardial damage	Myocardial damage	Psychological

Abl = ablation; Defib = implantable defibrillator; Pacing Dev = implantable pacing device; VT = ventricular tachycardia.

in patients with or without documented episodes of nonsustained ventricular tachycardia. A reentrant circuit (as demonstrated by the reproducible initiation of sustained ventricular tachycardia during programmed stimulation) was present in 93% of patients with documented spontaneous episodes of sustained ventricular tachycardia. These observations suggest that in a large number of patients a possible ventricular reentrant circuit is present after myocardial infarction *independent of the spontaneous occurrence of ventricular tachycardia.* Administration of an agent slowing conduction velocity without lengthening the refractory period may under those circumstances facilitate (as shown in Fig. 22.7 and 22.8) the occurrence of a more rapid ventricular tachycardia possibly leading to sudden cardiac death.

Implications. The marked differences in properties among antiarrhythmic drugs can make the selection of such drugs very difficult. This is reason for us to stress that 1) a physician treating arrhythmias should be really knowledgeable about a few antiarrhythmic drugs (and restrict himself or herself to those drugs); and 2) high risk patients should be referred to a center with expertise and equipment for treating arrhythmias.

Surgery

Identification of the site of origin of an arrhythmia (as in atrial or ventricular tachycardia) or the essential component in a tachycardia pathway (like the accessory AV pathway in the Wolff-Parkinson-White syndrome) was the basis for the development of new surgical methods for treating arrhythmias. At present, many different types of tachycardias can be approached surgically. In some types, surgical treatment is still in an experimental phase (as in atrial flutter or atrial fibrillation), in others (like the Wolff-Parkinson-White syndrome, AV node tachycardia and ventricular tachycardia) their value is well established (70–78). As pointed out in Table 22.3, by removing, isolating or interrupting the arrhythmia substrate, surgery offers curative treatment. It can only be done, however, in specialized centers having expertise in localizing the arrhythmia. Operative risk depends on the type of arrhythmia. Perioperative mortality varies from 10% to 15% for ventricular tachycardia to almost zero for the Wolff-Parkinson-White syndrome (77,78).

In ventricular tachycardia, operative mortality and long-term outcome can be improved by careful selection of

Figure 22.6. The mean half-life of several currently available antiarrhythmic drugs; marked differences exist among these drugs. Half-life is only one property of the drug. There are also differences in pharmacokinetics, breakdown, excretion, active metabolites, side effects, and so forth.

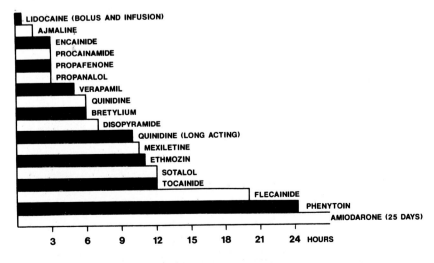

LIDOCAINE (BOLUS AND INFUSION)
AJMALINE
ENCAINIDE
PROCAINAMIDE
PROPAFENONE
PROPANALOL
VERAPAMIL
QUINIDINE
BRETYLIUM
DISOPYRAMIDE
QUINIDINE (LONG ACTING)
MEXILETINE
ETHMOZIN
SOTALOL
TOCAINIDE
FLECAINIDE
PHENYTOIN
AMIODARONE (25 DAYS)

3   6   9   12   15   18   21   24   HOURS

HALF LIFE OF ANTIARRHYTHMIC DRUGS

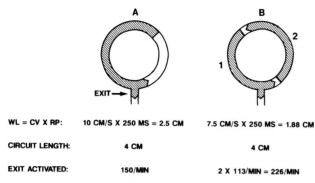

WL = CV X RP:	10 CM/S X 250 MS = 2.5 CM	7.5 CM/S X 250 MS = 1.88 CM
CIRCUIT LENGTH:	4 CM	4 CM
EXIT ACTIVATED:	150/MIN	2 X 113/MIN = 226/MIN

Figure 22.7. Possible mechanism of acceleration in rate of tachycardia by a drug that slows conduction velocity but does not prolong the refractory period. **Panel A** shows a reentrant circuit with a length of 4 cm and a single exit point. The wave length (WL) of the circulating impulse (the product of conduction velocity [CV] and the refractory period [RV]) measures 10 cm/s × 250 ms = 2.5 cm. Each minute, 150 impulses will leave the exit point. **Panel B** shows the situation after the administration of a drug (like a class Ic drug) that slows conduction without lengthening the refractory period (RP) within the circuit. The wave length (WL) now measures 7.5 cm/s × 200 ms = 1.88 cm. This means that two consecutive impulses can fit within the circuit of 4 cm. Each minute 2 × 113 = 226 impulses will reach the exit point of the circuit.

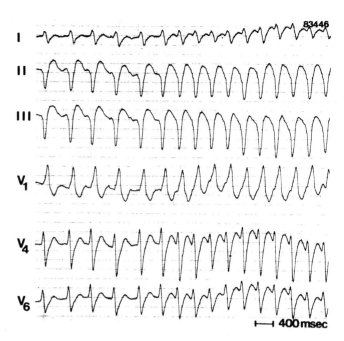

Figure 22.8. Possible clinical example of the situation in Figure 22.7. During intravenous administration of a class Ic drug a sudden acceleration in rate of ventricular tachycardia is observed without change in QRS configuration. The change in RR interval 500 ms to 380 ms can be explained by assuming a change from one to two circulating impulses within one reentrant circuit. Other possible mechanisms are a sudden change from a larger to a smaller reentrant circuit using the same exit point.

patients. Van Hemel et al. (79) recently reported on the use of a left ventricular segmental wall motion score for that purpose. They suggested nonsurgical therapy if less than three of nine segments of the left ventricle showed normal motion or slight hypokinesia.

Costs of surgery are high because of the detailed electrophysiologic studies required before, during and after operation, but as shown for the Wolff-Parkinson-White syndrome, surgical treatment can be cost effective (80).

Electrical Ablation or Fulguration

An electrical shock can destroy tissue in which an arrhythmia originates or a pathway that plays a role in conduction of the cardiac impulse. At present, it has been used successfully to interrupt conduction in the His bundle and accessory AV pathways and to treat patients with atrial, AV node and ventricular tachycardia (81–86). Its use for treating patients with atrial flutter is under investigation (87). Again, as with surgery, this treatment requires a specialized center. Good long-term results have been obtained in His bundle ablation. Because of a smaller series of patients long-term outcome is not yet clear for the different types of tachycardia treated with electrical ablation. Use of other techniques like radiofrequency and laser ablation is being studied (88,89).

Chemical Ablation

After experiments by Inoue et al. (90) that showed the possibility of destroying arrhythmogenic myocardial tissue

by injecting chemicals into the coronary artery supplying that area, arrhythmias have been successfully treated in humans by transcoronary chemical ablation of the arrhythmia substrate (91). In patients with ventricular tachycardia not responding to or not suitable for pharmacologic or nonpharmacologic intervention, selective injection of alcohol into the coronary artery branch supplying the arrhythmogenic area resulted in cure of the arrhythmia. The technique, which requires expertise in both "angiographic and electrophysiologic mapping" of the site of origin of the arrhythmia, results in a small amount of myocardial damage. We have also applied chemical ablation of AV node conduction by selective injection of alcohol in the AV node coronary artery in patients in whom electrical ablation of AV conduction was unsuccessful. At present, the technique should be considered experimental and long-term results are awaited.

Pacing and Defibrillation

Indications. The value of antitachycardia pacemakers in the management of supraventricular and ventricular reentrant tachycardia has been well demonstrated (92–95). Antitachycardia pacing may be the therapy of choice in patients who do not respond to or cannot tolerate drugs, patients who do not take the prescribed medication, are not suited for or refuse surgery or are not able to tolerate prolonged episodes of tachycardia because of the development of cardiac failure, angina pectoris or dizziness. Patients may prefer treatment with a small reliable pacemaker instead of the long-term intake of antiarrhythmic drugs with possible side effects and accumulating expense. Fully automatic pacemakers may terminate tachycardia so rapidly that the arrhythmia is not noticed or is experienced only as a premature beat.

Role of pacing. In recent years, research has been directed to identifying a single and simple mode of pacing that terminates tachycardia rapidly and safely, irrespective of rate, site of origin and body position. We believe that such a "universal" pacing mode can best be achieved by giving premature stimuli during the tachycardia with adaptive coupling intervals and an automatically increasing number of stimuli (96). Termination of tachycardia by pacing, especially at the ventricular level, carries the risk of tachycardia acceleration and ventricular fibrillation. In devices implanted for pacing termination of ventricular tachycardia, a back-up defibrillation mode should therefore be implemented.

The implantable automatic defibrillator. The value of the implantable automatic defibrillator in properly selected cases has been well documented (97–99). Candidates for implantation include patients with cardiac arrest, those with recurrent symptomatic episodes of ventricular tachycardia despite drug therapy and those with syncope. Most patients have underlying coronary artery disease or cardiomyopathy. A point of discussion is what should be considered an adequate antiarrhythmic trial before insertion of a defibrillator is advised. Our own approach to this problem will be discussed later.

The Practical Approach to Treatment

The decision to treat or not to treat an arrhythmia should be based on answers to two questions. Is the patient symptomatic during the arrhythmia? Has the arrhythmia prognostic significance (either because of structural cardiac disease or because the arrhythmia will lead to cardiac damage as in incessant tachycardia)? Four answers are possible.

1. The patient is symptomatic and the arrhythmia has prognostic significance. In these patients treatment of the arrhythmia is indicated. An example is the patient with sustained ventricular tachycardia and ventricular fibrillation after a previous myocardial infarction. Depending on the risk profile (Fig. 22.2 to 22.4) and after correction (as best as possible) of ischemia and pump failure, the patient with a small chance of dying suddenly is treated with an antiarrhythmic drug, preferably guided by results from programmed electrical stimulation of the heart. Inability to initiate a previously inducible arrhythmia after drug therapy definitely predicts a reduced chance of spontaneous recurrences of ventricular tachycardia (100–102).

There is a difference in opinion, however, on the effect of suppression of arrhythmia inducibility by drug therapy on the chance of dying suddenly (103–105). Therefore, in the patient with a high chance of an arrhythmic death (Fig. 22.2, left) in view of the poor outcome with antiarrhythmic drug treatment, nonpharmacologic treatment should be considered in an early stage. If destruction or isolation of the arrhythmia substrate is not possible or too risky, an electrical device able to pace and defibrillate should be implanted.

Another example of an arrhythmia that is symptomatic and of prognostic significance is found in the patient suffering from cardiomyopathy induced by a tachycardia. Typically, the arrhythmia is incessant (it can be atrial fibrillation, atrial flutter, atrial tachycardia, circus movement tachycardia using an accessory AV pathway with long conduction times or ventricular tachycardia) and cure of the arrhythmia is essential to interrupt a downhill course.

2. The patient is symptomatic but the arrhythmia has no prognostic significance. In this group we find patients who have a normal heart but arrhythmias leading to symptoms such as dizziness, syncope and dyspnea. Examples are the patients with circus movement tachycardia in the Wolff-Parkinson-White syndrome and the patient with idiopathic ventricular tachycardia. Treatment is selected depending on the incidence and severity of the arrhythmia and the age of the patient. A young patient with frequent episodes of circus movement tachycardia is preferably treated with surgical or electrical ablation of the accessory pathway, whereas a patient with idiopathic ventricular tachycardia should first receive antiarrhythmic drug therapy. In the symptomatic patient having no additional heart disease care should be taken not to prescribe an antiarrhythmic drug that, because of proarrhythmic or other side effects, worsens the situation.

3. The patient is asymptomatic but the arrhythmia has prognostic significance. In this category we find patients with a complex ventricular arrhythmia after myocardial infarction or in the presence of cardiomyopathy, hypertensive heart disease or congestive heart failure. In these patients the emphasis should primarily be on correction (if possible) of the contributing factors shown in Figure 22.1. Apart from treatment with beta-blocking agents and the possible exception of the use of amiodarone in hypertrophic cardiomyopathy (106), no convincing evidence has been presented that suppression of the spontaneously occurring arrhythmias by antiarrhythmic drug therapy leads to a decrease in arrhythmic death. The value of nonpharmcologic antiarrhythmic therapy in these patients is not clear.

4. The patient is asymptomatic and the arrhythmia has no prognostic significance. An example is the patient with a (complex) ventricular arrhythmia in the absence of structural heart disease. No antiarrhythmic treatment should be prescribed.

It is clear that the approach described requires ability to perform reliable risk classification of the patient. As pointed out, this is possible in some patients (for example the patient with ventricular tachycardia/fibrillation after myocardial infarction or the patient with hypertrophic cardiomyopathy) (106) but much more difficult or even impossible in others.

The Future

Better risk classification is one of the most important challenges of the "arrhythmology" of tomorrow. More precise and less costly methods are urgently needed. In risk classification, also, the role of the autonomic nervous system should be known better and methods to evaluate and correct abnormalities should be developed (107,108). It seems unlikely, in view of the different mechanisms of arrhythmias, that a universal antiarrhythmic drug will be developed. Because most clinically occurring arrhythmias seem to be based on a reentrant mechanism, the profile of an ideal antireentrant drug should include the ability to suppress triggering mechanisms, like premature beats, and to lengthen the refractory period of myocardial tissue without affecting conduction velocity. The drug should also prevent rate-related shortening of the refractory period of myocardial tissue, have anti-ischemic properties and reduce sudden oscillations in the balance of the autonomic nervous system. In addition, it should have a long half-life, no side effects and be inexpensive.

Theoretically, by using molecular biologic techniques, agents could be developed that are site specific, selectively inactivating cells in the arrhythmogenic area. These fascinating new possibilities have recently been discussed by Zipes (2). In the absence of antiarrhythmic "miracle" drugs, increasing use will be made of electrical devices in the high risk patient. Smaller, less expensive units not requiring thoracotomy will become available. Last but not least, an important aspect in arrhythmia management will be its prevention. In acute myocardial infarction, thrombolytic therapy by reducing infarct size has resulted in a decrease of both spontaneous and inducible ventricular arrhythmias (109,110). Primary prevention of coronary heart disease should lead to a further decrease in serious arrhythmias in the future (111).

References

1. Rosen MR. The links between basic and clinical cardiac electrophysiology. Circulation 1988;77:251–63.
2. Zipes DP. Cardiac electrophysiology: promises and contributions. J Am Coll Cardiol 1989;13:1329–52.
3. Hoffman BF, Cranefield PF. Electrophysiology of the Heart. New York: McGraw-Hill, 1960.
4. Cranefield PF. The Conduction of the Cardiac Impulse. Mt Kisco, NY: Futura, 1975.
5. Brugada P, Wellens HJJ. Cardiac Arrhythmias: Where to Go From Here? Mt Kisco, NY: Futura, 1987.
6. Cranefield PF, Aronson RS. Cardiac Arrhythmias: The Role of Triggered Activity and Other Mechanisms. Mt Kisco, NY: Futura, 1988.
7. Durrer D, Schoo L, Schuilenburg RM, Wellens HJJ. The role of premature beats in the initiation and termination of supraventricular tachycardia in the WPW syndrome. Circulation 1967;36:644–62.
8. Coumel PL, Cabrol C, Fabiato A, Gorgon R, Slama R. Tachycardie permanente par rythme réciproque. Arch Mal Coeur 1967;60:1830–54.
9. Wellens HJJ. Electrical Stimulation of the Heart in the Study and Treatment of Tachycardias. Baltimore: University Park Press, 1971.
10. Gallagher JJ, Sealy WC, Wallace AG, Kasell J. Correlation between catheter electrophysiologic studies and findings in mapping of ventricular excitation in the WPW syndrome. In: Wellens HJJ, Lie KI, Janse MJ, eds. The Conduction System of the Heart, Philadelphia: Lea & Febiger, 1976:588–612.
11. Josephson ME, Horowitz LN, Farshidi A, Spear JF, Kastor JA, Moore EN. Recurrent sustained ventricular tachycardia. 2. Endocardial mapping. Circulation 1978;57:440–7.
12. Scherlag BJ, Lau SH, Helfant RH, Berkowitz WD, Stein E, Damato AN. Catheter technique for recording His bundle activity in man. Circulation 1969;39:13–22.
13. Damato AN, Lau SH. The clinical value of the electrogram of the conducting system. Prog Cardiovasc Dis 1970;13:119–40.
14. Narula OS, Scherlag BJ, Samet P, Javier RP. Atrioventricular block: localization and classification by His bundle recordings. Am J Med 1971;50:146–61.
15. Rosen KM. Evaluation of cardiac conduction in the catheterization laboratory. Am J Cardiol 1972;30:701–3.
16. Puech P, Grolleau R. L'Activité du Faisceau de His Normale et Pathologique. Paris: Ed Sandoz, 1972.
17. Lie KI, Wellens HJJ, Schuilenburg RM. Factors influencing prognosis of bundle branch block complicating acute myocardial infarction. Circulation 1974;50:935–48.
18. Josephson ME, Waxman HL, Marchlinski FE, Horowitz LN, Spielman SR. Relation between site of origin and QRS configuration in ventricular rhythms. In: Wellens HJJ, Kulbertus HE, eds. What's New in Electrocardiography. The Hague: Martinus Nijhoff, 1981:200–28.
19. Wellens HJJ, Bär FWHM, Lie KI. The value of the electrocardiogram in the differential diagnosis of a tachycardia with a widened QRS complex. Am J Med 1978;64:27–33.
20. Wu D, Denes P, Amat-y-Leon F, et al. Clinical, electrocardiographic and electrophysiologic observations in patients with paroxysmal supraventricular tachycardia. Am J Cardiol 1978;41:1045–51.
21. Farshidi A, Josephson ME, Horowitz LN. Electrophysiologic characteristics of concealed bypass tracts: clinical and electrocardiographic correlates. Am J Cardiol 1978;41:1052–60.
22. Farré J, Wellens HJJ. The value of the electrocardiogram in diagnosing site of origin and mechanism of supraventricular tachycardia. In: Ref 18:131–71.
23. Coumel P. Junctional reciprocating tachycardia. The permanent and paroxysmal forms of AV nodal reciprocating tachycardias. J Electrocardiol 1975;8:79–90.
24. Kindwall KE, Brown J, Josephson ME. Electrocardiographic criteria for ventricular tachycardia in wide complex left bundle branch block morphology tachycardias. Am J Cardiol 1988;61:1279–83.
25. Gallagher JJ, Pritchett ELC, Sealy WC, Kasell J, Wallace AG. The pre-excitation syndromes. Prog Cardiovasc Dis 1978;20:285–327.
26. Milstein S, Sharma AD, Guiraudon GM, Klein GJ. An algorithm for the electrocardiographic location of the accessory pathway in the Wolff-Parkinson-White syndrome. PACE 1987;10:555–63.
27. Wellens HJJ. The electrocardiograms 80 years after Einthoven. J Am Coll Cardiol 1986;7:484–91.
28. Brugada P, Wellens HJJ. Early afterdepolarizations. Role in conduction block, prolonged repolarization dependent re-excitation and tachyarrhythmias in the human heart. PACE 1985;8:889–96.
29. Jackman WM, Friday KJ, Anderson JC, Aliot EM, Clark M, Lazzara R. The long QT syndromes: a critical review, new clinical observations and a unifying hypothesis. Prog Cardiovasc Dis 1988;31:115–72.
30. Gorgels APM, Beekman HDM, Brugada P, Dassen WRM, Richards DAB, Wellens HJJ. Extrastimulus-related shortening of the first post-pacing interval in digitalis-induced ventricular tachycardia: observations during programmed electrical stimulation in the conscious dog. J Am Coll Cardiol 1983;1:840–57.
31. Vos MA, Gorgels APM, Leunissen JDM, Wellens HJJ. Flunarizine allows differentiation between mechanisms of arrhythmias in the intact heart. Circulation 1990;81:343–349.

32. Franz MR. Longterm recording of monophasic action potentials from human endocardium. Am J Cardiol 1983;51:1629–34.

33. Messerli FH, Ventura HD, Elizardi DJ, Dunn FG, Frohlich ED. Hypertension and sudden death: increased ventricular ectopic activity in left ventricular hypertrophy. Am J Med 1984;77:18–22.

34. McLenachan JM, Henderson E, Morris KJ, Dajgie HJ. Ventricular arrhythmias in patients with left ventricular hypertrophy. N Engl J Med 1987;317:787–92.

35. Chakko Cs, Gheorgiade M. Ventricular arrhythmias in severe heart failure: incidence, significance and effectiveness of antiarrhythmic therapy. Am Heart J 1985;109:497–504.

36. Coumel PL, Leclercq JF, Zimmerman M, Funck-Brentano JI. Antiarrhythmic therapy: non-invasive guided strategy versus empirical or invasive strategies. In Ref 5: 403–19.

37. Kim SG. The management of patients with life-threatening ventricular arrhythmias: programmed stimulation or Holter monitoring (or both?). Circulation 1987;76:1–5.

38. Wellens HJJ. Value and limitations of programmed electrical stimulation of the heart in the study and treatment of tachycardias. Circulation 1978;57:845–53.

39. Mitchell LB, Duff HJ, Manyari DE, Wyse DG. A randomized clinical trial of the non-invasive and invasive approaches to drug therapy of ventricular tachycardia. N Engl J Med 1987;317:1681–7.

40. The ESVEM investigators. The ESVEM trial: electrophysiologic study versus electrocardiographic monitoring for selection of anti-arrhythmic therapy of ventricular tachyarrhythmias. Circulation 1989;79:1354–60.

41. Simson MB, Untereker WJ, Spielman SR, et al. The relationship between late potentials on the body surface and directly recorded fragmented electrograms in patients with ventricular tachycardia. Am J Cardiol 1983;51:105–12.

42. Gomes A, Winters SL, Stewart D, Horowitz S, Milner M, Barreca P. A new non-invasive index to predict sustained ventricular tachycardia and sudden death in the first year after myocardial infarction based on signal-averaged electrocardiogram, radionuclide ejection fraction and Holter monitoring. J Am Coll Cardiol 1987;10:349–19.

43. Denniss AR, Ross DL, Richards DA, et al. Differences between patients with ventricular tachycardia and ventricular fibrillation as assessed by signal-averaged electrocardiograms, radionuclide ventriculography and cardiac mapping. J Am Coll Cardiol 1988;11:276–83.

44. Lindsay BD, Markham J, Schechtman KB, Ambos HD, Cain ME. Identification of patients with sustained ventricular tachycardia by frequency analysis of signal-averaged electrocardiograms despite the presence of bundle branch block. Circulation 1988;77:120–30.

45. Worley SJ, Mark DB, Smith WM, et al. Comparison of time domain and frequency domain variables from the signal-averaged electrocardiogram. J Am Coll Cardiol 1988;11:1041–51.

46. Haberl R, Lilge G, Pulter R, Steinbeck G. Comparison of frequency and time domain analysis of the signal-averaged electrocardiogram in patients with ventricular tachycardia and coronary artery disease: methodologic validation and clinical relevance. J Am Coll Cardiol 1988;12: 150–8.

47. Anastasiou-Naza MJ, Anderson JL, Stewart JR, et al. Occurrence of exercise induced and spontaneous wide complex tachycardia during therapy with flecainide for complex ventricular arrhythmias: a probable proarrhythmic effect. Am Heart J 1987;113:1071–7.

48. Ranger S, Talajic M, Lemery R, Roy D, Nattel S. Amplification of flecaïnide-induced ventricular conduction slowing by exercise: a potentially significant clinical consequence of use-dependent sodium channel blockade. Circulation 1989;79:1000–6.

49. Brugada P, Wellens HJJ. Arrhythmogenesis of antiarrhythmic drugs. Am J Cardiol 1988;61:1108–11.

50. Brugada P, Talajic M, Smeets J, Mulleneers R, Wellens HJJ. Risk stratification of patients with ventricular tachycardia or ventricular fibrillation after myocardial infarction. The value of the clinical history. Eur Heart J 1989;10:747–52.

51. Ruberman W, Weinblatt E, Goldberg JD, et al. Ventricular premature beats after myocardial infarction. N Engl J Med 1977;297:750–7.

52. Moss AJ, Davis HT, DeCamilla J, Boyer LW. Ventricular ectopic beats and their relation to sudden and nonsudden cardiac death after myocardial infarction. Circulation 1979;60:998–1003.

53. Bigger JT, Fleiss JL, Kleiger R, et al. The relationship between ventricular arrhythmias, left ventricular dysfunction and mortality in the two years after myocardial infarction. Circulation 1984;69:250–8.

54. Mukharji J, Rude FE, Poole K, et al. Risk factors for sudden death following acute myocardial infarction: two-year follow-up. Am J Cardiol 1984;54:31–6.

55. Meinertz T, Hofmann J, Kasper W, et al. Significance of ventricular arrhythmias in idiopathic dilated cardiomyopathy. Am J Cardiol 1984; 53:902–7.

56. McKenna WJ, Krikler DM, Goodwin JF. Arrhythmias in dilated and hypertrophic cardiomyopathy. Med Clin North Am 1984;68:983–1000.

57. Holmes J, Kubo SJ, Cody RJ, Kligfield P. Arrhythmias in ischemic and nonischemic dilated cardiomyopathy: prediction of mortality by ambulatory electrocardiography. Am J Cardiol 1985;55:146–51.

58. Moss AJ, Bigger TJ, Case RB, et al. The Multicenter Postinfarction Research Group: risk stratification and survival after myocardial infarction. N Engl J Med 1983;390:331–6.

59. Richards D, Taylor A, Fahey P, et al. Identification of patients at risk of sudden death after myocardial infarction: the continued Australian experience. In Ref 5:329–41.

60. Marchlinski FE, Buxton AE, Waxmann HL, Josephson ME. Identifying patients at risk of sudden death after myocardial infarction: value of the response to programmed stimulation, degree of ventricular ectopic activity and severity of left ventricular dysfunction. Am J Cardiol 1983;52:1190–6.

61. Santarelli P, Belloci F, Loperfido F, et al. Ventricular arrhythmias induced by programmed ventricular stimulation after acute myocardial infarction. Am J Cardiol 1985;55:391–4.

62. Brugada P, Waldecker B, Kersschot Y, Zehender M, Wellens HJJ. Ventricular arrhythmias initiated by programmed electrical stimulation in four groups of patients with healed myocardial infarction. J Am Coll Cardiol 1986;8:1035–40.

63. Roy D, Arenal A, Godin D, et al. The Canadian experience on the identification of candidates for sudden cardiac death after myocardial infarction. In Ref 5:343–51.

64. The Cardiac Arrhythmia Suppression Trial (CAST) Investigators. Preliminary report: effect of encainide and flecainide on mortality in a randomized trial of arrhythmia suppression after myocardial infarction. N Engl J Med 1989;321:406–12.

65. May GS, Eberlein KA, Furberg CD, Passamani ER, Demets DL. Secondary preventation after myocardial infarction: a review of long term trials. Prog Cardiovasc Dis 1982;24:331–52.

66. Yusuf S, Peto R, Lewis J, Collins R, Sleight P. Betablockade during and after myocardial infarction: an overview of the randomized trials. Prog Cardiovasc Dis 1985;27:335–71.

67. Furberg CD, Morton-Hawkins C, Lichtstern E, for the Beta-blocker Heart Attack Trial Study Group. Effect of propranolol in post-infarction patients with mechanical and electrical complications. Circulation 1984; 69:761–7.

68. Nattel S, Pedersen DH, Zipes DP. Alterations in regional myocardial distribution and arrhythmogenic effects of aprinidine produced by coronary artery occlusions in the dog. Cardiovasc Res 1981;15:80–5.

69. Brugada J, Boersma L, Brugada P, Havenith M, Wellens HJJ, Allessie M. Double wave re-entry as a mechanism of acceleration of ventricular tachycardia. Circulation 1990;81:1633–1643.

70. Gallagher JJ, Sealy WC, Cox JL, et al. Results of surgery for preexcitation caused by accessory atrioventricular pathways in 267 consecutive cases. In: Josephson ME, Wellens HJJ, eds. Tachycardias, Mechanisms, Diagnosis, Treatment. Philadelphia: Lea & Febiger, 1984:259–69.

71. Klein GJ, Guiraudon GM, Sharma AD, Milstein S. Surgical treatment of tachycardias: indications and electrophysiologic assessment. Prog Cardiol 1987;15:139–53.

72. Cox JL. The status of surgery for cardiac arrhythmias. Circulation 1985;71:413–7.

73. Ross DL, Johnson DC, Denniss AR, Cooper MJ, Richards DA, Uther JB. Curative surgery for atrioventricular junctional ("AV nodal") reentrant tachycardia. J Am Coll Cardiol 1985;6:1383–92.

74. Cox JL, Holman WL, Cain ME. Cryosurgical treatment of atrioventricular node reentrant tachycardia. Circulation 1987;76:1329–6.

75. Josephson ME. Treatment of ventricular arrhythmias after myocardial infarction. Circulation 1986;74:653–8.

76. Borggrefe M, Podczek A, Ostermeyer J, Breithardt G, The Surgical Ablation Registry. Long-term results of electrophysiologically guided antitachycardia surgery and ventricular tachyarrhythmias: a collaborative report on 665 patients. In: Breithardt G, Borggrefe M, Zipes DP, eds. Nonpharmacological Therapy of Tachyarrhythmias. Mt Kisco, NY: Futura, 1987:109–32.

77. Miller J, Kienzle M, Harken A, Josephson ME. Subendocardial resection for ventricular tachycardia: predictors of surgical success. Circulation 1984;70:624–31.

78. Guiraudon GM, Klein GJ, Sharma AD, Yee R. Use of old and new anatomic, electrophysiologic, and technical knowledge to develop operative approaches to tachycardia. In Ref 5:639–52.

79. Van Hemel NM, Kingma JH, DeFauw JAM, et al. Left ventricular segmental wall motion score as a criterion for selecting patients for direct surgery in the treatment of postinfarction ventricular tachycardia. Eur Heart J 1989;9:304–15.

80. Lezaun R, Brugada P, Talajic M, et al. Cost-benefit analysis of medical versus surgical treatment of symptomatic patients with accessory atrioventricular pathways. Eur Heart J 1989;12:1105–1109.

81. Gallagher JJ, Svenson RH, Kasell JH, et al. Catheter technique for closed-chest ablation of the atrioventricular conduction system: a therapeutic alternative for the treatment of refractory supraventricular tachycardia. N Engl J Med 1982;306:194–200.

82. Scheinman MM, Morady F, Hess DS, et al. Catheter-induced ablation of the atrioventricular junction to control refractory supraventricular arrhythmias. JAMA 1982;248:851–7.

83. Evans GT Jr, Scheinman MM, Executive Committee of the Percutaneous Cardiac Mapping and Ablation Registry. Catheter ablation for control of ventricular tachycardia: a report of the Percutaneous Cardiac Mapping and Ablation Registry. PACE 1986;9:1391–5.

84. Evans GT Jr, Scheinman MM, Executive Committee of the Registry. The Percutaneous Cardiac Mapping and Ablation Registry: summary of results. PACE 1986;9:923–6.

85. Fontaine G, Tonet JL, Frank R, Gallais Y, et al. Electrode catheter ablation of resistant ventricular tachycardia by endocavitary fulguration associated with antiarrhythmic therapy: experience of 38 patients with mean follow-up of 23 months. In Ref 5:539–69.

86. Morady F, Scheinman MM, Kou WH, et al. Long term results of catheter ablation of a posteroseptal accessory atrioventricular connection in 48 patients. Circulation 1989;79:1160–70.

87. Saoudi N, Mouton-Schleifer D, Cribier A, Letac B. Direct entrainment guided catheter fulguration of atrial flutter in man. J Interv Cardiol 1988;1:273–276.

88. Shoei K, Huang SK, Graham AR, Wharton K. Radiofrequency catheter ablation of the left and right ventricles: anatomic and electrophysiologic observations. PACE 1988;11:449–55.

89. Kunze KP, Schluter M, Geiger M, Kuck KH. Modulation of atrioventricular nodal conduction using radiofrequency current. Am J Cardiol 1988;61:657–62.

90. Inoue H, Waller BF, Zipes DP. Intracoronary ethyl alcohol or phenol injection ablates aconitine-induced ventricular tachycardia in dogs. J Am Coll Cardiol 1987;10:1342–9.

91. Brugada P, de Swart H, Smeets JLRM, Wellens HJJ. Transcoronary chemical ablation of ventricular tachycardia. Circulation 1989;79:475–82.

92. Barold SS, Falkoff MD, Ong LS, Heinle RA. New pacing techniques for the treatment of tachycardias. In: Barold SS, Mugica JM, eds. The Third Decade of Cardiac Pacing. Mt Kisco, NY: Futura, 1982:309–32.

93. Fisher JD, Kim SG, Furman S, Matos JA. Role of implantable pacemakers in control of recurrent ventricular tachycardia. Am J Cardiol 1982;49:194–206.

94. Den Dulk K, Bertholet M, Brugada P, et al. A versatile pacemaker system for termination of tachycardias. Am J Cardiol 1983;52:731–8.

95. Den Dulk K, Bertholet M, Brugada P, et al. Clinical experience with implantable devices for control of tachyarrhythmias. PACE 1984;7:548–56.

96. Den Dulk K, Kersschot JE, Brugada P, Wellens HJJ. Is there a universal antitachycardia pacing mode? Am J Cardiol 1986;57:950–5.

97. Mirowski M. The automatic implantable cardioverter defibrillator: an overview. J Am Coll Cardiol 1985;6:461–6.

98. Tchou PJ, Kadri N, Anderson J, Caceres JA, Jazayeri M, Akhtar M. Automatic implantable cardioverter defibrillators and survival of patients with left ventricular dysfunction and malignant ventricular arrhythmias. Ann Intern Med 1988;109:529–34.

99. Winkle RA, Mead RH, Ruder MA, et al. Long-term outcome with the automatic implantable cardioverter defibrillator. J Am Coll Cardiol 1989;13:1353–61.

100. Fisher JD, Cohen HL, Mehra R, Altschuler H, Escher DJW, Furman S. Cardiac pacing and pacemakers. II. Serial electrophysiologic-pharmacologic testing for control of recurrent tachyarrhythmias. Am Heart J 1977;93:658–68.

101. Mason JW, Winkle RA. Electrode-catheter arrhythmia induction in selection and assessment of antiarrhythmic drug therapy for recurrent ventricular tachycardia. Circulation 1978;58:971–85.

102. Horowitz LN, Josephson ME, Farshidi A, Spielman SR, Michelson EL, Greenspan AM. Recurrent sustained ventricular tachycardia. 3. Role of the electrophysiologic study in selection of antiarrhythmic regimens. Circulation 1978;58:986–97.

103. Wilber DJ, Garan H, Finkelstein D, et al. Out-of-hospital cardiac arrest: use of electrophysiologic testing in the prediction of long-term outcome. N Engl J Med 1988;318:19–24.

104. Waller TJ, Kay HR, Spielman SR, Kutalek SP, Greenspan AM, Horowitz LN. Reduction in sudden death and total mortality by antiarrhythmic therapy evaluated by electrophysiologic drug testing: criteria of efficacy in patients with sustained ventricular tachyarrhythmia. J Am Coll Cardiol 1987;10:83–9.

105. Oyarzun R, Brugada P, Torner P, Wellens HJJ, Brachmann J, Kuebler W. Serial electrophysiologic testing guided versus empirical treatment of sustained ventricular arrhythmias in patients with coronary artery disease. The Heidelberg-Maastricht Study (abstr). PACE 1989;12:647.

106. McKenna WJ. Sudden death in hypertrophic cardiomyopathy: identification of the ''high risk'' patients. In Ref 5:353–66.

107. Schwartz PJ. Manipulation of the autonomic nervous system in the prevention of sudden cardiac death. In Ref 5:741–65.

108. Zipes DP, Inoue H. Autonomic neural control of cardiac excitable properties. In: Kulbertus H, Franck G, eds. Neurocardiology. Mt Kisco, NY: Futura: 1988:59–84.

109. Kersschot I, Brugada P, Ramentol M, et al. Effects of early reperfusion in acute myocardial infarction on arrhythmias induced by programmed stimulation: a prospective randomized study. J Am Coll Cardiol 1986;7:1234–42.

110. Vermeer F, Simoons ML, Lubsen J. Reduced frequency of ventricular fibrillation after early thrombolysis in acute myocardial infarction. Lancet 1986;2:1147–8.

111. Goldberg RJ. Declining out-of-hospital sudden coronary death rates: additional pieces of the epidemiologic puzzle. Circulation 1989;79:1369–73.

CHAPTER 23

Beat to Beat Variability in Cardiovascular Variables: Noise or Music?

MARVIN L. APPEL, MS, RONALD D. BERGER, MD, PhD, J. PHILIP SAUL, MD,
JOSEPH M. SMITH, MD, PhD, RICHARD J. COHEN, MD, PhD

Cardiovascular variables such as heart rate, arterial blood pressure, stroke volume and the configuration of electrocardiographic (ECG) complexes all fluctuate from beat to beat. The variation in pulse rate synchronous with respiration (respiratory sinus arrhythmia) was noted in ancient times and the respiratory variation in arterial blood pressure was documented by Hales in 1733 (1).

Beat to Beat Variation in Cardiovascular Signals

Despite the long-standing recognition of the presence of beat to beat variation in cardiovascular signals, physicians and physiologists have tended to overlook the possible significance of subtle beat to beat variability. The variability has generally been treated as *noise* that is to be either ignored or averaged out. Thus, one reports the *mean* heart rate averaged over many beats and the *typical* systolic or diastolic blood pressure. Electrocardiograms are similarly interpreted by analyzing the morphology of typical waveforms and identifying those waveforms that are grossly abnormal.

Part of the historical reason that subtle beat to beat variability in cardiovascular variables has received marginal attention is that it was difficult to characterize before digital computers became available. Although analog signal analyzers such as spectrum analyzers predated digital signal processing, their applicability to cardiovascular signals was limited. Analysis of beat to beat variability in cardiovascular signals often requires a flexible combination of feature recognition (e.g., R wave detection, interval measurement, determination of systolic or diastolic arterial blood pressure) with more traditional signal analysis techniques. Such an approach is enormously facilitated by digital processing and is cumbersome to achieve with analog processing.

Perhaps the area in which the potential clinical significance of beat to beat variability in cardiovascular signals was first recognized is obstetrics (2). With the advent of fetal monitoring, it was noted that the fetal heart rate fluctuated from beat to beat. This variability correlated with fetal viability; a diminution in this beat to beat variability indicated fetal compromise. The postulated mechanism for this observation was that the fetal heart rate is modulated on a beat to beat basis by the parasympathetic and sympathetic nervous systems. Depression of the central nervous system secondary to anoxia leads to a loss of this fine beat to beat

modulation of heart rate and, hence, to a more metronome-like heartbeat.

Indeed, beat to beat variability in cardiovascular variables often reflects an interplay between various perturbations to cardiovascular function and the response of the cardiovascular regulatory systems to these perturbations. The perturbations may be either exogenous or endogenous. For example, perturbations may result from environmental stress, changes in posture and the mechanical effects of respiratory variation in intrathoracic pressure on the filling and emptying of cardiovascular structures. Similarly, autoregulatory adjustments in local vascular resistance in different tissue beds lead to fluctuations in total vascular resistance, thus perturbing global cardiovascular function. Perturbation to cardiac electrical function may emanate from the variability inherent in such arrhythmias as atrial fibrillation or from subtle beat to beat variation in conduction times through regions of myocardial tissue. The response of the cardiovascular regulatory system may include, for example, the arterial baroreceptor reflex impinging on heart rate and peripheral vascular resistance, as well as the autonomic modulation of cardiac conduction processes.

Thus, by studying beat to beat variability one has the opportunity to study *homeodynamics*, the dynamic processes involved in the maintenance of *homeostasis*. One can glean information about the nature of the perturbations to which the cardiovascular system is exposed as well as the regulatory responses to these perturbations.

Heart Rate and Blood Pressure Variability

Heart rate power spectrum. Heart rate is perhaps the most easily accessible cardiovascular signal for analysis of variability. Spectral analysis involves decomposing a signal into a sum of sine waves of different amplitudes and frequencies. The power spectrum presents the squared amplitude of the sine waves as a function of frequency. Power spectra are familiar to us in the spectrometric analysis of the frequency content of light. Spectral analysis of heart rate variability is similar except that, in the case of visible light, the typical frequencies of interest are on the order of 10^{14} to 10^{15} Hz, whereas for heart rate variability analysis the frequencies of interest are <1 Hz.

Computation of the heart rate power spectrum involves detection of the QRS complexes of the ECG, defining an instantaneous heart rate signal (Fig. 23.1) and then applying filtering and spectral estimation techniques to the heart rate signal (Fig. 23.2) (3). From a 5-min epoch of heart rate one can compute a power spectrum for frequencies above roughly 0.01 Hz. Early investigators (4) identified peaks in the heart rate power spectrum located at approximately 0.04 and 0.10 Hz and the respiratory frequency, although in any given spectrum one or more of these peaks may not be present. Our laboratory (5,6) used pharmacologic blockade in the conscious dog to demonstrate the physiologic mechanisms involved in mediating heart rate fluctuations at these frequencies. Parasympathetic blockade, using the peripheral muscarinic blocking agent glycopyrrolate, abolished all heart rate fluctuations above 0.15 Hz and substantially reduced lower frequency heart rate fluctuations. Adding beta-sympathetic blockade with propranolol removed the residual low frequency fluctuations, leading to a metronome-like heartbeat. Thus, fluctuations above 0.15 Hz are purely parasympathetically mediated, whereas lower frequency fluctuations are jointly mediated by the sympathetic and parasympathetic nervous systems. Similar results have been observed in humans (7,8). The mechanism for this effect is revealed in the 1934 work of Rosenblueth and Simeone (9). They showed that the heart rate response to a change in parasympathetic efferent activity is extremely rapid, occurring usually within a single beat. The change in heart rate in response to changes in efferent sympathetic activity is much slower, occurring on a time scale up to 20 s. Thus, the sympathetic system is simply too sluggish to mediate fluctuations in heart rate at normal respiratory frequencies. The sympathetic system acts like a low-pass filter, whereas the parasympathetic system acts like a broad band-pass filter (Fig. 23.3). More recently, we have shown (10) that this filtering effect occurs at the sinoatrial node.

Blood pressure power spectrum. In addition to studying fluctuations in heart rate, one can similarly compute the power spectrum of fluctuations in arterial blood pressure. The power spectrum of blood pressure fluctuations is similar to that of heart rate at frequencies below the mean heart rate itself. One notes respiratory frequency fluctuations and lower frequency (Mayer wave) fluctuations in arterial blood pressure. Evidence from a number of sources suggests that the lower frequency (0.02 to 0.12 Hz) fluctuations in heart rate and blood pressure may result from a resonance in the baroreflex control of peripheral resistance at these frequencies, and that heart rate fluctuations at these frequencies represent a compensatory heart rate baroreflex response (6,11,12).

Clinical factors related to variability in heart rate and blood pressure spectral peaks. A number of studies have been conducted relating the size of spectral peaks to various physiologic and pathophysiologic states. Low frequency fluctuations are greatly enhanced by standing, hemorrhage, aortic constriction and hypotension (7,8,13,14). Respiratory frequency fluctuations are decreased by standing and exercise. The area of low and high frequency peaks decreases with aging (15). In a retrospective study, Gordon et al. (16)

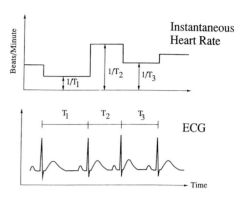

Figure 23.1. Derivation of instantaneous heart rate signal (heart rate tachogram) from the electrocardiographic (ECG) signal.

showed a decreased ratio of low frequency to respiratory frequency power in the heart rate power spectrum of pediatric patients after cardiac surgery, who subsequently died. Patients with heart failure have diminished power at all frequencies >0.02 Hz (17). Cardiac transplant patients have greatly diminished heart rate variability compared with control subjects, but during rejection may demonstrate a broad-band pattern of variability indicative of variable beat to beat supraventricular conduction (18) (Fig. 23.4).

Kleiger et al. (19) demonstrated that diminished heart rate variability (using nonspectral measures) in postmyocardial infarction patients is an extremely strong predictor of mortality. Myers et al. (20) found that decreased power in the heart rate power spectrum was also predictive of mortality.

Clinical interpretation. Although the areas of spectral peaks in heart rate and blood pressure do vary widely under varying pharmacologic and physiologic conditions, the significance of a change in a spectral peak area may be difficult to interpret diagnostically. For example, the area of the respiratory frequency peak in heart rate is often interpreted as a measure of vagal tone. However, the area of the respiratory peak in heart rate reflects the intensity of respiratory effort (the input) as well as the strength of the coupling between respiration and heart rate variation. This coupling largely reflects the incremental gain of the parasympathetic nervous system at this frequency. This frequency-dependent incremental gain may or may not be directly related to the mean level of vagal tone. Similarly, the amplitude of the low

Figure 23.2. Human heart rate signal and corresponding heart rate power spectrum. Notice the three peaks, one at the respiratory frequency near 0.2 Hz and two at lower frequencies centered near 0.1 and 0.04 Hz.

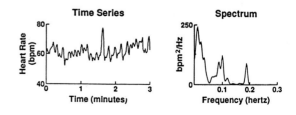

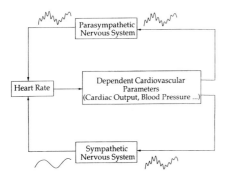

Figure 23.3. Simple model of heart rate control. Fluctuations in heart rate affect dependent cardiovascular variables (e.g. arterial blood pressure). Fluctuations in these variables are detected by sensors (e.g., baroreceptor), and reflex adjustments in heart rate are mediated by the parasympathetic and sympathetic nervous systems. The figure indicates the low-pass character of the sympathetic system relative to the parasympathetic system.

frequency peak in heart rate may reflect the amplitude of (peripheral, central or both) blood pressure oscillations at these frequencies, as well as the strength of the parasympathetically and sympathetically mediated coupling of blood pressure to heart rate fluctuations. Thus, a multitude of

factors might be expected to alter low frequency heart rate fluctuations, including interventions that alter the control of blood pressure fluctuations and those that alter coupling between blood pressure and heart rate fluctuations.

Transfer Function Analysis

To characterize directly the coupling between different physiologic variables, our laboratory has been developing methods for transfer function analysis. The transfer function is the incremental gain as a function of frequency between an input x and output y (Fig. 23.5). Thus, the transfer function evaluated at frequency f yields the amplitude of an output sine wave of frequency f divided by the amplitude of an input sine wave at the same frequency. Transfer function analysis is applicable to linear systems.

The transfer function can be measured by applying pure sinusoidal inputs to linear systems. This is time consuming and laborious, especially in a physiologic system whose state may change in time. Therefore, we have employed "white noise" stimulation techniques in which a known broad-band signal is applied to a system and the output is measured. The white noise technique enables one to measure the transfer

Figure 23.4. Heart rate traces and power spectra from a healthy control subject (**A**), a cardiac transplant recipient without rejection (**B**) and the same patient during a subsequent rejection episode (**C**). Note the different y axis scales for power spectral density (**PSD**) in each frame (reproduced from reference 18 with permission).

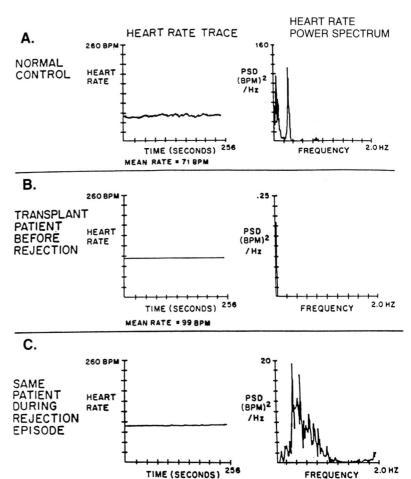

function at many different frequencies simultaneously. We (10) used this approach to demonstrate directly the low-pass character of sympathetic synaptic transmission and the more broad-band parasympathetic transfer function relation in the canine sinoatrial node.

Clinical application. The white noise technique can be used clinically by utilizing respiration as a controlled broadband input (21). Subjects are instructed to inspire in synchrony with randomly spaced audio "beeps" (Fig. 23.6). Depth of respiration is not controlled, thus leaving total ventilation unperturbed. Respiration is measured with a noninvasive volumetric transducer (Respitrace) and heart rate is determined from the ECG. The transfer function between the measured lung volume signal and the heart rate is determined (Fig. 23.7). In a pure sympathetic state, the transfer function is "low-pass," whereas in a parasympathetic state the transfer function is more broad-band. Although this coupling involves more than just the autonomic nervous system, the autonomic nervous system is the critical component (Fig. 23.8).

Linearity hypothesis. Transfer function analysis is applicable to linear systems. In linear systems a sinusoidal input will lead to a sinusoidal output at the same frequency. The cardiovascular system may demonstrate nonlinear behavior over large changes in state. We hypothesize, however, that for relatively small fluctuations of cardiovascular signals about their mean, the signals are linearly coupled—the system is thus linear about a given operating point. The white noise stimulation technique provides a direct means for testing this linearity hypothesis. Two different sequences of broad-stimulation will lead to the estimation of the same transfer function only if the system is indeed linear. Repeated measurements of the transfer functions do, in fact, lead to highly reproducible results, thus substantiating the linearity hypothesis. Although linear systems analysis applies here, nonlinear interactions may nonetheless play an important role in other aspects of cardiovascular signal variability.

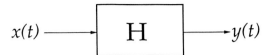

Figure 23.5. Transfer function H transforms input x(t) into output y(t).

System Identification Techniques

Analysis of multiple interacting cardiovascular signals. The use of controlled exogenous broad-band inputs enables one to directly measure coupling between signals. However, the coupling may not always be simple to interpret, particularly when feedback loops are involved. For example, consider the coupling between heart rate and arterial blood pressure. As a result of the pumping action of the heart and the impedance properties of the vasculature, fluctuations in heart rate are mechanically coupled to fluctuations in arterial blood pressure. In turn, fluctuations in arterial blood pressure are coupled to heart rate fluctuations through the baroreceptor reflex. A single transfer function measurement would intertangle these two physiologically distinct feedforward and feedback features. However, autoregressive moving average algorithms (22) are available that impose *causality* conditions on the measured transfer functions, allowing one to separately identify the feedforward and feedback transfer functions.

One can generalize this approach to analyze a multiplicity of interacting cardiovascular signals. In particular, if one measures n signals, one can construct as many as $n(n - 1)$ possible causal couplings between them, each of which might represent a distinct physiologic mechanism. In such a system model there may also be associated with each signal a noise source representing endogenous or exogenous perturbations. Efforts to estimate the transfer relations and power spectra of the noise sources by analyzing spontaneous fluctuations have been reported (11,23). Our laboratory has introduced the idea of using broad-band exogenous stimula-

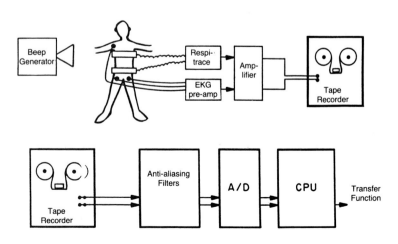

Figure 23.6. Assessment of respiration to heart rate transfer function in humans. Electrocardiogram and respiration are monitored during random interval breathing cued by a "beep" generator. Recorded signals are filtered, undergo analog to digital (A/D) conversion and are analyzed by a computer program (reproduced from reference 37 with permission).

Figure 23.7. Respiration to heart rate transfer function analysis during white noise breathing in man. The time series (**A and B**) and spectra (**C and D**) reveal the broad-band nature of the signals. The transfer function magnitude (**E**) during "vagal" conditions (β-sympathetic blockade with propranolol, position supine) rolls off gradually with frequency. The transfer function during "sympathetic" conditions (parasympathetic blockade with atropine, position standing) rolls off more abruptly, indicative of the low-pass nature of the β-sympathetic filter. The phase (**F**) remains near zero during "vagal conditions" and rolls off linearly under "sympathetic conditions," suggestive of a fixed time delay.

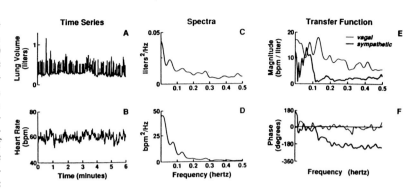

tion to achieve this system identification in a reliable way (24). Provided that the signals are sufficiently broad-band, it is possible to estimate each of the transfer relations and the power spectra of the noise sources.

Clinical application. A clinically applicable approach to system identification is shown in Figure 23.9. In this example, a subject performs "white noise" breathing while lung volume, arterial blood pressure and the ECG are recorded. The transfer function representing the arterial blood pressure response to a single heartbeat (circulatory mechanics) and the baroreceptor coupling between changes in arterial blood pressure and heart rate (HR baroreflex) are shown as well as the neurally mediated coupling between respiratory activity and heart rate (H_1) and the mechanical coupling between variations in lung volume and arterial blood pressure (H_2). The noise source (N_{ABP}) represents all fluctuations in arterial blood pressure not attributable to fluctuations in heart rate or respiratory activity. The noise source (N_{HR}) represents all fluctuations in heart rate not attributable to fluctuations in arterial blood pressure or respiratory activity. Thus, the noise sources represent the input of all physiologic mechanisms not expressly considered in the model.

In Figure 23.10 we show an example of the computed

values of these transfer relations and the spectra of the noise sources obtained during white noise breathing. (Here the transfer relations are shown in the time domain as impulse response functions. The impulse response function is the output y that results from an arbitrarily narrow impulse of unit area applied to the input x. The impulse response is the inverse Fourier transform of the transfer function.) Figure 23.10a demonstrates the heart rate response that would be obtained if one could deliver an impulse in arterial blood pressure; it shows that, after an initial rapid drop, the heart rate gradually returns to baseline. The heart rate and arterial blood pressure responses to an impulse in lung volume (Fig. 23.10b and c) are biphasic. The blood pressure response, however, is very short and very low in amplitude. Figure 23.10d shows the arterial blood pressure response to a single heartbeat (note the presence of a dicrotic notch). The noise spectra in Figures 23.10e and f constitute <1% of the energy in the raw heart rate and arterial blood spectra shown in Figures 23.10g and h. Thus, nearly all the heart rate and arterial pressure variability in this study can be ascribed to respiratory variation and the couplings between the signals.

The transfer relations shown here are all linear. However, this type of linear system identification scheme can incorporate nonlinearities. The signals whose interactions are analyzed can be derived from physiologic signals by means of nonlinear transformations. For example, the heart rate signal (Fig. 23.1) is a nonlinear transformation of the electrocardiogram signal. Thus, one can often incorporate the necessary nonlinearities into the definition of the signals themselves, leaving only linear relations to be analyzed.

The system identification approach shown here can be realized from 5 min of data collection. Using a noninvasive arterial blood pressure recording device (e.g., Colin noninvasive radial artery blood pressure monitor), these measurements can be achieved in a totally noninvasive fashion. This approach enables one to describe the principal mechanisms involved in short-term cardiovascular control with the rigorous mathematical techniques that an electrical engineer uses to describe feedback in an electronic circuit.

Figure 23.8. Model of respiratory modulation of heart rate. The "respiratory" center is centrally coupled with "vagal" and "sympathetic" centers. In addition, mechanical effects of respiration on hemodynamics lead to feedback input to autonomic centers by way of ("other inputs"). SA = sinoatrial.

Model of Respiratory Modulation of Heart Rate

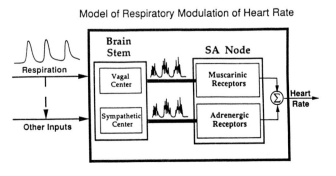

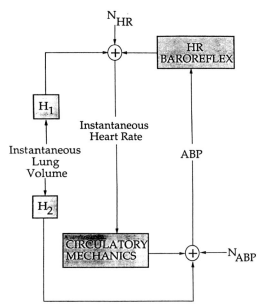

Figure 23.9. Identifiable closed loop model of short-term cardiovascular control. (See text for discussion.) ABP = arterial blood pressure; CIRCULATORY MECHANICS = transfer function representing blood pressure response to a single heartbeat; H_1 and H_2, respectively, are the neurally mediated coupling between respiratory activity and heart rate, and the mechanically mediated coupling between variations in lung volume and blood pressure. N_{ABP} and N_{HR} = noise sources (arterial blood pressure and heart rate, respectively).

Long-Term Heart Rate Fluctuations

Heart rate and blood pressure fluctuations over longer times. Up to now we have been discussing heart rate fluctuations on a time scale of seconds to minutes. However, the heart rate fluctuates with much longer periodicities as well. One can compute the heart rate power spectrum from a 24 h data record down to frequencies of 10^{-5} Hz (25). Kobayashi and Musha (26) first noted that over many decades of frequency the power spectrum decays as $1/f^\alpha$ where α is very close to unity. On a log-log scale (see Fig. 23.11) the heart rate power spectrum appears as a line with a slope close to -1 in value. The peaks in the range of 0.04 to 0.5 Hz are smeared out and appear diminutive on the larger landscape of heart rate variability on the 10^{-5} to 1 Hz range.

The fact that the heart rate spectrum follows this 1/f decay must reflect some fundamental principles of intermediate-term cardiovascular control. Goldberger and West (27) speculated that the 1/f decay could reflect the fractal nature of hemodynamic regulation. However, at this point the origin of the remarkably reproducible 1/f behavior must be considered as unexplained. Arterial blood pressure fluctuations have also been observed to follow a 1/f decay (Donald Marsh, personal communication). The interaction of long-term variability in heart rate, blood pressure and other cardiovascular signals remains an important area of investigation from a physiologic, pharmacologic and pathophysiologic perspective.

Estimates of heart rate variance. An important corollary to the observation that the heart rate power spectrum decays

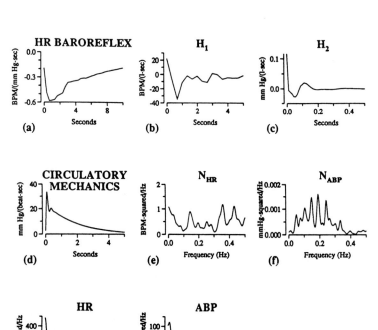

Figure 23.10. Impulse response functions and power spectra of noise sources, heart rate and arterial blood pressure of Figure 23.9 identified from a human subject during white noise breathing. (See text for discussion.) Abbreviations as in Figure 23.9.

NORMAL

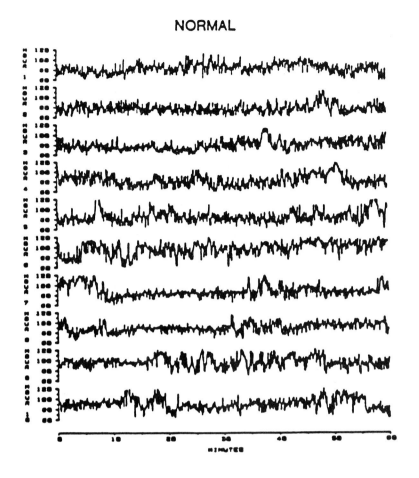

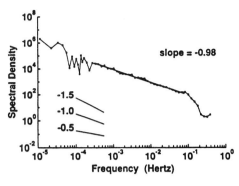

Figure 23.11. Ten hour heart rate tracing (**upper**) and corresponding power spectrum (**lower**) from a 24 h record of a normal subject.

as 1/f over a 24 h time period is that the variance of heart rate variability is not defined, at least on time scales of less than 24 h.

The variance (square of the standard deviation) is just equal to the area under the power spectrum. However, the integral for this area diverges for small f for a 1/f decay. From a practical point of view, this means that estimates of the heart rate variance (or standard deviation) will depend on the record length. The longer the record, the greater the estimated variance as more low frequency power is included. For example, Kleiger et al. (19) estimated RR interval standard deviation over a 24 h period as a predictor of mortality in postmyocardial infarction patients. This 24 h estimate reflects primarily the very low frequency power in heart rate variability, not the peaks above 0.01 Hz.

Variability in the Morphology of ECG Complexes

The morphologies of ECG complexes fluctuate from beat to beat. Some of this variability may reflect the mechanical rotation and translation of the heart in the thorax and the changes in transthoracic impedance, for example that result from respiratory movement. However, variability in ECG

configuration may also result from intrinsic beat to beat variability in cardiac conduction processes.

Relation of beat to beat variability in ECG complex morphology to ventricular arrhythmias. Our laboratory was intrigued by the question whether a ventricle in a state of enhanced susceptibility to fibrillation might by marked by an altered pattern of beat to beat variability in QRS and T wave morphology. Does an unstable state, which may give rise to a microscopically disorganized pattern of electrical activity, first manifest itself in terms of subtle beat to beat variability in excitation and repolarization processes? We approached this problem in two ways. One approach involved finite element model computer simulation of cardiac conduction incorporating the dispersion of refractoriness hypothesis (28,29). The second approach involved animal studies in which susceptibility to ventricular fibrillation was augmented by tachycardia, coronary artery ligation, or hypothermia, or combinations thereof (30).

The computer model was found to simulate a wide range of arrhythmias including reentrant premature depolarizations, tachycardia and fibrillation. When analyzing the computer simulation we observed a pattern of "electrical alternans" preceding the onset of reentrant rhythm disturbances in almost every instance (Fig. 23.12). Electrical alternans is

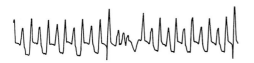

Figure 23.12. Simulated electrocardiogram of a paced ventricle showing the presence of electrical alternans before and after a burst of reentrant activity (reproduced from reference 28 with permission).

a conduction pattern involving an ECG complex configuration that alternates every other beat between two morphologies resulting in an ABABAB type of pattern. Electrical alternans in the computer model resulted from alternating conduction patterns attributable to regions of tissue with refractory periods longer than the interbeat interval.

Electrical alternans and ventricular fibrillation. Electrical alternans in humans often occurs in the setting of pericardial effusion (31) and, under such circumstances, is associated with mechanical alternation of the position of the heart, and would not be expected to be associated with arrhythmias per se. Accordingly, we developed computer algorithms to specifically identify alternation (QRS, ST or T wave) in the pattern of electrical conduction in the analysis of ECG recordings. These algorithms were designed specifically to reject variations attributable to mechanical alternation and can quantify electrical alternans generally not detectable by visual inspection. We found that susceptibility to ventricular fibrillation, as measured by the ventricular fibrillation threshold technique, correlated with the presence of electrical alternans in dogs. A similar correlation was also observed in a pilot study (30) of patients undergoing invasive electrophysiologic testing in which the presence of alternans correlated with inducibility of ventricular tachycardia or ventricular fibrillation under a standard protocol. Taken together, these results suggest that beat to beat variability in excitation and repolarization processes in the pattern of electrical alternans may reflect decreased electrical stability. Analysis of beat to beat variability in ECG complex morphology may provide a noninvasive means of assessing susceptibility to cardiac arrhythmias.

Beat to Beat Variability During Arrhythmias

This review has focused on beat to beat variability of cardiovascular signals during apparently normal conduction processes. Another whole range of analyses can be made to probe mechanisms of arrhythmias by analyzing variability in timing or morphology of complexes during frank arrhythmias. For example, analysis of RR interval variability during atrial fibrillation can provide insight into the electrical interaction of the atria and atrioventricular junction during atrial fibrillation and the effects of pharmacologic intervention (32,33). The occurrence of ventricular premature depolarizations can be treated as stochastic process reflective of the

underlying mechanisms involved with the generation of ventricular ectopic activity (34,35). Parasystolic mechanisms give rise to a rich range of dynamic behavior (36). A review of this fertile area of investigation is beyond the scope of this report.

Conclusions

Cardiovascular signals do indeed fluctuate on a beat to beat basis throughout one's lifetime. These fluctuations reflect the dynamic interplay of diverse physiologic processes. Traditionally, these fluctuations have escaped serious scrutiny. With modern techniques of analysis, such fluctuations can reveal the delicate dynamics involved in beat to beat cardiovascular control. Analysis of these fluctuations may provide a powerful, quantitative means of characterizing these physiologic processes. This approach may also provide a noninvasive or minimally invasive means for clinically assessing alterations in closed loop cardiovascular regulation and stability in a wide range of pathophysiologic states.

It may soon become common to assess autonomic function, baroreceptor function and cardiac electrical stability by mathematical analysis of commonly monitored signals such as heart rate, blood pressure and the ECG. Such an assessment could be used diagnostically as well as to guide and monitor therapeutic interventions. Fluctuations in cardiovascular signals should be considered not as noise but as music to be appreciated with a properly tuned mathematical ear.

References

1. Hales S. Haemastaticks. In: Hales S, ed. Statistical Essays. London: Innys and Manby, 1735;II:1–186.
2. Hon EH, Lee ST. Electronic evaluation of the fetal heart rate patterns preceding fetal death, further observations. Am J Obstet Gynecol 1965; 87:814–26.
3. Berger RD, Akselrod S, Gordon D, Cohen RJ. An efficient algorithm for spectral analysis of heart rate variability. IEEE Trans Biomed Eng 1986;33:900–4.
4. Hyndman BW, Gregory JR. Spectral analysis of sinus arrhythmia during mental loading. Ergonomics 1975;18:255–80.
5. Akselrod S, Gordon D, Ubel FA, Shannon DC, Barger AC, Cohen RJ. Power spectrum analysis of heart rate fluctuations: a quantitative probe of beat-to-beat cardiovascular control. Science 1981;213:220–2.
6. Akselrod S, Gordon D, Madwed JB, Snidman NC, Shannon DC, Cohen RJ. Hemodynamic regulation: investigation by spectral analysis. Am J Physiol 1985;249:H867–75.
7. Pomeranz B, Macaulay RJB, Caudill MA, et al. Assessment of autonomic function in man by heart rate spectral analysis. Am J Physiol 1985;248: H151–3.
8. Pagani M, Lombardi F, Guzzetti S, et al. Power spectral analysis of heart rate and arterial pressure as a marker of sympatho-vagal interaction in man and conscious dog. Circulation 1986;59:178–93.
9. Rosenblueth A, Simeone FA. The interrelations of vagal and accelerator effects on the cardiac rate. Am J Physiol 1934;110:42–55.
10. Berger RD, Saul JP, Cohen RJ. Transfer function analysis of autonomic regulation: I. The canine atrial rate response. Am J Physiol 1989;25:H142–H152.

11. Baselli G, Cerutti S, Civardi S, Malliani A, Pagani M. Cardiovascular variability signals: towards the identification of a closed-loop model of the neural control mechanisms. IEEE Trans Biomed Eng 1988;35:1033–46.
12. Madwed JB, Albrecht P, Mark RG, Cohen RJ. Low-frequency oscillations in arterial pressure and heart rate: a simple computer model. Am J Physiol 1989;25:H1573–9.
13. Madwed JB, Sands KEF, Saul JP, Cohen RJ. Spectral analysis of beat-to-beat variability in HR and ABP during hemorrhage and aortic constriction. In: Lown B, Malliani A, Prosdocimi M, eds. Neural Mechanisms and Cardiovascular Disease. Fidia Research Series, Padova: Liviana Press, 1986;5:291–301.
14. Taratuta E, Albrecht P, Dennis R, Akselrod S, Valeri CR, Cohen RJ. Analysis of blood pressure in conscious baboons. Proceedings of the 9th Annual Conference of the IEEE Engineering in Medicine and Biology Society 1987:94–5.
15. Shannon DC, Carley DW, Benson H. Aging of modulation of heart rate. Am J Physiol 1987;253:H874–7.
16. Gordon D, Herrera VL, McAlpine L, et al. Heart rate spectral analysis: a noninvasive probe of cardiovascular regulation in critically ill children with heart disease. Pediatr Cardiol 1988;9:69–77.
17. Saul JP, Arai Y, Berger RD, Lilly LS, Colucci WS, Cohen RJ. Assessment of autonomic regulation in chronic congestive heart failure by heart rate spectral analysis. Am J Cardiol 1988;61:1292–9.
18. Sands KEF, Appel ML, Lilly LS, Schoen FJ, Mudge GH, Cohen RJ. Assessment of heart rate variability in human cardiac transplant recipients using power spectrum analysis. Circulation 1989;79:76–82.
19. Kleiger RE, Miller JP, Bigger JT, Moss AJ. Decreased heart rate variability and its association with increased mortality after acute myocardial infarction. Am J Cardiol 1987;59:256–62.
20. Myers GA, Martin GJ, Magid NM, et al. Power spectral analysis of heart rate variability in sudden cardiac death: comparison to other methods. IEEE Trans Biomed Eng 1986;33:1149–65.
21. Saul JP, Berger RD, Chen MH, Cohen RJ. Transfer function analysis of autonomic regulation: II. Respiratory sinus arrhythmia. Am J Physiol 1989;25:H153–61.
22. Ljung L. System Identification: Theory for the User. Englewood Cliffs, NJ: Prentice Hall, 1987.
23. Kalli S, Suoranta R, Jokipii M, Turjanmaa V. Analysis of blood pressure and heart rate variability using multivariate autoregressive modelling. Computers in Cardiology 1986;13:427–30.
24. Appel ML, Saul JP, Berger RD, Cohen RJ. Closed-loop identification of cardiovascular regulatory mechanisms. Computers in Cardiology 1989; 15 (in press).
25. Saul JP, Albrecht P, Berger RD, Cohen RJ. Analysis of long term heart rate variability: methods, 1/f scaling and implications. Computers in Cardiology 1987;14:419–22.
26. Kobayashi M, Musha T. 1/f fluctuation of heartbeat period. IEEE Trans Biomed Eng 1982;29:456–7.
27. Goldberger AL, West BJ. Applications of nonlinear dynamics to clinical cardiology. Ann NY Acad Sci 1987;504:195–213.
28. Smith JM, Cohen RJ. Simple finite element model accounts for wide range of cardiac dysrhythmias. PNAS 1984;81:233–7.
29. Kaplan DT, Smith JM, Saxberg BEH, Cohen RJ. Nonlinear dynamics in cardiac conduction. Math Biosci 1988;90:19–48.
30. Smith JM, Clancy EA, Valeri CR, Ruskin JN, Cohen RJ. Electrical alternans and cardiac electrical instability. Circulation 1988;77:110–21.
31. Goldberger AL, Shabetai R, Bhargava V, West BJ, Mandell AJ. Nonlinear dynamics, electrical alternans and pericardial tamponade. Am Heart J 1984;107:1297–9.
32. Cohen RJ, Berger RD, Dushane TE. A quantitative model for the ventricular response during atrial fibrillation. IEEE Trans Biomed Eng 1983;30:769–81.
33. Berger RD, Bailin MT, Pollick F, Cohen RJ. Experimental application of a computer model for atrial fibrillation. Computers in Cardiology 1983; 10:197–200.
34. Lovelace DE, Knoebel SB. Time series analysis in predicting ventricular arrhythmias. Computers in Cardiology 1982;9:45–7.
35. Albrecht P, Cohen RJ, Mark R. Stochastic characterization of chronic ventricular ectopic activity. IEEE Trans Biomed Eng 1988;35:539–50.
36. Glass L, Goldberger AL, Belair J. Dynamics of pure parasystole. Am J Physiol 1986;20:H841–7.
37. Chen MH, Berger RD, Saul JP, Stevenson K, Cohen RJ. Transfer function analysis of the autonomic response to respiratory activity during random interval breathing. Computers in Cardiology 1987;14:149–52.

CHAPTER 24

Molecular Cardiology: New Avenues for the Diagnosis and Treatment of Cardiovascular Disease

DAVID R. HATHAWAY, MD, KEITH L. MARCH, PhD, MD

Historical Perspective

An early appreciation of the importance of molecules to overall function of the cardiovascular system may be ascribed to Ringer (1), who in 1882 recognized the key role of calcium ions in cardiac muscle contraction. Only recently, however, has a more comprehensive understanding of the many molecules that constitute the cardiovascular system been made possible as a result of major advances in several disciplines, most notably, cellular and molecular biology.

In the beginning years of this century and even earlier, therapy of cardiovascular diseases was largely empiric and applied symptomatically with little ability to target treatments to the underlying pathophysiologic process. Such treatments included digitalis leaf and phlebotomy for symptoms now understood to be the result of heart failure, amyl nitrite and narcotic analgesia for angina pectoris and activity restriction for both. The soundness of the principles underlying these interventions has been borne out and modern analogs of each exist. Nevertheless, a wider range of therapeutic approaches has gradually been developed. In the last several decades, elucidation of both normal and abnormal physiologic mechanisms involving the cardiovascular system has made more precise and targeted therapeutic interventions possible. Pertinent examples include the use of diuretic agents for heart failure and bypass grafting and, more recently, angioplasty to remedy the mechanical obstructions of blood vessels that result in angina pectoris and myocardial infarction. Such attention to mechanisms has required greater emphasis on quantitative anatomic and physiologic measurements and the use of some of the most advanced technology to make these measurements with increasing precision. This has allowed recognition of the relations between asymptomatic abnormalities such as hypertension and symptomatic diseases such as dilated cardiomyopathy and coronary atherosclerosis and has provided the rationale for the development of preventive therapy.

Most recently, investigation of some of the molecular processes that underlie mechanical abnormalities has suggested new approaches to therapeutics that target basic mechanisms of disease. Extrapolation of this trend into the future promises further evolution of diagnosis and treatment to more basic levels and to application progressively earlier in time and in the chain of events that lead to disease. Understanding the genetic mechanisms that predispose to disease and the environmental influences that modify the genetic substrate can lead to prevention or cure of many cardiovascular diseases.

A review on the current status of molecular cardiology and the areas in which elucidation of basic mechanisms will improve future diagnosis and treatment of cardiovascular disease can provide only highlights of some of the more important developments. Accordingly, we have divided the review into four major sections that will cover 1) cardiac muscle; 2) the primary components of the blood vessel, smooth muscle and endothelium; 3) the multifactorial disease, atherosclerosis, which involves interaction between several cell types; and 4) thrombosis and thrombolysis.

Cardiac Muscle

Mechanisms regulating adrenergic receptor sensitivity or density. The cardiac muscle cell possesses an array of hormone receptors that are coupled to ionic and metabolic pathways that modulate overall contractile and electrophysiologic function of the heart. There has always been particular interest in the role of the autonomic nervous system in regulation of cardiac function and this interest continues at the most basic levels.

The development of specific radioligands for measurement of the number and affinity of alpha- and beta-adrenergic receptors and muscarinic cholinergic receptors has provided the necessary methodology for assessing changes in receptor density associated with pathophysiologic states. Thus, thyroid hormone has been shown to increase cardiac beta-receptors (2), whereas heart failure has been associated with a decrease in these receptors (3). Moreover, ischemia has been linked to an increase in both beta- (4) and alpha- (5) adrenergic receptors.

An important development has been the recognition and characterization of changes in adrenergic receptor function or density that occur after lengthy exposure of tissues to catecholamines. Several mechanisms appear to account for adrenergic receptor desensitization. Desensitization not associated with a decrease in receptor number is due to uncoupling of agonist binding to the receptor from the stimulation of adenylate cyclase. The specific blockade in this coupling is at the level of G_s, the guanine nucleotide-binding protein that couples beta-receptor stimulation to activation of adenylate cyclase (6). Recent studies (7) have shown that a specific protein kinase, beta-adrenergic receptor kinase or beta-ARK, phosphorylates the $beta_2$-receptor initiating the uncoupling process from G_s. Beta-ARK can only phosphorylate the beta$_2$-adrenergic receptor when catecholamine is bound (6). Therefore, with sustained receptor occupation, a feedback mechanism to attenuate or dampen beta-adrenergic stimulation supervenes. In similar fashion, the target protein kinase of beta-adrenergic receptor stimulation, namely, cAMP cyclic adenosine monophosphate-dependent protein kinase, can phosphorylate and desensitize the alpha$_1$- and beta-adrenergic receptors, and both the beta$_2$- and alpha$_1$-adrenergic receptors are substrates for protein kinase C (8), which is the target enzyme for diacylglycerol, a second messenger derived from phosphatidylinositol metabolism (see later). In all cases examined to date, receptor phosphorylation appears to mediate desensitization (6). Most recently, a protein phosphatase activity that dephosphorylates the beta$_2$-adrenergic receptor has been identified (8a). Therefore, desensitization as a result of phosphorylation can be reversed.

Down-regulation of beta-adrenergic receptors requires much longer periods of exposure to catecholamines, is associated with complete loss of receptors and appears to involve an actual decrease in the synthesis of receptor protein (9). The recent cloning of complementary deoxyribonucleic acid (cDNA) for the adrenergic receptors (10,11) and beta-adrenergic receptor genes (12,13) opens new possibilities for more sensitive detection of receptor message and for determining how receptor expression is regulated at the gene level.

In summary, adrenergic receptors are modulated by a variety of molecular processes that serve to dampen effects of sustained catecholamine stimulation. There is "crosstalk" among receptor populations with, for example, desensitization of alpha$_1$-receptors by the beta-adrenergic system and vice versa. Selective agents for modulation of adrenergic receptor function in the future may be targeted at the desensitization processes when a more thorough understanding of their contribution to pathophysiology is attained.

Guanine nucleotide regulatory proteins: coupling receptors to effectors. Beyond adrenergic and cholinergic receptors are the guanine nucleotide regulatory proteins or G-proteins. The G-proteins reside within the sarcolemma and are composed of three subunits (alpha, beta and gamma). G-proteins couple several hormone receptors to ion channels or enzymes (14). The coupling process requires 1) binding of the hormone to its receptor, 2) binding of guanosine-5'-triphosphate (GTP) by the alpha subunit of the G-protein, 3) liberation of the alpha subunit from the complex, and 4) binding of the alpha subunit to an effector system (for beta-adrenergic receptors, this would be adenylate cyclase) followed by activation. Activation is terminated by conversion of GTP to guanosine-5'-diphosphate (GDP) and rebinding of the alpha subunit to the corresponding complex. Modulation of the function of G-proteins occurs at several levels. First, there are multiple genes encoding different subunit types (15). Second, coupling can be affected by

nicotinamide-adenine dinucleotide (ADP)-ribosylation catalyzed by extrinsic agents such as pertussis and cholera toxins (14). Finally, G-proteins are substrates for protein kinases, most notably protein kinase C (see later) and phosphorylation may serve to desensitize the coupling mechanism (16).

In cardiac muscle, stimulatory G-proteins (G_s) couple beta-adrenergic (both beta$_1$ and beta$_2$) receptors to adenylate cyclase (17). Muscarinic cholinergic (M$_2$) receptors are coupled to atrial potassium ion channels (18) by different G-proteins (G$_k$), whereas alpha$_1$-adrenergic receptors are coupled to phospholipase C (19). When considering pathophysiologic modulation (enhancement or dampening) of a particular receptor-effector pathway, it has, therefore, become necessary to investigate receptor–G-protein coupling. For example, as beta$_1$-adrenergic receptors numerically decline in the failing human heart (20), beta$_2$-receptors uncouple from G-protein activation of adenylate cyclase (21). Recently, an increase in measurable G-protein has been reported (22) in membranes from failing human hearts. Moreover, several noncardiac diseases have been shown to be associated with alterations in the amount of a particular G-protein (23,24). At present, other than the microbial toxins, there are no agents that specifically enhance or inhibit function of guanine nucleotide regulatory proteins. The quest for such agents, as well as continued examination of the role of G-proteins in molecular pathophysiology, will require considerable emphasis in the future.

The phosphoinositide pathway: a new second messenger system. In the 1960s, investigation of the cyclic nucleotides adenosine and guanosine monophosphates (cAMP and cGMP) as second messengers yielded immense information about biochemical regulatory mechanisms in virtually all tissues. In a similar fashion, the discovery in the 1970s of calmodulin and its role as an intracellular calcium ion (Ca^{2+}) receptor facilitated the development of new ideas about intracellular enzyme regulation (25). Although pathways of phosphoinositide metabolism have been elucidated over several years, only recently has liberation of specific phosphoinositide metabolites been linked to hormone receptor systems (26). The phosphoinositide pathway is summarized in Figure 24.1.

An important site for hormonal regulation of phosphoinositide metabolism is the enzyme phospholipase C (PLC), which catalyzes the conversion of L-alpha-phosphatidylinositol diphosphate (PIP$_2$) to inositol-1, 4, 5-triphosphate (IP$_3$) and diacylglycerol (27). Recent studies (19) of several tissues have provided evidence for hormonal receptor (for example, alpha$_1$-adrenergic, muscarinic-1 and angiotensin) modulation of phospholipase C. Moreover, G-proteins appear to couple these receptors to phospholipase C activation (19). In cardiac muscle, the alpha$_1$ receptor is linked to this pathway, but the predominant muscarinic cholinergic receptor, which is the M$_2$ type, is not (28).

Two products of phosphoinositide metabolism are particu-

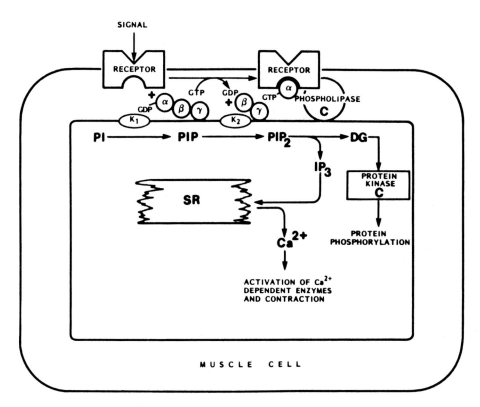

Figure 24.1. *Activation of the phospho-inositide pathway by hormones.* In this simplified scheme, a hormone (for example, alpha-adrenergic receptor agonist, M_1-muscarinic cholinergic agonist) activates the enzyme phospholipase C through guanine nucleotide regulatory proteins, or G-proteins. The latter consists of three subunits (alpha, beta and gamma). The alpha subunit is liberated by binding of guanosine-5′-triphosphate (GTP) and this activated form increases the activity of phospholipase C. Phospholipase C catalyzes the formation of inositol-1,4,5-triphosphate (IP_3) and diacylglycerol (DG) from L-alpha-phosphatidylinositol diphosphate (PIP_2). The latter is produced by sequential phosphorylation of L-alpha-phosphatidylinositol (PI) and L-phosphatidylinositol phosphate (PIP) by membrane-bound kinases (K_1 and K_2). IP_3 can stimulate release of Ca^{2+} from sarcoplasmic reticulum (SR) of smooth muscle and may serve a similar function in cardiac muscle. Increases in intracellular Ca^{2+} activate the contractile mechanism. Diacylglycerol, in concert with Ca^{2+} and other phospholipids, activates protein kinase C. A variety of cellular proteins (for example, adrenergic receptors, Na^+/H^+ antiporter) can be phosphorylated by protein kinase C resulting in modulation of activity.

larly important: diacylglycerol and inositol phosphates. Diacylglycerol, in concert with Ca^{2+} and phosphatidylserine, activates protein kinase C (29). As indicated in the discussion of adrenergic receptor desensitization, protein kinase C can phosphorylate both alpha- and beta-adrenergic receptors, uncoupling them from their respective G-proteins. This might be an especially important feedback mechanism to attenuate the increase in intracellular Ca^{2+} that occurs in response to alpha$_1$-adrenergic receptor stimulation. Protein kinase C also phosphorylates cardiac sarcolemmal proteins (30) and activates the sodium/hydrogen (Na^+/H^+) antiporter leading to intracellular alkalinization (31).

Of the several inositol phosphates and cyclic inositol phosphate derivatives identified to date, inositol-1, 4, 5-triphosphate (IP_3) has engendered the most attention. As indicated, it is generated by the action of phospholipase C on L-alpha-phosphatidylinositol diphosphate and a major pathway for degradation involves conversion of IP_3 to inositol-1, 4-diphosphate by the enzyme, 5-phosphomonoesterase (27). IP_3 appears to release Ca^{2+} from sarcoplasmic reticulum of smooth muscle (32) and may mediate a similar action in cardiac and skeletal muscle (33).

Regulation of intracellular ions: pumps, channels and antiporters. A variety of processes operate in the cardiac myocyte to maintain electrochemical gradients and to regulate the intracellular concentration and movements of Ca^{2+} (Fig. 24.2). However, elaboration of some of the more important mechanisms regulating levels of intracellular Ca^{2+} is especially relevant to such disease processes as ischemia and heart failure.

The principal entry sites for Ca^{2+} are the sarcolemmal Ca^{2+} channels that are concentrated in T-tubules and opened by membrane depolarization (34). Two sorts of Ca^{2+} channels have been identified, T-type and L-type. The L-type Ca^{2+} channel that binds dihydropyridines and other Ca^{2+} channel blocking drugs has been isolated and cloned from skeletal muscle (35). The prevailing thought is that Ca^{2+} entry through sarcolemmal Ca^{2+} channels induces the release of much larger amounts of Ca^{2+} from the sarcoplasmic reticulum (36). A particularly exciting development (37) has been the recent identification of a major Ca^{2+}-release channel in the sarcoplasmic reticulum. These structures appear to open in response to Ca^{2+} (38) and can be blocked by the drug ryanodine (37); hence, the name "ryanodine

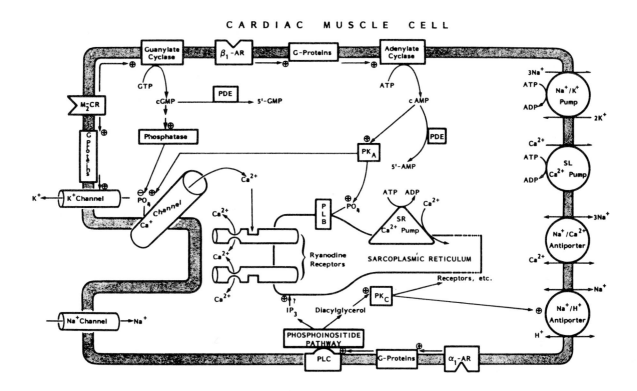

Figure 24.2. *Biochemical mechanisms modulating intracellular ion fluxes and Ca²⁺ homeostasis in cardiac muscle.* The opening of Na⁺ channels by depolarization and subsequent influx of Na⁺ leads to opening of voltage sensitive Ca²⁺ channels in the sarcolemma. The influx of Ca²⁺ stimulates release of Ca²⁺ from sarcoplasmic reticulum through Ca²⁺ release channels ("ryanodine receptors"). This mechanism can be augmented by beta-adrenergic receptor activation of cAMP(adenosine monophosphate)-dependent protein kinase (PK$_A$), which phosphorylates the sarcolemmal Ca²⁺ channel. cAMP is inactivated by conversion to 5'-adenosine monophosphate (5'-AMP) by action of a phosphodiesterase (PDE). Alpha-adrenergic receptor stimulation may increase intracellular Ca²⁺ through activation of phospholipase c(PLC) as described in Figure 24.1. Muscarinic cholinergic agonists (M₂-CR) diminish intracellular Ca²⁺ levels by antagonizing cAMP-mediated protein phosphorylation and by membrane hyperpolarization. Ca²⁺ uptake by a sarcoplasmic reticulum (SR) pump is enhanced by phosphorylation of the protein, phospholamban (PLB). In addition, Ca²⁺ efflux from cardiac myocytes occurs through a sarcolemmal Ca²⁺ pump.

receptors." Both the L-type Ca²⁺ channels of the sarcolemma and the Ca²⁺-release channels of the sarcoplasmic reticulum are substrates for protein kinases (39). Moreover, the sarcoplasmic reticulum Ca²⁺-release channels are highly sensitive to Ca²⁺-dependent proteolysis (39). The latter process may be one of the mechanisms accounting for Ca²⁺ overload in myocardial ischemia because proteolysis of the channel greatly increases its open time (40). On the other hand, phosphorylation of the sarcolemmal L-type Ca²⁺ channel by cAMP-dependent protein kinase is the mechanism accounting for the increase in inward Ca²⁺ current observed in response to catecholamine stimulation of cardiac muscle. The molecular mechanism appears to be an increase in the probability of the open state of individual channels (41).

In addition to the intracellular Ca²⁺ overload state of myocardial ischemia (see later), abnormal Ca²⁺ transients and Ca²⁺ overload have been observed to occur in failing human myocardium (42). The latter could be improved by administration of ryanodine to isolated muscle strips (42). Such experiments suggest that development of pharmacologic agents directed at the Ca²⁺ release channel of sarcoplasmic reticulum might be useful therapeutically.

There is another pathway for Ca²⁺ influx into cardiac myocytes. Sodium ion (Na⁺) plays a central role in this pathway through a Na⁺/Ca²⁺ antiporter localized to the cardiac sarcolemma (43). Antiporters do not require adenosine triphosphate (ATP) for translocation of ions. Inhibition of the Na⁺/K⁺ pump by cardiac glycosides (44) or by depletion of ATP in ischemia (45) may lead to increases in

intracellular Na⁺ and thereby increase intracellular Ca²⁺ through Na⁺/Ca²⁺ exchange. Moreover, intracellular acidosis (for example, ischemia) or activation of the Na⁺/H⁺ antiporter by pharmacologic agonists may enhance Ca²⁺ entry through Na⁺/Ca²⁺ exchange due to a rise in intracellular Na⁺.

The levels of intracellular Ca²⁺ in cardiac myocytes are reduced during diastole by an ATP-dependent Ca²⁺ pump located in the sarcoplasmic reticulum (46). Inside the sarcoplasmic reticulum, Ca²⁺ may remain in solution or be bound to the protein calsequestrin (47). Earlier studies provided evidence for beta-adrenergic stimulation of Ca²⁺ uptake by sarcoplasmic reticulum mediated by phosphorylation (that is, by cAMP-dependent protein kinase) of the protein phospholamban (48). The mechanism presumably involves enhanced affinity of the sarcoplasmic reticulum Ca^{2+} pump for Ca^{2+} and the predominant physiologic consequence is enhanced relaxation rate of the muscle (49). Recent studies (50) have shown that phospholamban possesses Ca^{2+} channel activity as well. Therefore, more than one pathway for Ca^{2+} efflux from the sarcoplasmic reticulum may exist. Finally, Ca^{2+} may exit the cardiac myocyte through a sarcolemmal Ca^{2+} pump that is stimulated by Ca^{2+} plus calmodulin and by cAMP-mediated phosphorylation (51).

In summary, the elucidation of specific pathways for Ca^{2+} movement in cardiac myocytes and the channels and enzyme systems responsible for this movement provides a rich framework for developing pharmacologic agents that enhance or attenuate levels of intracellular Ca^{2+}. Given the important role that Ca^{2+} serves in both normal and pathophysiologic states, such as heart failure and ischemia, the development of new kinds of Ca^{2+} antagonists and agonists seems well justified.

Molecules mediating myocardial injury or repair. The recent development of thrombolytic agents and the use of balloon angioplasty to alleviate the constricting lesions of coronary atherosclerosis in the setting of myocardial infarction has created a need for new therapy directed at the adverse consequences of reperfusion (52). The phenomenon of continued myocardial cell death after reperfusion following a period of ischemia appears to be due to molecular alterations brought about by the transient accumulation of free radicals both within ischemic myocardium and from neutrophils that localize to areas of ischemic myocardium after reperfusion. Such "reperfusion injury" does not occur to nearly the same extent in the presence of free radical scavengers (N-2-mercaptoproprionyl glycine) (53) or enzymes involved in free radical degradation (superoxide dismutase, catalase) (54), or if the heart is reperfused with blood that has been depleted of oxygen or neutrophils (55,56). The free radicals originating from the myocardium itself arise from the action of xanthine oxidase formed from xanthine dehydrogenase in endothelial cells possibly by the pH and Ca^{2+}-related activation of a Ca^{2+}-dependent protease (57,58). This source of radicals thus could be blocked by inhibitors of xanthine oxidase (allopurinol, oxypurinol) or the Ca^{2+}-dependent protease. Treatment with xanthine oxidase inhibitors has been demonstrated to be effective but also rather impractical because these must be administered for 12 to 18 h before ischemia occurs.

A more fruitful area of therapeutic research has targeted the other source of free radicals, the neutrophil, at the level of the cell-cell interactions that enable recognition of and localization to areas of recent ischemia. This recognition is mediated by the neutrophil membrane antigen complex CD_W 18 (LFA-1/Mac-1/p150, 95), which associates with one or more endothelial surface antigens variously called ELAM-1

(endothelium-leukocyte adhesion molecule-1) (59) and ICAM-1 (intercellular adhesion molecule-1) (60). Expression of these endothelial antigens is enhanced in the presence of inflammatory cytokines such as tumor necrosis factor (TNF-alpha), lymphotoxin (TNF-beta) and interleukin-1 (61,62). Neutrophil attachment and subsequent free radical related injury may be prevented to a great extent by blocking antibodies to either of these surface antigens (63), or theoretically by blocking peptides made to correspond to the binding portions of either.

Expression of the "heat shock" series of proteins can occur under a variety of cellular stresses including myocardial ischemia (64). Although the function and regulation of this class of proteins is unknown, it is presumed that they play some role in protection or restitution of an injured cell. Further information regarding the expression and function of these proteins holds promise for understanding the basic mechanisms of cellular response to injury.

Cardiac growth and regulation of gene expression. Understanding the mechanisms that regulate the expression of genes that encode the many proteins that constitute cardiac muscle is an important objective of molecular cardiology. In the adult, cardiac myocytes have reached a state of terminal differentiation, such that, despite the presence of nuclei, the ability for actual cellular division (and therefore replacement of dead tissue) is lost. Although this occurrence suggests the appearance of genetic inactivity in the heart, more recent studies have shown that a variety of genetic processes are involved constantly in regulating adaptation of the heart to normal and abnormal physical states. At present, relatively little is known about the reasons for the protein phenotypic changes that occur during development, under hemodynamic stresses such as congestive heart failure or under hormonal influences such as that of hyper- or hypothyroidism. The latter include major shifts in the predominantly expressed isoforms of contractile proteins (65,66), the Na^+/K^+ adenosine triphosphatase (ATPase) (67), and in the distribution of atrial natriuretic factor (ANF) (68,69), and several other proteins. The relative quantity of classes of translated proteins also changes with stress, with the proportion of myofibrillar elements increasing under pressure overload (70) and decreasing with overt congestive heart failure (71). At present, it is not known which of these well described alterations in protein content constitute physiologic adaptation and which, if any, constitute the basis for pathology. Discovery of the proximate stimuli for these changes, the controls of the promoter and enhancer DNA sequences responsible for regulation of these genes in a physiologically coordinated fashion, and the physiologic role played by each protein change will be necessary to allow identification of appropriate targets for therapeutic intervention.

Proto-oncogenes are believed to regulate cell differentiation, growth and replication (72). It has been found that the level of the proto-oncogene c-fos decreases suddenly, and afterward the level of c-myc decreases more gradually during embryonic development of the rat heart (73). On the contrary, pressure overload-induced hypertrophy is associated with early expression of c-myc and c-fos as well as heat shock protein hsp 70 (73,74); c-myc expression has also been noted after stimulation of cardiac myocyte growth by alpha-adrenergic agents, phorbol esters and serum (75). Effects of various oncogenes on expression of muscle-related genes including ion channels as well as contractile elements have been studied in noncardiac cells derived from muscle (76), but such studies have not yet been fully extended to cardiac myocytes. A knowledge of the mechanisms controlling cardiac myocyte proliferation and terminal differentiation may lead to the development of interventions directed toward stimulation of regrowth and regeneration after cell death such as that due to myocardial infarction. A transgenic mouse that expresses the c-myc oncogene constitutively in the heart has been developed (77). Moreover, a transgenic mouse transfected with the promotor region of DNA from the atrial natriuretic factor gene ligated to an oncogene, the SV40 large T-antigen, has been shown to develop massive right atrial hyperplasia accompanied by supraventricular arrhythmias (77a). Such approaches to investigation of the mechanisms of action of proto-oncogenes may suggest various therapeutic modalities applicable to cardiac hypertrophy or toward regeneration.

The importance of genetic influences on the myocardium is also apparent through the variety of cardiomyopathies that have a familial component. Some of these include hypertrophic obstructive cardiomyopathy, the dilated cardiomyopathy that is X-linked (78), several autosomal dominant cardiomyopathic kindreds (79,80) and the cardiomyopathies that manifest themselves as the full expression of a genetic defect involving both skeletal and cardiac muscle, such as Duchenne and Becker muscular dystrophy and myotonic dystrophy. The long QT syndromes variously referred to as Lange-Nielsen, Jervell and Romano-Ward may involve inherited abnormalities most prominently affecting cardiac conduction tissue. The underlying genetic abnormality has been described for relatively few of these human diseases with the exception of the recent discovery (81) of dystrophin as the protein that is greatly reduced in Duchenne and Becker muscular dystrophies. This protein was found with use of the techniques of "reverse genetics," which could isolate the unique genetic abnormality repeatedly associated with the disease before any knowledge of the associated protein. Current evidence suggests that dystrophin is a component of the transverse tubular membranes (82). The T-tubules are involved in excitation-contraction coupling, and dystrophin appears to anchor these structures to cytoplasmic elements (83). This anchoring may be important for proper alignment of the major membrane components mediating excitation-contraction coupling.

Similar techniques are being applied to some of the other diseases mentioned and should lead to understanding of their molecular bases as well. Familial hypertrophic obstructive cardiomyopathy is a particularly important disease for investigation, as it is a major cause of sudden death in young adults (84,85). Given that its major histologic abnormality is myocardial disorganization at each of the levels of fiber bundles, fibers and myofibrils (86), it is not surprising that recent studies have identified an abnormality in the heavy chain of cardiac myosin (87).

Endocrine functions of the heart. Recently the capacity of the heart to function as a volume monitor and endocrine organ that secretes atrial natriuretic factor in response to increased intravascular volume has been appreciated (88). Although the majority of secretory activity typically takes place in the atria, it has been noted more recently that a remarkably high degree of induction of atrial natriuretic factor expression occurs in the ventricles in the setting of significant hemodynamic stress (89). The function of this latter expression is unknown at present. The classic endocrine function of atrial natriuretic factor, to enhance natriuresis while reducing blood pressure, is mediated by a receptor that activates guanylate cyclase (90). Moreover, a receptor has been cloned that may represent a distinct subtype (91) among the three receptors for which evidence currently exists (91a). Formation of cGMP and subsequent activation of cGMP-dependent protein kinase (Fig. 24.3) results in smooth muscle relaxation (92). Efforts to discover agents that function to elevate cGMP in a similar way either through the atrial natriuretic factor receptor or independently of it are underway and should lead to useful agents for reducing systemic resistance without increasing sodium retention. A peptide analog of atrial natriuretic factor, anaritide, has been developed for this purpose and is currently undergoing clinical trials (93). The mode of regulation of atrial natriuretic factor synthesis and release is not well understood but would presumably involve a pressure- or stretch-sensitive receptor in myocardium. The identity of these receptors has yet to be established.

The Blood Vessel: Smooth Muscle and Endothelium

Regulation of blood vessel tone. The source of muscular force in vasculature is smooth muscle that constitutes the medial layer of the vessel. The molecular mechanisms that account for the generation and maintenance of tone by smooth muscle are different from those in cardiac muscle. Teleologically, the task of the blood vessel is to maintain tone for protracted periods of time. It is not surprising, then, that the contractile mechanism in vascular muscle is energy efficient (94). The molecular nature of this mechanism is only partially characterized but appears to involve attached cross-bridges that cycle very slowly (95). To some extent sustained tension in vascular muscle resembles the rigor state in cardiac or skeletal muscle and has at least one analogy in nature, the "catch state" of the mollusk (96). The

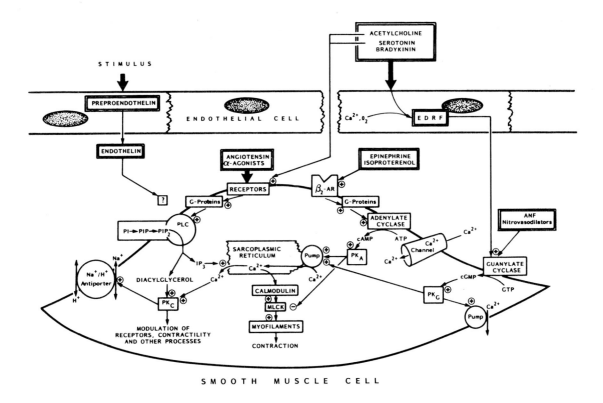

Figure 24.3. *Major pathways influencing contractility of smooth muscle of the blood vessel wall.* Ca^{2+} can enter smooth muscle cells through voltage-sensitive sarcolemmal Ca^{2+} channels. Moreover, a variety of hormones or pharmacologic agents can activate the phosphoinositide pathway as described in Figure 24.1 leading to release of Ca^{2+} from sarcoplasmic reticulum. Ca^{2+} bound to calmodulin initiates contraction by activating myosin light chain kinase (MLCK). Activation of cAMP-dependent protein kinase (PK_A) or cyclic guanosine monophosphate (cGMP) dependent protein kinase (PK_G) through their respective pathways leads to smooth muscle relaxation. Atrial natriuretic factor (ANF) and endothelium-derived relaxation factor (EDRF) activate the cGMP pathway. The divergent effects of certain agents (serotonin, acetylcholine) that can stimulate either contraction or relaxation of smooth muscle depends on whether a normal endothelium is present or not. Normally, these agonists stimulate release of EDRF from endothelium inducing relaxation. Endothelin is a vasoconstrictor released from endothelium.

energy efficiency of the mechanism is the direct result of slow cross-bridge cycling. Cross-bridge cycling consumes ATP and the slower the cycling, the less ATP that is needed to maintain tone.

The generation and maintenance of tone by vascular muscle requires Ca^{2+} (97). Some of the molecular pathways involved in regulating intracellular Ca^{2+} as well as mediators of contraction and relaxation are summarized in Figure 24.3. The initial molecular events involved in force generation have been extensively described and involve activation of an enzyme, myosin light chain kinase, by Ca^{2+} and the Ca^{2+}-binding protein, calmodulin (98). The latter binds certain classes of drugs such as phenothiazines and the Ca^{2+} chan-

nel blocker verapamil (99). This interaction may account, in part, for the vasodilating effects of these agents. Myosin light chain kinase activates cross-bridge cycling in smooth muscle by phosphorylating the regulatory light chain subunits of myosin and the cycling of cross-bridges is the mechanism for development of tone (100). With prolonged contraction, a second mechanism is activated that appears to capture cross-bridges in a "latch state." This mechanism requires only very low levels of Ca^{2+} and most likely operates by inhibiting the detachment of cross-bridges (101). Recently, an actin-binding protein, caldesmon, has been implicated in the formation of the "latch state" in vascular muscle and phosphorylation of this protein in response to selective agonists may account for latching (102,103). Elucidation of the molecular mechanism(s) accounting for the "latch state" in vascular muscle may lead to the development of newer agents for controlling blood vessel tone or preventing vasospasm.

Interactions between blood vessels and endothelium. Blood vessel tone results from the interaction of autonomic, endothelial, autacoid and hormonal influences. Prostaglandins (104), leukotrienes (105), peptide hormones (106), platelet factors (107), catecholamines and various neurotransmitters (108) are the specific substances that mediate vasomotion. Segmental vasospasm is an important pathologic concomitant of atherosclerosis. Under these circumstances, abnormal endothelium, activated platelets (109) and accumulations of certain neurotransmitter substances (that is, serotonin, histamines) in adventitial mast cells or nerve endings (110) are especially important cofactors in the pathogenesis of vasospasm.

The role of the endothelium in modulation of blood vessel tone has achieved considerable prominence. An important discovery was the finding that endothelium releases endothelium-derived relaxation factor (EDRF) (111), most likely nitric oxide (NO) (112), in response to several pharmacologic agents including bradykinin (113) and acetylcholine. EDRF is a potent vasodilator that activates the enzyme guanylate cyclase in vascular muscle, increasing the levels of cGMP (114). Although the intracellular site or sites of action of cGMP-dependent protein kinase, the target enzyme for cGMP, is unknown, increases in cGMP are associated with a decrease in intracellular Ca^{2+} (115), which in turn results in relaxation of the muscle.

Injury, hyperlipidemia (116) and atherosclerosis (117) impair EDRF release by many agents. Therefore the release of serotonin by activated platelets, which normally results in vasodilation through EDRF, causes vasoconstriction (109). Moreover, the effect of platelet factor 4, an EDRF-dependent vasodilator, is blunted (107).

Investigation of the nature and mechanism of action of EDRF has additionally stimulated new efforts to understand the molecular pharmacology of nitrate tolerance (118). Nitrates activate smooth muscle guanylate cyclase directly. However, the active form of the nitrate is a nitrosothiol (119). Tolerance may be associated with depletion of sulfhydryl compounds by excess nitrates. Clinical studies have shown that intravascular administration of N-acetylcysteine inhibits the development of tolerance (120).

Quite recently endothelium has been shown to be the source of another vasoactive substance, endothelin (121). Endothelin is a 21 amino acid peptide that is synthesized as preproendothelin (122). The active peptide is released by proteolytic processing of the precursor form. Although the physiologic and pharmacologic agents that can release endothelin are not yet known, the peptide is a potent vasoconstrictor (123). Moreover, the potential role of endothelin in such disorders as vasospasm and hypertension remains to be explored. Nevertheless, the recent discovery of this naturally occurring vasoconstrictor serves to emphasize the considerable work required to understand the many factors that are involved in regulating blood vessel tone.

Atherosclerosis

Atherosclerosis is a disease that involves complex interplay of all the components of the blood vessel wall with each other as well as with both soluble and formed blood elements. In recent years, much has been learned about the specific secreted and membrane-bound molecules involved in normal cell-cell communications and the perturbations in these that underlie atherosclerosis. The variety of these agents, ranging from small molecules derived from amino acids, nucleotides or lipids (for example, serotonin, adeno-sine diphosphate (ADP), thromboxane A_2, prostacyclin) to peptides and large protein complexes (for example, platelet-derived growth factor, transforming growth factor-beta, von Willebrand factor, low density lipoprotein), provides for many possible negative and positive feedback loops among the elements of the blood vessel wall (Fig. 24.4). Several reviews have outlined various perspectives on atherosclerosis with particular focus on various of these communication pathways (124–127).

Initiation and progression of atherosclerosis. The typical initiation and progression of atherosclerosis have been observed to have certain characteristic features occurring in sequence: 1) the attraction of circulating monocytes to an area of endothelium followed by passage between cells to form a subendothelial layer of activated macrophages; 2) the gradual uptake of lipid by these macrophages to form foam cells; 3) the migration from the media and progressive replication of smooth muscle cells in the intima to form crescentic masses; 4) the conversion of some of these myocytes to form foam cells; 5) the secretion of extracellular matrix in and around the lesion; and 6) necrosis and calcification of cells and matrix within the lesion. At some point concomitant with these events, gaps in the endothelial layer are observed and localization of degranulating platelets is noted adherent to such areas. These structural changes set the stage for the functional changes recognized as contributing to a majority of sudden cardiac events (128–131): loss of the nonthrombogenic property of the normal intact endothelial lining, leading to thrombosis, and the exaggerated tendency to vasospasm that has been shown in atherosclerotic arteries (110,116,117,132).

Endothelial cell injury. The theory of Ross and Glomset (127,133,134) focuses on endothelial cell injury as the cause for monocyte adhesion and the progression described. These changes may occur in the absence or the presence of endothelial separation or regional "denudation." Many investigators (135–137) have focused on the role of elevated circulating lipids as one of the known primary risk factors that operate in the absence of endothelial denudation. The mechanism by which hyperlipidemias cause the initial endothelial injury is not clear but may involve either uptake of oxidized LDL (low density lipoprotein), discussed later (138), or changes in physicochemical membrane properties (135,136). The mechanical stimuli of both hypertension and turbulent flow are sensed by endothelium and alter endothelial metabolism and ion fluxes. Turbulence induces a mitogenic response that could explain its atherogenicity (139,140). Later in the disease, the separation or loss of endothelium causes exposure of the thrombogenic subendothelium and resultant platelet attraction and aggregation.

Injury to endothelium by any of these means causes binding of blood monocytes, possibly by enhanced expression on the endothelial surface of association molecules similar to the intercellular adhesion molecules mentioned previously (141), as well as secretion of various cytokines

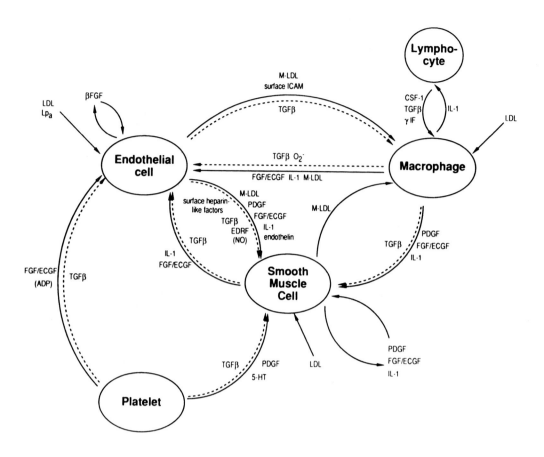

Figure 24.4. *Paracrine and autocrine interactions in atherosclerosis.*
This figure illustrates some of the complex paracrine and autocrine
interactions that occur between and among the cells playing major
roles in atheroma formation. It has been simplified by eliminating
coagulation factors and arachidonic acid derivatives. Molecules
with predominantly stimulatory function, which here may refer
either to growth, contraction, adhesion, secretion or gene expression, are depicted with solid lines. Molecules with inhibitory function with regard to any of the above are depicted with broken lines
among the endothelium, smooth muscle, macrophages and platelets.
Interactions with other cells and autocrine interactions are all shown
with solid lines for simplicity.

The figure suggests the many possibilities for counterproductive
positive feedback loops when the balances of stimulation and inhibition
are disturbed. Moreover, it highlights the centrality of the bidirectional
interactions between the smooth muscle cell and the endothelial cell,
and suggests the wide importance of the growth factors platelet-derived
growth factor (PDGF) and the ECGF/FGF (endothelial cell growth
factor) group, the interleukin (IL-1) that functions particularly as a
switch to turn on (or off) other genes and the growth inhibitor
TGF-beta. The small vasoactive molecules serotonin (5-HT) and
endothelial-derived relaxation factor (EDRF) (nitric oxide, NO), which
are stimulatory and inhibitory, respectively, to smooth muscle growth
are depicted. Endothelin, a powerful vasoconstrictor, also possesses
mitogenicity (127a). Adenosine-5 diphosphate (ADP) is shown paren-
thetically as a molecule important in causing EDRF release from
endothelial cells. The role in cell injury of low density lipoproteins
(LDL) Lp(a), oxygen radicals, and M-LDL, the oxidatively modified
LDL, are represented. Finally are shown the surface molecules of
endothelial cells that mediate macrophage/monocyte attachment (the
intercellular adhesion molecules [ICAM]) and those that suppress
smooth muscle growth (the heparin-like molecules).

that are chemotactic for monocytes. The mechanism of
conversion to foam cells likely involves uptake of LDL that
has been oxidatively modified by endothelial cells to modified-LDL (142), a form with much diminished binding to the
classic LDL receptor but with avid binding to a distinct high
affinity receptor on endothelial cells and macrophages. This
receptor is termed the scavenger acetyl-LDL or modified
LDL receptor (143,144). Bound modified-LDL appears to be
internalized through receptor-coated pits (145), after which
cholesterol is esterified by acyl-CA:cholesterol acyltrans-
ferase (ACAT) and may tend to accumulate because lack of
down regulation of uptake by esterified cholesterol (146).
The major component of LDL in atherosclerotic plaque is
modified-LDL (147,148), which is toxic to proliferating cells
(141,149) and may thus create a vicious cycle of injury,
macrophage invasion and modified-LDL accumulation.
Modification of VLDL (very low density lipoprotein) by
oxidation followed by receptor-mediated uptake may play a
similar role in macrophage cholesterol ester overload and
injury (150).

Abnormal LDL metabolism. Several atherogenic inherited abnormalities in LDL metabolism have been identified,
the classic example being the group of abnormalities in the
LDL receptor associated with familial hypercholesterolemia
(151). Others are due to abnormal LDL constituent apoproteins, such as apo B (152) or apo E and have been extensively reviewed (153,154). The atherogenicity of all these

diseases is presumably referable to increased interaction of LDL with endothelial cells or macrophages, or both, as a result of either elevated levels or affinities, then leading to increased accumulation of modified-LDL and the attendant damage.

Abnormalities in the normal removal of cholesterol from cholesterol ester-laden macrophages by high density lipoprotein (155) caused by mutations in its constituents such as apo A (156) can also lead to atherosclerosis, again presumably due to resulting elevated local concentrations of modified-LDL and its associated toxicity.

Neointimal hyperplasia and monoclonal proliferation. The next phase of atherosclerosis involving smooth muscle cell migration to and growth in the subendothelial region, termed neointimal hyperplasia, has been viewed as the primary problem in the monoclonal proliferation hypothesis of Benditt and Benditt (157), thus considering the atherosclerotic plaque as analogous to a benign tumor. Such loss of regulation of this process, normally involved in healing, has been suggested to be due to expression of abnormal transforming genes (158), but might alternatively be seen as a consequence of an inappropriate shift in the dynamic equilibrium of normal vascular myocyte populations between a "contractile phase" and a "proliferative phase" (124), toward the latter. This action might occur by loss of regulation of normal proto-oncogenes or growth factors. Interconversion between two such phenotypes of vascular myocytes would involve concerted up-regulation and down-regulation of the multiple genes required for determining each phenotype. Although such conversions are difficult to demonstrate in vivo, they are readily observable in cell culture (124). It is interesting to note that the contraction, migration and replication responses of the respective cell types are regulated in parallel by many factors, such that those species directly favoring contraction will often be chemotactic and mitogenic (that is, serotonin, platelet-derived growth factor); the converse is also often true (for example, prostacyclin).

Such concepts of hyperproliferation due either to expression of an abnormal gene or to abnormal expression of a normal gene have precedents in oncology; many human cancers are caused by single amino acid mutations of the ras proto-oncogene to a transforming protein (159–162), whereas Burkitt's lymphoma is caused by abnormal regulation of a normal myc proto-oncogene (163,164). Smooth muscle hyperplasia by either of these mechanisms could be mediated intracellularly by autocrine hyperstimulation in which individual cells both synthesize and respond to a mitogenic stimulus. They could also be stimulated by intercellular mechanisms involving paracrine response to the secretion by neighboring cells of either elevated levels of growth factors or insufficient growth inhibiting factors (chalones). Evidence for each of these mechanisms exists, and recognition of the remarkable homology between the oncogene v-sis and the B-chain of the platelet-derived growth factor (165,166) in conjunction with the discovery of

expression of significantly elevated amounts of both the A and B chains of platelet-derived growth factor in atherosclerotic lesions (167,168) has implicated this factor as one of the more important in their etiology.

Platelet derived growth factor. This factor is one of the primary constituents of the platelet alpha-granule, but one or both of its chains can also be synthesized and generated by several other cells, including endothelial cells, macrophages and even smooth muscle in early stages of development when stressed (169). It is a powerful chemotactic agent as well as the major mitogen for smooth muscle (170). There is evidence that it serves as a vasoconstrictor as well (171). Although human platelet-derived growth factor is a hetrodimer of the homologous A and B chains, other cells may secrete instead or in addition a homodimeric protein (that is, AA or BB). Macrophages appear to strongly favor B chains, smooth muscle cells favor A chains, and endothelial cells exhibit independent regulation of the two by agents such as thrombin and transforming growth factor-beta (TGF-beta) (172–175). All forms are mitogenic with greater potency of the B-chain (176,177). A platelet-derived growth factor receptor was cloned in 1986 (178), and recently two receptors have been described with differing specificities (176,179,180). Paracrine stimulation by these chains from platelets and arterial cells under the abnormal conditions predisposing to atherosclerosis likely accounts for a major proportion of the dysfunctional muscular proliferation (Fig. 24.4). Although expression in vascular myocytes normally seems reserved to early stages of vascular development (181), its presence in neointimal muscle suggests that a vicious cycle of autocrine self-stimulation may have occurred with expression of the factor and receptor in the same cell, much as is seen in cells that are transformed by the homologous v-sis oncogene (182). As noted, such expression might represent that of a normal gene or an altered, transforming gene (183); the reason for such a mutation in the gene or its controlling element is unclear but could reflect injury by free radicals induced by macrophages or endothelial cells. It could also be caused by lipid-soluble carcinogens delivered by LDL (184), which is believed to be important in effecting delivery to cells of several lipid-soluble species such as cyclosporine (185).

Many other paracrine and autocrine factors present in platelets and atheroma cells are mitogenic toward vascular myocytes and also lead to other contractile or metabolic changes (Fig. 24.4); these include endothelial cell growth factor, interleukin-1 (186a), its derivative alpha-fibroblast growth factor (alpha-FGF) and its homolog beta-fibroblast growth factor (beta-FGF) (186), serotonin (187) and thrombospondin (188). Various neurotransmitters and hormones such as catecholamines (189) and angiotensin II (190) are likewise implicated in myocyte growth regulation. The endothelial cell growth factor group of factors is mitogenic in a paracrine and autocrine fashion for both endothelium and smooth muscle (191,192) and induce angiogenesis. These factors are beneficial in helping repair endothelial breaks that could lead to thrombogenesis and the described series of events; but might also be detrimental by their stimulation of endothelial cells and by induction of neovascularization of plaques with the possibility of subsequent intraplaque hemorrhage and rupture (193). Angiogenin is another, unrelated angiogenic factor, but it is not a strong mitogen (194).

A final contribution to unregulated smooth muscle proliferation might be deficiency of local growth inhibitors such as prostacyclin and the heparin-like molecules on the endothelial surface after endothelial injury (195,196). Changes in the heparan component of atheroma matrix could have a similar effect (197,198).

Other contributing agents and mechanisms in atheroma formation. The accumulation of additional lipid to form the neointimal foam cells of smooth muscle, rather than macrophage origin as identified by typical antibody staining (199), may occur by somewhat different mechanisms involving either oncogenic transformation (200) after many cycles of replication or transfer of lipid from macrophage-derived foam cells (201), because the smooth muscle cells do not possess the scavenger LDL receptor. Conversely, endothelial cells appear to stimulate hydrolysis of cholesterol esters by smooth muscle cells (202).

Observations of lipid accumulations in conjunction with herpes viruses frequently detected in plaque myocytes have suggested viruses as additional possible contributing agents to atheroma formation (203,204). Yet another molecular mechanism for atherosclerosis has been suggested by the recent cloning of the apo(a) component of the lipoprotein Lp(a), a little known variant of LDL that is characterized by the presence of the protein apo(a) in disulfide linkage to apo-B-100 (205). Elevations of Lp(a) have been associated in many studies with atherosclerosis as a risk factor independent of the typical lipoprotein profile (206). The apo(a) component is characterized by multiple repetitions of a "kringle" structure similar to that employed by plasminogen and tissue plasminogen activator (t-PA) for fibrin binding, but the mechanism by which elevated Lp(a) predisposes to atherogenesis has not been elucidated.

Diagnostic methods and therapeutic interventions. Understanding of the specific autocrine and paracrine interactions mediated by the numerous growth factors depicted in Figure 24.4 should afford many opportunities for development of diagnostic methods as well as therapeutic interventions for early detection and treatment of atherosclerosis. The immediate diagnostic possibilities are likely to include evaluations for genetic predispositions to atherosclerotic and other diseases by methods of restriction fragment length polymorphisms (207). Detection of areas of endothelial denudation or platelet activation by appropriate radiolabeled monoclonal antibodies could allow local mechanical interventions such as laser "sealing" (208,209) or use of antibodies to deliver in a targeted fashion drugs such as growth factor modulators or antimitotic agents.

Administration of n-3 fatty acids has been successful recently in reduction of postangioplasty restenosis (210) and several other methods for interfering with the pathways depicted in Figure 24.4 are also being considered as ways to avoid this cause of much morbidity (211,212). The known effects of n-3 fatty acids to diminish intimal hyperplasia may relate to their capacity to inhibit endothelial secretion of platelet-derived growth factor homologs (213). The preliminary use of cyclosporine to prevent immune-mediated components of vascular injury observed in the post-transplant setting has been promising in animals (214) and may reflect the beginning of an era of atherosclerosis treatment with the use of agents designed to suppress or mimic various biologic cytokines as directed by understanding of their roles.

Selected areas for research might include blockade of the expression of platelet derived growth factor or its receptor; or the platelet-derived growth factor-receptor interaction itself by inhibitors such as suramin (215) or antibodies or peptide fragments intended to compete for binding. Conversely, antibody-directed delivery of endothelial growth-stimulating agents to promote coverage of denuded areas of endothelium might be promising, as could some means of modulation of the genes expressed on the endothelial surface that govern interactions with blood elements. Along similar lines, it is exciting to note the recent treatment of LDL receptor-deficient fibroblasts by transfer of the LDL receptor gene, which successfully resulted in expression of functional LDL receptors (215a).

Thrombosis and Thrombolysis

Antithrombotic properties of endothelium. The process of intravascular thrombosis, like that of atherosclerosis, is complex and requires the cooperative interaction of several elements. That coronary occlusion is a result of thrombus formation, and causes myocardial infarction are not new ideas (216), but the strongest supporting evidence has been obtained in more recent years (128). Both myocardial infarction and unstable angina pectoris are associated with ulceration of atherosclerotic plaques (130), thus underscoring the importance of endothelium as an important line of defense against arterial thrombosis. Some of the antithrombotic properties of endothelium include production of prostacyclin and endothelial-derived relaxation factor (EDRF) that inhibit platelet aggregation (217), the presence of heparin-like polysaccharides on the cell surface (218), the presence on the surface of thrombomodulin, which participates in generation of anticoagulants (132), and an affinity for tissue plasminogen activator as well as plasminogen (219). The antithrombotic properties of the endothelium can be diminished by a wide range of factors. Hypercholesterolemia (116), immune injury as in transplantation (220) and circulating factors such as cytokines (221) can impair normal endothelial function. Moreover, the injured endothelium has the capacity to facilitate thrombosis by binding factor VII(a) (132) and expressing tissue factor activator (132) and by secreting platelet activating factor (107) and plasminogen activator inhibitor (222).

Tissue plasminogen activator. The two major constituents of the thrombus, fibrin and platelets, continue to receive considerable attention. The isolation, DNA cloning and large scale production of tissue plasminogen activator (t-PA) by recombinant DNA technology has opened a new era in the treatment of myocardial infarction (223,224). Although intravenous t-PA has proved effective in clinical studies and is available for broad usage, much current research is directed to improving several features of the molecule on the basis of sound principles of protein structure-function. Attempts to engineer the molecule are aimed at enhancing affinity for fibrin, improving specificity, lengthening half-life and reducing interaction with endogenous inhibitors. Such strategies as modifying the glycosylation state for prolonging the half-life (225) and covalently linking t-PA to fibrin-specific monoclonal antibodies (226) are only two examples of attempts to improve clinical efficacy.

Plasminogen activator inhibitors. There are at least three types of plasminogen activator inhibitors (PAI). Serum levels of these inhibitors have been shown to be elevated in patients with thrombotic disorders and atherosclerosis (227) and are increased with inflammation or infection (228). Plasminogen activator inhibition is important not only because of the potential problem it poses for t-PA treatment of patients with myocardial infarction but also because it may be one component in the overall pathogenesis of vascular disease. It is not surprising, therefore, that efforts to understand the tissue expression and regulation of secretion of plasminogen activator inhibitors are especially intense. In addition, at the protein structural level, genetic engineering strategies to produce a synthetic t-PA devoid of affinity for such inhibitors may be especially fruitful.

Platelet aggregation inhibitors. The platelet is not only a major constituent of the thrombus but also the source of powerful vasoconstrictors that can cause vasospasm and enhance coagulation by diminished blood flow (132). Platelet aggregation and re-thrombosis after recanalization of arteries by t-PA is a significant drawback for present thrombolytic therapy. Thus, the development of more efficacious agents (both potent and selective) to inhibit the cyclooxygenase (229) and lipoxygenase (105) pathways that produce platelet-aggregating prostaglandins, thromboxanes and leukotrienes is needed. Moreover, the recent demonstration that antibodies directed against platelet surface glycoproteins expressed on activation (that is, thrombospondin and GIIb/IIIa) effectively inhibit aggregation suggests new possibilities for preventing the platelet aggregates enmeshed in fibrin that are resistant to thrombolysis (230).

Conclusions

The major advances in understanding the cellular and molecular bases of normal and abnormal cardiovascular function now provide a useful paradigm for future investigation of specific disease entities. New insights into the causes of atherosclerosis and specific application of molecular biologic methodologies to the common problem, myocardial infarction, have drawn sharp attention to the utility of molecules as clinical tools for cardiologists (231). This review has highlighted some of the exciting areas of investigation in molecular cardiology; the future shows great promise.

We thank Nils Bang, MD, Larry R. Jones, MD, Jon Lindemann, MD and Suzanne B. Knoebel, MD, Department of Medicine, Indiana University School of Medicine, for helpful suggestions and critiques. In addition, we are grateful to Linda Bethuram for editorial assistance.

References

1. Ringer S. A further contribution regarding the influence of the different constituents of the blood of the contraction of the heart. J Physiol (Lond) 1882;4:30.
2. Williams LT, Lefkowitz RJ, Watanabe AM, Hathaway DR, Besch HR. Thyroid hormone regulation of beta-adrenergic receptor number. J Biol Chem 1977;252:2787–9.
3. Bristow MR, Ginsberg R, Minobe WA, et al. Decreased catecholamine sensitivity and β_1-adrenergic receptor density in failing human hearts. N Engl J Med 1982;307:205–11.
4. Maisel AS, Motulsky HJ, Insel PA. Externalization of β-adrenergic receptors promoted by myocardial ischemia. Science 1985;230:183–6.
5. Heathers GP, Yamada KA, Kanter EM, Corr PB. Long-chain acylcarnitines mediate the hypoxia-induced increase in α-adrenergic receptors in adult canine cardiac myocytes. Circ Res 1987;61:735–76.
6. Lefkowitz RJ, Caron MG. Adrenergic receptors: models for the study of receptors coupled to guanine nucleotide regulatory proteins. J Biol Chem 1988;263:4993–6.
7. Benovic JL, Kuhn H, Weyand I, et al. Functional sensitization of the isolated β-adrenergic receptor by the β-adrenergic kinase: potential role of an analog of the retinal protein arrestin (48kDa protein). Proc Natl Acad Sci USA 1987;8:8879–82.
8. Bouvier M, Leeb-Lundberg LMF, Benovic JL, Caron MG, Lefkowitz RJ. Regulation of adrenergic receptor function by phosphorylation. J Biol Chem 1987;262:3106–13.
8a. Yang SD, Fong YL, Benovic JL, et al. Dephosphorylation of the β_2-adrenergic receptor and rhodopsin by latent phosphatase 2. J Biol Chem 1988;263:8856–8.
9. Hadcock JR, Malbon CC. Down-regulation of β-adrenergic receptors: agonist-induced reduction in receptor mRNA levels. Proc Natl Acad Sci USA 1988;85:5021–5.
10. Dixon RAF, Kobilka BK, Strader DJ, et al. Cloning of the gene and cDNA for mammalian β-adrenergic receptor and homology with rhodopsin. Nature 1986;321:75–9.
11. Frielle T, Collins S, Daniel KW, et al. Cloning of the cDNA for the human β-adrenergic receptor. Proc Natl Acad Sci USA 1987;84:7920–4.
12. Kobilka BK, Frielle T, Dohlman HG, et al. Delineation of the intronless nature of the genes for the human and hamster β-adrenergic receptor and their putative promotor regions. J Biol Chem 1987;262:7321–7.
13. Kobilka BK, Dixon RAF, Frielle T, et al. cDNA for the human β-adrenergic receptor: a protein with multiple membrane-spanning domains and encoded by a gene whose chromosomal location is shared with that of the receptor for platelet-derived growth factor. Proc Natl Acad Sci USA 1987;84:46–50.
14. Gilman AG. G-proteins: transducers of receptor-generated signals. Annu Rev Biochem 1987;56:615–49.

15. Lochrie MA, Simon MI. G-protein multiplicity in eukaryotic signal transduction systems. Biochem 1988;27:4957–65.

16. Zick Y, Sagi-Eisenberg R, Pines M, et al. Multisite phosphorylation of the α-subunit of transducin by the insulin receptor kinase and protein kinase C. Proc Natl Acad Sci USA 1986;83:9294–7.

17. Dohlman HG, Caron MC, Lefkowitz RJ. A family of receptors coupled to guanine nucleotide regulatory proteins. Biochem 1987;26:2658–64.

18. Neer EJ, Clapman DE. Roles of G-proteins in transmembrane signaling. Nature 1988;333:129–34.

19. Fain JN, Wallace MA, Wajcikiewicz RJH. Evidence for involvement of guanine nucleotide-binding regulatory proteins in the activation of phospholipases by hormones. FASEB J 1988;2:2569–74.

20. Bristow MR, Ginsburg R, Umans V, et al. β₁- and β₂-adrenergic receptor subpopulations in nonfailing and failing human ventricular myocardium: coupling of both receptor subtypes to muscle contraction and selective β₁-receptor down-regulation in heart failure. Circ Res 1986;59:297–309.

21. Port JD, Bristow MR. Myocardial β₂-receptor subsensitivity in the failing human heart (abstr). J Am Coll Cardiol 1988;11:117A.

22. Feldman AM, Cates AE, Veazey WB, et al. Increase in the 40,000-mol wt pertussis toxin substrate (G-protein) in the failing heart. J Clin Invest 1988;82:189–97.

23. Heinsimer JA, Davies AO, Downs RW, et al. Impaired formation of β-adrenergic receptor-nucleotide binding protein complexes in pseudohypoparathyroidism. J Clin Invest 1984;68:1450–5.

24. Gawler D, Milligan G, Spiegel AM, Unson CG, Houslay MD. Abolition of the expression of inhibitory guanine nucleotide regulatory protein G₁ activity in diabetes. Nature 1987;327:229–31.

25. Means AR, Dedman JR. Calmodulin—an intracellular calcium receptor. Nature 1980;285:73–7.

26. Berridge MJ. Inositol triphosphate and diacylglycerol: two interacting second messengers. Annu Rev Biochem 1987;53:159–93.

27. Majerus PW, Connolly TM, Bansal VS, et al. Inositol phosphates: synthesis and degradation. J Biol Chem 1988;263:3051–4.

28. Ashkenazi A, Winslow JW, Peralta EG, et al. An M₂ muscarinic receptor subtype couples to both adenylyl cyclase and phosphoinositide turnover. Science 1987;238:672–5.

29. Nishizuka Y. Studies and perspectives of protein kinase C. Science 1986;233:305–12.

30. Preseti CF, Scott BT, Jones LR. Identification of an endogenous protein kinase C activity and its 15-kilodalton substrate in purified canine cardiac sarcolemmal vesicles. J Biol Chem 1985;260:13879–89.

31. Seifter JL, Aronson PS. Properties and physiologic roles of the plasma membrane sodium-hydrogen exchanger. J Clin Invest 1986;78:859–64.

32. Somlyo AV, Bond M, Somlyo AP, Scarpa A. Inositol trisphosphate-induced calcium release and contraction in vascular smooth muscle. Proc Natl Acad Sci USA 1985;82:5231–5.

33. Nosek TM, Williams MF, Zeigler ST, Godt RE. Inositol triphosphate enhances calcium release in skinned cardiac and skeletal muscle. Am J Physiol 1986;250:C807–11.

34. Tsien RW, Hess P, McCleskey EW, Rosenberg RL. Calcium channels: mechanisms of selectivity, permeation, and block. Ann Rev Biophys Biophys Chem 1987;16:265–90.

35. Ellis SB, Williams ME, Ways NR, et al. Sequence and expression of mRNAs encoding the α₁ and α₂ subunits of a dihydropyridine-sensitive calcium channel. Science 1988;241:1661–4.

36. Hathaway DR, Watanabe AM. Biochemical basis for cardiac and vascular smooth muscle contraction. In: Textbook of Internal Medicine. Kelley WN, ed. Philadelphia: Harper & Row, 1989 (in press).

37. Inui M, Wang S, Saito A, Fleischer S. Characterization of junctional and longitudinal sarcoplasmic reticulum from heart muscle. J Biol Chem 1988;263:10843–50.

38. Horne WA, Abdul-Ghany E, Racker E, et al. Functional reconstitution of skeletal muscle Ca²⁺ channels: separation of regulatory and channel components. Proc Natl Acad Sci USA 1988;85:3718–22.

39. Seiler S, Wegener AD, Whang DD, Hathaway DR, Jones LR. High molecular weight proteins in cardiac and skeletal muscle junctional sarcoplasmic reticulum vesicles bind calmodulin, are phosphorylated and are degraded by Ca²⁺-activated protease. J Biol Chem 1984;259:8550–7.

40. Rardon DP, Cefali DC, Mitchell RD, Seiler SM, Hathaway DR, Jonas LR. Digestion of cardiac and skeletal muscle junctional sarcoplasmic reticulum vesicles with calpain II. Circ Res 1990;67:84–96.

41. Tsien RW. Calcium channels in excitable cell membranes. Annu Rev Physiol 1983;45:341–58.

42. Gwatmey JK, Copelas L, MacKinnon R, et al. Abnormal intracellular calcium handling in myocardium from patients with end-stage heart failure. Circ Res 1987;61:70–6.

43. Reeves JP. The sarcolemmal sodium-calcium exchange system. Cur Top Membr Trans 1985;25:77–127.

44. Akera T, Brody TM. Myocardial membranes: regulation and function of the sodium pump. Annu Rev Physiol 1982;44:375–88.

45. Jennings RB, Steenbergen C. Nucleotide metabolism and cellular damage in myocardial ischemia. Annu Rev Physiol 1985;47:729–49.

46. Tada M, Yamamota T, Tonomura Y. Molecular mechanism of active calcium transport by sarcoplasmic reticulum. Physiol Rev 1978;58:1–79.

47. Scott BT, Simmerman HKB, Collins JH, Nadal-Ginard B, Jones LR. Complete amino acid sequence of canine cardiac calsequestrin deduced by cDNA cloning. J Biol Chem 1988;263:8958–64.

48. Tada M, Inui M. Regulation of calcium transport by the ATPase-phospholamban system. J Mol Cell Cardiol 1983;15:565–75.

49. Lindemann JP, Jones LR, Hathaway DR, Henry BG, Watanabe AM. Beta-adrenergic stimulation of phospholamban phosphorylation and Ca²⁺-ATPase activity in guinea pig ventricles. J Biol Chem 1983;258:464–81.

50. Kovacs RJ, Nelson MT, Simmerman HKB, Jones LR. Phospholamban forms Ca²⁺-selective channels in lipid bilayers. J Biol Chem 1988;263:18364–68.

51. Caroni P, Carafoli E. An ATP-dependent Ca²⁺ pumping system in dog heart sarcolemma. Nature 1980;283:765–7.

52. Bolli R. Oxygen-derived free radicals and postischemic myocardial dysfunction ("stunned myocardium"). J Am Coll Cardiol 1988;12:239–49.

53. Mitsos SE, Fantone JC, Gallagher KP, et al. Canine myocardial reperfusion injury: protection by a free radical scavenger, N-Z-mercaptopropionyl glycine. J Cardiovasc Pharmacol 1986;8:978–88.

54. Werns SW, Shea MJ, Mitsos SE, et al. Reduction of the size of infarction by allopurinol in the ischemic-reperfused canine heart. Circulation 1986;73:518–24.

55. Romson JL, Hook BG, Kunkel SL, et al. Reduction of the extent of ischemic myocardial injury by neutrophil depletion in the dog. Circulation 1983;67:1016–23.

56. Mitsos SE, Askew JE, Fantone JC, et al. Protective effects of N-2-mercaptopropionyl glycine against myocardial reperfusion injury after neutrophil depletion in the dog: evidence for the role of intracellular-derived free radicals. Circulation 1986;73:1077–86.

57. Battelli MG. Enzymatic conversion of rat liver xanthine oxidase from dehydrogenase (D-form) to oxidase (O-form). FEBS Lett 1980;113:47–51.

58. Korthius RJ, Granger DN, Townsley MI, Taylor AE. The role of oxygen-derived free radicals in ischemia-induced increases in canine skeletal muscular vascular permeability. Circ Res 1985;57:599–609.

59. Bevilacqua MP, Pober JS, Mendrick DL, Cotran RS, Gimbrone MA. Identification of an inducible endothelial-leukocyte adhesion molecule. Proc Natl Acad Sci USA 1987;84:9238–42.

60. Dustin ML, Springer TA. Lymphocyte function-associated antigen-1 (LFA-1) interaction with intercellular adhesion molecule-1 (ICAM-1) is one of at least three mechanisms for lymphocyte adhesion to cultured endothelial cells. J Cell Biol 1988;107:321–31.

61. Pohlman TH, Stanness KA, Beatty PG, Ochs HD, Harlan JM. An endothelial cell surface factor(s) induced in vitro by lipopolysaccharide, interleukin-1 and tumor necrosis factor-alpha increases neutrophil adherence by a CDw18-dependent mechanism. J Immunol 1986;136:4548–53.

62. Broudy VC, Harlan JM, Adamson JW. Disparate effects of tumor necrosis factor-alpha/cachectin and tumor necrosis factor-beta/lymphotoxin on hematopoietic growth factor production and neutrophil adhesion molecule expression by cultured human endothelial cells. J Immunol 1987;138:4298–302.

63. Simpson PJ, Todd RF, Fantone JC, Mickelson JK, Griffin JD, Lucchesi BR. Reduction of experimental canine myocardial reperfusion injury by a monoclonal antibody (anti-Mol, anti-CD11b) that inhibits leukocyte adhesion. J Clin Invest 1988;81:624–9.

64. Dillmann WH, Mehta HB, Barrieux A, Guth BD, Neeley WE, Ross J Jr. Ischemia of the dog heart induces the appearance of a cardiac mRNA coding for a protein with migration characteristics similar to heat-shock/stress protein 71. Circ Res 1986;59:110–4.

65. Morkin E. Chronic adaptations in contractile proteins: genetic regulation. Annu Rev Physiol 1987;49:545–54.

66. Emerson C, Fischman D, Nadal-Ginard B, Siddiqui MAQ, eds. Molecular Biology of Muscle Development. New York: Alan R. Liss, 1986: 773–863.

67. Orlowski J, Lingrel JB. Tissue-specific and developmental regulation of rat Na,K-ATPase catalytic α isoform and α^1 subunit mRNAs. J Biol Chem 1988;263:10436–42.

68. Bloch KD, Seidman JG, Naftilan JD, Fallon JT, Seidman CE. Neonatal atria and ventricles secrete atrial natriuretic factor via tissue-specific secretory pathways. Cell 1986;47:695–702.

69. Ladenson PW, Bloch KD, Seidman JG. Modulation of atrial natriuretic factor by thyroid hormone: mRNA and peptide levels in hypothyroid, euthyroid and hyperthyroid rat atria and ventricles. Endocrinology 1988;123:652–7.

70. Page E, McCallister LP. Quantitative electron microscopic description of heart muscle cells. Application to normal, hypertrophied and thyroxine-stimulated hearts. Am J Cardiol 1973;31:172–81.

71. Schwartz F, Schaper J, Kittstein D, et al. Reduced volume fraction of myofibrils in myocardium of patients with decompensated pressure overload. Circulation 1981;63:1299–304.

72. Varmus HE. The molecular genetics of cellular oncogenes. Annu Rev Genet 1984;18:553–612.

73. Schneider MD, Payne PA, Ueno H, Perryman MB, Roberts R. Dissociated expression of c-myc and a-fos related competence gene during cardiac myogenesis. Mol Cell Biol 1986;6:4140–3.

74. Komuro I, Kurabayashi M, Takaku F, Yazaki Y. Expression of cellular oncogenes in the myocardium during the developmental stage and pressure-overloaded hypertrophy of the rat heart. Circ Res 1988;62: 1075–9.

75. Starksen NF, Simpson PC, Bishopric N, et al. Cardiac myocyte hypertrophy is associated with c-myc protooncogene expression. Proc Natl Acad Sci USA 1986;83:8348–50.

76. Schneider MD, Olson EN. Control of myogenic differentiation by cellular oncogenes. Mol Neurobiol 1988;2:1–39.

77. Swain JL, Stewart TA, Leder P. Parental legacy determines methylation and the expression of an autosomal transgene: a molecular mechanism for parental imprinting. Cell 1987;50:719–27.

77a.Field LJ. Atrial natriuretic factor-SV40 T antigen transgenes produce tumors and cardiac arrhythmias in mice. Science 1988;239:1029–33.

78. Berko BA, Swift M. X-linked dilated cardiomyopathy. N Engl J Med 1987;316:1186–91.

79. Gardner RJ, Hanson JW, Ionasescu VV, et al. Dominantly inherited dilated cardiomyopathy. Am J Med Genet 1987;27:61–73.

80. Greaves SC, Roche AH, Neutze JM, Whitlock RM, Veale AM. Inheritance of hypertrophic cardiomyopathy: a cross sectional and M mode echocardiographic study of 50 families. Br Heart J 1987;58:259–66.

81. Hoffman EP, Brown RH, Kunkel LM. Dystrophin: the protein product of the Duchenne muscular dystrophy locus. Cell 1987;51:919–28.

82. Knudson CM, Hoffman EP, Kahl SD, Kunkel LM, Campbell KP. Evidence for the association of dystrophin with the transverse tubular system in skeletal muscle. J Biol Chem 1988;263:8480–4.

83. Zubrzycka-Gaarn EE, Bulman DE, Karpati G, et al. The Duchenne muscular dystrophy gene product is localized in sarcolemma of human skeletal muscle. Nature 1988;333:466–9.

84. Maron BJ, Bonow RO, Cannon RO, Leon MB, Epstein SE. Hypertrophic cardiomyopathy: interrelations of clinical manifestations, pathophysiology and therapy. N Engl J Med 1987;316:780–9.

85. Maron BJ, Bonnow RO, Cannon RO, Leon MB, Epstein SE. Hypertrophic cardiomyopathy: interrelations of clinical manifestations, pathophysiology and therapy. N Engl J Med 1987;316:844–52.

86. Davies MJ. Current status of myocardial disarray in hypertrophic cardiomyopathy. Br Heart J 1984;51:361–3.

87. Tanigawag G, Jarcho JA, Kass S, Solomon SD, Vosberg HP, Seidman JG, Seidman CE. A molecular basis for familial hypertrophic cardiomyopathy: An α/β cardiac myosin heavy chain hybrid gene. Cell 1990;62: 991–98.

88. Genest J, Cantin M. Atrial natriuretic factor. Circulation 1987;75(suppl I):I-118–I-24.

89. Lee RT, Bloch KD, Pfeffer JM, et al. Atrial natriuretic factor gene expression in ventricles of rats with spontaneous biventricular hypertrophy. J Clin Invest 1988;81:431–4.

90. Waldman SA, Rapoport RM, Murad F. Atrial natriuretic factor selectively activates particulate guanylate cyclase and elevates cyclic GMP in rat tissues. J Biol Chem 1984;259:14332–4.

91. Fuller F, Porter JG, Arfsten AE, et al. Atrial natriuretic peptide clearance receptor. Complete sequence and functional expression of cDNA clones. J Biol Chem 1988;263:9395–401.

91a.Pandey KN, Pavlou SN, Inagami T. Identification and characterization of three distinct atrial natriuretic factor receptors. J Biol Chem 1988;263: 13406–13.

92. Rashatwar SS, Cornwell TL, Lincoln TM. Effects of 8-bromo-cGMP on Ca^{2+} levels in vascular smooth muscle cells: possible regulation of Ca^{2+}-ATPase by cGMP-dependent protein kinase. Proc Natl Acad Sci USA 1987;84:5685–9.

93. Herrmann HC, Palacios IF, Dec GW, Sheer JM, Fifer MA. Effects of atrial natriuretic factor on coronary hemodynamics and myocardial energetics in patients with heart failure. Am Heart J 1988;115:1232–8.

94. Siegman MJ, Butler TM, Mooers SU, Davies RE. Chemical energetics of force development, force maintenance and relaxation in mammalian smooth muscle. J Gen Physiol 1980;79:609–9.

95. Dillon PF, Aksoy MO, Driska SP, Murphy RA. Myosin phosphorylation and the crossbridge cycle in arterial smooth muscle. Am Science 1981;211:495–7.

96. Cohen C. Matching molecules in the catch mechanism. Proc Natl Acad Sci USA 1982;79:3176–8.

97. Rembold CM, Murphy RA. Myoplasmic calcium, myosin phosphorylation, and regulation of the crossbridge cycle in swine arterial smooth muscle. Circ Res 1986;58:803–15.

98. Adelstein RS, Sellers JR. Effects of calcium on vascular smooth muscle contraction. Am J Cardiol 1987;59:4B–10B.

99. Triggle DJ, Swamy VC. Pharmacology of agents that affect calcium: agonists and antagonists. Chest 1980;78(suppl):174–9.

100. Haeberle JR, Hathaway DR, DePaoli-Roach AA. Dephosphorylation of myosin by the catalytic subunit of a type-2 phosphatase produces relaxation of chemically skinned uterine smooth muscle. J Biol Chem 1985;260:9965–8.

101. Lash JA, Sellers J, Hathaway DR. The effects of caldesmon on smooth muscle acto-HMM ATPase activity and binding of HMM to actin. J Biol Chem 1986;261:16155–60.

102. Sobue K, Kanda K, Tanake T, Uek N. Caldesmon: a common actin-linked regulatory protein in the smooth muscle and non muscle contractile system. J Cell Biochem 1988;37:317–25.

103. Adam LP, Haeberle JR, Hathaway DR. Phosphorylation of caldesmon in arterial smooth muscle. J Biol Chem 1988 (in press).

104. Majerus PW. Arachidonate metabolism in vascular disorders. J Clin Invest 1983;72:1521–5.

105. Feuerstein G, Hallenbeck JM. Leukotrienes in health and disease. FASEB J 1987;1:186–92.

106. Lynch DR, Snyder SH. Neuropeptides: multiple molecular forms, metabolic pathways, and receptors. Ann Rev Biochem 1986;55:773–99.

107. O'Flaherty JT, Wykle RL. Biology and biochemistry of platelet-activating factor. Clin Rev Allergy 1983;1:353–67.

108. Vanhoutte PM, Verbeuren TJ, Webb RC. Local modulation of adrenergic neuro effector. Interaction in the blood vessel wall. Physiol Rev 1981;61:151–247.

109. Vanhoutte PM, Houston DS. Platelets, endothelium and vasospasm. Circulation 1985;72:728–34.

110. Kalsner S, Richards R. Coronary arteries of cardiac patients are hyperreactive and contain stores of amines: a mechanism for coronary spasm. Science 1984;30:1435–7.

111. Furchgott RF. Role of endothelium in responses of vascular smooth muscle. Circ Res 1983;53:557–73.

112. Palmer RMJ, Ferrige AG, Moncada S. Nitric oxide release accounts for the biological activity of endothelium-derived relaxing factor. Nature 1987;327:524–6.

113. Griffith TM, Lewis MJ, Newby AC, Henderson AH. Endothelium-derived relaxing factor. J Am Coll Cardiol 1988;12:797–806.

114. Murad F, Rapoport RM, Fiscus R. Role of cyclic GMP in relaxations of vascular smooth muscle. J Cardiovasc Pharmacol 1985;7:111–8.

115. Collius P, Griffith TM, Henderson AH, Lewis MJ. Endothelium-derived relaxing factor alters calcium fluxes in rabbit aorta: a cyclic guanosine monophosphate-mediated effect. J Physiol (Lond) 1986;381:427–37.

116. Heistad DD, Armstrong ML, Marcus ML, Piegors DJ, Mark AL. Augmented responses to vasoconstrictor stimuli in hypercholesteralemic and atherosclerotic monkeys. Circ Res 1984;54:711–8.

117. Bossaller C, Habib GB, Yamamoto H, Williams C, Wells S, Henry P. Impaired muscarinic endothelium-dependent relaxation and cyclic guanosine-5-monophosphate formation in atherosclerotic human coronary artery and rabbit aorta. J Clin Invest 1987;79:170–4.

118. Abrams J. Tolerance to nitrates. Circulation 1986;74:1181–5.

119. Ignarro LJ, Lippton H, Edwards JC, et al. Mechanism of vascular smooth muscle relaxation by organic nitrates, nitroprusside and nitric oxide: evidence for the involvement of S-nitrosothiols as active intermediates. J Pharmacol Exp Ther 1981;218:739–49.

120. May DC, Popma JJ, Black WH, et al. In vivo induction and reversal of nitroglycerin tolerance in human coronary arteries. N Engl J Med, 1987;31:805–9.

121. Yanagisawa M, Karihara H, Kimura S, et al. A novel potent vasoconstrictor peptide produced by vascular endothelial cells. Nature 1988;332:411–5.

122. Yanagisawa M, Inoue A, Ishikawa T, et al. Primary structure, synthesis and biological activity of rat endothelin, an endothelial-derived vasoconstrictor peptide. Proc Natl Acad Sci USA 1988;85:6964–7.

123. Hirata Y, Yoshima H, Takata S, et al. Cellular mechanism of action by a novel vasoconstrictor endothelin in cultured rat vascular smooth muscle cells. Biochem Biophy Res Commun 1988;154:868–75.

124. Campbell GR, Chamley-Campbell JH. Invited review: the cellular pathobiology of atherosclerosis. Pathology 1981;13:423–40.

125. Niewiarowski S, Rao AK. Contribution of thrombogenic factors to the pathogenesis of atherosclerosis. Prog Cardiovasc Dis 1983;26:197–222.

126. Schwartz SM, Campbell GR, Campbell JH. Replication of smooth muscle cells in vascular disease. Circ Res 1986;58:427–44.

127. Ross R. The pathogenesis of atherosclerosis—an update. N Engl J Med 1986;314:488–500.

127a.Komuro I, Kurihara H, Sugiyama T, Takaku F, Yazaki Y. Endothelin stimulates c-fos and c-myc expression and proliferation of vascular smooth muscle cells. FEBS Lett 1988;238:249–52.

128. DeWood MA, Spores J, Notske R, et al. Prevalence of total coronary artery occlusion during the early hours of transmural myocardial infarction. N Engl J Med 1980;303:897–902.

129. Falk E. Unstable angina with fatal outcome: dynamic coronary thrombosis leading to infarction and/or sudden death. Circulation 1985;71:699–708.

130. Sherman CT, Litvack F, Grundfest W, Lee M, et al. Coronary angioscopy in patients with unstable angina pectoris. N Engl J Med 1986;315:913–8.

131. Brown BG, Bolson EL, Dodge HT. Dynamic mechanisms in human coronary stenosis. Circulation 1984;70:917–22.

132. Rodger GM. Hemostatic properties of normal and perturbed vascular cells. FASEB J 1988;2:116–23.

133. Ross R, Glomset JA. The pathogenesis of atherosclerosis. I. N Engl J Med 1976;295:369–77.

134. Ross R, Glomset JA. The pathogenesis of atherosclerosis. II. N Engl J Med 1976;295:420–5.

135. Papahadjopoulos O. Cholesterol and cell membrane function: a hypothesis concerning the etiology of atherosclerosis. J Theor Biol 1974;43:329–41.

136. Jackson RL, Gotto AM Jr. Hypothesis concerning membrane structure, cholesterol, and atherosclerosis. In: Paoletti R, Gotto AM Jr, eds. Atherosclerosis Reviews, Vol. 1. New York: Raven Press, 1976:1.

137. Bondjers G, Brattsand R, Hansson GK, Bjorkerud S. Cholesterol transfer and content in aortic regions with defined endothelial integrity from rabbits with moderate hypercholesterolemia. Nutr Metab 1976;20:452–60.

138. Cathcart MK, Morel DW, Chisolm GM III. Monocytes and neutrophils oxidize low-density lipoprotein making it cytotoxic. J Leuk Biol 1985;38:341–50.

139. Davies PF, Remuzzi A, Gordon EJ, Dewey CF, Gimbrone MA. Turbulent fluid shear stress induces vascular endothelial cell turnover in vitro. Proc Natl Acad Sci USA 1986;83:2114–7.

140. Lansman JB. Going with the flow. Nature 1988;331:481–2.

141. DiCorleto PE, Chisolm GM. Participation of the endothelium in the development of the atherosclerotic plaque. Prog Lipid Res 1986;25:365–74.

142. Parthasarathy S, Steinbrecher UP, Barnett J, Witztum JL, Steinberg D. Essential role of phospholipase A_2 activity in endothelial cell-induced modification of low density lipoprotein. Proc Natl Acad Sci USA 1985;82:3000–4.

143. Goldstein JL, Ho YK, Basu SK, Brown MS. Binding site on macrophages that mediates uptake and degradation of acetylated low density lipoprotein, producing massive cholesterol deposition. Proc Natl Acad Sci USA 1979;76:333–7.

144. Via DP, Dresel HA, Gotto AM. Isolation and assay of the Ac-LDL receptor. Methods Enzymol 1986;129:216–26.

145. Fukuda S, Horiuchi S, Tomita K, et al. Acetylated low-density lipoprotein is endocytosed through coated pits by rat peritoneal macrophages. Virchows Arch 1986;52:1–13.

146. Tabas I, Weiland DA, Tall AR. Metabolism of low-density lipoprotein-proteoglycan complex by macrophages: further evidence for a receptor pathway. J Biol Chem 1986;261:3147–55.

147. Hoff HF, O'Neil J. Extracts of human atherosclerotic lesions can modify low density lipoproteins leading to enhanced uptake by macrophages. Atherosclerosis 1988;70:29–41.

148. Shaikh M, Martini S, Quiney JR, et al. Modified plasma-derived lipoproteins in human atherosclerotic plaques. Atherosclerosis 1988;69:165–72.

149. Jurgens G, Hoff HF, Chisholm GM, Esterbauer H. Effect of butyrate on thyroid hormone-mediated gene expression in rat pituitary tumor cells. Chem Phys Lipids 1987;45:315–36.

150. Mazzone T, Lopez C, Bergstraesser L. Metabolism of low-density lipoprotein-proteoglycan complex by macrophages: further evidence for a receptor pathway. Arteriosclerosis 1987;7:191–6.

151. Russell DW, Lehrman MA, Sudhof TC, et al. The LDL receptor in familial hypercholesterolemia: use of human mutations to dissect a membrane protein. Cold Spring Harbor Symp Quant Biol 1986;51:811–9.

152. Hegele RA, Huang LS, Herbert PN, et al. Apolipoprotein B-gene DNA polymorphisms associated with myocardial infarction. N Engl J Med 1986;315:1509–15.

153. Goldstein JL, Brown MS. Genetics and cardiovascular disease. In: Braunwald E, ed. Heart Disease: A Textbook of Cardiovascular Medicine. 3rd ed. Philadelphia: WB Saunders, 1988:1617–49.

154. Gotto AM, Farmer J. Risk factors for coronary artery disease. In: Ref. 153:1153–90.

155. Schmitz G, Robenek H, Lojman U, Assmann G. Interaction of high-density lipoproteins with cholesteryl ester-laden macrophages: biochemical and morphological characterization of cell surface receptor binding, endocytosis, and resecretion of high-density lipoproteins by macrophages. EMBO J 1985;4:613–22.

156. Ordovas JM, Schaefer EJ, Salem D, et al. Apolipoprotein AI gene polymorphism associated with premature coronary artery disease and familial hypoalphalipoproteinemia. N Engl J Med 1986;314:671–7.

157. Benditt EP, Benditt JM. Evidence for a monoclonal origin of human atherosclerotic plaques. Proc Natl Acad Sci USA 1973;70:1753–6.

158. Penn A, Garte SJ, Warren L, Nesta D, Mindich B. Transforming gene in human atherosclerotic plaque DNA. Proc Natl Acad Sci USA 1986;83:7951–5.

159. Seeburg PH, Colby WW, Capon DJ, Goeddel DV, Levinson AD. Biological properties of human c-Ha-ras1 genes mutated at codon 12. Nature 1984;312:71–5.

160. Fasano O, Aldrich T, Tamanoi F, et al. Analysis of the transforming potential of the human H-ras gene by random mutagenesis. Proc Natl Acad Sci USA 1984;81:4008–12.

161. Varmus HE. The molecular genetics of cellular oncogenes. Annu Rev Genet 1984;18:553–612.

162. Gibbs JB, Sigal IS, Scolnick EM. Biochemical properties of normal and oncogenic ras p21. TIBS 1985;10:350–3.

163. Leder P, Battey J, Lenoir G, et al. Translocations among antibody genes in human cancer. Science 1983;222:765–71.

164. Taub R, Moulding C, Battey J, et al. Activation and somatic mutation of the translocated c-myc gene in Burkitt lymphoma cells. Cell 1984;36: 339–48.

165. Waterfield MD, Scrace GT, Whittle N, et al. Platelet-derived growth factor is structurally related to the putative transforming protein p28 of simian sarcoma virus. Nature 1983;304:35–9.

166. Doolittle RF, Hunkapiller MW, Hood LE. Simian sarcoma virus onc gene, v-sis, is derived form the gene (or genes) encoding platelet-derived growth factor. Science 1983;221:275–7.

167. Barrett TB, Benditt EP. sis(platelet-derived growth factor B chain) gene transcript levels are elevated in human atherosclerotic lesions compared to normal artery. Proc Natl Acad Sci USA 1987;84:1099–103.

168. Libby P, Warner SJC, Salomon RN, Birinyi LK. Production of platelet-derived growth factor-like mitogen by smooth muscle cells from human atheroma. N Engl J Med 1988;318:1493–8.

169. Ross R. Platelet-derived growth factor. Annu Rev Med 1987;38:71–9.

170. Williams LT. Stimulation of paracrine and autocrine pathways of cell proliferation by platelet-derived growth factor. Clin Res 1987;36:5–10.

171. Berk BC, Alexander RW, Brock TA, Gimbrone MA, Webb RC. Vasoconstriction: a new activity for platelet-derived growth factor. Science 1986;232:87–90.

172. Benditt TB, Benditt EP. Platelet-derived growth factor gene expression in human atherosclerotic plaques and normal artery wall. Proc Natl Acad Sci USA 1988;85:2810–4.

173. Sejersen T, Betsholtz C, Sjolund M, et al. Rat skeletal myoblasts and arterial smooth muscle cells express the gene for the A chain but not the gene for the B chain (c-sis) of platelet-derived growth factor. Proc Natl Acad Sci USA 1986;83:6844–8.

174. Majesky MW, Benditt EP, Schwartz SM. Expression and developmental control of platelet-derived growth factor A-chain and B-chain/Sis genes in rat aortic smooth muscle cells. Proc Natl Acad Sci USA 1988;85:1524– 8.

175. Starksen NF, Harsh GR, Gibbs VC, Williams LT. Regulated expression of the platelet-derived growth factor A chain in microvascular endothelial cells. J Biol Chem 1987;262:14381–4.

176. Escobedo JA, Navankasatussas S, Cousens LS, et al. A common PDGF receptor is activated by homodimeric A and B forms of PDGF. Science 1988;240:1532–4.

177. Beckmann MP, Betsholtz C, Heldin CH, et al. Comparison of biological properties and transforming potential of human PDGF-A and PDGF-B chains. Science 1988;241:1346–9.

178. Yarden Y, Escobedo JA, Kuang WJ, et al. Structure of the receptor for platelet-derived growth factor helps define a family of closely related growth factor receptors. Nature 1986;323:226–32.

179. Gronwald RGK, Grant FJ, Haldeman BA, et al. Cloning and expression of a cDNA coding for the human platelet-derived growth factor: evidence for more than one receptor class. Proc Natl Acad Sci USA 1988;85:3435–9.

180. Hart CE, Forstrom JW, Kelly JD, et al. Two classes of PDGF receptor recognize different isoforms of PDGF. Science 1988;240:1529–31.

181. Seifert RA, Schwartz SM, Bowen-Pope DF. Developmentally regulated production of platelet-derived growth factor-like molecules. Nature 1984;311:669–71.

182. Keating MT, Williams LT. Autocrine stimulation of intracellular receptors in v-sis-transformed cells. Science 1988;239:914–6.

183. Evered D, Whelan T, eds. Symposium on Growth Factors. London: Pitman Publishing, 1985:261–9.

184. Majesky MW, Reidy MA, Benditt EP, Juchau MR. Focal smooth muscle proliferation in the aortic intima produced by an initiation-promotion sequence. Proc Natl Acad Sci USA 1985;82:3450–4.

185. deGroen PC. Cyclosporine, low-density lipoprotein and cholesterol. Mayo Clin Proc 1988;63:1012–21.

186. Thomas KA, Gimenez-Gallego G. Fibroblast growth factors: broad spectrum mitogens with potent angiogenic activity. In: Bradshaw RA, Prentis S, eds. Oncogenes and Growth Factors. Amsterdam: Elsevier Science Publishing, 1987:149–56.

187. Nemecek GM, Coughlin SR, Handley DA, Moskowitz MA. Stimulation of aortic smooth muscle cell mitogenesis by serotonin. Proc Natl Acad Sci USA 1986;83:674–8.

188. Majack RA, Goodman LV, Dixit VM. Cell surface thrombospondin is functionally essential for vascular smooth muscle cell proliferation. J Cell Biol 1988;106:415–22.

189. Blaes N, Boissel JP. Growth-stimulating effect of catecholamines on rat aortic smooth muscle cells in culture. J Cell Physiol 1983;116:167–72.

190. Geisterfer AA, Peach MJ, Owens GK. Angiotensin II induces hypertrophy, not hyperplasia, of cultured rat aortic smooth muscle cells. Circ Res 1988;62:749–56.

191. Schweigerer L, Neufeld G, Friedman J, et al. Capillary endothelial cells express basic fibroblast growth factor, a mitogen that promotes their own growth. Nature 1987;325:257–9.

192. Winkles JA, Friesel R, Burgess WH, et al. Human vascular smooth muscle cells both express and respond to heparin-binding growth factor I (endothelial cell growth factor). Proc Natl Acad Sci USA 1987;84: 7124–8.

193. Gospodarowicz D, Neufeld G, Schweigerer L. Fibroblast growth factor. Mol Cell Endocrin 1986;46:187–204.

194. Weiner HL, Weiner LH, Swain JL. Tissue distribution and developmental expression of the messenger RNA encoding angiogenin. Science 1987;237:280–2.

195. Castellot JJ Jr, Favreau LV, Karnovsky MJ, Rosenberg RD. Inhibition of vascular smooth muscle cell growth by endothelial cell-derived heparin. J Biol Chem 1982;257:11256–60.

196. Grunwald J. Effects of anti-atherosclerotic substances on smooth muscle cell migration and proliferation analyzed by time-lapse video microscopy. Int Angiol 1987;6:59–64.

197. Schwartz SM, Reidy MA. Common mechanisms of proliferation of smooth muscle in atherosclerosis and hypertension. Hum Pathol 1987; 18:240–7.

198. Radhakrishnamurthy B, Srinivasan SR, Eberle K, et al. Composition of proteoglycans synthesized by rabbit aortic explants in culture and the effect of experimental atherosclerosis. Biochim Biophys Acta 1988;964: 231–43.

199. Roessner A, Herrera A, Honing HJ, et al. Identification of macrophages and smooth muscle cells with monoclonal antibodies in the human atherosclerotic plaque. Virchows Arch 1987;412:169–74.

200. Nachtigal M, Greenspan P, Terracio L, Fowler SD. Transformation of rabbit arterial smooth muscle cells with simian virus 40. Arch Virol 1987;95:225–35.

201. Wolfbauer G, Glick JM, Minor LK, Rothblat GH. Development of the smooth muscle foam cell: uptake of macrophage lipid inclusions. Proc Natl Acad Sci USA 1986;83:7760–4.

202. Hajjar DP, Marcus AJ, Hajjar KA. Interactions of Arterial Cells: studies on the mechanisms of endothelial cell modulation of cholesterol metabolism in co-cultured smooth muscle cells. J Biol Chem 1987;262:6976– 81.

203. Cunningham MJ, Pasternak RC. The potential role of viruses in the pathogenesis of athersclerosis. Circulation 1988;77:964–6.

204. Hajjar DP, Pomerantz KB, Falcone DJ, Weksler BB, Grant AJ. Herpes simplex virus infection in human arterial cells: implications in arteriosclerosis. J Clin Invest 1987;80:1317–21.

205. McLean JW, Tomlinson JE, Kuang WJ, et al. cDNA sequence of human apolipoprotein(a) is homologous to plasminogen. Nature 1987;330:132–7.

206. Dahlen GH, Guyton JR, Attar M, et al. Association of levels of lipoprotein Lp(a), plasma lipids, and other lipoproteins with coronary artery disease documented by angiography. Circulation 1986;74:758–65.

207. Caskey CT. Disease diagnosis by recombinant DNA methods. Science 1987;236:1223–9.

208. White RA. Technical frontiers for the vascular surgeon: laser anastomotic welding and angioscopy-assisted intraluminal instrumentation. J Vasc Surg 1987;5:673–80.

209. Jenkins RD, Sinclair IN, Anand R, et al. Laser balloon angioplasty: effect of tissue temperature on weld strength of human postmortem intima-media separations. Lasers Surg Med 1988;8:30–9.

210. Dehmer GJ, Popma JJ, Egerton K, et al. Reduction in the rate of early restenosis after coronary angioplasty by a diet supplemented with n-3 fatty acids. N Engl J Med 1988;319:733–40.

211. McBride W, Lange RA, Hillis LD. Restenosis after successful coronary angioplasty: pathophysiology and prevention. N Engl J Med 1988;318:1734–7.

212. Harker LA. Role of platelets and thrombosis in mechanisms of acute occlusion and restenosis after angioplasty. Am J Cardiol 1987;60:20B–8B.

213. Fox PL, DiCorleto PE. Fish oils inhibit endothelial cell production of platelet-derived growth factorlike protein. Science 1988;241:453–6.

214. Jonasson L, Holm J, Hansson GK. Cyclosporin A inhibits smooth muscle proliferation in the vascular response to injury. Proc Natl Acad Sci USA 1988;85:2303–6.

215. Huang SS, Huang JS. Rapid turnover of the platelet-derived growth factor receptor in sis-transformed cells and reversal by suramin. J Biol Chem 1988;263:12608–18.

215a. Miyanohara A, Sharkey MF, Witztum JL, Steinberg D, Friedmann T. Efficient expression of retroviral vector-transduced human low density lipoprotein (LDL) receptor in LDL receptor-deficient rabbit fibroblasts in vitro. Proc Natl Acad Sci USA 1988;85:6538–42.

216. Duguid JB. Thrombosis as a factor in the pathogenesis of coronary atherosclerosis. J Pathol 1946;58:207–12.

217. Cohen RA, Shepherd JT, Vanhoutte PM. Inhibitory role of the endothelium in the response of isolated coronary arteries to platelets. Science 1983;221:273–4.

218. Rosenberg RD. Role of heparin and heparin like molecules in thrombosis and atherosclerosis. Fed Proc 1985;44:404–9.

219. Beebe DP. Binding of tissue plasminogen activator to human umbilical vein endothelial cells. Thromb Res 1987;46:241–4.

220. Billingham ME. Cardiac transplant atherosclerosis. Transplant Proc 1987;19(suppl 5):19–25.

221. Bevilacqua MD, Pober SJ, Majeau GR, et al. Recombinant tumor necrosis factor induced procoagulant activity in cultured human vascular endothelium: characterization and comparison with the actions of interleukin-1. Proc Natl Acad Sci USA 1986;83:4533–7.

222. Collen D. Mechanisms of inhibition of tissue-type plasminogen activator in blood. Thromb Haemost 1986;53:415.

223. Marder VJ, Sherry S. Thrombolytic therapy: current status. N Engl J Med 1988;318:1512–20.

224. Ref. 223:1585–95.

225. Collen D, Stassen JM, Larsen G. Pharmacokinetics and thrombolytic properties of deletion mutants of human tissue-type plasminogen activator in rabbits. Blood 1988;71:216–9.

226. Runge MS, Bode C, Matsueda GR, Haber E. Antibody-enhanced thrombolysis: targeting of tissue plasminogen activator in vivo. Proc Natl Acad Sci USA 1987;84:7659–62.

227. Lucore CL, Sobel BE. Interactions of tissue-type plasminogen activator with plasma inhibitors via their pharmacological imprecations. Circulation 1988;77:660–9.

228. Colucci M, Paramo JA, Collen D. Generation in plasma of a fast-acting inhibitor of plasminogen activator in response to endotoxin stimulation. J Clin Invest 1985;75:818–24.

229. Hirsh PD, Campbell WB, Willerson JT, Hillis LD. Prostaglandins and ischemic heart disease. Am J Med 1981;71:1009–26.

230. Gold HK, Coller B, Yasuda T, et al. Rapid and sustained coronary artery recanalization with combined bolus injection of recombinant tissue-type plasminogen activator and monoclonal antiplatelet GPIIb/IIIa antibody in a canine preparation. Circulation 1988;77:670–7.

231. Braunwald E. On future directions for cardiology: the Paul D. White Lecture. Circulation 1988;77:13–31.

CHAPTER 25

Decision Analysis in Clinical Cardiology: When Is Coronary Angiography Required in Aortic Stenosis?

STEVEN GEORGESON, MD, KLEMENS B. MEYER, MD, STEPHEN G. PAUKER, MD

Introduction

When making medical decisions, physicians use trained intuition, informed by professional experience, to solve complex problems. For the conscientious clinician, the haphazard growth of medical knowledge has made this task more difficult. As the qualitative, categorical, evocative description of natural history and prognosis is rewritten in various quantitative dialects, it becomes harder to defend instinct and authority in clinical debate. Nor are our colleagues the only skeptics and critics of our decisions. Whether because they are informed, perceptive or just anxious, our patients challenge us. Insurers challenge us. Professional review organizations, malpractice tribunals and the courts challenge us. We are required to explain and often defend our choices.

Despite its limitations, an experienced and responsible physician's clinical judgment remains the best tool for making a medical decision. However, neither intuition nor the catechisms of medical education equip us to revise understanding and practice rationally in response to new information. We find ourselves touting and clinging to isolated statistics, as if any one of these could capture the complexity of a clinical situation. Various emerging techniques can support the physician's decision making. Decision analysis is one such method, one that can help us to make sensible choices and make sense of those choices to our professional constituencies.

Decision Analysis

Originating in game theory and operations research in the 1940s (1,2), over the past 17 years, decision analysis has been applied to questions of clinical medicine and health policy (3–8). Decision analysis is *explicit*: the strategies from among which the decision maker must choose are listed, the possible results of each of those strategies are enumerated and both the probability and the value that the decision maker attaches to each outcome are specified. Decision analysis is *reproducible*: the analyst records the strategies, results and values in the form of a tree. Using this record, the analyst, his or her colleagues and skeptics can examine the influence of the data on the results. They can distinguish important points of uncertainty from those that have little influence, reformulate the structure of the problem, revise the estimates used and examine the effect of these changes on the decision.

In this report, we present a tutorial introduction to clinical decision analysis and show how it can illuminate a difficult, controversial question. Clinical decision analysis consists of 1) problem formulation, 2) tree construction, 3) probability assessment, 4) utility assessment, 5) strategy evaluation, 6) sensitivity analysis, and 7) interpretation. We illustrate this process with an example.

Problem formulation. The first step in decision analysis is to formulate the clinical problem as a choice among several alternative strategies that the clinician is considering.

The structure of a tree. Using either pencil and paper or microcomputer software (9), the second step is to represent the strategies as a decision tree consisting of 1) decision nodes, 2) chance nodes, and 3) terminal nodes. A *decision* (square) node is a point in the tree where a choice must be made (such as between medical or surgical therapy). Each branch emanating from a decision node represents a different strategy. A *chance* (circular) node is a point in the tree where the laws of probability determine the outcome of events or the true state of the world. Examples of chance events include the result of a test, the outcome of a treatment and whether or not a patient has a disease. The branches of both decision and chance nodes are assumed to be both exhaustive and mutually exclusive, specifying all relevant options and representing them explicitly. A *terminal* node represents the consequence of one sequence of events of a given strategy. Each terminal branch represents a unique outcome state, which is assigned a value or utility. How each state is valued depends on who the decision maker is and what criteria he or she wants to use in selecting a strategy.

Probabilities. Each chance node represents the circumstance that one of several mutually exclusive chance events has occurred or will occur. The analyst estimates the likelihood or probability of each of these chance events. At any chance node, the sum of these probabilities must, by definition, be unity. To specify the probabilities, we usually turn first to the medical literature. If published data do not yield usable data, if their applicability is uncertain or if the urgency of the analysis precludes detailed review of the literature, we then estimate probabilities subjectively or ask an expert's opinion.

Utilities. Just as we must make explicit the probability of clinical events, so too we must specify their relative value, or more precisely their utility, on some consistent scale. First we determine from whose perspective we are performing the analysis. Is it the patient's, the doctor's or the payor's? We then choose the scale on which we will rate the different outcomes. In medical decision analysis, quality-adjusted survival has become a popular utility scale: life expectancy, or average survival, is adjusted for short- and long-term morbidity. In our example, we consider results on three utility scales: short-term (1 month) survival; long-term survival and then two simultaneous scales—long-term survival and cost—from which we calculate a cost/effectiveness ratio. In this analysis, we do not adjust for the quality of the patient's life under different circumstances. Specifically, we do not consider the effect of subsequent angina, should it develop, on the quality of life.

Strategy evaluation. To compare strategies, we calculate the value of each strategy by applying two simple rules. At a decision node, the value of the node is the value of the best strategy. At a chance node, the value is a weighted average of the value of each outcome state (utility), where the weight assigned to each state is the probability of arriving at that state.

Sensitivity analysis. Although choosing the best strategy is important, decision analysis also allows us to ask "what if?", substituting a range of values for one or more probability or utility parameters. Repeated recalculation of results, which can be done very rapidly by a microcomputer, shows how the expected utility of each strategy changes as the value of these parameters change and whether the choice among strategies is sensitive to the value of these parameters.

Dual utilities. When one performs a decision analysis from the perspective of an institution or individual who pays for the treatment involved or from the perspective of society (in which case we all pay), the analysis usually must consider economic cost. When both costs and health outcome benefits are considered together, there are two common approaches: *cost-benefit* analysis and *cost-effectiveness* analysis. In cost-benefit analysis, all costs and benefits are expressed in a single unit, usually in monetary units. In cost-effectiveness analysis, costs (in dollars) and effectiveness (typically, in life-years) are considered separately and a marginal ratio is calculated (i.e., how much it will cost to buy an additional unit of effectiveness or health output). Some clinicians consider cost-effectiveness analysis more congenial and intuitively more appealing than cost-benefit analysis. A comparison of the marginal cost-effectiveness ratios with an explicit or implied willingness to pay allows one to choose among alternative uses of limited health care resources and decide if a given strategy is reasonable.

An Example: Is Coronary Angiography Necessary Before Aortic Valve Replacement?

A 63 year old woman presents with exertional syncope. She has no history of chest pain, myocardial infarction or congestive heart failure and has typical physical, electrocar-

Table 25.1. Prevalence of Coronary Artery Disease (CAD) in Patients With Aortic Stenosis But No Angina

Reference	No. of Pts.	Definition of Significant CAD (% stenosis)	No. of Pts. Without Angina	No. (%) Without Angina But With CAD
Chobadi et al. (34)	146	>50%	39	9(23)
Exadactylos et al. (35)	88	>50%	88	0 (0)
Bermudez et al. (36)	64	>75%	13	7(54)
Miller et al. (37)	91	>60%	91	34(37)
Graboys and Cohn (38)	19	>75%	19	0 (0)
Hancock (39)	173	>50%	173	15 (9)
Paquay et al. (40)	76	>75%	19	1 (5)
Moraski et al. (11)	88	>50%	20	9(45)
Total	745		462	75(16)

diographic (ECG) and echocardiographic findings of severe aortic stenosis. Aortic valve replacement is recommended. Should she undergo preoperative coronary angiography?

Brief review of published studies. Hemodynamically significant aortic stenosis and coronary artery disease often coexist. Among patients with aortic stenosis and angina pectoris, the prevalence of coronary artery disease is 40% to 80% (10,11). Because coronary artery disease increases the operative mortality rate associated with aortic valve replacement and shortens long-term survival, there is general agreement that angina is an indication for performing coronary angiography in preparation for aortic valve replacement. However, in the absence of angina, the issue is less clear. In adults with aortic stenosis, aortic valve replacement is typically performed in the sixth or seventh decade of life, when the prevalence of coronary artery disease in the general population is 10% to 15% among men and 5% to 10% among women (12). Table 25.1 summarizes data regarding the prevalence of coronary artery disease in patients with aortic stenosis who do not have angina.

Coexisting coronary artery disease raises the operative mortality rate in aortic valve replacement for aortic stenosis (13–16). Although this increased risk persists even with cold cardioplegia, concomitant coronary artery bypass grafting modulated surgical mortality in several series (Table 25.2). Myocardial revascularization also improves long-term survival (13,14,16), but patients without significant coronary artery disease will not benefit from a policy of universal coronary angiography before aortic valve replacement. Recent American College of Cardiology and American Heart Association guidelines suggest coronary angiography before aortic valve replacement 1) in a patient with angina or ECG evidence of coronary artery disease, 2) in all men >35 years of age, and 3) in all postmenopausal women (17). Conversely, at least one study (18) found no increase in operative mortality despite omission of coronary angiography in

Table 25.2. Operative Mortality Rates (with the use of cold cardioplegia)

	No CAD		CAD			
	AVR		AVR/No CABG		AVR + CABG	
Reference	No.	Deaths (%)	No.	Deaths (%)	No.	Deaths (%)
Mullany et al. (13)	73	1 (1.4)	32	3 (9.3)	99	4 (4.0)
Jones et al. (14)	428	18 (4.2)	51	9 (17.6)	68	9 (13.2)
Lytle et al. (15)	272	3 (1.1)	23	1 (4.3)		
Lytle et al. (16)					375	20 (5.3)
Total	773	22 (2.8)	106	13 (12.2)	542	33 (6.1)

AVR = aortic valve replacement; CABG = coronary artery bypass grafting; CAD = coronary artery disease.

patients with valvular heart disease, and some authors (19) argue that angiography is not universally necessary.

History, physical examination and electrocardiography do not reliably differentiate patients with aortic stenosis and coronary artery disease from those with aortic stenosis alone. In theory, noninvasive testing might allow one to identify patients likely to have coronary artery disease. However, because of the risk of hemodynamic collapse, the suspicion of severe aortic stenosis is regarded as a contraindication to stress testing (20). Nonetheless, such tests have been performed with low complication rates (21). However, the ECG response to exercise does not discriminate well between patients with aortic stenosis alone and those with aortic stenosis and concomitant coronary artery disease (22,23).

A report from Finland (24) describes the use of thallium imaging after dipyridamole injection and handgrip exercise to detect coronary artery disease in patients with aortic stenosis. The presence of perfusion defects could predict $\geq 50\%$ stenosis of at least one coronary artery with a sensitivity of 85% and a specificity of 86%. These performance characteristics are very similar to those of dipyridamole thallium testing in the absence of aortic stenosis (25). Two of 27 patients with aortic stenosis experienced symptomatic hypotension after dipyridamole infusion, which resolved during handgrip exercise. During handgrip exercise, two others had chest pain that responded to treatment. There were no deaths.

Problem formulation. In a 63 year old woman with characteristic findings of aortic stenosis, no angina and no special risk factors for coronary artery disease, should coronary angiography be performed before aortic valve replacement?

Structure of the model. Figure 25.1 shows the structure of the decision tree. The "No Catheterization" and "Catheterization" strategies are represented as branches emanating from the square decision node on the left. For the "No Catheterization" strategy, the first circular chance node represents the possibility that the patient has coronary artery disease. This chance node thus represents the current state of the patient. Both the "Coronary Artery Disease" and the "No Coronary Artery Disease" branches themselves lead to

chance nodes that represent whether or not the patient will survive aortic valve replacement. The terminal nodes at the extreme right represent possible consequences of the strategy. The patient can be dead, alive with coronary artery disease (but without coronary artery bypass grafting) or alive without coronary artery disease.

In the "Catheterization" branch, the first chance node represents the possibility of death at catheterization. If the patient survives, the angiographic results (denoted by a second chance node) will determine whether or not she has coronary artery disease. (In this case, we can consider coronary angiography a "gold standard" test because published reports about prognosis in coronary artery disease have used angiography as a point of reference.) Patients shown to have coronary artery disease undergo coronary artery bypass grafting as well as aortic valve replacement.

Probabilities (Table 25.3). We based the *probability of coronary artery disease* in this asymptomatic 63 year old woman on the compilation by Diamond and Forrester (12) of autopsy findings in patients who died of noncardiac causes. They noted a close correlation between the autopsy prevalence data and Framingham Study findings on the 6 year incidence of symptomatic coronary artery disease. Figure 25.2 summarizes both data sets and regressions on the autopsy data (linear for men, exponential for women).

Short-term survival. Severe aortic stenosis slightly increases the risk of coronary angiography (26,27). We used a value of 0.002, twice the overall mortality of coronary angiography. Operative risks were based on the data in Table 25.2. *Efficacy* is a number between 0 and 1, which represents the extent to which an intervention prevents an undesired event. We define efficacy as the quantity:

$$1 - \frac{\text{Frequency of event with treatment}}{\text{Frequency of event without treatment}}.$$

If the treatment is completely effective, the event will not occur with treatment and efficacy will be 1. If the treatment is completely ineffective, the event will occur with the same frequency with and without treatment and efficacy will be 0. In Table 25.3, we calculate the efficacy of coronary bypass

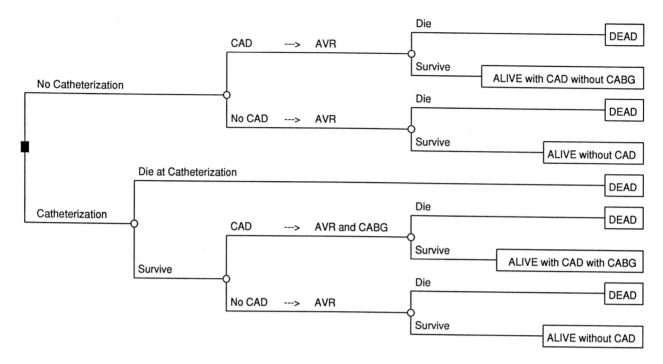

Figure 25.1. Decision tree including "No Catheterization" and "Catheterization" strategies. AVR = aortic valve replacement; CABG = coronary artery bypass grafting; CAD = coronary artery disease.

surgery in reducing the mortality of aortic valve replacement in the presence of coronary artery disease.

Utilities. We initially consider only short-term survival, assigning a utility of 1 to patients alive after 1 month and a utility of 0 to patients who die within 1 month. On this scale, the calculated expected utility corresponds to the likelihood of surviving the perioperative period.

Results of the short-term model. The "No Catheterization" strategy has an expected utility of 0.966; the "Catheterization" strategy gives an expected utility of 0.968. On the

basis of a 0.2% difference in survival alone, it would be hard to recommend either strategy with great conviction in this 63 year old woman. However, plausible changes in our baseline assumptions might cause the expected utilities of the two strategies to diverge substantially. This brings us to sensitivity analysis.

Sensitivity analyses: short-term survival. Although we estimated the probability of asymptomatic coronary artery disease in this patient to be 0.067, that value might substantially differ for several reasons. For example, she might have smoked, have been hyperlipidemic or hypertensive, or both, or had a strong family history of coronary artery disease. Figure 25.3 shows how a change in our estimate of the probability of coronary artery disease would affect the choice between the two strategies. This sensitivity analysis shows the relation between the probability of 1 month survival (vertical axis) and the probability of coronary artery disease (uppermost scale on the horizontal axis). As the probability that coronary artery disease is present increases, the expected survival rates for *both* strategies decline because coronary artery bypass grafting reduces but does not eliminate the increase in operative mortality attributable to coronary artery disease. Note that if the probability of coronary artery disease is 0.032, the two strategies have the same expected utility. We refer to the value of a variable at which two strategies yield the same expected utility as a *threshold*. If the probability of coronary artery disease is less than the threshold, "No Catheterization" is slightly better; if the probability is higher than the threshold, "Catheterization" is slightly better.

What if we erred in estimating the efficacy of coronary artery bypass grafting in decreasing the operative mortality

Table 25.3. Probability of Short-Term Events

Variable	Baseline Value
Probability of dying at angiography	0.002
Probability of CAD in a 63 year old woman	0.067
Probability of perioperative death	
AVR alone, no CAD	0.028
AVR with CAD, without CABG	0.122
Excess AVR mortality attributable to CAD without CABG (0.122 − 0.028)	0.094
AVR with CAD and CABG	0.061
Excess AVR mortality attributable to CAD with CABG (0.061 − 0.028)	0.033
Efficacy of CABG in decreasing probability of perioperative death (1 − 0.033/0.094)	0.65

Abbreviations as in Table 25.2.

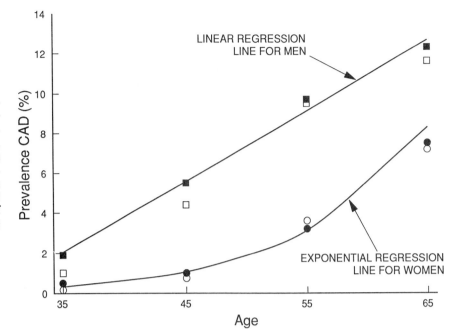

Figure 25.2. Prevalence of coronary artery disease (CAD) as a function of age. For individuals dying a noncardiac death (compiled by Diamond and Forrester [12]), **closed squares** represent men, **closed circles** represent women. **Regression lines** are plotted on the autopsy prevalence data. **Open squares** (men) and **open circles** (women) represent Framingham Study predictions of the incidence of coronary artery disease over 6 years (12).

attributable to coronary artery disease? The threshold value of efficacy at which "Catheterization" and "No Catheterization" have the same short-term survival rate is about 0.31, less than half our baseline value of 0.65. In contrast, even if the efficacy of coronary artery bypass grafting were 1, (i.e., if it eliminated excess operative mortality attributable to coronary artery disease), the difference in expected utility between the two strategies would only be about 0.004. Again, in a short-term analysis for this patient, the difference in survival is small.

Age and gender. So far, we have analyzed this problem with reference to a 63 year old woman. Using the regression analysis shown in Figure 25.2, we extend the decision analysis to men and women of other ages (Fig. 25.3). The two lower scales on the horizontal axis show the ages for men and women, respectively, which correspond to prevalence of coronary artery disease shown on the upper scale. "Catheterization" is the preferred strategy in women >57 years of age and men >39 years of age. For neither men nor women is the difference in 1 month survival >1% at any age.

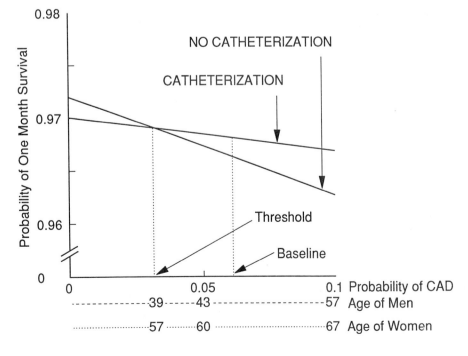

Figure 25.3. Sensitivity analysis for the short-term model showing 1 month survival as a function of the probability of coronary artery disease and age for men and women, respectively. CAD = coronary artery disease.

Table 25.4. Long-Term Survival for a 63 Year Old Woman

Step 1: calculate average base annual mortality rate from life expectancy

$$\frac{1}{\text{Life expectancy}} = \frac{1}{19.8} = 0.05/\text{year}$$

Step 2: calculate efficacy of CABG in decreasing excess annual CAD mortality

Patient characteristics	Excess mortality rates (calculated from observed survival and expected survival based on age, gender, race)		Weighted Average
AS, CAD, CABG	0.032*	0.040†	0.039
AS, CAD, no CABG	0.085*	0.089†	0.087

$$\text{Efficacy of CABG} = 1 - \frac{0.039}{0.087} = 0.55$$

Step 3: calculate compound mortality rates for all possible outcomes

	Aortic stenosis without CAD	Aortic stenosis with CAD	
		CABG No	CABG Done
Mortality rate			
Average base annual rate	0.05	0.05	0.05
Excess with aortic valve prosthesis	0.025*	0.025*	0.025*
Excess with CAD	0	0.087	0.039
Total	0.075/yr	0.162/yr	0.114/yr
Step 4: calculate life expectancies as reciprocals of compound annual mortality rates			
Life expectancy (1/total)	13.3 yr	6.2 yr	8.8 yr

*Jones et al. (14); †Czer et al. (40). AS = aortic stenosis; other abbreviations as in Table 25.2.

Operative mortality may be substantially lower for younger patients than for our index patient. Data from the Coronary Artery Surgery Study (CASS) (28) show that the operative mortality for coronary artery bypass grafting in a 35 year old woman is about one-third that for a patient in her 60s. Diminishing operative mortality by a factor of 3 for patients in their 40s does not affect the ranking of strategies or significantly change short-term survival.

Long-term survival: representing life expectancy. Short-term survival may not capture all of the potential benefit that a patient with significant coronary artery disease may derive from concomitant coronary artery bypass grafting. By revascularizing potentially ischemic myocardium, coronary artery bypass grafting could diminish long-term excess annual mortality from coronary artery disease. Of course, this additional benefit is speculative because we are considering patients without angina.

To incorporate long-term survival into our model, we must estimate the patient's life expectancy for each outcome. Although this estimate can be made in several ways, we used the Declining Exponential Approximation of Life Expectancy (DEALE) (29,30). The DEALE combines 1) the base case average mortality rate (determined by the patient's age, gender and race), and 2) the excess mortality rate imposed by each of the patient's diseases. The DEALE

estimates of long-term survival for our index case are presented in Table 25.4.

Results of the long-term model. "No Catheterization" has an expected utility of 12.37 years and "Catheterization" has an expected utility of 12.53 years. On average, performing coronary angiography will be expected to lengthen this patient's life by 1.9 months or 1.3%.

Sensitivity analysis: long-term survival. Although there is little difference between the two strategies, for men "Catheterization" is favored over the entire age range, whereas for women it is favored only in those >45 years of age. Because of the potential long-term survival benefit of coronary artery bypass grafting, there is no longer a threshold excess operative mortality below which "No catheterization" is preferred. Similarly, there is no threshold for the efficacy of coronary artery bypass grafting in decreasing the excess operative mortality.

To this point, we have presented "one-way" sensitivity analyses that show utility as a function of one variable. In a "two-way" sensitivity analysis, we examine the consequences of simultaneous variation of two variables. For example, what if both the short- and long-term efficacy of bypass surgery differed from our base case? Might there be some plausible combinations for which "No Catheterization" would be better? Figure 25.4 explores this issue. The

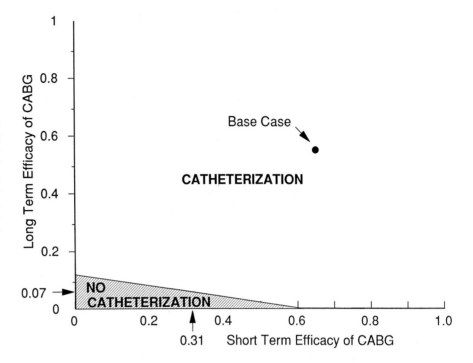

Figure 25.4. "Two-way" sensitivity analysis for the long-term model showing effect of simultaneous changes in estimates of the short- and long-term efficacy of coronary artery bypass grafting (CABG). Short-term efficacy is the efficacy in reducing operative mortality. Long-term efficacy is the efficacy in reducing excess annual mortality attributable to coronary artery disease.

horizontal axis shows short-term efficacy, the vertical axis long-term efficacy. Every possible combination corresponds to a point in the plane. In effect, we calculate the expected utility of both strategies for each such combination and draw a line separating the region in which "Catheterization" has the higher expected utility from the shaded area in which "No Catheterization" has the higher expected utility. Notice that even if the short-term efficacy of coronary artery bypass grafting were 0.31 (the threshold value we determined in our short-term analysis), long-term efficacy would have to be <0.07 for "No Catheterization" to be the strategy of choice (arrows).

We can add one more dimension, performing a "three-way" sensitivity analysis. Figure 25.5 has the same axes, but instead of one threshold line, we show a family of lines, each corresponding to a different age. For example, for a 40-year-old woman, "Catheterization" would be preferred to "No Catheterization" only for efficacies corresponding to points above the top line; for a 50 year old woman, "Catheterization" would be preferred for points above the second line from the top.

Dipyridamole/thallium testing: Bayes' rule. Even when we take the long-term benefit of revascularization into account, the gain from catheterization is small. Perhaps a strategy that includes a noninvasive diagnostic test to stratify patients by likelihood of coronary artery disease before catheterization would be better. Although physicians sometimes think of a diagnostic test as indicating the presence or the absence of a disease, tests are imperfect and can produce false negative and false positive results. If we estimate the likelihood of disease in a given patient before knowing test results (the prior probability) and if we know the likelihood

of observing a test result in patients with and without the disease (the conditional probabilities), we can revise our

Figure 25.5. "Three-way" sensitivity analysis for the long-term model. Lines representing women 40, 50, 60 and 70 years of age have been substituted for the single line representing a 63 year old woman in Figure 25.4. CABG = coronary artery bypass grafting.

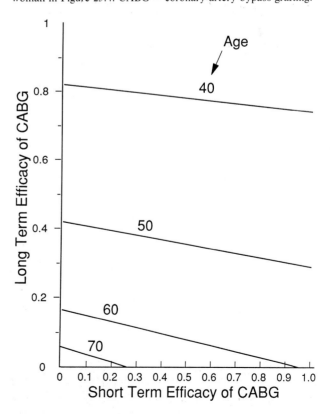

Table 25.5. Effect of Dipyridamole/Thallium Test on the Probability of Coronary Artery Disease

A: Diagnosis	B: Prior Probability	C: Conditional Probability of Test Result	D: Product (B × C)	E: Posterior or Revised Probability (D/sum)
Positive test				
CAD	0.067	0.85*	0.057	0.057/0.188 = 0.303
No CAD	0.933	0.14†	0.131	0.131/0.188 = 0.697
			Sum = 0.188	
Negative test				
CAD	0.067	0.15‡	0.010	0.010/0.812 = 0.012
No CAD	0.933	0.86§	0.802	0.802/0.812 = 0.988
			Sum = 0.812	

*Sensitivity or true positive rate; †false positive rate (1−specificity); ‡false negative rate (1−sensitivity); §specificity or true negative rate. Abbreviations as in Table 25.2.

belief about the probability of disease on the basis of the test result. A positive result revises the probability upward, a negative result downward. The result is the posterior probability of disease, posterior with respect to the test.

Bayes' rule (8) formulates these relations precisely. It allows us to combine the prior probability of disease with test sensitivity (the probability that the test will give a positive result in someone with disease) and test specificity (the probability that the test will give a negative result in someone without disease).

Consider the dipyridamole/thallium test. The probability of a positive result in a patient with aortic stenosis and substantial coronary artery disease (the sensitivity) is 0.85. The probability of a negative test in a patient with aortic stenosis but without substantial coronary artery disease (the specificity) is 0.86. Table 25.5 shows how Bayes' rule can be applied. The upper half of the table applies to a positive test result; the lower half applies to a negative result. The table is organized into five columns. Column A lists the diagnostic possibilities. Column B specifies the prior probabilities. Column C specifies the conditional probability of the observed finding given each diagnosis: in the case of a positive result, the sensitivity and the false positive rate; in the case of a negative result, the false negative rate and the specificity. Column D is simply the product of columns B and C. Finally, column D is summed and column E calculated as the quotient of each entry in column D and that sum. The dipyridamole/thallium test, if positive, revises the probability of coronary artery disease upward from 0.067 to 0.303 in our patient. The lower half of the table shows that a negative result would revise the probability of coronary artery disease downward from 0.067 to 0.012.

Having interpreted the results of a dipyridamole/thallium test in the setting of aortic stenosis, we must decide whether or not a strategy that stratifies patients on the basis of those results is reasonable. We modify our decision tree (Fig. 25.1) by adding a third strategy: dipyridamole/thallium screening.

Figure 25.6 shows the third strategy, incorporating information from dipyridamole/thallium testing with handgrip exercise. If the patient has a positive test, she will undergo catheterization, but the probability that substantial coronary artery disease is present will increase from 0.067 to 0.3. If the dipyridamole/thallium results are negative, she will undergo aortic valve replacement without catheterization, but the probability that coronary artery disease is present will decrease from 0.067 to 0.01. Utility is once again measured in terms of long-term survival.

Dipyridamole/thallium testing: results. In the base case, "Dipyridamole/Thallium" has an expected utility of 12.51 years, still not quite as good as that of "Catheterization" (12.53 years). Although the testing strategy spares 86% of the patients without coronary artery disease the small risk of catheterization (0.002), that benefit is outweighed by its failure to detect 15% of the patients who do have significant coronary artery disease, who would then be exposed to a substantial excess risk (0.061) during aortic valve replacement. "Catheterization" is preferred in men >36 years of age. For women, however, there is a decade (between 43 and 53 years of age) for which "Dipyridamole/Thallium" yields the longest life expectancy. For women 35 to 43 years of age, "No Catheterization" is preferable; for women >53 years, "Catheterization" is best.

Cost-effectiveness analysis. Whether we consider short- or long-term survival, the expected gain associated with "Catheterization" is small, even if a noninvasive test was used to stratify patients. If resources were unlimited, perhaps we should pursue the practice that maximizes expected survival. In 1990, however, resources available for health care are limited. In the context of that limitation, are these small gains worth the price? Although we cannot answer this question in any absolute sense, cost-effectiveness analysis puts the additional cost of catheterization in perspective.

We examined the three strategies from a hospital's perspective, using life expectancy in years as our measure of

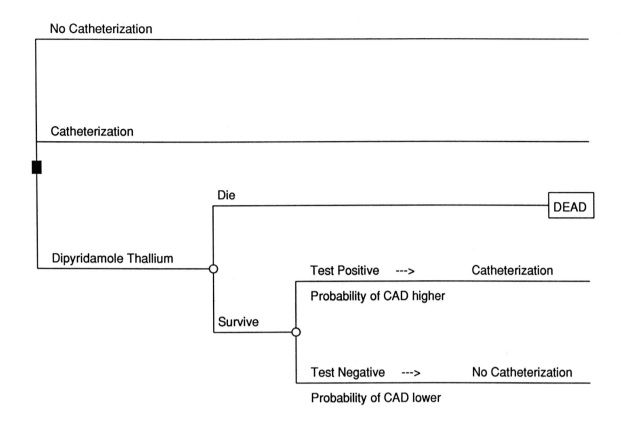

Figure 25.6. Decision tree with the addition of the "Dipyridamole/Thallium" strategy. Details of "No Catheterization" and "Catheterization" are as in Figure 25.1. CAD = coronary artery disease.

effectiveness and using variable costs (*not* charges). At our hospital, the average variable costs are approximately $250 for dipyridamole/thallium testing, $1,000 for catheterization, $10,000 for aortic valve replacement without coronary artery bypass grafting and $11,000 for aortic valve replacement with coronary artery bypass grafting. Table 25.6 shows the calculations for our index case. First, we order the strategies (column A) by cost (column B), listing the effectiveness of each (column C). Next, we calculate the additional, or marginal, cost and effectiveness of each strategy (columns D and E, respectively) and the marginal cost/effectiveness ratio (column F). "Dipyridamole/Thallium" costs $480 more than "No Catheterization" and provides 0.14 years (7 weeks) of additional life expectancy for a marginal cost/effectiveness ratio of $3400 per life year gained. "Catheterization" costs $570 more than "Dipyridamole/Thallium" and provides a

survival benefit of 0.02 years (1.5 weeks) for a marginal cost-effectiveness ratio of $29,000 per year of life saved.

Figure 25.7 shows marginal cost/effectiveness ratios for men and women as a function of age. Each graph has two curves, one comparing "Dipyridamole/Thallium" and "No Catheterization" and a higher one comparing "Catheterization" and "Dipyridamole/Thallium." The curves for men and women are similar, but those for men are shifted to the left; for any age, the cost-effectiveness ratio is lower for men than women. For each gender, as patients become younger and approach the threshold age at which marginal effective-

Table 25.6. Cost Effectiveness (C/E): Baseline Results for a 63 Year Old Woman

Strategy	Cost ($)	Survival (yr)	Marginal Cost ($)	Marginal Survival (yr)	Marginal C/E Ratio ($/year gained)*
No Catheterization	10,000	12.37	—	—	—
Dipyridamole/Thallium	10,480	12.51	480	0.14	3,400
Catheterization	11,050	12.53	570	0.02	29,000

*Calculated as: Marginal cost/Marginal effectiveness (rounded off).

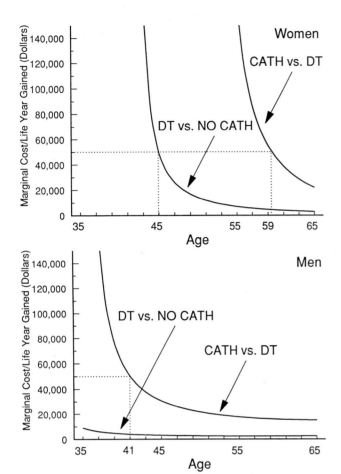

Figure 25.7. Marginal cost-effectiveness of "Catheterization" (CATH) and "Dipyridamole/Thallium" (DT) compared with "No Catheterization" (NO CATH) and with each other for women (**upper panel**) and men (**lower panel**).

Table 25.7. Relation Between Willingness to Pay and Patient Age

Willingness to Pay ($/extra life-year)	No Catheterization	Dipyridamole/ Thallium	Catheterization
Men (yr)			
$20,000	—	35–52	> 52
$50,000	—	35–41	> 41
$100,000	—	35–39	> 39
Women (yr)			
$20,000	< 49	49–65	> 65
$50,000	< 45	45–59	> 59
$100,000	< 44	44–56	> 56

Discussion

In this tutorial, we have outlined the technique of clinical decision analysis, beginning with a specific patient and generalizing to a clinical strategy. Because the data supporting several assumptions were uncertain, we used sensitivity analyses to examine the quantitative importance of simultaneous uncertainty regarding these variables.

At the most general level, decision analysis represents the study of decision making under uncertainty. It allows us to explore the possible implications of data despite uncertainty regarding their precision. It gives us a consistent reproducible method by which to integrate information regarding the conflicting considerations that influence our decisions. It allows us to structure problems. Most importantly, it forces us to be *explicit*.

This analysis was developed as a didactic exercise and is not sufficiently detailed to form the basis for a policy regarding coronary angiography or noninvasive testing in patients who are to undergo replacement of stenotic aortic valves. Although careful, our review of the medical literature was not exhaustive, and our model involves some obvious simplifications. For example, we did not perform quality adjustment for life with angina, if and when it begins, and we did not represent the possibility that the patient might subsequently require reoperation or percutaneous transluminal coronary angioplasty for coronary artery disease.

However, even this simplistic but explicit model does provide insights into the dynamics of the problem of aortic stenosis and possible coronary artery disease. Except among the youngest of the 35 to 65 year old men and women to whom we generalized the analysis, coronary angiography provides a very modest increase in long-term survival. However, even for 65 year old men, average survival with "Catheterization" would be only 3 months longer than with "No Catheterization." This 2.7% prolongation for a life expectancy of 9.5 years is surely a "close call" (31).

Introducing a dual utility scale that incorporates cost offers several new perspectives on these small survival gains. First, it offers another criterion by which to distinguish small survival differences. For some patients, the small

ness is 0, the marginal cost per each life-year gained by pursuing "Dipyridamole/Thallium" rather than "No Catheterization" or "Catheterization" rather than "Dipyridamole/Thallium" increases sharply.

Strategies with lower cost/effectiveness ratios are not necessarily better strategies. To use the analyses summarized in Figure 25.7 to choose a strategy, the decision maker must specify a maximum "willingness to pay." If resources were unlimited, "Catheterization" should be used in all men >36 years and all women >53 years. Suppose, however, that society chose to spend no more than $50,000 to save a year of life (broken lines). In that case, "Catheterization" should be used only in men >41 years and "Dipyridamole/Thallium" for men 35 to 41 years of age (lower panel). For women (upper panel), "Dipyridamole/Thallium" should be used between 45 and 59 years of age and "Catheterization" should be used in those >59 years. Similar threshold ages could be calculated for different "willingness to pay" levels (Table 25.7).

Table 25.8. Marginal Cost Effectiveness*

Clinical Scenario (reference)	Marginal Cost Effectiveness ($/year gained)
Treatment of high risk postmyocardial infarction patient with a beta-blocker (41)	$ 2,500
CABG for left main CAD (42)	$ 4,900
Treatment of male smokers with nicotine gum (43)	$ 7,900
Treatment of low risk postmyocardial infarction patient with a beta-blocker (40)	$ 13,600
Kidney transplantation (44)	$ 18,600
Treatment of middle age males with moderate hypertension (45)	$ 29,600
Heart transplantation (44)	$ 30,700
CABG for single vessel CAD (43)	$ 38,800
Use of coronary care unit to rule out myocardial infarction in low probability patient (46)	$249,900

*Inflated to 1988 dollars using the consumer price index. Abbreviations as in Table 25.2.

survival gains cost a few thousand dollars per additional life-year; for others, they will cost tens or hundreds of thousands of dollars.

Second, cost-effectiveness analysis shows that a strategy that provides intermediate benefit at intermediate cost may be worth further study. Although "Dipyridamole/Thallium" does not provide a survival advantage *over* "Catheterization," it may provide a substantial part of the survival advantage *of* "Catheterization" at a lower cost. A third and corollary observation is that introducing "Dipyridamole/Thallium" into the cost-effectiveness analysis increases the marginal cost/effectiveness ratio of the more expensive and more effective strategy of "Catheterization." If we compare only "Catheterization" and "No Catheterization," the marginal cost of an additional year of life gained by performing coronary angiography on a 40 year old man would be $9,300. If "Dipyridamole/Thallium" is an option, the marginal cost of a year of life gained by angiography would be almost $61,000.

Fourth, cost-effectiveness analysis shows the relation between the "willingness to pay" (32) (i.e., the maximal acceptable cost/effectiveness ratio) and threshold ages for "Catheterization" and "Dipyridamole/Thallium." One could set such payment levels by direct questioning, by consensus or by using the Delphi technique (33). Alternatively, one can examine currently accepted therapies and tests to see what the implied "willingness to pay" threshold might be (Table 25.8). For example, a $20,000/year threshold would endorse neither coronary artery bypass grafting for single vessel disease nor cardiac transplantation, but would allow renal transplantation, coronary artery bypass grafting for left main coronary artery disease and coronary angiography in asymptomatic men >52 years old as a prelude to aortic valve replacement.

In our illustrative problem, analysis using the dual utility scales of cost and effectiveness yielded results more striking than analysis of survival alone. Although it is not the only voice we should hear, cost-effectiveness analysis has much to tell us about the rational allocation of limited resources. It does not follow, however, that a cost-effectiveness analysis is more important or more correct than an analysis that examines survival or cost alone. Furthermore, an economic perspective is neither appropriate nor required in every clinical decision analysis. Although decision analysis can recommend strategies, it is the decision maker who prescribes the perspective and the utility scale. In making explicit our choice among perspectives and the tradeoffs which that choice implies, clinical decision analyses can help us articulate the contradictions in society's expectations of medical care.

References

1. Von Neumann J, Morgenstern O. Theory of Games and Economic Behavior. Princeton: Princeton University Press, 1944.
2. Raiffa H. Decision Analysis: Introductory Lectures on Choices Under Uncertainty. New York: Random House, 1968.
3. Schwartz WB, Gorry GA, Kassirer JP, Essig A. Decision analysis and clinical judgment. Am J Med 1973;55:459–72.
4. McNeil BJ, Keeler E, Adelstein SJ. Primer on certain elements of medical decision making. N Engl J Med 1975;293:211–5.
5. Weinstein MC, Fineberg HV. Clinical Decision Analysis. Philadelphia: WB Saunders, 1980.
6. Sox HC Jr, Blatt MA, Higgins MC, Marton KI. Medical Decision Making. Boston: Butterworths, 1988.
7. Kassirer JP, Moskowitz AJ, Lau J, Pauker SG. Decision analysis: a progress report. Ann Intern Med 1987;106:275–91.
8. Pauker SG, Kassirer JP. Decision analysis. N Engl J Med 1987;316:250–8.
9. Wong JB, Moskowitz AJ, Pauker SG. Clinical decision analysis using microcomputers: a case of coexistent hepatocellular carcinoma and abdominal aortic aneurysm. West J Med 1986;145:805–15.
10. Basta LL, Raines D, Najjar S, Kioschos JM. Clinical, hemodynamic and coronary angiographic correlates of angina pectoris in patients with severe aortic valve disease. Br Heart J 1975;37:150–7.
11. Moraski RE, Russell RO Jr, Mantle JA, Rackley CE. Aortic stenosis, angina pectoris, coronary artery disease. Cathet Cardiovasc Diagn 1976;2:157–64.
12. Diamond GA, Forrester JS. Analysis of probability as an aid in the clinical diagnosis of coronary artery disease. N Engl J Med 1979;300:1350–8.
13. Mullany CJ, Elveback LR, Frye RL, et al. Coronary artery disease and its management: influence on survival in patients undergoing aortic valve replacement. J Am Coll Cardiol 1987;10:66–72.
14. Jones M, Schofield PM, Brooks NH, et al. Aortic valve replacement with combined myocardial revascularisation. Br Heart J 1989;62:9–15.
15. Lytle BW, Cosgrove DM, Taylor PC, et al. Primary isolated aortic valve replacement: early and late results. J Thorac Cardiovasc Surg 1989;97:675–94.
16. Lytle BW, Cosgrove DM, Loop FD, et al. Replacement of aortic valve combined with myocardial revascularization: determinants of early and late risk for 500 patients, 1967–1981. Circulation 1983;68:1149–62.
17. Ross J, Brandenburg RO, Dinsmore RE, et al. Guidelines for coronary angiography: a report of the American College of Cardiology/American Heart Association task force on assessment of diagnostic and therapeutic cardiovascular procedures (subcommittee on coronary angiography). J Am Coll Cardiol 1987;10:935–50.
18. St. John Sutton MG, St. John Sutton M, Oldershaw P, et al. Valve replacement without preoperative cardiac catheterization. N Engl J Med 1981;305:1233–8.

19. Brandenburg RO. No more routine catheterization for valvular heart disease? N Engl J Med 1981;305:1277–8.

20. Schlant RC, Blomqvist CG, Brandenburg RO, et al. Guidelines for exercise testing: a report of the American College of Cardiology/American Heart Association task force on assessment of cardiovascular procedures (subcommittee on exercise testing). J Am Coll Cardiol 1986; 8:725–38.

21. Atwood JE, Kawanishi S, Myers J, Froelicher VF. Exercise testing in patients with aortic stenosis. Chest 1988;93:1083–7.

22. Bailey IK, Come PC, Kelly DT, et al. Thallium-201 myocardial perfusion imaging in aortic valve stenosis. Am J Cardiol 1977;40:889–99.

23. Pfisterer M, Muller-Brand J, Brundler H, Cueni T. Prevalence and significance of reversible radionuclide ischemic perfusion defects in symptomatic aortic valve disease patients with or without concomitant coronary artery disease. Am Heart J 1982;103:92–6.

24. Huikuri HV, Korhonen UR, Ikaheimo MJ, Heikkila J, Takkunen JT. Detection of coronary artery disease by thallium imaging using a combined intravenous dipyridamole and isometric handgrip test in patients with aortic valve stenosis. Am J Cardiol 1987;59:336–40.

25. Ruddy TD, Dighero HR, Newell JB, et al. Quantitative analysis of dipyridamole-thallium images for the detection of coronary artery disease. J Am Coll Cardiol 1987;10:142–9.

26. Kennedy JW, Baxley WA, Bunnel IL, et al. Mortality related to cardiac catheterization and angiography. Cathet Cardiovasc Diagn 1982;8:323–40.

27. Folland ED, Oprian C, Giacomini J, et al. Complications of cardiac catheterization and angiography in patients with valvular heart disease. Cathet Cardiovasc Diagn 1989;17:15–21.

28. Kennedy JW, Kaiser GC, Fisher LD, et al. Clinical and angiographic predictors of operative mortality from the collaborative study in coronary artery surgery (CASS). Circulation 1981;63:793–802.

29. Beck JR, Kassirer JP, Pauker SG. A convenient approximation of life expectancy (the "DEALE"): I. Validation of the method. Am J Med 1982;73:883–8.

30. Beck JR, Pauker SG, Gottlieb JE, Klein K, Kassirer JP. A convenient approximation of life expectancy (the "DEALE"): II. Use in medical decision making. Am J Med 1982;73:889–97.

31. Kassirer JP, Pauker SG. The toss-up. N Engl J Med 1981;305:1467–9.

32. Thompson M. Benefit-Cost Analysis for Program Evaluation. Beverly Hills, CA: Sage Publications, 1980:52.

33. Milholland AV, Wheeler SG, Heieck JJ. Medical assessment by a Delphi group opinion technic. N Engl J Med 1973;288:1272–5.

34. Chobadi R, Wurzel M, Teplitsky, Menkes H, Tamari I. Coronary artery disease in patients 35 years of age or older with valvular aortic stenosis. Am J Cardiol 1989;64:811–2.

35. Exadactylos N, Sugrue DD, Oakley CM. Prevalence of coronary artery disease in patients with isolated aortic valve stenosis. Br Heart J 1984;51:121–4.

36. Bermudez GA, Abdelnur R, Midell A, DeMeester T. Coronary artery disease in aortic stenosis: importance of coronary arteriography and surgical implications. J Vasc Dis 1983:591–6.

37. Miller DC, Stinson EB, Oyer PE, Rossiter SJ, Reitz BA, Shumway NE. Surgical implications and results of combined aortic valve replacement and myocardial revascularization. Am J Cardiol 1979;43:494–501.

38. Graboys TB, Cohn PF. The prevalence of angina pectoris and abnormal coronary arteriograms in severe aortic valve disease. Am Heart J 1977; 93:683–6.

39. Hancock EW. Aortic stenosis, angina pectoris and coronary artery disease. Am Heart J 1977;93:382–93.

40. Czer LS, Gray RJ, Stewart ME, DeRobertis M, Chaux A, Metcalf JM. Reduction in late sudden death by concomitant revascularization with aortic valve replacement. J Thorac Cardiovasc Surg 1988;95:390–401.

41. Goldman L, Benjamin Sia ST, Cook EF, Rutherford JD, Weinstein MC. Costs and effectiveness of routine therapy with long-term beta-adrenergic antagonists after acute myocardial infarction. N Engl J Med 1988;319: 152–7.

42. Weinstein MC, Stason WB. Cost-effectiveness of coronary artery bypass surgery. Circulation 1982;66(suppl III):III-56–66.

43. Oster G, Huse DM, Delea TE, Colditz GA. Cost-effectiveness of nicotine gum as an adjunct to physician's advice against cigarette smoking. JAMA 1986;256:1315–8.

44. Evans RW. Cost-effectiveness analysis of transplantation. Surg Clin North Am 1986;66:603–16.

45. Weinstein MC, Stason WB. Hypertension: a policy perspective. Cambridge, MA: Harvard University Press, 1976.

46. Fineberg HV, Scadden D, Goldman L. Care of patients with a low probability of acute myocardial infarction: cost effectiveness of alternatives to coronary-care-unit admission. N Engl J Med 1984;310:1301–7.

CHAPTER 26

Clinical Judgment and Therapeutic Decision Making

MARK A. HLATKY, MD, ROBERT M. CALIFF, MD, FRANK E. HARRELL JR, PHD, KERRY L. LEE, PHD, DANIEL B. MARK, MD, MPH, LAWRENCE H. MUHLBAIER, PHD, DAVID B. PRYOR, MD

A clinician makes hundreds of decisions every day, some mundane, others concerning matters of life and death. The sum of these decisions by the half million physicians in the United States profoundly affects the health of the country, as well as controls the bulk of medical care costs (1) ($500 billion dollars in 1987 [2]). Because cardiovascular disease is the leading cause of death and a major cause of morbidity, disability and health care costs in the United States (3), the decisions made by cardiovascular specialists have particular prominence.

Clinicians once made decisions with virtual autonomy, but that freedom is quickly eroding. Individual clinicians increasingly must justify their therapeutic choices to review panels and third party payors. The profession itself must demonstrate that technologically sophisticated and expensive modes of therapy are worthwhile. Clinical decision making is under scrutiny, and pressures are increasing to improve both the process by which clinical decisions are made and the data on which they are based.

This review examines selected aspects of the clinical decision-making process. We first discuss how physicians make decisions. Next, we review the methods of prognostic stratification, with emphasis on the use of the Cox proportional hazards model. We then examine the relative strengths of various designs for clinical research studies, particularly the use of randomized trials and observational analyses. Finally, we outline some future trends for clinical trials, meta-analysis and data base research.

Clinical Decision Making

In principle, physicians should use the linear, logical reasoning processes exemplified by decision analysis (4,5) to make therapeutic recommendations. First, the patient's diagnosis and underlying prognosis are established accurately. Second, the possible therapeutic alternatives are identified, and the effect of each alternative on patient outcome is estimated. Not only is the effect on survival assessed, but many additional factors are also taken into account, such as the effect on quality of life, functional capacity, employment status, medical costs and the patient's values and preferences. Finally, the benefits, risks and costs of each alternative are weighed, and the best course of action is undertaken.

Although the process just described is highly rational, clinicians do not usually make decisions in this fashion (6). It appears that experts in a variety of fields make decisions using a more intuitive process of recognizing patterns and applying heuristics ("rules of thumb") (7–9). In cardiovascular medicine, for instance, a rule of thumb might be that "patients with significant left main coronary artery disease should have coronary bypass surgery." This particular heuristic is generally accepted, but many of the rules of thumb used by individual clinicians are more personal and idiosyncratic. The process by which new data are absorbed and formulated into heuristics remains poorly understood. In varying proportions, pathophysiologic reasoning, personal clinical experience, published research and the opinion of experts in the field each play a role in the development of a clinical rule of thumb.

Selection of therapy depends critically on an underlying model of the disease process because the pathophysiology of disease often suggests a method for its treatment. Antibiotic therapy for endocarditis is rational, based on the current concepts of bacterial pathogenesis and specific experimental models of endocarditis. Coronary angioplasty has been widely used, in large part because of the perception that it corrects the immediate cause of myocardial ischemia. Nonetheless, knowledge of pathophysiology is far from complete, and for some disorders it may be rudimentary. Advances in pathophysiologic understanding may suggest new approaches to therapy or, alternatively, may undermine the rationale for previously accepted techniques (e.g., pericardial poudrage for the treatment of coronary artery disease or prolonged bedrest after myocardial infarction).

In addition to pathophysiologic reasoning, physicians apply their personal experience and information from clinical research to arrive at therapeutic recommendations. The physician's recall of personal clinical experience is notoriously selective, however, being too heavily influenced by recent cases or particularly bad or good outcomes (10). Computerized clinical data bases were developed in part to overcome these recognized deficiencies in human memory by providing a complete and unbiased picture of clinical experience. Clinical research reports should be the soundest basis for therapeutic decisions because they aim to evaluate the efficacy of therapy directly. The quality of this evidence, however, varies among studies, and much of it is open to several interpretations. Although forums such as the National Institutes of Health Consensus Development Conferences may foster more uniform therapeutic recommendations, legitimate differences of opinion about proper clinical management are likely to remain (10).

The variability in physician decision making is evident from recent studies documenting substantial geographic differences in the use of various cardiac procedures. Coronary artery bypass graft surgery has one of the highest rates of variation of any surgical procedure (11). One study (11) among Medicare beneficiaries found that the rate of bypass surgery in different areas of the United States varied threefold from a low of 7 per 10,000 to a high of 23 per 10,000. The use of cardiac catheterization also showed substantial variation, from a low of 22 per 10,000 to a high of 51 per 10,000 Medicare beneficiaries (12). Wennberg et al. (13) compared hospitalization rates for a variety of diagnoses in the cities of Boston and New Haven. These investigators (13) found that the rate of hospital admission for atherosclerosis and coronary bypass surgery varied two-fold between these two cities, whereas the rate of admission for acute myocardial infarction varied only slightly. One important difference among these conditions is that widespread consensus exists that patients with acute myocardial infarction should be admitted to the hospital, but there is far less consensus about when patients need to be admitted for bypass surgery or treatment of chronic coronary artery disease. "Black and white" decisions exhibit little variability among physicians, whereas "gray zone" decisions are highly variable.

Variability in decision making has attracted the attention of health care policy makers and those concerned about high medical costs. It will be increasingly important for cardiovascular specialists to attempt to define the appropriate indications for procedures and base these recommendations on data from clinical research studies whenever possible.

Estimation of Prognosis

Therapeutic decision making requires an appreciation of the prognosis of disease and methods of risk stratification because therapeutic recommendations should be quite different for a patient with a good prognosis than for a patient with a very poor prognosis. Outcomes are not uniform, even in a group of patients with the same disease; some patients may live for years, while others may die quickly. Because prognostic statements for any one patient cannot be made with certainty, an understanding of probability and statistics is essential for the use of information concerning prognosis.

The survival probability is one of the simplest descriptors of prognosis. This statistic represents the probability that a patient with a given diagnosis will survive longer than a specified period of time. For example, the 1 year survival probability after myocardial infarction can be estimated by collecting a large cohort of patients with acute myocardial infarction, observing their outcomes during follow-up study and dividing the number of patients who died within a year of their myocardial infarction by the total number of patients who had been followed up for ≥ 1 year (assuming no one has been lost to follow-up study). The advantages of this statistic are that it summarizes an important outcome of the disease in a single number, confidence limits can be easily calculated and survival rates can readily be compared between therapies and among diseases.

Unfortunately, calculating crude survival probabilities using the approach just described sacrifices much important information. For instance, patients who died at 10 days after myocardial infarction and 11 months after myocardial infarction are considered equivalently, whereas a patient who died 13 months after the index infarction would be considered alive for the purposes of calculating the 1 year survival rate. Furthermore, a patient who was known to be alive at 8 months after myocardial infarction would not be included at all because he or she had not been followed up for the required 1 year. The technique of Kaplan-Meier life table analysis overcomes these limitations (14–16). In the construction of a life table, each patient contributes information from the time of study entry until either the time of death or last follow-up contact. This information is then combined using special techniques to estimate the probability of a patient's being alive at any point in time after study entry. This powerful technique includes observations from all patients, regardless of their length of follow-up study. This information is often presented graphically in the form of a survival curve, which displays the likelihood of survival at any time point, rather than only at a single arbitrary point in time. More detailed descriptions of life table methods can be found in standard statistics references (14–16).

One important assumption in the use of survival rates is that the underlying probability of death for all patients in the cohort is the same. In fact, prognosis is generally affected by a large number of factors, including the patient's age, gender, symptom severity, extent of disease and coexisting medical disorders. Consequently, techniques are needed to identify prognostic factors, quantify their strength and assess their relative importance. These techniques must handle variable lengths of patient follow-up evaluation and provide estimates of survival probability that apply to individual patients. If the shapes of survival curves are either known or reasonably approximated by a mathematical function (e.g., as an exponential curve), powerful specialized techniques can be applied. More often, however, survival curves do not correspond to simple mathematical functions, so it is best to use analytic techniques that can accommodate survival curves of any shape. The Cox proportional hazards model (17) has been used extensively in cardiovascular studies because of its flexibility in analyzing survival curves of arbitrary shape.

The Cox model assumes that the hazard, which equals the instantaneous death rate, is given by the formula: $h_i(t) = h(t) C_i$, where $C_i = \exp(B_1 X_{1i} + B_2 X_{2i} + ... + B_p X_{pi})$. The model assumes that the hazard of death for patient "i" at time "t"

($h_i[t]$) equals the hazard of death for an "average patient" at the same time ($h[t]$) multiplied by a factor (C_i) that is a function of the prognostic profile of patient "i"; this is the proportional hazards assumption that gives the model its name. The proportional hazard coefficient for patient "i" (C_i) is, in turn, a function of the values for that patient of a set of prognostic factors ($X_{1i};...,X_{pi}$), multiplied by a corresponding set of regression coefficients ($B_1;...,B_p$) that measure the strength of the association between the prognostic factor and outcome. These coefficients must be estimated from observations of the outcomes of large numbers of patients with the same disorder.

Practical Considerations in Prognostic Studies

Identification and quantification of prognostic factors are the major goals of the Cox proportional hazards model. A number of computer programs perform the necessary calculations simply and easily (18,19). The ready availability of such statistical software packages has allowed many researchers to use the Cox model without necessarily appreciating its assumptions and limitations. For instance, the strength of a prognostic factor may be greater during one period of time than another. A prominent example of such a factor is surgical therapy, which entails a short-term risk of operative death, yet offers long-term benefit in terms of survival. In comparing a therapy such as surgery with another therapy that is not associated with a period of early high risk, a standard Cox model must be used with considerable caution because the survival curves have different shapes and the proportional hazards assumption is violated (20).

The Cox model also assumes that the effect of a prognostic factor on outcome is linear. The validity of this assumption should be checked in the analysis. For example, left ventricular ejection fraction is a strong prognostic factor among patients with coronary artery disease. An ejection fraction >60%, however, is not associated with any lower hazard of death than an ejection fraction of 60% (20). In the model, therefore, the value of ejection fraction should be truncated at 60% to indicate its effect on prognosis accurately.

The importance of statistical power and the type II error in the interpretation of randomized trials are now widely appreciated (21). The concept of statistical power is less frequently applied to prognostic studies, but remains just as relevant. In survival analyses, the statistical power for detecting a prognostic factor is chiefly determined by the number of outcome events, not by the total number of patients. For example, a study with 100 patients and 25 deaths has greater statistical power for analysis of prognosis than a study with 500 patients and 10 deaths, all other aspects of the studies being equal. Another important aspect of prognostic analysis is the problem of a "false positive"

(i.e., identifying a factor as a significant predictor of prognosis that has no real effect on outcome) or type I error. This problem is particularly important when more than one potential prognostic factor is analyzed per 10 outcome events in the sample (22). For instance, a study with 30 outcome events can afford examination of only three *candidate* prognostic factors. If a larger number of factors was analyzed, the likelihood of spurious associations would be increased.

In attempting to increase the number of outcome events, some clinical studies combine diverse end points such as death, nonfatal myocardial infarction and coronary bypass surgery. Such compound end points can be very useful for comparing different therapies when they are used to summarize the proportion of patients with a predefined "poor outcome." Compound end points should be interpreted with great caution in prognostic studies, however, because the mechanisms and risk factors for the individual outcomes are likely to be quite different. For instance, an analysis of 50 events consisting of 4 deaths, 10 nonfatal myocardial infarctions and 36 surgeries will primarily identify the factors clinicians use to select patients for surgery, not the determinants of the "natural history" of disease.

Regression modeling techniques for prognostic analysis can be enhanced by the use of clinical indexes (22) that combine several clinical variables measuring different aspects of the same underlying pathophysiologic phenomenon. For instance, the presence of cardiomegaly, an S3 gallop, a history of myocardial infarction and Q waves on the electrocardiogram all measure different aspects of the extent of myocardial damage. The full importance of myocardial damage as a prognostic factor might be overlooked by placing each of these variables separately in a stepwise regression analysis, particularly if there are relatively few outcome events. A clinical index that combines the information provided from several related variables is a more powerful prognostic factor than any individual variable, improves the reproducibility of the prognostic model and more closely stimulates the clinician's "gestalt" impression of the patient's illness (22).

Variables of prognostic importance may be discrete (e.g., male, female) or continuous (e.g., ejection fraction). Many studies analyze the strength of a continuous prognostic factor by setting an arbitrary "cut point" and dividing the patients into subgroups with values above and below the cut point. Although this technique is helpful to illustrate findings and facilitate drawing survival curves, it discards valuable prognostic information and may weaken the apparent prognostic significance of a continuous variable. For instance, ejection fraction is often described as being > or <40%. It is important to recognize that dividing patients by this criterion implicitly assumes that an ejection fraction of 39% has the same prognostic importance as an ejection fraction of 12%. The value of ejection fraction as a prognostic factor would be

Table 26.1. Clinical Research Designs in Increasing Order of Rigor

No controls (case reports, case series)
Literature controls
Historic controls
Concurrent controls
Concurrent controls with multivariable analysis
Randomized controlled clinical trials

considerably underestimated by an analysis that lumps together patients with such markedly different prognoses.

Clinical Research Design

Although pathophysiologic insight may be necessary for the development of medical therapeutics, empiric testing remains essential. The history of medicine is filled with examples of seemingly rational therapies that have failed the empiric test. In 1989, for instance, the hypothesis that antiarrhythmic drug therapy after myocardial infarction would reduce sudden death was forcefully rejected by the observation that flecainide and encainide actually increased the incidence of sudden death (23). The hypothesis that coronary angioplasty immediately after thrombolysis for acute myocardial infarction would improve outcome has been tested in three randomized controlled clinical trials (24–27) without evidence for efficacy. The failure of a seemingly rational therapy to work as planned leads to refinement of the initial hypothesis and, hopefully, improvement in the underlying pathophysiologic model. Such failures dramatically illustrate the need for rigorous empiric testing of therapeutic hypotheses.

Clinical research regarding various therapies may be classified within a hierarchy of increasing rigor (Table 26.1). Clinical observations such as case reports and case series are the least rigorous design. However, virtually all therapeutic innovations begin with the report of a few cases. The power of a key observation may be sufficient to alter an entire paradigm for treatment because it takes only a few cases to demonstrate the potential of a new technique. Electrical defibrillation, angioplasty and valvuloplasty were remarkable advances that initiated entirely new eras of treatment by demonstrating powerful therapeutic principles. Although additional studies of more stringent design are generally needed to measure the effectiveness of a novel therapy accurately and test it in relation to standard therapy, most innovations are first reported as uncontrolled observations (28).

The degree of rigor in clinical research design depends in large part on the quality of the control group (Table 26.1). The most accessible standard of comparison is the experience of other institutions with treatment of patients with the same illness, as reported in the literature. A large number of factors differ among institutions, however, including differences in disease incidence and severity, referral patterns, standards of diagnosis, ancillary therapy and selection of patients for alternative therapies, so that controls from the literature are not definitive. Historic controls of previously treated patients from the same institution are an improvement over literature controls because variability in some of these factors is eliminated. Nevertheless, changes in patient selection and supportive care can lead to better outcomes in more recently treated patients. A few diseases, however, have such a uniform and predictable clinical course that the use of literature or historic controls may be sufficient. Ventricular fibrillation and infective endocarditis were essentially 100% fatal before the introduction of electrical defibrillation and antibiotics, respectively. Given the uniformly dismal prognosis, the effect of potential confounding factors was not an issue, so that the striking effects of the new therapy were obvious. There are very few conditions today for which either literature or historic controls would be adequate.

Concurrent controls from the same institution assure greater comparability of patients than do historic controls because patient referral patterns and supportive care are similar. However, a concurrent control group may differ from treated patients in many ways. In particular, low risk patients may be selected for the new therapy, whereas high risk patients might receive the older control therapy. This problem can be partially alleviated through the use of multivariable analysis to correct for imbalances in prognostic factors between treatment groups, as discussed in detail in a later section of this review. Assignment of therapy randomly, as is done in a randomized controlled clinical trial, represents the ultimate method of assuring that patient groups are comparable for all other factors except that of treatment.

Randomized Trials

The prospective randomized controlled clinical trial represents a major development in the evaluation of medical therapeutics. This study design was initially used by the father of modern statistics, R.A. Fisher, in agricultural experiments during the 1920s (29). The first use of randomization in medical experimentation occurred in the 1930s and the first multicenter controlled clinical trials began in the 1940s. The importance of clinical trials was increased after amendments to the charter of the Food and Drug Administration in 1962 required that drug approval be based on evidence from controlled investigations (29). As a result of the rigor of the experimental design, randomized controlled clinical trials have had particular impact on therapeutic decision making. A selected number of major clinical trials in cardiovascular disease are listed in Table 26.2 (30–78).

The impact of a randomized clinical trial is greatest when it can establish a broad therapeutic principle. For example, the lipid hypothesis of coronary atherosclerosis was based

Table 26.2. Selected Major Randomized Clinical Trials in Cardiovascular Disease

Primary prevention
  Lipid Research Clinics Coronary Primary Prevention Trial (30,31)
  Multiple Risk Factor Intervention Trial (32)
  Physicians' Health Study (33)
  Helsinki Heart Study (34)
  Oslo Study of Diet and Smoking Intervention (35)
Hypertension
  Veterans Administration Cooperative Study (36,37)
  U.S. Public Health Service Trial (38)
  Hypertension Detection and Follow-up Program (39–42)
  Australian Therapeutic Trial (43,44)
  Medical Research Council Trial (45)
Coronary artery bypass surgery
  Veterans Administration Cooperative Study (46–49)
  European Coronary Surgery Study (50–52)
  Coronary Artery Surgery Study (53–55)
  National Cooperative Unstable Angina Study (56,57)
Thrombolysis for acute myocardial infarction
  Thrombolysis in Myocardial Infarction Study, Phase I (TIMI-I) (58–60)
  Gruppo Italiano per lo Studio della Streptochinasi Nell'Infarcto Miocardico (GISSI) (61)
  Second International Study of Infarct Survival (ISIS-2) (62)
  European Cooperative Studies (63–65)
Congestive heart failure
  Cooperative North Scandinavian Enalapril Survival Study (66)
  Veterans Administration Study of Vasodilator Therapy (67)
Secondary prevention after myocardial infarction
  Coronary Drug Project (68,69)
  Beta-Blocker Heart Attack Trial (70–72)
  Aspirin Myocardial Infarction Study (73)
  Multicenter Diltiazem Postinfarction Trial (74)
  Persantine-Aspirin Reinfarction Study (75)
Unstable angina
  Canadian Multicenter Study (76)
  Veterans Administration Cooperative Study (77)
  Montreal Study (78)

on pathologic observations of coronary arteries, as well as consistent epidemiologic evidence linking serum cholesterol to coronary heart disease. Nevertheless, pathophysiologic reasoning and statistical associations of elevated serum cholesterol with coronary heart disease did not constitute convincing proof of the hypothesis that lowering serum cholesterol would reduce coronary heart disease. The Lipid Research Clinics Coronary Primary Prevention Trial (30,31) was designed to test the lipid hypothesis directly. It used cholestyramine to treat men 35 to 59 years of age with serum cholesterol levels ≥265 mg/dl. This study (30) demonstrated a significant 19% reduction in coronary heart disease end points (coronary death or nonfatal myocardial infarction) over a 7 year follow-up period. Evidence from this trial has been considered to be the "keystone" joining evidence from basic sciences, epidemiology and clinical investigation to establish the lipid hypothesis.

Some of the controversy regarding clinical trials relates to the question of whether a trial should be subject to "narrow interpretation" or "broad interpretation." The controversy over the Lipid Research Clinics Coronary Primary Prevention Trial is less over the validity of the findings in the randomized subjects than whether those findings can be generalized to other groups of patients. A very narrow interpretation would be that only patients similar to those enrolled in the trial (middle-aged men) with cholesterol elevated to similar levels (≥265 mg/dl) and treated with the same drug (cholestyramine) would receive benefit. The trial has received a broader interpretation as proving an important therapeutic principle, namely that lowering cholesterol leads to a reduction in death from coronary heart disease. This interpretation relies on additional evidence to lead to the more extensive recommendations regarding cholesterol lowering that have now been promulgated as part of the National Cholesterol Education Program (79).

In a strict sense, the results of a randomized trial apply only to the patients who were enrolled or perhaps to patients meeting the study entry criteria and given identical treatment. It is a "leap of faith" to expand the results of a trial into a broad therapeutic principle. Trial evidence has been used to establish widely accepted principles regarding the treatment of mild hypertension, thrombolytic therapy for acute myocardial infarction and the use of beta-adrenergic blocking agents after myocardial infarction.

It is simpler to demonstrate that a therapy works for some patients than it is to define precisely which patients benefit and which do not. The number of patients that must be enrolled in a trial becomes much greater as lower risk patients are included. Trials of mild disease are therefore more difficult to conduct and may not be practical. Because a randomized trial will not be done for every subgroup of patients, the extrapolation of findings from trials conducted in severely diseased patients to the treatment of less severely affected patients will always be an issue for debate.

Observational Data Bases

Although the randomized controlled clinical trial is the best method for testing therapeutic hypotheses, it is also a difficult, expensive and time-consuming exercise. The Lipid Research Clinic Coronary Primary Prevention Trial, for instance, lasted 15 years and cost $142,250,000. In an era of fiscal limits, the ability to plan and fund large clinical trials is much more restricted than in the 1960s and 1970s. It is simply not practical to perform randomized studies to answer every question. As a result, there is considerable interest in targeting randomized trials to the topics most likely to require this definitive form of study and developing alternatives to the traditional randomized controlled clinical trial. The use of clinical data bases and registries to address therapeutic questions can provide a complementary approach to the randomized trial (80).

Modern observational data bases share many methodologic strengths with randomized studies, including standard

Table 26.3. Major Data Bases in Cardiovascular Disease

Duke Cardiovascular Disease Databank (20,81–93)
Seattle Heart Watch (94–97)
Coronary Artery Surgery Study Registry (98–106)
NHLBI PTCA Registry (107–113)
Percutaneous Cardiac Mapping and Ablation Registry (114)
Valvuloplasty Registry (114a,114b)

NHLBI PTCA = National Heart, Lung and Blood Institute Percutaneous Transluminal Coronary Angioplasty.

definitions for data, complete and prospective data collection, use of computerized data management, comprehensive patient follow-up and multidisciplinary research teams (80). Examples of modern data bases are provided in Table 26.3 (20,81–114).

Even though there is little doubt that observational data bases can characterize trends in management and patient outcome and identify prognostic factors, it remains controversial whether they can be used to evaluate therapy (80). Our view is that observational databases can and should play an important role in the evaluation of therapy. By design, a data base is relatively nonselective, so that the entire spectrum of patients with a disease is represented. Many patients included in a clinical data base would not be included in a randomized trial. For instance, only 13% of patients in the Coronary Artery Surgery Study (CASS) screened for entry met the criteria for randomization (53), and 4.2% of patients in the Duke Cardiovascular Disease Databank (115) fulfilled the eligibility criteria for randomization in CASS. The broad spectrum of patients in a clinical data base permits analysis of subgroups excluded from or poorly represented in randomized studies. A number of observational studies have been published from the Coronary Artery Surgery Study Registry that have considerably enhanced the value of the overall investigation, including examinations of the efficacy of coronary bypass surgery in the elderly (104) and those with poor left ventricular function (101) or severe angina (106).

An observational data base is also helpful in providing corroborative evidence when randomized trial data are relatively sparse. Coronary bypass surgery for left main coronary artery disease has been shown to prolong life significantly in only one small randomized study (47), but the value of surgery in such patients is widely accepted. We believe this consensus is due to the confluence of pathophysiologic considerations (the large amount of the left ventricle supplied by the left main coronary artery that is jeopardized by a significant lesion in this location), the evidence that left main coronary artery disease is associated with a poor prognosis (99,116), the observational studies that suggested that surgery increases survival (98), and finally the randomized trial data (47). Observational data bases can provide key contextual data for identifying patients with poor outcomes likely to benefit from therapy, as well as providing initial estimates of the efficacy of therapy.

The major limitation of observational data in the evaluation of therapy is the possibility of selection bias because patients chosen to receive one therapy may differ in a number of prognostic factors from those chosen for an alternative therapy. Multivariable analysis of observational data can be used to adjust for the *known* imbalances between patient groups in clinical characteristics of prognostic importance. Regardless of the number of factors used in statistical adjustments and the care with which the analyses are performed, there will always be concerns about the potential effects of confounding factors. To test the extent to which statistical models could remove the influence of selection bias from estimates of the effects of therapy, we used multivariable prediction models developed in the Duke Cardiovascular Disease Databank (115) to predict the results of the three major randomized controlled clinical trials of coronary artery bypass surgery. Predictions of the Duke model were within the 95% confidence limits of the observed results in 24 of 26 subgroups from the Veterans Administration Cooperative Study, the European Cooperative Surgery Study and the Coronary Artery Surgery Study (115). Although this result applies to one statistical model from a particular data base, it does suggest that carefully performed observational studies can be used to make treatment comparisons and can complement information from randomized trials in assisting clinical decision making.

Earlier, we alluded to the difficulty in defining which patients are likely to benefit from a specific therapy, even one shown to be effective in randomized studies. Randomized studies are generally conducted in a large group of patients who meet specific entry criteria, and it is not always clear whether all patients enrolled experience the same treatment effect. Results are often reported separately for several relevant subgroups, but these are much smaller than the trial as a whole, with consequently less precise estimates of the treatment effect. Observational analyses can be a useful complement to randomized studies in several respects. First, the lack of selection criteria provides a broader spectrum of patients and allows better representation of the effect of therapy across the spectrum of patients. Second, multivariable modeling can be of particular value in assessing whether a therapy works better for some types of patients than others. The formal multivariable assessment of "treatment by covariate interactions" can be used to provide insight into the therapeutic principles underlying the application of therapy (20). In a study of patients treated with bypass surgery or medical therapy over a 15 year period, we (20) found that coronary artery bypass surgery generally increased patient survival. Perhaps most importantly, the magnitude of this effect was related in a systematic fashion to three factors: the number of diseased vessels, the year of catheterization and the underlying medical risk. The impact of the number of diseased vessels was not surprising, considering the major effect of bypass surgery is to correct the abnormalities in coronary anatomy. The therapeutic effect of bypass surgery compared with medical therapy improved during each year of the study, probably because of incremental improvements in surgical technique, cardiac anesthesia and supportive care. Finally, the overall benefit from surgery was consistently related to the underlying risk of medical therapy: the greater the chance of death on medical therapy, the greater the absolute survival benefit from bypass surgery. Importantly, the risk reduction was not dependent on the specific factor that elevated the risk. Thus, patients at high risk as a result of severe myocardial ischemia, age or reduced ejection fraction had a similar risk reduction after bypass surgery. These observations suggest that the effect of coronary bypass surgery on survival should be viewed as a continuum, with the magnitude of benefit depending on the patient's underlying risk (20). This conclusion contrasts with the prevailing view that the beneficial effect of surgery is limited to specific subgroups of patients.

Future Developments

Advances in therapeutic decision making will depend on progress in several areas, including development of new pathophysiologic insights, clinical observations and analysis and randomized controlled clinical trials.

One important source of improved decision making is a better understanding of disease processes. The advances in molecular biology, for instance, may affect therapy for atherosclerosis through insights in metabolism by pinpointing sites of action for drugs, as well as by providing tools to epidemiologists. New drugs are also being made by genetic engineering techniques. In addition to basic research, clinical observations and epidemiologic analyses will be essential sources of the insights needed to advance both therapeutics and clinical decision making.

Clinical trials. There are a number of major clinical trials underway or being planned that will expand the knowledge base for clinical decision making (Table 26.4). The treatment of acute myocardial infarction is under intensive investigation, and the array of clinical trials should provide large amounts of data. Six trials of coronary angioplasty are also underway or in the planning stages. These studies will be completed between 1989 and the mid 1990s and should provide data for decision making into the 21st century.

One development that has enhanced the conduct of randomized trials is the emergence of relatively stable multicenter collaborative groups that perform a series of studies. This model for clinical trials has long been used by cancer investigators, in part because no one clinical center treated enough patients with a particular form of cancer to perform therapeutic studies. With the increased recognition of the need for large sample sizes and timely data to address pressing clinical questions, the value of stable multicenter collaborative arrangements is becoming recognized by cardiovascular investigators. Two major advantages of ongoing collaborations are that the establishment of a communica-

Table 26.4. Selected Ongoing Trials in Cardiovascular Disease

Coronary angioplasty
  Bypass Angioplasty Revascularization Investigation (BARI)
  Emory Angioplasty Surgery Trial (EAST)
  Randomized Interventional Treatment of Angina (RITA)
  German Angioplasty Bypass Interventional Trial (GABI)
  Coronary Angioplasty Bypass Revascularization Investigation (CABRI)
  Angioplasty Compared Medicine (ACME)
Thrombolysis for acute ischemic syndromes
  Gruppo Italiano per lo Studio Della Supravivenza Nell'Infarto
    Miocardico (GISSI-2)
  International Study of Infarct Survival, Phase 3 (ISIS-3)
  Thrombolysis and Angioplasty in Myocardial Infarction Studies (TAMI-5,
    TAMI-6)
  Thrombolysis in Myocardial Infarction Study, Phase 3 (TIMI-3)
  Late Assessment of Thrombolytic Efficacy (LATE)
  Estudio Multicentrico Estreptoquinasa Republica Argentina (EMERA)
Hypertension
  Systolic Hypertension in the Elderly (SHEP)
Atherosclerosis
  Stanford Coronary Risk Intervention Project (SCRIP)
  Post Coronary Artery Bypass Graft Study
  Program on Surgical Control of Hyperlipidemias (POCOSH)
Congestive heart failure
  Studies of Left Ventricular Dysfunction (SOLVD)
  Survival and Ventricular Enlargement (SAVE)
  Immunosuppressive Therapy for Biopsy Proven Myocarditis
Arrhythmias
  Cardiac Arrhythmia Suppression Trial (CAST)
  Electrophysiologic Study Versus Electrocardiographic Monitoring for
    Selection of Antiarrhythmic Therapy of Ventricular Tachyarrhythmias
    (ESVEM)

tions infrastructure, including standardization of methods, terminology and procedures, need not be repeated for each study and that the talented interdisciplinary team necessary for such trials can be maintained intact.

Meta-analysis. Clinical decision makers need to synthesize information from a variety of sources to arrive at management strategies. The data from the literature vary in study design, quality, accessibility and impact. Reviews by experts can place findings from disparate studies within a conceptual framework for consistent interpretation, but such reviews rely heavily on the reviewer's judgment to weigh evidence from distinct studies appropriately (117–119).

The technique of meta-analysis has been increasingly applied in recent years. Meta-analysis was originally developed in the social sciences (120,121) and achieved prominence in the medical literature in 1977 when Chalmers et al. (122) pooled the results of several small randomized trials of anticoagulant therapy for acute myocardial infarction. Although the legitimacy of the technique has been challenged (118,120,123,124), meta-analysis has been extensively applied to cardiovascular disease (125,126). Meta-analyses have been published, combining data from randomized trials in acute myocardial infarction of thrombolytic therapy (127,128), beta-blockade (129), lidocaine (130) and nitrates

(131), as well as trials of secondary prevention after myocardial infarction using antiarrhythmic agents (132), beta-blockers (129,132), aspirin (133), anticoagulants (122,132) and exercise training (132,134). Other meta-analyses have examined the treatment of congestive heart failure (135,136) and hypertension (137,138). A summary of meta-analysis results in cardiovascular disease has been recently published (125,126).

The technique of meta-analysis have been criticized on a variety of grounds (120,123,124). Although seemingly simple to perform, meta-analysis is actually a fairly demanding and complex technique. The quality of meta-analyses varies considerably (121), and several interested investigators (117,121) have proposed methodologic standards to ensure the technical quality of analysis. Philosophic issues regarding meta-analysis cannot be resolved as simply. Many observers remain concerned about the heterogeneity among studies in terms of patient characteristics, treatments, regimens and overall study quality. Should more weight be given to "good" studies? Does a meta-analysis of small studies eliminate the need for a large randomized trial? These and other questions about meta-analysis will be discussed extensively during the next few years.

Outcomes in cardiovascular disease. Clinical research in cardiovascular disease has tended to emphasize objective "hard end points," such as mortality, myocardial infarction or physiologic measures such as ejection fraction. The need for additional measures of "soft end points," such as functional capacity, quality of life, satisfaction with care and work status, has been increasingly recognized. One important barrier to inclusion of such end points has been a lack of accepted standardized measurement techniques. Methodologic studies (139,140) have been completed to develop brief instruments to measure several of these key aspects of outcome. The National Heart, Lung and Blood Institute has convened two workshops on quality of life measurement (141,142), which should be of considerable assistance to investigators in the design and conduct of future investigations. Quality of life measures have been incorporated into several ongoing clinical trials, including the Bypass Angioplasty Revascularization Investigation (BARI), the Cardiac Arrhythmia Suppression Trial (CAST), Studies of Left Ventricular Dysfunction (SOLVD), the Systolic Hypertension in the Elderly Program (SHEP) and the Thrombolysis and Angioplasty in Myocardial Infarction Study, Phase 5 (TAMI-5).

Administrative data bases. The large administrative data bases generated in the process of health care delivery have become increasingly more important sources of information relevant to clinical decision making. In general, these data bases provide a limited set of information concerning hospitalizations, physician claims (including physician visits, services provided in outpatient departments, treadmill testing, angiography, etc.) and registration histories (dates of eligibility, mortality and residence) (143). Considerable care

is required in analyzing the data and assessing their quality (144). These data bases include information from large groups of patients and provide a unique perspective on the results of therapy as provided in the community setting. In contrast, data from clinical trials and observational data bases usually reflect the efficacy of specific therapies provided in ideal settings. This difference between effectiveness and efficacy is relevant not only to policy planners, but also to physicians recommending specific therapies. Differences between "ideal" results reported in the literature and results in a specific setting may alter therapeutic recommendations for individual patients, as well as highlight opportunities to improve the delivery of care. Examples of large administrative data bases include the Medicare Provider and Analysis and Review (MEDPAR) files, which contain 11 million records per year; the Manitoba Claims Data Base, which covers all adults in the province since 1972; the New York State Department of Health's Statewide Planning and Research Cooperative System (SPARCS), which includes discharge abstract data since 1980 and the California discharge abstract data maintained by the Office of Statewide Health Planning and Development.

The information from these large administrative data bases provides an overview of the effectiveness of specific procedures. Their value for providing data for therapeutic decision making is considerably enhanced when linked with much more detailed clinical information for specific subgroups of patients. The Medicare data, for example, have been supplemented by data on key clinical findings for a random sample of approximately 3,100 cases of coronary revascularization from eight peer review organizations in seven states. The extraction of data from the medical record, which was performed by a modification of the Medis-Groups abstraction technique, provided clinical details, including admission diagnosis, aspects of the medical history, physical examination, laboratory and specialized diagnostic tests, up to 30 diagnostic codes, up to 36 procedure codes and untoward hospital events.

Analyses of the effectiveness of different therapies for patients with coronary artery disease have been performed using administrative data bases. For example, coronary bypass surgery and coronary angioplasty results have been compared in the Medicare population (145). Unadjusted 3 month mortality rates were significantly higher among patients undergoing surgery (8.6% versus 5.8%), and both rates were considerably higher than the corresponding rates from the literature. After adjustment for 5 baseline characteristics, mortality rates were still significantly different; however, when 37 variables were used in the adjustment process, mortality rates were equivalent (145). Although these particular results need additional confirmation, they demonstrate the potential application of large computerized administrative data bases.

Clearly, considerable methodologic research is necessary to determine the best ways to use administrative data bases.

For instance, prognosis in coronary heart disease can be quite sensitive to a number of clinical factors, most of which are not available in claims data bases (146). Methods to ensure the quality of data that were not collected for research purposes must also be carefully considered. Imaginative methodologic approaches involving linkage of administrative data to select clinical data may be able to overcome the limitations of the data contained in these large data bases. Nevertheless, population-based data sources such as the Medicare claims data base provide a much broader look at the effectiveness of therapy in general practice as opposed to the experience of academic medical centers in highly selected patient populations.

Clinical data bases. Clinical data bases will likely become an increasingly more important means of providing data for clinical decision making. A clinical data base can provide valuable information to individual physicians about the delivery of care at their hospital and allow extrapolation of information reported in the medical literature from clinical trials or observational studies.

A number of trends are driving the development of clinical data bases. Dramatic increases in microcomputer capabilities coupled with decreasing costs now make clinical data bases financially feasible for even small practices. Physicians are becoming more computer literate as newly trained physicians enter practice and established physicians "retrain" themselves. Increasing medical costs have put enormous pressure on physicians to account for the quality and cost of care provided. Increased paperwork will require efficient methods for information management. The practice of medicine has become more competitive, encouraging physicians and hospital administrators to "market" their services. There is also a growing body of evidence to suggest that computer-aided decision making is superior to more traditional approaches (147–150). In response to these trends, it seems inevitable that local data bases will continue to proliferate.

Large collaborative data bases can be developed to link information from a variety of practice settings in geographically dispersed areas. Such data bases could provide information more representative of clinical practice than current data bases from individual hospitals that have relatively homogeneous practice patterns. To realize the potential for collaborative clinical data bases, a number of problems must be overcome (151). Before information from a number of diverse practice settings can be shared to perform observational research studies, a common terminology must be developed, as well as similar approaches for collecting and ensuring the quality of data. New biostatistical methods must be developed to analyze the increasingly more complex practice of cardiology. A sound financial base is required for the installation and maintenance of a collaborative data base for it to be feasible to collect long-term outcome information. Financial support will likely be realized not only from the physician, but from hospital administrators as well. Conse-quently, the implementation strategy, focus and function of the data base will need to meet a variety of objectives. Successful development of large-scale collaborative clinical data bases will require considerable input and communication among all parties with a "stake" in their development, namely, the physician, hospital administrator, third party payor, policy planner and researcher.

It is unlikely that the potential of clinical data bases to improve the practice of medicine will be realized without the physician playing a prominent role in their development. The challenge to the cardiologist practicing in the 1990s is to recognize that fundamental changes in the practice environment provide opportunities to improve the quality of care. Physicians will need to understand how to use computers to practice more efficiently and support the development of clinical data bases that not only will allow others to monitor the quality and cost of care provided, but enable all physicians to improve the quality of care.

Conclusions

Physicians will continue to face difficult decisions about the choice of therapy, but there will be better information in the future to guide such decisions. There will be a number of randomized controlled clinical trials, new data base techniques, and most importantly, new pathophysiologic insights from both basic research and keen clinical observations that will create paradigms for therapy.

We thank Drs. Thomas Robertson and Eric Topol for information concerning ongoing trials, and Alexandria Lubans and Melissa Hurt for assistance in preparing the manuscript.

References

1. Eisenberg JM. Doctor's Decisions and the Cost of Medical Care: The Reasons for Doctors' Practice Patterns and the Ways to Change Them. Ann Arbor: Health Administration Press Perspectives, 1986.
2. Letsch SW, Levit KR, Waldo DR. National health expenditures, 1987. Health Care Financ Rev 1988;10:109–22.
3. National Heart Lung and Blood Institute. Heart and vascular disease: magnitude of the problem. In: National Heart Lung and Blood Institute. Tenth Report of the Directory. Bethesda, MD: National Heart, Lung, and Blood Institute, 1982.
4. Sox HC Jr, Blatt MA, Higgins MC, Marton KI. Medical Decision Making. Stoneham, MA: Butterworth, 1988.
5. Weinstein MC, Fineberg HV, Elstein AS, et al. Clinical Decision Analysis. Philadelphia: WB Saunders, 1980.
6. Detsky AS, Redelmeier D, Abrams HB. What's wrong with decision analysis? Can the left brain influence the right? J Chronic Dis 1987;40:831–6.
7. Eraker SA, Politser P. How decisions are reached: physician and patient. Ann Intern Med 1982;97:262–8.
8. Larkin J, McDermott J, Simon DP, Simon HA. Expert and novice performance in solving physics problems. Science 1980;208:1335–42.
9. Szolovits P, Patil RS, Schwartz WB. Artificial intelligence in medical diagnosis. Ann Intern Med 1988;108:80–7.
10. Eddy DM. Variations in physician practice: the role of uncertainty. Health Affairs 1984;3:74–89.

11. Chassin MR, Kosecoff J, Winslow CM, et al. Does inappropriate use explain geographic variations in the use of health care services? A study of three procedures. JAMA 1987;258:2533–7.

12. Chassin MR, Brook RH, Park RE, et al. Variations in the use of medical and surgical services by the medicare population. N Engl J Med 1986;314:285–90.

13. Wennberg JE, Freeman JL, Culp WJ. Are hospital services rationed in New Haven or over-utilised in Boston? Lancet 1987;1:1185–9.

14. Lee ET. Statistical Methods for Survival Data Analysis. Belmont, CA: Lifetime Learning Publications, 1980.

15. Ingelfinger JA, Mosteller F, Thibodeau LA, Ware JH. Biostatistics in Clinical Medicine. New York: Macmillan, 1987.

16. Matthews DE, Farewall VT. Using and Understanding Medical Statistics. Basel: S Karger, 1985.

17. Cox DR. Regression models and life-tables (with discussion). J R Stat Soc B 1972;34:187–220.

18. Harrell FE Jr. The PHGLM procedure. In: SUGI Supplemental Library Users Guide. Cary, NC: SAS Institute, 1986:437–66.

19. Dixon WN, Brown MB, Engelman L, et al. Survival analysis with covariates—Cox models. In: Dixon WJ, ed. BMDP Statistical Software. Berkeley: University of California Press, 1985:576–94.

20. Califf RM, Harrell FE Jr, Lee KL, et al. The evolution of medical and surgical therapy for coronary artery disease: a 15-year perspective. JAMA 1989;261:2077–86.

21. Frieman JA, Chalmers TC, Smith H Jr, Kuebler RR. The importance of beta, the type II error, and sample size in the design and interpretation of the randomized controlled trial. N Engl J Med 1978;299:690–4.

22. Harrell FE Jr, Lee KL, Califf RM, Pryor DB, Rosati RA. Regression modelling strategies for improved prognostic prediction. Stat Med 1984; 3:143–52.

23. Nightingale SL. From the Food and Drug Administration: flecainide and encainide not to be used in non-life-threatening arrhythmias. JAMA 1989;261:3368.

24. Topol EJ, Califf RM, George BS, et al. A randomized trial of immediate versus delayed elective angioplasty after intravenous tissue plasminogen activator in acute myocardial infarction. N Engl J Med 1987;317:581–8.

25. Simoons ML, Arnold AER, Betriu A, et al. Thrombolysis with tissue plasminogen activator in acute myocardial infarction: no additional benefit from immediate percutaneous coronary angioplasty. Lancet 1988;1:197–203.

26. TIMI Research Group. Immediate vs delayed catheterization and angioplasty following thrombolytic therapy for acute myocardial infarction: TIMI II A results. JAMA 1988;260:2849–58.

27. TIMI Study Group. Comparison of invasive and conservative strategies after treatment with intravenous tissue plasminogen activator in acute myocardial infarction: results of the Thrombolysis in Myocardial Infarction (TIMI) Phase II Trial. N Engl J Med 1989;320:618–27.

28. Lederman LM. Observations in particle physics from two neutrinos to the standard model. Science 1989;244:664–72.

29. Meinert CL. Clinical Trials: Design, Conduct, and Analysis. New York: Oxford University Press, 1986.

30. Lipid Research Clinics Program. The Lipid Research Clinics Coronary Primary Prevention Trial results. I. Reduction in incidence of coronary heart disease. JAMA 1984;251:351–64.

31. Lipid Research Clinics Program. The Lipid Research Clinics Coronary Primary Prevential Trial results. II. The relationship of reduction in incidence of coronary heart disease to cholesterol lowering. JAMA 1984;251:365–74.

32. Multiple Risk Factor Intervention Trial Research Group. Multiple Risk Factor Intervention Trial. JAMA 1982;248:1465–77.

33. Steering Committee of the Physicians' Health Study Research Group. Preliminary report: findings from the aspirin component of the ongoing Physicians' Health Study. N Engl J Med 1988;318:262–4.

34. Frick MH, Elo O, Haapa K, et al. Helsinki Heart Study: primary-prevention trial with gemfibrozil in middle-aged men with dyslipidemia. N Engl J Med 1987;317:1237–45.

35. Hjermann I, Velve Byre K, Holme I, Leren P. Effect of diet and smoking intervention on the incidence of coronary heart disease: report from the Oslo Study Group of a randomized trial in healthy men. Lancet 1981;2:1303–10.

36. Veterans Administration Cooperative Study Group on Antihypertensive Agents. Effects of treatment on morbidity in hypertension: results in patients with diastolic blood pressures averaging 115 through 129 mm Hg. JAMA 1967;202:1028–34.

37. Veterans Administration Cooperative Study Group on Antihypertensive Agents. Effects of treatment on morbidity in hypertension. II. Results in patients with diastolic blood pressure averaging 90 through 114 mm Hg. JAMA 1970;213:1143–52.

38. Smith WM. Treatment of mild hypertension: results of a ten-year intervention trial. Circ Res 1977;40(suppl I):I-98–105.

39. Hypertension Detection and Follow-up Program Cooperative Group. Five-year findings of the Hypertension Detection and Follow-up Program. I. Reduction in mortality of persons with high blood pressure, including mild hypertension. JAMA 1979;242:2562–71.

40. Hypertension Detection and Follow-up Program Cooperative Group. Five-year findings of the Hypertension Detection and Follow-up Program. II. Mortality by race, sex and age. JAMA 1979;242:2572–7.

41. Hypertension Detection and Follow-up Program Cooperative Group. Five-year findings of the Hypertension Detection and Follow-up Program. III. Reduction in stroke incidence among persons with high blood pressure. JAMA 1982;247:633–8.

42. Hypertension Detection and Follow-up Program Cooperative Group. The effect of treatment on mortality in "mild" hypertension. N Engl J Med 1982;307:976–80.

43. Management Committee. The Australian Therapeutic Trial in Mild Hypertension. Lancet 1980;2:1261–7.

44. Management Committee of the Australian Therapeutic Trial in Mild Hypertension. Untreated mild hypertension. Lancet 1982;2:185–91.

45. Medical Research Council Working Party. MRC Trial of Treatment of Mild Hypertension: principal results. Br Med J 1985;291:97–104.

46. Murphy ML, Hultgren H, Detre KM, Thomsen J, Takaro T, Participants of the Veterans Administration Cooperative Study. Treatment of chronic stable angina. N Engl J Med 1977;297:621–7.

47. Takaro T, Hultgren H, Lipton MJ, Detre KM, Participants in the Study Group. The VA cooperative randomized study of surgery for coronary arterial occlusive disease: II. subgroup with significant left main lesions. Circulation 1976;54:107–17.

48. Veterans Administration Coronary Artery Bypass Surgery Cooperative Study Group. Eleven-Year survival in the Veterans Administration randomized trial of coronary bypass surgery for stable angina. N Engl J Med 1984;311:1333–9.

49. Takaro T, Hultgren HN, Detre KM, Peduzzi P. The Veterans Administration cooperative study of stable angina: current status. Circulation 1982;65:(suppl II):II-60–6.

50. European Coronary Surgery Study Group. Long-term results of prospective randomized study of coronary artery bypass surgery in stable angina pectoris. Lancet 1982;2:1173–80.

51. Varnauskas E, European Coronary Surgery Study Group. Twelve-year follow-up of survival in the randomized European Coronary Surgery Study. N Engl J Med 1988;319:332–7.

52. European Coronary Surgery Study Group. Prospective randomized study of coronary artery bypass surgery in stable angina pectoris: a progress report on survival. Circulation 1982;65(suppl II):II-67–71.

53. CASS Principal Investigators and Their Associates. Coronary Artery Surgery Study (CASS): a randomized trial of coronary artery bypass surgery: survival data. Circulation 1983;68:939–50.

54. CASS Principal Investigators and Their Associates. Coronary Artery Surgery Study (CASS): a randomized trial of coronary artery bypass surgery: quality of life in patients randomly assigned to treatment groups. Circulation 1983;68:951–60.

55. CASS Principal Investigators and Their Associates. Myocardial infarction and mortality in the Coronary Artery Surgery Study (CASS) randomized trial. N Engl J Med 1984;310:750–8.

56. Russell RO, Moraski RE, Kouchoukos N, et al. Unstable angina pectoris: National Cooperative Study Group to compare medical and surgical therapy. I. Report of protocol and patient populations. Am J Cardiol 1976;37:896–902.

57. Russell RO Jr, Moraski RE, Kouchoukos N, et al. Unstable angina pectoris: National Cooperative Study Group to compare surgical and medical therapy. II. In-hospital experience and initial follow-up results in patients with one, two and three vessel disease. Am J Cardiol 1978;42:839–48.

58. TIMI Study Group. Special report: the Thrombolysis in Myocardial Infarction (TIMI) Trial, Phase I findings. N Engl J Med 1985;312:932–6.

59. Chesebro JH, Knatterud G, Roberts R, et al. Thrombolysis in Myocardial Infarction (TIMI) Trial, Phase I: a comparison between intravenous tissue plasminogen activator and intravenous streptokinase. Circulation 1987;76:142–54.

60. Dalen JE, Gore JM, Braunwald E, et al. Six- and twelve-month follow-up of the Phase I Thrombolysis in Myocardial Infarction (TIMI) Trial. Am J Cardiol 1988;62:179–85.

61. Gruppo Italiano per lo Studio Della Streptochinasi Nell'infarto Miocardico (GISSI). Effectiveness of intravenous thrombolytic treatment in acute myocardial infarction. Lancet 1986;1:397–402.

62. ISIS-2 (Second International Study of Infarct Survival) Collaborative Group. Randomised trial of intravenous streptokinase, oral aspirin, both, or neither amount 17,187 cases of suspected acute myocardial infarction: ISIS-2. Lancet 1988;2:349–60.

63. Verstraete M, Bleifeld W, Brower RW, et al. Double-blind randomised trial of intravenous tissue-type plasminogen activator versus placebo in acute myocardial infarction. Lancet 1985;2:842–7.

64. Verstraete M, Bernard R, Bory M, et al. Randomised trial of intravenous recombinant tissue-type plasminogen activator versus intravenous streptokinase in acute myocardial infarction. Lancet 1985;1:965–9.

65. de Bono DP. Thrombolysis with intravenous human recombinant tissue-type plasminogen activator in acute myocardial infarction: the European experience. J Am Coll Cardiol 1987;10:75B–8B.

66. CONSENSUS Trial Study Group. Effects of enalapril on mortality in severe congestive heart failure. N Engl J Med 1987;316:1429–35.

67. Cohn JN, Archibald DG, Ziesche S, et al. Effect of vasodilator therapy on mortality in chronic congestive heart failure: results of a Veterans Administration Cooperative Study. N Engl J Med 1986;314:1547–52.

68. Coronary Drug Project Research Group. Implications of findings in the Coronary Drug Project for secondary prevention trials in coronary heart disease. Circulation 1981;63:1342–50.

69. Canner PL, Berge KG, Wenger NK, et al. Fifteen year mortality in Coronary Drug Project patients: long-term benefit with niacin. J Am Coll Cardiol 1986;8:1245–55.

70. Beta-Blocker Heart Attack Trial Research Group. A randomized trial of propranolol in patients with acute myocardial infarction. I. Mortality results. JAMA 1982;247:1707–14.

71. Beta-Blocker Heart Attack Trial Research Group. A randomized trial of propranolol in patients with acute myocardial infarction. II. Morbidity results. JAMA 1983;250:2814–9.

72. Furberg CD, Hawkins CM, Lichstein E, Beta-Blocker Heart Attack Trial Study Group. Effect of propranolol in postinfarction patients with mechanical or electrical complications. Circulation 1984;69:761–5.

73. Aspirin Myocardial Infarction Study Research Group. A randomized, controlled trial of aspirin in persons recovered from myocardial infarction. JAMA 1980;243:661–9.

74. Multicenter Diltiazem Postinfarction Trial Research Group. The effect of diltiazem on mortality and reinfarction after myocardial infarction. N Engl J Med 1988;319:385–92.

75. Persantine-Aspirin Reinfarction Study Research Group. Persantine and aspirin in coronary heart disease. Circulation 1980;62:449–61.

76. Cairns JA, Gent M, Singer J, et al. Aspirin, sulfinpyrazone, or both in unstable angina: results of a Canadian multicenter trial. N Engl J Med 1985;313:1369–75.

77. Lewis HD Jr, Davis JW, Archibald DG, et al. Protective effects of aspirin against acute myocardial infarction and death in men with unstable angina: results of a Veterans Administration Cooperative Study. N Engl J Med 1983;309:396–403.

78. Theroux P, Ouimet H, McCans J, et al. Aspirin, heparin, or both to treat acute unstable angina. N Engl J Med 1988;319:1105–11.

79. Expert Panel. Report of the National Cholesterol Education Program Expert Panel on detection, evaluation, and treatment of high blood cholesterol in adults. Arch Intern Med 1988;148:36–69.

80. Hlatky MA, Lee KL, Harrell FE Jr, et al. Tying clinical research to patient care by use of an observational database. Stat Med 1984;3:375–84.

81. Harris PJ, Harrell FE Jr, Lee KL, Behar VS, Rosati RA. Survival in medically treated coronary artery disease. Circulation 1979;60:1259–69.

82. Harris PJ, Lee KL, Harrell FE Jr, Behar VS, Rosati RA. Outcome in medically treated coronary artery disease. Ischemic events: nonfatal infarction and death. Circulation 1980;62:718–26.

83. Harris PJ, Harrell FE Jr, Lee KL, Rosati RA. Nonfatal myocardial infarction in medically treated patients with coronary artery disease. Am J Cardiol 1980;46:937–42.

84. Califf RM, Tomabechi Y, Lee KL, et al. Outcome in one-vessel coronary artery disease. Circulation 1983;67:283–90.

85. Califf RM, Conley MJ, Behar VS, et al. "Left main equivalent" coronary artery disease: its clinical presentation and prognostic significance with nonsurgical therapy. Am J Cardiol 1984;53:1489–95.

86. Califf RM, Phillips HR III, Hindman MC, et al. Prognostic value of a coronary artery jeopardy score. J Am Coll Cardiol 1985;5:1055–63.

87. Califf RM, Harrell FE Jr, Lee KL, et al. Changing efficacy of coronary revascularization: implications for patient selection. Circulation 1988;78(suppl I):I-185–91.

88. Califf RM, Mark DB, Harrell FE Jr, et al. Importance of clinical measures of ischemia in the prognosis of patients with documented coronary artery disease. J Am Coll Cardiol 1988;11:20–6.

89. Hlatky MA, Califf RM, Kong Y, Harrell FE Jr, Rosati RA. Natural history of patients with single-vessel disease suitable for percutaneous transluminal coronary angioplasty. Am J Cardiol 1983;52:225–9.

90. Pryor DB, Harrell FE Jr, Lee KL, Califf RM, Rosati RA. Estimating the likelihood of significant coronary artery disease. Am J Med 1983;75:771–80.

91. Pryor DB, Harrell FE Jr, Lee KL, Califf RM, Rosati RA. An improving prognosis over time in medically treated patients with coronary artery disease. Am J Cardiol 1983;52:444–8.

92. Pryor DB, Harrell FE Jr, Lee KL, et al. Prognostic indicators from radionuclide angiography in medically treated patients with coronary artery disease. Am J Cardiol 1984;53:18–22.

93. Pryor DB, Harrell FE Jr, Rankin JS, et al. The changing survival benefits of coronary revascularization over time. Circulation 1987;76:(suppl V):V-13–21.

94. Hammermeister KE, DeRouen TA, Dodge HT. Variables predictive of survival in patients with coronary disease: selection by univariate and multivariate analyses from the clinical electrocardiographic, exercise, arteriographic and quantitative angiographic evolution. Circulation 1979;59:421–30.

95. Hammermeister KE, DeRouen TA, Murray JA, Dodge HT. Comparison of survival of medically and surgically treated coronary disease patients in Seattle Heart Watch: nonrandomized study. Circulation 1982;65:(suppl II):II-53–9.

96. Hammermeister KE. The effect of coronary bypass surgery on survival. Prog Cardiovasc Dis 1983;25:297–334.

97. Hammermeister KE, DeRouen TA, Zia M, Dodge HT. Survival of medically treated coronary artery disease patients in the Seattle Heart Watch Angiography Registry. In: Hammermeister KE, ed. Coronary Bypass Surgery: the Late Results. New York: Praeger, 1983:167–94.

98. Chaitman BR, Fisher LD, Bourassa MG, et al. Effect of coronary artery bypass surgery on survival patterns in subsets of patients with left main coronary artery disease. Am J Cardiol 1981;48:765–77.

99. Mock MB, Ringquist I, Fisher LD, et al. Survival of medically treated patients in the Coronary Artery Surgery Study (CASS) Registry. Circulation 1982;66:562–8.

100. Ringqvist I, Fisher LD, Mock M, et al. Prognostic value of angiographic indices of coronary artery disease from the Coronary Artery Surgery Study (CASS). J Clin Invest 1983;71:1854–66.

101. Alderman EL, Fisher LD, Litwin P, et al. Results of coronary artery surgery in patients with poor left ventricular function (CASS). Circulation 1983;68:785–95.

102. Gersh BJ, Kronmal RA, Schaff HV, et al. Long-term (5 year) results of coronary bypass surgery in patients 65 years old or older: a report from the Coronary Artery Surgery Study. Circulation 1983;68(suppl II):II-190–9.

103. Chaitman BR, Davis K, Fisher LD, et al. A life table and Cox regression analysis of patients with combined proximal left anterior descending and proximal left circumflex coronary artery disease: nonleft main equivalent lesions (CASS). Circulation 1983;68:1163–70.

104. Gersh BJ, Kronmal RA, Schaff HV, et al. Comparison of coronary artery bypass surgery and medical therapy in patients 65 years of age or older: a nonrandomized study from the Coronary Artery Surgery Study (CASS) Registry. N Engl J Med 1985;313:217–24.

105. Ellis S, Alderman E, Cain K, et al. Prediction of risk of anterior myocardial infarction by lesion severity and measurement method of stenoses in the left anterior descending coronary distribution: a CASS Registry Study. J Am Coll Cardiol 1988;11:908–16.

106. Kaiser GC, Davis KB, Fisher LD, et al. Survival following coronary artery bypass grafting in patients with severe angina pectoris (CASS). J Thorac Cardiovasc Surg 1985;89:513–24.

107. Kent KM, Bentivoglio LG, Block PC, et al. Percutaneous transluminal coronary angioplasty: report from the Registry of the National Heart, Lung, and Blood Institute. Am J Cardiol 1982;49:2011–20.

108. Mullin SM, Passamani ER, Mock MB. Historical background of the National Heart, Lung, and Blood Institute Registry for Percutaneous Transluminal Coronary Angioplasty. Am J Cardiol 1984;54:3C–6C.

109. Detre KM, Myler RK, Kelsey SF, Van Raden M, To T, Mitchell H. Baseline characteristics of patients in the National Heart, Lung, and Blood Institute Percutaneous Transluminal Coronary Angioplasty Registry. Am J Cardiol 1984;54:7C–11C.

110. Faxon DP, Kelsey SF, Ryan TJ, McCabe CH, Detre K. Determinants of successful percutaneous transluminal coronary angioplasty: report from the National Heart, Lung, and Blood Institute Registry. Am Heart J 1984;108:1019–23.

111. Cowley MJ, Mullin SM, Kelsey SF, et al. Sex differences in early and long-term results of coronary angioplasty in the NHLBI PTCA Registry. Circulation 1985;71:90–7.

112. Reeder GS, Holmes DR Jr, Detre K, Costigan T, Kelsey SF. Degree of revascularization in patients with multivessel coronary disease: a report from the National Heart, Lung, and Blood Institute Percutaneous Transluminal Coronary Angioplasty Registry. Circulation 1988;77:638–44.

113. Detre K, Holubkov R, Kelsey S, et al. Percutaneous transluminal coronary angioplasty in 1985–1986 and 1977–1981. N Engl J Med 1988;318:265–70.

114. Scheinman MM, Evans-Bell T, Executive Committee of the Percutaneous Cardiac Mapping and Ablation Registry. Catheter ablation of the atrioventricular junction: a report of the Percutaneous Mapping and Ablation Registry. Circulation 1984;70:1024–9.

114a. Bashore TM, Berman AD, Davidson CJ, Kennedy JW, Davis K. NHLBI balloon valvuloplasty registry. Percutaneous balloon aortic valvuloplasty: The acute and 30 day outcome in 671 patients. Circulation 1990; 82(Suppl II):II-79(Abstr).

114b. McKay CR, Otto C, Block P, et al. Immediate results of mitral balloon commissurotomy in 737 patients. Circulation 1990;82(Suppl II)II-545 (Abstr).

115. Hlatky MA, Califf RM, Harrell FE Jr, Lee KL, Mark DB, Pryor DB. Comparison of predictions based on observational data with the results of randomized controlled clinical trials of coronary artery bypass surgery. J Am Coll Cardiol 1988;11:237–45.

116. Conley MJ, Ely RL, Kisslo JA, Lee KL, McNeer JF, Rosati RA. The prognostic spectrum of left main stenosis. Circulation 1978;57:947–52.

117. L'Abbe KA, Detsky AS, O'Rourke K. Meta-analysis in clinical research. Ann Intern Med 1987;107:224–33.

118. Gerbarg ZB, Horwitz RI. Resolving conflicting clinical trials: guidelines for meta-analysis. J Clin Epidemiol 1988;41:503–9.

119. Thacker SB. Meta-analysis: a quantitative approach to research integration. JAMA 1988;259:1685–9.

120. Wachter KW. Disturbed by meta analysis? Science 1988;241:1407–8.

121. Sacks HS, Berrier J, Reitman D, Ancona-Berk VA, Chalmers TC. Meta-analyses of randomized controlled trials. N Engl J Med 1987;316:450–5.

122. Chalmers TC, Matta RJ, Smith H Jr, Kunzler AM. Evidence favoring the use of anticoagulants in the hospital phase of acute myocardial infarction. N Engl J Med 1977;297:1091–6.

123. Goldman L, Feinstein AR. Anticoagulants and myocardial infarction: the problems of pooling, drowning, and floating. Ann Intern Med 1979;90:92–4.

124. Anonymous. Whither meta-analysis? Lancet 1987;1:897–8.

125. Yusuf S, Wittes J, Friedman L. Overview of results of randomized clinical trials in heart disease. I. Treatments following myocardial infarction. JAMA 1988;260:2088–93.

126. Yusuf S, Wittes J, Friedman L. Overview of results of randomized clinical trials in heart disease. II. Unstable angina, heart failure, primary prevention with aspirin, and risk factor modification. JAMA 1988;260:2259–63.

127. Stamper MJ, Goldhaber SZ, Yusuf S, Peto R, Hennekens CH. Effect of intravenous streptokinase on acute myocardial infarction: pooled results of randomized trials. N Engl J Med 1982;307:1180–2.

128. Yusuf S, Collins R, Peto R, et al. Intravenous and intracoronary fibrinolytic therapy in acute myocardial infarction: overview of results on mortality, reinfarction and side-effects from 33 randomized controlled trials. Eur Heart J 1985;6:556–85.

129. Yusuf S, Peto R, Lewis J, Collins R, Sleight P. Beta blockade during and after myocardial infarction: an overview of the randomized trials. Prog Cardiovasc Dis 1985;27:335–71.

130. MacMahon S, Collins R, Peto R, Koster RW, Yusuf S. Effects of prophylactic lidocaine in suspected acute myocardial infarction: an overview of results from the randomized controlled trials. JAMA 1988;260:1910–6.

131. Yusuf S, Collins R, MacMahon S, Peto R. Effect of intravenous nitrates on mortality in acute myocardial infarction: an overview of the randomised trials. Lancet 1988;1:1088–92.

132. May GS, Eberlein KA, Furberg CD, Passamani ER, DeMets DL. Secondary prevention after myocardial infarction: a review of long-term trials. Prog Cardiovasc Dis 1982;24:331–52.

133. Antiplatelet Trialists' Collaboration. Secondary prevention of vascular disease by prolonged antiplatelet treatment. Br Med J 1988;296:320–31.

134. Oldridge NB, Guyatt GH, Fischer ME, Rimm AA. Cardiac rehabilitation after myocardial infarction: combined experience of randomized clinical trials. JAMA 1988;260:945–50.

135. Furberg CD, Yusuf S. Effect of drug therapy on survival in chronic congestive heart failure. Am J Cardiol 1988;62:41A–5A.

136. Mulrow CD, Mulrow JP, Linn WD, Aguilar C, Ramirez G. Relative efficacy of vasodilator therapy in chronic congestive heart failure. JAMA 1988;259:3422–6.

137. Cutler JA, Furberg CD. Drug treatment trials in hypertension: a review. Prev Med 1985;14:499–518.

138. MacMahon S, Cutler JA, Furberg CD, Payne GH. The effects of drug treatment for hypertension on morbidity and mortality from cardiovascular disease: a review of randomized controlled trials. Prog Cardiovasc Dis 1986;29:99–118.

139. Stewart AL, Hays RD, Ware JE Jr. The MOS short-form general health survey: reliability and validity in a patient population. Med Care 1988;26:724–35.

140. Hlatky MA, Boineau RE, Higginbotham MB, et al. A brief self-administered questionnaire to determine functional capacity (The Duke Activity Status Index). Am J Cardiol 1989;64:651–54.

141. Wenger NK, Mattson ME, Furberg CD, Elinson J. Assessment of Quality of Life in Clinical Trials of Cardiovascular Therapies. New York: Le Jacq, 1984.

142. Shumaker SA, Furberg CD. Research on quality of life in cardiovascular disease. J Prev Med (in press).

143. Roos LL, Roos NP. Using Large Data Bases for Research on Surgery. St. Louis: CV Mosby, 1989.

144. Roos LL, Sharp SM, Wajda A. Assessing data quality: a computerized approach. Soc Sci Med 1989;28:175–82.

145. Roper WL, Winkenwerder W, Hackbarth GM, Krakauer H. Effectiveness in health care: an initiative to evaluate and improve medical practice. N Engl J Med 1988;319:1197–202.

146. Califf RM, Pryor DB, Greenfield JC Jr. Beyond randomized clinical trials: applying clinical experience in the treatment of patients with coronary artery disease. Circulation 1986;74:1191–4.

147. Lee KL, Pryor DB, Harrell FE Jr, et al. Predicting outcome in coronary disease: statistical models versus expert clinicians. Am J Med 1986;80: 553–60.

148. Kong DF, Lee KL, Harrell FE Jr, et al. Clinical experience and predicting survival in coronary disease. Arch Intern Med 1989;149:1177–81.

149. McDonald CJ. Protocol-based computer reminders: the quality of care and the non-perfectability of man. N Engl J Med 1976;295: 1351–5.

150. DeDombal FT, Clamp SE, Leaper DJ, Stomeland JR, Haricks JC. Computer-aided diagnosis of lower gastrointestinal tract disorder. Gastroenterology 1975;68:252–60.

151. Pryor DB, Califf RM, Harrell FE Jr, et al. Clinical data bases: accomplishments and unrealized potential. Med Care 1985;23:623–47.

CHAPTER 27

Risk Factors for Cardiovascular Disease and Death: A Clinical Perspective

HENRY D. McINTOSH, MD

> There are many simple solutions to complex problems, and most of them are wrong.
>
> *H.L. Mencken*

Historical Background

In 1948, Congress authorized the National Heart Institute (1). Back then, patients diagnosed as having an acute myocardial infarction were frequently treated at home; if hospitalized, they were confined for up to 6 weeks. Whether they were cared for at home or in the hospital, the physician usually told patients to stay in bed for 2 weeks and ". . . not move even a muscle. The heart has to have time to heal." During that period, the patient was fed by a care-giver or family member.

Fellow classmates and I used the seventh edition of Cecil's *Textbook of Medicine*, published in 1947, as our clinical bible (2). Only 6½ of its 1,703 pages were devoted to the topic of acute myocardial infarction, and only 10 pages to the subject of coronary artery disease. The reader of Cecil's *Textbook* was informed that during convalescence from an acute myocardial infarction, "after the third week has passed, the patient may begin to feed himself, may turn in bed without help, and may have an occasional visitor." The section closed with the advice, "Throughout the entire course, every effort should be made to maintain high morale and an optimistic attitude on the part of the patient, and prevent venous thrombosis of the legs."

Many patients developed a painful condition in the left arm called the shoulder-hand syndrome (3). The condition, rarely seen today, was considered a complication of acute infarction. It was reasoned that the infarction reduced blood flow to the left arm and shoulder and the resulting ischemia caused pain in that limb. As the practice of prolonged inactivity was abandoned, the shoulder-hand syndrome became a topic of only historic interest. However, its occurrence established a myth, without scientific basis, that is accepted by many to this day: pain in the left arm is most likely due to ischemia of the heart.

Liberation of the patient with an acute infarction from prolonged immobility was stimulated by observations by Levine and Lown (4). They found that cardiac output was less in the sitting than in the recumbent position, and in 1951 they proposed the "chair treatment." However, they were careful to recommend that two robust orderlies lift the patient from the bed to the chair. It seems a bit prophetic that they suggested that "no one is blamed if the coronary patient died in bed; but if he had been out of bed, the physician is likely to be held responsible."

Also in 1948, Irving Wright and his colleagues (5) initiated the first large multicenter randomized trial ever conducted. The study was designed to evaluate the use of the anticoagulant warfarin in patients with acute infarction. It was completed in 1954. After collecting and analyzing voluminous data without the assistance of a computer, the investigators concluded that the mortality rate from acute myocardial infarction could be reduced from 23% to 16% by the use of anticoagulant therapy. It is indicative of the care that patients received in those days to appreciate that some years after the report was published, the method of randomizing the patients who entered the study was questioned. The study was designed so that patients admitted on odd days were given anticoagulant therapy; those admitted on even days were not. At that time, many doctors had reservations about prescribing "rat poison," as warfarin was referred to by many. Allegedly, when evaluating a patient with symptoms suggesting an acute myocardial infarction, some physicians participating in the study appeared to have little hesitation about making the admitting diagnosis final only on an even day!

Such actions should not be surprising because, at that time, most physicians believed that coronary artery disease was an inevitable manifestation of aging and that little could be done by specific therapy to alter its course. A sense of optimism, much less urgency, in the treatment of acute myocardial infarction had not been introduced into the therapeutic practice of medicine.

It is doubtful that many of the cardiologists of the first half of this century appreciated that they were treating patients who were a part of what was to be recognized as the greatest epidemic of modern civilization: Coronary Artery Disease. In 1910, coronary artery disease caused only 10% of the deaths in the United States, but by 1948, it accounted for 50% of deaths. This increase continued until 1962, when coronary disease accounted for 56.1% of deaths. Since then, the incidence of death due to coronary disease has declined. Coronary artery disease accounted for <50% of deaths in 1981 (1,6). Despite the unequivocal decline in the incidence of death, however, coronary disease is still the most common cause of death in this country, resulting in almost 1 million deaths each year.

Progress: 1962 to 1980

In retrospect, 1962, the year the incidence of death from coronary artery disease peaked, was a signal year. That year, Stamler (7) reported that "overwhelming evidence indicates that the disease is multifactorial in causation, with diet as a key essential etiologic factor, accounting for the occurrence of coronary artery disease in the middle-aged population of the economically more developed countries, particularly the United States. This is a far cry from the intellectual atmosphere of only a few years ago when these diseases (coronary artery disease, hypertensive cardiovascular disease and cerebrovascular disease) were regarded as the inevitable consequences of aging." However, these observations did not excite the cardiological world to action as much as the report the next year by Day (8) on the establishment of the first coronary care unit, or the report in 1969 by Favaloro (9) on the use of saphenous vein grafting in the treatment of coronary artery disease.

Gradually, thoughtful cardiologists and internists accepted the conclusions reached by worldwide epidemiologists: *coronary artery disease was indeed an epidemic disease*. They accepted the century-old teaching of Virchow: "When the frequency of occurrence of a disease increases to epidemic proportions in the population, it reflects disturbances in human culture." Stamler (10) identified the disturbances of human culture contributing to this modern day epidemic of coronary artery disease as "a rich diet and cigarette smoking and possibly sedentary habits and psychosocial stresses and tensions leading to incongruent behavior patterns." Increasing numbers of clinicians wondered, if these observations were accurate, was it possible that coronary artery disease could be prevented?

In 1964, Luther Terry released the first U.S. Public Health Surgeon General's Report on the adverse effects of smoking on health. The American Heart Association was directing and has continued to direct attention to the desirability of consuming a more prudent diet and of attaining and maintaining an ideal body weight and normal blood pressure. In 1972, the National Heart Institute released the first of four reports of the National High Blood Pressure Education Program. Exercise became a way of life for many. In 1974, early morning jogging became an integral part of the Annual Scientific Sessions of the American College of Cardiology. Finally, in 1980, the topic for discussion at the 11th Bethesda Conference of the College was the Prevention of Coronary Artery Disease (11).

Increasing numbers of individuals began to modify their life-style favorably; they accepted that "it is what you do, hour by hour, day by day, that largely determines the state of your health, whether you get sick, what you get sick with, and perhaps when you shall die" (12). At the same time, there was an explosion of things that could be done for the patient with coronary artery disease: surgery, new diagnostic tests, new drugs. Furthermore, systems were developed to assist and bring patients with symptomatic coronary artery disease into the health care network rapidly. Much more recently, angioplasty and related procedures directed at the obstructing coronary artery lesion were introduced.

Declining Mortality From Coronary Artery Disease: Role of Prevention

Because or in spite of these frequently aggressive efforts, during the last quarter of a century there has been a gratifying decline in the percent and total number of deaths due to cardiovascular disease in this country (Fig. 27.1). Although it appears unlikely that the decline can be attributed to a single cause, if coronary artery disease is indeed an epidemic disease, efforts at both primary and secondary prevention must have been important. How important has been difficult to determine. In 1984, Goldman and Cook (13) made an attempt. They accepted that from 1968 to 1976, 630,000 more premature deaths from coronary artery disease would have been expected had not the decline occurred. From a careful review of published reports, they tried to determine the relative contribution to the decline of various treatment efforts and changes in life-style (Table 27.1). They concluded that 30% of the "anticipated" premature deaths were postponed by a reduction in serum cholesterol, 24% by a reduction in cigarette smoking and 8.6% by medical treatment of hypertension. Thus, 62.5%—roughly two-thirds—of the anticipated 630,000 premature deaths were postponed because of modification of life-style and the control of three risk factors. As indicated, these data referred to the years 1968 to 1976. The decline continues. In 1982 alone, it was estimated that 680,000 premature coronary deaths were postponed. Between 1976 and 1986, the death rate from all forms of heart disease declined by 24%, and that for ischemic heart disease by 28%.

This decline in mortality is all the more remarkable because it occurred after a sustained period of increasing death rates due to coronary artery disease. In the late 1960s, the United States had the second highest death rate from coronary artery disease; only the death rate in Finland was higher. By the early 1980s, the United States ranked eighth among 27 economically developed countries. Only Australia has approached this rate of decline in mortality from the disease. However, the decline in the death rate from coronary artery disease was and is not universal. Therefore, it cannot be considered a contemporary "cohort" effort for the human species (14).

Role of changes in life-style. Data from Dupont Company employees showed that from 1957 to 1983, there was a 28% decline in the incidence rate of first major cardiac events (15). A decline in the incidence of the first major cardiac event due to coronary artery disease was also reported by investigators at the Mayo Clinic in Rochester, Minnesota (16). They reported that the incidence of first clinical manifestations of coronary artery disease peaked during 1955 to

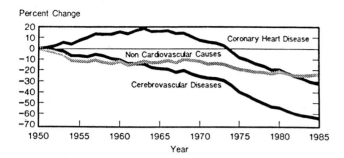

Figure 27.1. Percent changes in age-adjusted death rates for coronary heart disease, cerebrovascular diseases and noncardiovascular causes of death in the United States from 1950 to 1985. *Source*: Vital Statistics of the United States, National Center for Health Statistics.

Table 27.1. Factors Contributing to the Decline in Coronary Artery Disease: 1968 to 1976*

Medical Interventions	Estimated No. of Lives Saved	Estimated Decline in Mortality (%)
Coronary care units	85,000	13.5
Prehospital resuscitation	25,000	4.0
Coronary artery bypass surgery	23,000	3.5
Medical treatment of ischemic heart disease	61,000	10.0
Treatment of hypertension	55,000	8.5
Total	249,000	39.50
Life-style changes		
Reduction in serum cholesterol	190,000	30.0
Reduction in cigarette smoking	150,000	24.0
Total	340,000	54.00
Unexplained or errors in previous estimates	41,000	6.5
Total lives saved	630,000	100.00

*Adapted from Goldman and Cook (13).

1957. By 1975, the incidence had declined 15% among men and 18% among women. This decline parallels many changes of life-style, such as changes in diet and diet-dependent serum cholesterol, attaining an ideal body weight, abstaining from smoking, avoiding secondhand smoke, exercising and obtaining better control of hypertension.

The U.S. Department of Agriculture reported that the mean serum cholesterol level in this country declined in the early 1960s from 235–245 mg/dl to 210–215 mg/dl in the late 1970s (17). Furthermore, the prevalence of smoking among adults decreased from 40% in 1965 to 29% in 1987. By that year, nearly half of all living adults who had ever smoked had stopped smoking (18). The public had become more knowledgeable about high blood pressure and accepted therapy directed toward control of hypertension. Furthermore, millions in our society took up leisure time exercise.

Careful analysis of the data relating life-style changes to the decline in the incidence of coronary artery disease, as well as morbidity from the disease, reveals evidence of a socioeconomic connection. The more educated have changed their life-style more favorably than have the less educated (14). The incidence rate of the first major cardiac event among salaried employees of Dupont fell twice as steeply as that among hourly wage workers (38% and 18%, respectively) (15). These observations support the conclusion that the major cause of the decline in the occurrence of premature death from coronary artery disease has been a downward trend in the appearance of the first clinical manifestation of the disease. The most likely explanation for the decline in this incidence appears to be primary prevention as a result of efforts by doctors and health care workers to educate the public about a heart-healthy life-style (19).

Role of the physician. How important is the doctor compared with other health care workers in fostering prevention? If physicians are important, how compulsively do they encourage their patients to adopt a preventive and prudent life-style? In opening the 11th Bethesda Conference of the American College of Cardiology devoted to the prevention of coronary artery disease at Heart House in 1980, Robert I.

Levy, then the Director of the National Heart, Lung, and Blood Institute stated (11),

We learned, from the National High Blood Pressure Education Program, that the public feels strongly that medical advice about changes in lifestyle habits would be most positively responded to if it came from the physician! We also learned from the public that they feel that less than half of the physicians spend any considerable time providing them with information dealing with prevention.

With the passage of time, however, there was a perception that the public was abandoning the physician as a source of information regarding prevention and health maintenance. In 1985, at another conference held at Heart House, it was concluded (20):

The physician's office should be synonymous with a learning center. This is not presently the case, and there is a fear that it might not become such in the future because of physician inertia and fear of change. Indeed, time may be running out for the physician to remain the prime educator of individuals about health and hygiene matters in general. There is concern that the principal educator in the 21st century may not be the physician.

Role of coronary intervention procedures. Clearly, the incidence of the appearance or clinical recognition of coronary artery disease and premature death as a result of the disease is responding to changes in life-style by the individual and society, that is, "disturbances of human culture," as would be expected for an epidemic disease. As indicated, however, while these changes were occurring, many new invasive therapeutic efforts have become available for the treatment of coronary artery disease (for example, aortocoronary bypass grafting, thrombolytic therapy, angioplasty and a myriad of pharmacologic agents). It is likely that each of these techniques was anticipated by its advocates and large segments of society to have life-saving benefits in selected patients. Several have been demonstrated to salvage myocardium and prolong life, but none has been demonstrated to be a cure. They would appear to be at best only representatives of still developing technology.

For example, the long-term benefits of bypass surgery are compromised by progression of coronary artery disease, not only in the native circulation, but also in the bypass grafts. At the Montreal Heart Institute, Bourassa et al. (21) reported that extensive progression of atherosclerosis leading to occlusion of the aortocoronary saphenous vein grafts was not uncommon. Only about 60% of grafts remained patent as long as 10 to 12 years after implantation; 45% of grafts that were patent showed angiographic evidence of atherosclerosis; in 70% of the grafts the luminal diameter was reduced by >50%.

Would the long-term patency results of aortocoronary bypass grafting or angioplasty and other invasive efforts be improved if more effort was made by the surgeon and the invasive cardiologist to persuade patients of the value of life-style changes at the time of the procedure and to reinforce these efforts for years after the event? Would the long-term patency of grafts be improved if the surgeon saw the patient at 3 to 6 month intervals to determine if any "disturbances of human culture" were having an adverse effect on the implanted grafts and to make an effort to correct them (19)? At least one study (22) suggests that graft patency might be prolonged. It seems likely that the surgeon could have a great influence on his or her patients. The surgeon should maintain personal contact with the patient for years after the procedure is performed to reinforce in the patient's mind the importance of abstaining from smoking and avoiding secondhand smoke, of a prudent diet, of regular exercise and active life-style and of maintaining normal blood pressure. Too often, procedure-oriented physicians only give lip service to the more mundane efforts of risk modification, and the patient concludes that such advice is not important.

Ivan Illich (23) attempted to emphasize, possibly a bit cynically, the importance of recognizing and modifying "disturbances of human culture" in a probing analysis of the health care in this country. In 1976, 7 years after the introduction of coronary bypass grafting, he concluded that "the study of the evolution of disease patterns provides evidence that during the last century, doctors have affected epidemics no more profoundly than did priests during earlier times. Epidemics came and went, imprecated by both, but touched by neither. They are not modified any more decisively by the rituals performed in medical clinics than those customary at religious shrines."

Sudden Cardiac Death

Elveback et al. (16) reported that in Rochester, Minnesota during the 15 year period from 1959 to 1975, the incidence of death due to myocardial infarction declined by 12% and that due to angina pectoris by 10%, whereas the incidence of sudden unexpected cardiac death due to coronary artery disease declined by 40%. Kuller et al. (24) reported that the coronary artery disease death rate in Allegheny County, Pennsylvania declined by 53% between 1970 and 1984. The dramatic decrease in the incidence of sudden cardiac death accounted for two-thirds of the observed decline. There was a particularly sharp decline in the rate of sudden unexpected cardiac death in men with no history of coronary artery disease. The Framingham study (25) reported that 50% of the sudden unexpected cardiac deaths in men and 64% in women occurred in persons without prior manifestations of coronary artery disease. It would appear that the changes in life-style that have contributed to the overall decline in death from coronary artery disease during the last quarter of a century were particularly beneficial in reducing the incidence of sudden cardiac death. Yet, sudden cardiac death remains a major challenge for cardiologists to this day.

Coronary anatomic basis for sudden death. Recent studies (26,27) have cast new light on the pathophysiologic changes leading to sudden cardiac death; 95% of patients who died suddenly of coronary artery disease had an acute evolving coronary artery lesion. Virtually all lesions were related to rupture or fissuring of atheromatous plaques. Such rupture of a plaque led to a free communication between the lipid content of the plaque and the blood flowing within the arterial lumen. Dissection by blood from the lumen into the plaque, in many cases, resulted in a large platelet-rich intraintimal thrombus. Over the site of the rupture, thrombus developed in many instances and projected into the lumen and propagated distally into segments of the artery that did not have significant initial disease. In the remainder, an intraintimal thrombus formed within the fissure. Davis and Thomas (26,27) reported that plaque fissures and intraintimal thrombosis without an intraluminal thrombotic component were observed more commonly in patients with sudden ischemic disease. It was suggested that in some instances, death might have resulted from a large intimal dissection that bulged into the lumen and produced short-term obstruction. In others, the dissection might tear away a flap of the intima, which could obstruct the lumen. Furthermore, such an intimal rupture could produce local vascular spasm.

Some investigators reported a high incidence of platelet emboli within the myocardium distal to the site of plaque rupture. Sudden cardiac death might be the myocardial equivalent of the "transitory ischemic attack" due to platelet emboli arising from fissured or ulcerated atheromatous plaques, or both, in the carotid artery (28). Although the presence of such thrombi was not restricted to individuals who had experienced sudden cardiac death, within that subgroup, thrombi were more common in those <45 years than in those >45 years.

Studies (29) elucidating the mechanism for sudden cardiac death indicate that the disease process resulting in death need not be advanced, and that the occurrence of death is almost a matter of chance. However, for a death to be considered a sudden cardiac death, there has to have been some involvement of the intima of the coronary arteries in the atherosclerotic process. Despite countless advances in diagnosis and therapy, sudden cardiac death frequently occurs in persons without prior symptoms attributed to coronary artery disease, and thus is frequently unexpected.

Angiographic prediction of new and sudden critical coronary lesions. Serial studies of coronary arteriograms in the same individuals have demonstrated that coronary artery disease does not progress in a linear manner. The progression is quite unpredictable, frequently occurring at previously normal sites. Singh (30) reported that repeat coronary arteriograms separated by a mean of 51 months in 52 patients receiving medical therapy showed that two-thirds of the lesions were stable; only one-third showed progression. Thirty-seven new lesions developed during the period of observation.

Little et al. (31) studied coronary arteriograms obtained before and up to 1 month after acute myocardial infarction in 42 consecutive patients. Of the 42 patients, 29 had a newly occluded coronary artery, and experience suggests that the 13 who did not have an occluded artery at the time of study might have had one demonstrated had they been studied earlier. Twenty-five of these 29 patients had had at least one artery with >50% stenosis on the initial angiogram. In 19 (63%) of the 29 patients, the artery that was subsequently occluded had <50% stenosis on the first arteriogram; in 28 (97%) of the 29, the stenosis was <70% and in only 10 (34%) of the 29 did the infarct occur because of occlusion of the artery that previously contained the most severe stenosis. Furthermore, no correlation existed between the severity of the initial coronary stenosis and the time from the first cardiac catheterization to infarction. These studies strongly indicate that in most instances, the cardiologist reviewing the coronary arteriogram of a patient in stable condition cannot with confidence predict which lesions are critical and which vessels are likely to become suddenly occluded in the near future. One can hardly escape wondering how accurately a "culprit artery" may be identified, especially without demonstration of recent thrombosis.

Clinical implications: role of surgery and angioplasty. It would appear that the thoughtful cardiologist in 1989 must accept that 1) sudden unexpected cardiac death is still common and frequently is the first clinical manifestation of coronary artery disease; and 2) although the coronary arte-

riogram is considered the "gold standard," one usually cannot predict with confidence the rate of progression of the disease, or the lesions that are likely to progress and cause a myocardial infarction or death, by analyzing the angiogram the time of such progression.

Clearly, there are several life-threatening lesions or combinations of lesions that can be demonstrated to have a significantly improved prognosis if operated on or in selected cases treated with angioplasty. Such lesions include >60% left main stenosis, >70% stenosis of the left anterior descending coronary artery disease proximal to the first septal perforator, total occlusion of the right coronary artery and >70% stenosis of a left anterior descending artery distal to the first septal perforator and a lesion in the artery responsible for an incomplete non-Q wave infarction (32,33). It was possibly because of the uncertainty as to the significance of one lesion versus another in situations less critical than those just listed that the philosophy of complete revascularization evolved . . . "while you are there, bypass them all." Also, when the disease has progressed to advanced stages, and the ejection fraction is significantly reduced, bypass surgery or angioplasty can be life-saving. At that stage, efforts to prevent life-threatening disease are too late, but progression can possibly be slowed.

Conclusion

It seems that without more confidence in the long-term outcome of invasive procedures, the major therapeutic effort of cardiovascular physicians (whether using invasive or noninvasive techniques) and cardiovascular surgeons should be directed toward the complete modification of the adverse life-styles that have been demonstrated to be responsible for the increase in coronary artery disease to epidemic proportions (29). The patient's commitment to life-style modification, except in emergency or emergent situations, is best acquired before an invasive or operative procedure is performed. Once a procedure is performed, the patient, and frequently the physician, tends to assume that the process has been arrested. Such is obviously not true. The patient must aggressively work to attain a healthy life-style. Efforts at risk control are quite rational for the patient who has undergone bypass graft surgery because there is increasing evidence that regression of lesions is possible (22,34). All efforts to get the patient to adopt a heart-healthy life-style are more successful if the physician "practices what he or she preaches." Behavior modification depends on the physician truly saying, "Do as I do, rather than as I say" (19).

A caveat is necessary. Preventive efforts, whether individually initiated or physician-stimulated, have already contributed to increasing the aging population of the United States (35). A larger elderly population can cause striking socioeconomic problems. For example, if campaigns to eliminate smoking are successful, the cost to Social Security will escalate by billions of dollars to pay the benefits of people living longer. Shoven et al. (36), economists at Stanford University, recently reported that every man born in 1920 who smokes saves Social Security approximately $20,000 by dying earlier than an individual who does not smoke. For women born in 1923, the typical smoker saves Social Security $10,000. If none of these people had smoked, these investigators estimated that Social Security would have to pay out $14.5 billion in extra benefits.

These observations should not deter physicians from efforts to foster prevention. As leaders of society, physicians cannot ignore the warning that we must reexamine attitudes toward retirement and aging in the United States. Who will pay the bill required to support an ever increasing array of healthy older individuals who it is hoped will be the product of a total commitment to prevention of disease (35)?

I thank Suzie Burnette and Adrienne Southerland of the Watson Clinic for their untiring assistance in preparation of the manuscript.

References

1. McIntosh HD. The maturation of a cardiologist with reflections on the "passing sands of time." Ann Emerg Med 1986;15:1101–10.
2. Cecil RL, ed. Textbook of Medicine. 7th ed. Philadelphia: WB Saunders, 1947:1226.
3. Russek HI. Shoulder-hand syndrome following myocardial infarction. Med Clin North Am 1968;52:155–60.
4. Levine SA, Lown B. The "chair" treatment of coronary thrombosis. Trans Assoc Am Phys 1957;65:316–23.
5. Wright IS, Marple CH, Beck DF. Myocardial Infarction: Its Clinical Manifestations and Treatment With Anticoagulants. New York: Grune & Stratton, 1954.
6. McIntosh HD. From academia to private practice or the maturation of a physician. Int J Cardiol 1984;5:260–8.
7. Stamler J. Cardiovascular disease in the United States. Am J Cardiol 1962;10:319–40.
8. Day HW. Preliminary studies in an acute coronary care cardiac resuscitation program. Lancet 1963;1:53–9.
9. Favaloro RG. Saphenous vein graft in the surgical treatment of coronary artery disease. J Thorac Cardiovasc Surg 1969;58:179–90.
10. Stamler J. Review of primary prevention trials of coronary heart disease. Acta Med Scand (Suppl) 1985;701:100–28.
11. Eleventh Bethesda Conference: Prevention of Coronary Heart Disease, September 27–28, 1980, Bethesda, Maryland. Am J Cardiol 1981;47:713–76.
12. Breslow L. University of California, Los Angeles Graduate School of Public Health: Quoted in Holistic Health. Revolution or revivalism. Forbes 1977;Oct 1:44.
13. Goldman L, Cook EF. The decline of ischemic heart disease mortality rates: an analysis of the comparative efforts of medical intervention and changes in lifestyle. Ann Intern Med 1984;101:825–36.
14. Stamler J. Coronary heart disease: doing the "right things." N Engl J Med 1985;312:1053–5.
15. Pell S, Fayerweather WE. Trends in the incidence of myocardial infarction and in associated mortality and morbidity in a large employed population, 1957–1983. N Engl J Med 1985;312:1005–11.
16. Elveback LR, Connolly DC, Kurland LT. Coronary heart disease in residents of Rochester, Minnesota. II. Mortality, incidence, and survivorship, 1950–1975. Mayo Clin Proc 1981;56:665–72.
17. Working Group on Arteriosclerosis of the National Heart, Lung, and Blood Institute, Vol 2. Bethesda, Maryland: National Institutes of Health. 1981:265–426, DHHS publication no. (NIH) 82-2035.
18. Reducing the Health Conspiracy of Smoking: 25 Years of Progress. A Report of the Surgeon General. Washington, D.C.: U.S. Department of Health and Human Services. January 11, 1989: DHHS publication no. [CDC]89-8411 (prepublication version).
19. McIntosh HD. Office strategies to reduce the risk of coronary heart disease. J Am Coll Cardiol 1988;12:1095–7.
20. Wenger NK, Cheeman JI, Herd JA, McIntosh HD. Education of the patient with cardiac disease in the 21st century: an overview. Am J Cardiol 1986;1187–9.
21. Bourassa MG, Fisher LD, Campeau L, Gillespie MJ, McConney M, Lespenance J. Long term fate of bypass grafts: the Coronary Artery Surgery Study (CASS) and Montreal Heart Institute experience. Circulation 1985;72(suppl V):V-71–8.
22. Blankenhorn DH, Nessim SA, Johnson RL, et al. Beneficial effects of combined colestipol-niacin therapy on coronary atherosclerosis and coronary venous bypass grafts. JAMA 1987;257:3233–40.
23. Illich I. Medical Nemesis: The Expropriation of Health. New York: Pantheon Books, 1976:15.
24. Kuller L, Traven N, Perper J, Rutan G. The disappearance of coronary heart deaths, aged 35–44, 1970–1986 (abstr). Circulation 1988;78(suppl II):II-89.
25. Kannel WB, Schatzkin A. Sudden death: lesions from subsets of population studies. J Am Coll Cardiol 1985;5:141B–9B.
26. Davis MJ, Thomas A. Thrombosis and acute coronary artery lesions in sudden cardiac ischemic death. N Engl J Med 1984;310:1137–40.
27. Davis MJ, Thomas AC. Plaque fissuring: the course of acute myocardial infarction, sudden ischemic death, and crescendo angina. Br Heart J 1985;53:363–73.
28. El Maraghi N, Genton E. The relevance of platelet and fibrin thromboembolism of the coronary microcirculation, with special reference to sudden cardiac death. Circulation 1980;62:936–44.
29. McIntosh HD. The stabilizing and unstabilizing influence of neurogenic and vascular activities of the heart related to sudden cardiac death. J Am Coll Cardiol 1985;5:105B–10B.
30. Singh RN. Progression of coronary atherosclerosis. Clues to pathologies from serial coronary arteriography. Br Heart J 1984;52:451–61.
31. Little WC, Constantinescu M, Applegate RJ, et al. Can coronary angiography predict the site of a subsequent myocardial infarction in patients with mild-to-moderate coronary artery disease? Circulation 1988;78:1157–66.
32. McIntosh HD, Garcia JA. The first decade of aortocoronary bypass grafting. Circulation 1978;57:405–31.
33. McIntosh HD. Second opinions for aortocoronary bypass grafting are beneficial. JAMA 1987;258:1644–5.
34. Ornish DM, Scherwitz LW, Brown SE, et al. Can lifestyle changes reverse atherosclerosis? (abstr). Circulation 1988;78(suppl II):II-11.
35. McIntosh HD. Perspectives, epilogue and caveat. J Am Coll Cardiol 1988;12:1119–21.
36. Shoven J, Sundberg JO, Bunker P. Social security cost of smoking. In: Wise DA, ed. Economics of Aging. Chicago: University of Chicago Press, 1989:231–50.

CHAPTER 28

An Era in Cardiology: A Clinician's View

SYLVAN L. WEINBERG, MD

To grasp the magnitude of the progress that cardiology has made during the past four plus decades, one has only to browse through the *American and British Heart Journals* of the late 1940s. These journals were the only English language cardiology journals at that time.

To most cardiologists practicing today, the cardiology literature of the 1940s must seem like ancient history. This is not surprising. The average age of cardiologists attending the 40th Anniversary Meeting of the American College of Cardiology in Anaheim, California was 35 years. Nearly half were born in 1949 or later.

In 1949, electrocardiography dominated the pages of both heart journals. There were some 60 articles on electrocardiography in the *American Heart Journal* that year, more than a third of all papers published. The lead article in 1949 was titled "The Ventricular Gradient in Doubtful Electrocardiograms." That subject might not be of great interest today, but at the time, it was part of great excitement and ferment in electrocardiography. Articles by Gordon Myers correlating electrocardiographic (ECG) findings with the location of myocardial infarction were studied avidly. Patterns of left ventricular hypertrophy were defined. In one of the great debates of the day, Louis N. Katz and Frank Wilson disagreed on the significance of unipolar precordial leads versus the CF leads. The 12 lead ECG was not yet standard. Most ECGs consisted of three limb and three chest leads. The augmented unipolar leads of Goldberger were yet to be accepted.

Much of what we take for granted in electrocardiography today was being developed 40 years ago. The QT interval, for example, was studied in such conditions as hypocalcemia and rheumatic fever. The variability of the ECG in normal young men was defined. Ventricular fibrillation was recorded rarely enough to warrant publication. Its occurrence was just being recognized in patients with Adams Stokes attacks. Transient ventricular fibrillation was induced experimentally by gradual oxygen deprivation. Electrocardiograms of transient ventricular fibrillation were unique because continuous monitoring was not yet possible.

The next most common subject in both the *American and British Heart Journals* in 1949 was congenital heart disease. These papers consisted primarily of case reports and anatomic descriptions.

Although cardiologists and investigators in the 1940s lacked the electronic, nuclear, radiologic and invasive technology of today, there was no shortage of academic and intellectual activity. Even a cursory study of the cardiology literature of that time shows that the stage was being set for the cardiology of today.

Then, as now, there was great interest in atherosclerosis. Lesions were produced in chickens and dogs by feeding diets high in fat and cholesterol. One article suggested that although "restriction of fat and cholesterol in the diet of chickens to very low levels did not prevent the development of spontaneous atherosclerosis, [there was] suggestive evidence that the severity of lesions is less than when fat is restricted." These issues are not yet resolved.

Heparin was already being studied in the management of coronary artery thrombosis. Streptomycin was new in treating tuberculous pericarditis, as was penicillin in syphilitic heart disease and bacterial endocarditis.

Articles on surgical treatment were rare, but not entirely absent. One paper suggested the possibility of creating a venous shunt between the pulmonary vein and superior vena cava to palliate patients with mitral stenosis.

Phonocardiography and auscultation of the heart were in fashion. For those interested in high technology, there was radiokymography. Studies in hypertension included the use of rauwolfia and the measurement of renin in blood. Radioactive sodium was used to measure regional circulation.

Not many authors who published in the late 1940s are active today. One is Eliot Corday, who wrote even then on the coronary circulation in an article titled "The Effect of Shock on the Heart and Its Treatment."

No one could have predicted the dizzying pace of progress in cardiology that the next 40 years would bring. A new era was about to begin. Although many papers published in the 1940s signaled the coming change, as often happens, significant events are fully appreciated only in retrospect.

An article in the *British Heart Journal* described the use of angiography to diagnose transposition of the aorta and pulmonary artery. In the same volume, Cournand and Richard described the relation between electrical and mechanical events of the cardiac cycle using intravascular and intracardiac recordings. These Nobel Laureates had already performed intracardiac catheterization in the mid-1940s. Bing and Kety wrote about "the measurement of coronary blood flow, oxygen consumption and efficiency of the left ventricle in man." Irvine Page discussed "certain aspects of the nature and treatment of oligemic shock." A case report from Sweden was titled "A Case of Angina Pectoris Precipitated Chiefly by Tobacco Smoking and Meals." John Hickam, then in Durham, North Carolina, described intracardiac shunts, ventricular output and the pulmonary pressure gradient in atrial septal defect.

Cardiology was about to move from an era that had been largely descriptive and contemplative to one dominated by an invasive and interventional approach. This was triggered by an explosion of post World War II technology and bold physician investigators who took innovations from the laboratory to the bedside. Perhaps the new era was epitomized by Dwight Harken, who had removed missile fragments from the hearts of soldiers in London during World War II and later performed mitral valvuloplasty. Harken was not alone. It is not possible to mention all of those who contributed to the surgical revolution that took place in the late 1940s and early 1950s. Bailey, Brock, Lillehei, DeBakey, Cooley and others made innovations in cardiovascular surgery seem almost commonplace. In the early 1950s, Gibbon successfully used a mechanical heart and lung apparatus and the heart suddenly became an organ accessible to the surgeon.

It would be nearly a decade after 1950 before Mason Sones introduced selective coronary cineangiography and nearly two decades until Vineberg implanted a left internal mammary artery into the myocardium, a radical procedure at the time. Skeptics became believers when Mason Sones, using his coronary angiography, proved that Vineberg's technique could indeed bring blood into the myocardium. Nearly another decade passed before Favaloro and Effler showed that saphenous vein bypass surgery was feasible and effective, and the new era was in high gear.

During the 1970s, coronary artery bypass surgery became one of the most frequently performed operations in the United States. However, myocardial revascularization did not long remain the exclusive domain of the surgeon. Greuntzig pioneered percutaneous balloon dilation of the coronary arteries. As the 1980s ended, coronary angioplasty challenged bypass surgery as an alternative to revascularize the myocardium.

Meanwhile, valvular surgery had kept pace with a variety of prosthetic devices and repair techniques. In 1968, Christian Barnard startled the world with what had been unthinkable in previous decades—cardiac transplantation. And what was to become the pattern of an era, the unthinkable became the commonplace.

In the early 1960s, the coronary care unit would transform the treatment of acute myocardial infarction from bedrest and passive observation to one of the most dynamic therapeutic adventures in all of medicine. Monitoring of the ECG, the use of lidocaine, closed chest cardiac massage, defibrillation and cardioversion would largely control the early rhythm disturbances of acute myocardial infarction and sharply reduce the incidence of in-hospital death. Coronary care units proliferated throughout the country and were followed by stepdown units. Monitoring became widespread, even though a reduction in mortality outside of the coronary care unit was difficult to prove. There was no

resting on any laurels. By the early 1970s, hemodynamic monitoring came to the bedside with the Swan-Ganz catheter.

Invasive cardiologists and surgeons became ever more bold. Patients with acute myocardial infarction and unstable coronary syndromes found themselves moved directly from the emergency room to the catheterization laboratory. Thrombolysis, streptokinase and recombinant tissue-type plasminogen activator (rt-PA) brought medical revascularization to the earliest stages of myocardial infarction. The use of thrombolysis and coronary angioplasty became the subject of extensive worldwide clinical trials. The ultimate interrelation of thrombolysis, coronary artery dilation and surgical revascularization is still uncertain.

One thing is certain. As the 1990s begin, anginal syndromes, acute and chronic, will be defined, usually by coronary angiography, and revascularization will be considered.

Although less visible and dramatic than invasive and interventional techniques, pharmacology did not fail to keep step with cardiology's triumphal march. In the 1940s, cardiologists relied primarily on digitalis, mercurial diuretic drugs, nitroglycerin and quinidine. Since then, beta-adrenergic blocking agents, calcium antagonists, angiotensin converting enzyme inhibitors, furosemide and thiazide diuretic drugs have revolutionized the treatment of anginal syndromes, congestive failure and hypertension, to say nothing of the role of antiplatelet agents, anticoagulants and a spectrum of inotropic and cholesterol-lowering drugs.

Each new drug and intervention spawned what surely must rival cardiology's great technical advances as the hallmark of the age—the randomized, double-blind, multicenter clinical trial. As cardiologists tried to sort out their many therapeutic options, clinical trials began to take precedence over experience, clinical judgment and, at times, common sense. The results of these trials dominated not only scientific meetings and journals, but were important news in the lay press and media. The influence of clinical trials became paramount in clinical decision making. Clinical trials determined the choice of specific medications, such as thrombolysis, and whether or not a drug should be used at all, as in the current cholesterol controversy. Drug companies, suddenly a dominant source of funds as support from the National Institutes of Health began to dwindle, influenced not only the nature of clinical research, but also its reporting to both medical and lay communities. Pharmaceutical houses allocated huge sums to present clinical trials of their products in the most favorable light through extensive advertising campaigns and, more subtly, in the guise of support for medical education. Drug house influence on clinical research and the dissemination of results has become an alarming problem that is not yet resolved. Ethics in cardiology and the relation of practicing cardiologists and research scientists to industry are a continuing concern.

During the past two decades, perhaps no facet of cardiology has seen more progress than the field of imaging. Two-dimensional echocardiography, rapid computed tomography, magnetic resonance and nuclear imaging ever more successfully pursued the goal of visualizing the heart noninvasively, including the coronary arteries by angioscopy and ultrasound.

Forty years ago, it was well known that an ECG at rest might be normal in a patient with advanced coronary disease. The provocative test at that time was the Master two-step test. Cardiology fellows today are often unaware of that incredibly simple technique of walking up and down two steps for several minutes, followed by an ECG to bring out latent abnormalities. The Master two-step test was replaced by computerized treadmills and bicycle ergometers, with ECGs and often oxygen consumption recorded during exercise. Thallium and other imaging techniques may pinpoint areas of the heart that show exercise-induced reversible ischemia.

Intracardiac pacemakers were introduced toward the end of the 1950s. From relatively primitive devices to treat bradycardia, pacing technology has evolved into complex arrhythmia control devices. Pacemakers can synchronize atrial and ventricular activity and respond to stimuli such as exercise and physiologic changes. Implantable defibrillators offer new hope to survivors of ventricular fibrillation and sustained ventricular tachycardia.

Forty years of progress is not, in itself, an era. An era occurs when the times and people of vision conspire to create a milieu of change. An era may be a period of intellectual ferment and revolution such as occurred in the American Colonies in the late 18th century. The flowering of the Dublin School in the 19th century might be called an era in Irish medicine, produced by such figures as Corrigan, Graves and Stokes. It was a time of clinical excellence unexplained and unequalled in Dublin before or since.

An era is finite only in retrospect.

If the past four decades do constitute an era in cardiology, it was one marked by the integration of science and technology into clinical practice. It was an era when the cardiac catheterization unit, the coronary care unit and the operating room became physiologic laboratories.

Cardiology, once a contemplative and descriptive discipline, has evolved during the past four decades as a highly mechanistic and invasive practice that alters anatomy and physiology almost at will. Without minimizing developments in biochemistry and physiology, it is fair to say that progress in cardiology in the past four decades has been largely technological and interventional. The coronary arteries and chambers of the heart have been entered and visualized.

Blood flow, intracardiac pressures and heart muscle movement have been measured. Valves have been entered and visualized. Blood flow, intracardiac pressures and heart muscle movement have been measured. Valves have been replaced and repaired. The heart's electrical activity has been monitored, restored mechanically and arrhythmias terminated automatically. Some arrhythmias were cured by direct surgical assault on conduction pathways. Blocked arteries were bypassed, the failed ventricle supported and the heart itself replaced. Total artificial hearts are on the horizon. All these techniques have in common a mechanical and macroscopic approach—the hallmark of an era.

Every era, like every empire, contains at its crest irrevocable elements of change. This is true of cardiology even at the flood tide of a dramatic era of repair and restoration of cardiovascular form and function. These successes, magnificent as they are, have been achieved without full understanding of tissues and structures, however effectively they may have been manipulated. Mechanical interventions such as vein bypass surgery and angioplasty have reached an impasse. Progressive atherosclerosis, intimal proliferation and thrombus formation continued to frustrate doctors and patients alike. The successes of the era, though great, are incomplete. Empires rise and fall. One era gives way to another.

Cardiology's new frontier will be molecular. Many of the studies included in this book describe changes in cardiology that seem to presage the end of an era and the beginning of a new one. The new thinking is apparent in reports on congestive heart failure, cardiomyopathy and pulmonary hypertension. Molecular science may modify even congenital heart disease before it evolves, rather than rely on techniques of repair, however sophisticated. Our approach to arrhythmias will move beyond displaying, counting and suppressing. Molecular biology will bring new understanding to cardiac muscle function, atherosclerosis, thrombosis and thrombolysis and to the long-neglected endothelium.

Some day, cardiologists will look back on the last four decades as an era when cardiology evolved from a descriptive and contemplative practice to one of invasion and intervention—and the present remembered as the dawning of cardiology's molecular era. It will revolutionize our understanding and approach to cardiology's greatest problems—from congenital heart disease to myocardial contractility and hypertrophy, to clotting and ultimately to atherosclerosis.

If the promise of the molecular era is fulfilled, many of the brilliant interventions of an era now at its zenith may become unnecessary and obsolete.

◆ INDEX ◆